Infectious Diseases:
In Context

Infectious Diseases: In Context

Brenda Wilmoth Lerner & K. Lee Lerner, Editors

VOLUME 1

AIDS TO LYME DISEASE

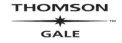

THOMSON
★
GALE

Detroit • New York • San Francisco • New Haven, Conn. • Waterville, Maine • London

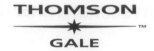

Infectious Diseases: In Context

Brenda Wilmoth Lerner and K. Lee Lerner, Editors

Project Editor
Madeline S. Harris

Editorial
Kathleen Edgar, Debra Kirby, Kristine Krapp, Paul Lewon, Elizabeth Manar, Kimberley McGrath, Jennifer Stock

Production Technology
Paul Lewon

Indexing Services
Factiva, Inc.

Rights and Acquisitions
Lisa Kincade, Ronald Montgomery, Tracie Richardson, Robyn Young

Imaging and Multimedia
Lezlie Light

Product Design
Jennifer Wahi

Product Management
Janet Witalec

Composition
Evi Seoud, Mary Beth Trimper

Manufacturing
Wendy Blurton, Dorothy Maki

LIBRARY OF CONGRESS CATALOGING-IN-PUBLICATION DATA

Infectious diseases: in context / Brenda Wilmoth Lerner & K. Lee Lerner, editors.
   p. cm.
  Includes bibliographical references and index.
  ISBN-13: 978-1-4144-2960-1 (set hardcover)–
  ISBN-13: 978-1-4144-2961-8 (vol. 1 hardcover)–
  ISBN-13: 978-1-4144-2962-5 (vol. 2 hardcover)–
  ISBN-13: 978-1-4144-2963-2 (set ebook)
  1. Communicable diseases–Encyclopedias.
  I. Lerner, Brenda Wilmoth. II. Lerner, K. Lee.
  RC111.I516 2008
  616.003–dc22

2007019024

This title is also available as an e-book.
ISBN 978-1-4144-2963-2
Contact your Gale sales representative for ordering information.

Printed in Canada
10 9 8 7 6 5 4 3 2 1

Contents

Contents

Contents

VOLUME 2

Contents

Advisors and Contributors

While compiling this volume, the editors relied upon the expertise and contributions of the following scientists, scholars, and researchers, who served as advisors and/or contributors for *Infectious Diseases: In Context*:

Susan Aldridge, Ph.D.
Independent scholar and writer
London, United Kingdom

William Arthur Atkins, M.S.
Independent scholar and writer
Normal, Illinois

Stephen A. Berger, M.D.
Director, Geographic Medicine
Tel Aviv Medical Center
Tel Aviv, Israel

L.S. Clements, M.D., Ph.D.
Assistant Professor of Pediatrics
University of South Alabama
College of Medicine
Mobile, Alabama

Bryan Davies, L.L.B.
Writer and journalist
Ontario, Canada

Paul Davies, Ph.D.
Director, Science Research Institute
Adjunct Professor Université
Paris - La Sorbonne.
Paris, France

Antonio Farina, M.D., Ph.D.
Department of Embryology, Obstetrics, and Gynecology
University of Bologna
Bologna, Italy

Larry Gilman, Ph.D.
Independent scholar and journalist
Sharon, Vermont

Tony Hawas, M.A.
Writer and journalist
Brisbane, Australia

Brian D. Hoyle, Ph.D.
Microbiologist
Nova Scotia, Canada

Kenneth T. LaPensee, Ph.D., MPH
Epidemiologist and Medical Policy Specialist
Hampton, New Jersey

Agnieszka Lichanska, Ph.D.
Institute for Molecular Sciences
University of Queensland
Brisbane, Australia

Adrienne Wilmoth Lerner, J.D.
Independent scholar
Jacksonville, Florida

Eric v.d. Luft, Ph.D., M.L.S.
Adjunct Lecturer, Center for Bioethics and Humanities
SUNY Upstate Medical University
Syracuse, New York

Caryn Neumann, Ph.D.
Visiting Assistant Professor
Denison University
Granville, Ohio

Anna Marie Roos, Ph.D.
Research Associate, Wellcome Unit for the History of Medicine
University of Oxford
Oxford, United Kingdom

Constance K. Stein, Ph.D.
Director of Cytogenetics, Associate Professor
SUNY Upstate Medical University
Syracuse, New York

Jack Woodall, Ph.D.
Director, Nucleus for the Investigation of Emerging Infectious Diseases
Institute of Medical Biochemistry, Center for Health Sciences
Federal University of Rio de Janeiro
Rio de Janeiro, Brazil

Melanie Barton Zoltán, M.S.
Independent scholar
Amherst, Massachusetts

Acknowledgments

The editors are grateful to the truly global group of scholars, researchers, and writers who contributed to *Infectious Diseases: In Context.*

The editors also wish to thank copyeditors Christine Jeryan, Kate Kretchmann, and Alicia Cafferty Lerner, whose keen eyes and sound judgments greatly enhanced the quality and readability of the text.

The editors gratefully acknowledge and extend thanks to Janet Witalec and Debra Kirby at the Gale Group for their faith in the project and for their sound content advice and guidance. Without the able guidance and efforts of talented teams in IT, rights and acquisition management, and imaging at the Gale Group, this book would not have been possible. The editors are especially indebted to Kim McGrath, Elizabeth Manar, Kathleen Edgar, Kristine Krapp, and Jennifer Stock for their invaluable help in correcting copy. The editors also wish to acknowledge the contributions of Marcia Schiff at the Associated Press for her help in securing archival images.

Deep and sincere thanks and appreciation are due to Project Manager Madeline Harris who, despite a myriad of publishing hurdles and woes, managed miracles with skill, grace, and humor.

Introduction

Humanity shares a common ancestry with all living things on Earth. We often share especially close intimacies with the microbial world. In fact, only a small percentage of the cells in the human body are human at all. "We" are vastly outnumbered, even within our bodies, by microbial life that can only be counted on the same scale as the vast numbers of stars in the universe. This is also an essential relationship, because humanity could not survive without an array of microflora that both nourish us and that provide needed enzymes for life processes.

Yet, the common biology and biochemistry that unites us also makes us susceptible to contracting and transmitting infectious disease.

Throughout history, microorganisms have spread deadly diseases and caused widespread epidemics that have threatened and altered human civilization. In the modern era, civic sanitation, water purification, immunization, and antibiotics have dramatically reduced the overall morbidity and the mortality rates of infectious disease in more developed nations. Yet, much of the world is still ravaged by disease and epidemics; new threats constantly appear to challenge the most advanced medical and public health systems.

Although specific diseases may be statistically associated with particular regions or other demographics, disease does not recognize social class or political boundary. In our intimately connected global village, an outbreak of disease in a remote area may quickly transform into a global threat. Given the opportunity, the agents of disease may spread across the globe at the speed of modern travel, and also leap from animals to humans.

The articles presented in these volumes, written by some of the world's leading experts, are designed to be readable and to instruct, challenge, and excite a range of student and reader interests while, at the same time, providing a solid foundation and reference for more advanced students and readers. It speaks both to the seriousness of their dedication to combating infectious disease and to the authors' great credit that the interests of younger students and lay readers were put forefront in preparation of these entries.

The editors are especially pleased to have contributions and original primary source essays within the volumes by experts that are currently in the forefront of international infectious disease research and policy. Jack Woodall, Ph.D., recounts memories of belonging to a team that identified and determined the cause of Machupo hemorrhagic fever in "Virus Hunters" and of his association with the developer of the yellow fever vaccine in "Yellow Fever." He also explains "ProMED," a disease-reporting system (of which Woodall is a founder) that allows scientists around the world, whether in the hospital, laboratory, or the field, to share real-time information about outbreaks of emerging infectious diseases. Jack Woodall now serves as the director of the Nucleus for the Investigation of Emerging Infectious Diseases at the Federal University of Rio de Janeiro in Brazil.

Stephen A. Berger, M.D., Ph.D., Director of Geographic Medicine at Tel Aviv Medical Center in Tel Aviv, Israel, served as a contributing advisor for *Infectious Diseases: In Context* and was the developer of GIDEON (Global Infectious Disease and Epidemiology Network), the world's premier global infectious diseases database. Dr. Berger explains the Web-based tool that helps physicians worldwide diagnose infectious diseases. Dr. Berger also contributes "Travel and Infectious Disease" and a special introduction. Dr. Berger's contributions reflect a dedication to teaching that has five times earned him the New York Medical College Teaching Award. Dr. Berger, author of numerous articles and books, including *Introduction to Infectious Diseases*, *The Healthy Tourist*, and *Exotic Viral Diseases: A Global Guide,* was gracious with his time, writing, and advice.

The editors are indebted to both of these distinguished scientists for their generous contributions of time and compelling material.

Readers interests were are also well-served by Anthony S. Fauci, M.D., Director of the National Institutes of Allergy and Infectious Diseases, for what was, at the time *Infectious Diseases: In Context* went to press, a preview of his latest version of the map of emerging and re-emerging infectious diseases, and also by L. Scott Clements, M.D., Ph.D., for his advice and articles, including "Childhood Infectious Diseases: Immunization Impacts."

Space limitations of this volume force the editors to include only those infectious diseases that directly affect human health. It is important to note, however, that diseases affecting plants and animals can have a significant indirect impact on the lives of humans. The 2001 outbreak of foot and mouth disease in the United Kingdom, for example, resulted in the slaughter of over six million pigs, sheep, and cattle, crippling farmers, tourism, and other commerce, and ultimately costing an estimated four billion dollars to the U.K. economy. At press time, the cocoa industry in Ghana is threatened by the Cocoa Swollen Shoot Virus, where farmers are reluctant to cut down their infected mature cocoa trees and plant healthy seedlings. Ghana is among the leading exporters worldwide of cocoa for chocolate. Scientists are also concerned about a lack of forthcoming information from the Chinese government concerning an epidemic virus among pigs in China that is contributing to a pork shortage and the strongest inflation in China in a decade. Although these diseases cannot inflict illness in humans, they can ultimately affect the nutritional, social, economic, and political status of a nation and its people.

Despite the profound and fundamental advances in science and medicine during the last fifty years, there has never been a greater need for a book that explains the wide-ranging impacts of infectious disease. It is hubris to assume that science alone will conquer infectious diseases. Globally, deaths due to malaria alone may double over the next twenty years and ominous social and political implications cannot be ignored when death continues to cast a longer shadow over the poorest nations.

The fight against infectious disease depends on far more than advances in science and public health. The hope that threats and devastation of infectious diseases could be eliminated for all humankind have long since been dashed upon the hard realities that health care is disproportionately available, and cavernous gaps still exist between health care in wealthier nations as opposed to poorer nations. Victory in the "war" against infectious disease will require advances in science and advances in our understanding of our fragile environment and common humanity.

K. Lee Lerner & Brenda Wilmoth Lerner, editors

DUBLIN, IRELAND, JULY 2007

Brenda Wilmoth Lerner and K. Lee Lerner were members of the International Society for Infectious Disease and delegates to the 12th International Congress on Infectious Disease in Lisbon, Portugal, in June 2006. Primarily based in London and Paris, the Lerner & Lerner portfolio includes more than two dozen books and films that focus on science and science-related issues.

"…any man's death diminishes me, because I am involved in mankind, and therefore never send to know for whom the bells tolls; it tolls for thee." —John Donne, 1624 (published) *Devotions upon Emergent Occasions*, no. 17 (Meditation)

The book is respectfully dedicated to Dr. Carlo Urbani and those who risk—and far too often sacrifice—their lives in an attempt to lessen the toll of infectious diseases.

A Special Introduction by Stephen A. Berger, M.D.

The Burden of Infectious Disease in Our Changing, Globalizing World

As we move into the twenty-first century, we continue to exist in a sea of ancient, hostile adversaries that threaten our very existence—both as individuals, and as a race of medium-sized mammals. The good news is that modern technology allows us to understand, diagnose, and treat an expanding number of infectious diseases. The bad news is that this same modern technology increasingly places us at risk for those same diseases.

For the purpose of clarity, I will classify the infectious diseases of humans into six broad categories: traditional, new, emerging, re-emerging, disappearing, and extinct. The latter category is depressingly small, and in fact contains only a single disease. The last case of smallpox was reported in Somalia in 1977, and the viral agent hibernates (as far as we know) in secure freezers located in the United States and Russian Federation. The few disappearing diseases include measles, leprosy, guinea worm, and poliomyelitis—conditions whose numbers have decreased in recent years, but which could suddenly blossom into outbreaks when the political and social climate permits.

One must distinguish between "new diseases" and "newly discovered" diseases. The former category includes conditions that had never before affected mankind: AIDS, SARS, Ebola. In contrast, Legionnaire's disease, Chlamydial infection, and Lyme disease appear to have affected man for many centuries, but were only "discovered" when appropriate technology permitted.

Emerging diseases such as West Nile fever and Dengue are certainly not new, but expand both geographically and numerically with the advent of mass tourism and the dispersal of mosquitoes in suitable animals or other vehicles. As the term implies, "re-emerging" diseases such as malaria repopulate areas from which they had been eliminated, often as the result of man-made alteration of the environment, elimination of natural predators, global warming, deforestation, and crowding. The best-known disease in this category is influenza, which is caused by a virus that seems to evolve and mutate continually into agents that are not recognized by the human host. Even this phenomenon is largely driven by the practice of some human populations to raise swine and ducks in crowded, unsanitary conditions that promote interchange of viral material.

The vast majority of infectious diseases might be classified as "traditional," forever with us and largely unchanged: the common cold, chickenpox, urinary tract infection, pneumonia, typhoid, gonorrhea, meningitis, and hundreds of others. In some cases, vaccines have altered the incidence of some traditional diseases among select populations. In other cases, increasing life span and advances in medical and surgical intervention have actually created a favorable ecological niche for heretofore non-pathogenic microbes.

Sadly, several new and distressing disease patterns have been the direct result of advances in managing the infection itself. Tuberculosis has been a largely treatable disease since the 1940's; but as of 2007, strains of the causative agent are increasingly resistant to all known drugs. Highly resistant microbes are now commonplace in cases of AIDS, malaria, and gonorrhea, as well as many of the traditional bacteria for which antibiotics were primarily developed: staphylococci, pneumococci and *E. coli*.

Hopefully, the seemingly self-destructive aspect of mankind will be overtaken by continued advances in the treatment, prevention, and understanding of the microbes that share our world.

Stephen A. Berger, M.D.
Director of Geographic Medicine
Tel Aviv Medical Center
Tel Aviv, Israel

About the *In Context* Series

Written by a global array of experts yet aimed primarily at high school students and an interested general readership, the *In Context* series serves as an authoritative reference guide to essential concepts of science, the impacts of recent changes in scientific consensus, and the effects of science on social, political, and legal issues.

Cross-curricular in nature, *In Context* books align with, and support, national science standards and high school science curriculums across subjects in science and the humanities, and facilitate science understanding important to higher achievement in the No Child Left Behind (NCLB) science testing. Inclusion of original essays written by leading experts and primary source documents serve the requirements of an increasing number of high school and international baccalaureate programs, and are designed to provide additional insights on leading social issues, as well as spur critical thinking about the profound cultural connections of science.

In Context books also give special coverage to the impact of science on daily life, commerce, travel, and the future of industrialized and impoverished nations.

Each book in the series features entries with extensively developed words-to-know sections designed to facilitate understanding and increase both reading retention and the ability of students to understand reading in context without being overwhelmed by scientific terminology.

Entries are further designed to include standardized subheads that are specifically designed to present information related to the main focus of the book. Entries also include a listing of further resources (books, periodicals, Web sites, audio and visual media) and references to related entries.

In addition to maps, charts, tables and graphs, each *In Context* title has approximately 300 topic-related images that visually enrich the content. Each *In Context* title will also contain topic-specific timelines (a chronology of major events), a topic-specific glossary, a bibliography, and an index especially prepared to coordinate with the volume topic.

About This Book

The goal of *Infectious Diseases: In Context* is to help high-school and early college-age students understand the essential facts and deeper cultural connections of topics and issues related to the scientific study of infectious disease.

The relationship of science to complex ethical and social considerations is evident, for example, when considering the general rise of infectious diseases that sometimes occurs as an unintended side effect of the otherwise beneficial use of medications. Nearly half the world's population is infected with the bacterium causing tuberculosis (TB); although for most people the infection is inactive, yet the organism causing some new cases of TB is evolving toward a greater resistance to the antibiotics that were once effective in treating TB. Such statistics also take on added social dimension when considering that TB disproportionately impacts certain social groups (the elderly, minority groups, and people infected with HIV).

In an attempt to enrich the reader's understanding of the mutually impacting relationship between science and culture, as space allows we have included primary sources that enhance the content of *In Context* entries. In keeping with the philosophy that much of the benefit from using primary sources derives from the reader's own process of inquiry, the contextual material introducing each primary source provides an unobtrusive introduction and springboard to critical thought.

General Structure

Infectious Diseases: In Context is a collection of 250 entries that provide insight into increasingly important and urgent topics associated with the study of infectious disease.

The articles in the book are meant to be understandable by anyone with a curiosity about topics related to infectious disease, and the first edition of *Infectious Diseases: In Context* has been designed with ready reference in mind:

- Entries are arranged alphabetically, rather than by chronology or scientific subfield.
- The **chronology** (timeline) includes many of the most significant events in the history of infectious disease and advances of science. Where appropriate, related scientific advances are included to offer additional context.
- An extensive glossary section provides readers with a ready reference for content-related terminology. In addition to defining terms within entries, specific Words-to-Know sidebars are placed within each entry.
- A bibliography section (citations of books, periodicals, websites, and audio and visual material) offers additional resources to those resources cited within each entry.
- A **comprehensive general index** guides the reader to topics and persons mentioned in the book.

Entry Structure

In Context entries are designed so that readers may navigate entries with ease. Toward that goal, entries are divided into easy-to-access sections:

- **Introduction**: A opening section designed to clearly identify the topic.
- **Words-to-know** sidebar: Essential terms that enhance readability and critical understanding of entry content.
- Established but flexible **rubrics** customize content presentation and identify each section, enabling the reader to navigate entries with ease. Inside *Infectious Diseases: In Context* entries readers will find two key schemes of organization. Most entries contain internal discussions of **Disease History, Characteristics, and Transmission**, followed by **Scope and Distribution**, then a summary of **Treatment and Prevention**. General social or science topics may have a simpler structure discussing, for example, **History and Scientific Foundations**. Regardless, the goal of *In Context* entries is a consistent, content-appropriate, and easy-to-follow presentation.
- **Impacts and Issues**: Key scientific, political, or social considerations related to the entry topic.
- **Bibliography:** Citations of books, periodicals, web sites, and audio and visual material used in preparation of the entry or that provide a stepping stone to further study.
- **"See also" references** clearly identify other content-related entries.

Infectious Diseases: In Context special style notes

Please note the following with regard to topics and entries included in *Infectious Diseases: In Context*:

- Primary source selection and the composition of sidebars are not attributed to authors of signed entries to which the sidebars may be associated. In all cases, the sources for sidebars containing external content (e.g., a CDC policy position or medical recommendation) are clearly indicated.
- The Centers for Disease Control and Prevention (CDC) includes parasitic diseases with infectious diseases, and the editors have adopted this scheme.
- Equations are, of course, often the most accurate and preferred language of science, and are essential to epidemiologists and medical statisticians. To better serve the intended audience of *Infectious Diseases: In Context*, however, the editors attempted to minimize the inclusion of equations in favor of describing the elegance of thought or essential results such equations yield.
- A detailed understanding of biology and chemistry is neither assumed nor required for *Infectious Diseases: In Context*. Accordingly, students and other readers should not be intimidated or deterred by the sometimes complex names of chemical molecules or biological classification. Where necessary, sufficient information regarding chemical structure or species classification is provided. If desired, more information can easily be obtained from any basic chemistry or biology reference.

Bibliography citation formats (How to cite articles and sources)

In Context titles adopt the following citation format:

Books

Magill, Gerard, ed. *Genetics and Ethics: An Interdisciplinary Study*. New York: Fordham University Press, 2003.

Verlinsky, Yury, and Anver Kuliev. *Practical Preimplantation Genetic Diagnosis*. New York: Springer, 2005.

Web Sites

ADEAR. Alzheimer's Disease Education and Referral Center. National Institute on Aging. <http://www.alzheimers.org/generalinfo.htm> (accessed January 23, 2006).

Genetics and Public Policy Center. <http://dnapolicy.org/index.jhtml.html> (accessed January 23, 2006).

Human Genetics in the Public Interest. The Center for Genetics and Society. <http://www.genetics-and-society.org> (accessed January 26, 2006).

PGD: Preimplantation Genetic Diagnosis. "Discussion by the Genetics and Public Policy Center." <http://dnapolicy.org/downloads/pdfs/policy_pgd.pdf> (accessed January 23, 2006).

Alternative citation formats

There are, however, alternative citation formats that may be useful to readers and examples of how to cite articles in often used alternative formats are shown below.

APA Style

Books: Kübler-Ross, Elizabeth. (1969) *On Death and Dying.* New York: Macmillan. Excerpted in K. Lee Lerner and Brenda Wilmoth Lerner, eds. (2006) *Medicine, Health, and Bioethics: Essential Primary Sources*, Farmington Hills, Mich.: Thomson Gale.

Periodicals: Venter, J. Craig, et al. (2001, February 16). "The Sequence of the Human Genome." *Science*, vol. 291, no. 5507, pp. 1304–51. Excerpted in K. Lee Lerner and Brenda Wilmoth Lerner, eds. (2006) *Medicine, Health, and Bioethics: Essential Primary Sources*, Farmington Hills, Mich.: Thomson Gale.

Web Sites: Johns Hopkins Hospital and Health System. "Patient Rights and Responsibilities." Retrieved January 14, 2006 from Http://www.hopkinsmedicine.org/patients/JHH/patient_rights.html. Excerpted in K. Lee Lerner and Brenda Wilmoth Lerner, eds. (2006) *Medicine, Health, and Bioethics: Essential Primary Sources*, Farmington Hills, Mich.: Thomson Gale.

Chicago Style

Books: Kübler-Ross, Elizabeth. *On Death and Dying.* New York: Macmillan, 1969. Excerpted in K. Lee Lerner and Brenda Wilmoth Lerner, eds. *Medicine, Health, and Bioethics: Essential Primary Sources*, Farmington Hills, MI: Thomson Gale, 2006.

Periodicals: Venter, J. Craig, et al. "The Sequence of the Human Genome." *Science* (2001): 291, 5507, 1304–1351. Excerpted in K. Lee Lerner and Brenda Wilmoth Lerner, eds. *Medicine, Health, and Bioethics: Essential Primary Sources*, Farmington Hills, MI: Thomson Gale, 2006.

Web Sites: *Johns Hopkins Hospital and Health System.* "Patient Rights and Responsibilities." <http://www.hopkinsmedicine.org/patients/JHH/patient_rights.html.> (accessed January 14, 2006). Excerpted in K. Lee Lerner and Brenda Wilmoth Lerner, eds. *Medicine, Health, and Bioethics: Essential Primary Sources*, Farmington Hills, MI: Thomson Gale, 2006.

MLA Style

Books: Kübler-Ross, Elizabeth. *On Death and Dying,* New York: Macmillan, 1969. Excerpted in K. Lee Lerner and Brenda Wilmoth Lerner, eds. *Medicine, Health, and Bioethics: Essential Primary Sources*, Farmington Hills, Mich.: Thomson Gale, 2006.

Periodicals: Venter, J. Craig, et al. "The Sequence of the Human Genome." *Science*, 291 (16 February 2001): 5507, 1304–51. Excerpted in K. Lee Lerner and Brenda Wilmoth Lerner, eds. *Terrorism: Essential Primary Sources*, Farmington Hills, Mich.: Thomson Gale, 2006.

Web Sites: "Patient's Rights and Responsibilities." Johns Hopkins Hospital and Health System. 14 January 2006. <http://www.hopkinsmedicine.org/patients/JHH/patient_rights.html.> Excerpted in K. Lee Lerner and Brenda Wilmoth Lerner, eds. *Terrorism: Essential Primary Sources*, Farmington Hills, Mich.: Thomson Gale, 2006.

Turabian Style (Natural and Social Sciences)

Books: Kübler-Ross, Elizabeth. *On Death and Dying*, (New York: Macmillan, 1969). Excerpted in K. Lee Lerner and Brenda Wilmoth Lerner, eds. *Medicine, Health, and Bioethics: Essential Primary Sources*, (Farmington Hills, Mich.: Thomson Gale, 2006).

Periodicals: Venter, J. Craig, et al. "The Sequence of the Human Genome." *Science*, 291 (16 February 2001): 5507, 1304–1351. Excerpted in K. Lee Lerner and Brenda Wilmoth Lerner, eds. *Medicine, Health, and Bioethics: Essential Primary Sources*, (Farmington Hills, Mich.: Thomson Gale, 2006).

Web Sites: Johns Hopkins Hospital and Health System."Patient's Rights and Responsibilities." available from http://www.hopkinsmedicine.org/patients/JHH/patient_rights.html; accessed14 January 2006. Excerpted in K. Lee Lerner and Brenda Wilmoth Lerner, eds. *Medicine, Health, and Bioethics: Essential Primary Sources*, (Farmington Hills, Mich.: Thomson Gale, 2006).

Using Primary Sources

The definition of what constitutes a primary source is often the subject of scholarly debate and interpretation. Although primary sources come from a wide spectrum of resources, they are united by the fact that they individually provide insight into the historical *milieu* (context and environment) during which they were produced. Primary sources include materials such as newspaper articles, press dispatches, autobiographies, essays, letters, diaries, speeches, song lyrics, posters, works of art—and in the twenty-first century, web logs—that offer direct, first-hand insight or witness to events of their day.

Categories of primary sources include:

- Documents containing firsthand accounts of historic events by witnesses and participants. This category includes diary or journal entries, letters, email, newspaper articles, interviews, memoirs, and testimony in legal proceedings.
- Documents or works representing the official views of both government leaders and leaders of other organizations. These include primary sources such as policy statements, speeches, interviews, press releases, government reports, and legislation.
- Works of art, including (but certainly not limited to) photographs, poems, and songs, including advertisements and reviews of those works that help establish an understanding of the cultural milieu (the cultural environment with regard to attitudes and perceptions of events).
- Secondary sources. In some cases, secondary sources or tertiary sources may be treated as primary sources. For example, if an entry written many years after an event, or to summarize an event, includes quotes, recollections, or retrospectives (accounts of the past) written by participants in the earlier event, the source can be considered a primary source.

Analysis of primary sources

The primary material collected in this volume is not intended to provide a comprehensive or balanced overview of a topic or event. Rather, the primary sources are intended to generate interest and lay a foundation for further inquiry and study.

In order to properly analyze a primary source, readers should remain skeptical and develop probing questions about the source. Using historical documents requires that readers analyze them carefully and extract specific information. However, readers must also read "beyond the text" to garner larger clues about the social impact of the primary source.

In addition to providing information about their topics, primary sources may also supply a wealth of insight into their creator's viewpoint. For example, when reading a news article about an outbreak of disease, consider whether the reporter's words also indicate something about his or her origin, bias (an irrational disposition in favor of someone or something), prejudices (an irrational disposition against someone or something), or intended audience.

Students should remember that primary sources often contain information later proven to be false, or contain viewpoints and terms unacceptable to future generations. It is important to view the primary source within the historical and social context existing at its creation. If for example, a newspaper article is written within hours or days of an event, later developments may reveal some assertions in the original article as false or misleading.

Test new conclusions and ideas

Whatever opinion or working hypothesis the reader forms, it is critical that they then test that hypothesis against other facts and sources related to the incident. For example, it might be wrong to conclude that factual mistakes are deliberate unless evidence can be produced of a pattern and practice of such mistakes with an intent to promote a false idea.

The difference between sound reasoning and preposterous conspiracy theories (or the birth of urban legends) lies in the willingness to test new ideas against other sources, rather than rest on one piece of evidence such as a single primary source that may contain errors. Sound reasoning requires that arguments and assertions guard against argument fallacies that utilize the following:

- false dilemmas (only two choices are given when in fact there are three or more options);
- arguments from ignorance (*argumentum ad ignorantiam*; because something is not known to be true, it is assumed to be false);
- possibilist fallacies (a favorite among conspiracy theorists who attempt to demonstrate that a factual statement is true or false by establishing the possibility of its truth or falsity. An argument where "it could be" is usually followed by an unearned "therefore, it is.");
- slippery slope arguments or fallacies (a series of increasingly dramatic consequences is drawn from an initial fact or idea);
- begging the question (the truth of the conclusion is assumed by the premises);
- straw man arguments (the arguer mischaracterizes an argument or theory and then attacks the merits of their own false representations);
- appeals to pity or force (the argument attempts to persuade people to agree by sympathy or force);
- prejudicial language (values or moral goodness, good and bad, are attached to certain arguments or facts);
- personal attacks (*ad hominem*; an attack on a person's character or circumstances);
- anecdotal or testimonial evidence (stories that are unsupported by impartial observation or data that is not reproducible);
- *post hoc* (after the fact) fallacies (because one thing follows another, it is held to cause the other);
- the fallacy of the appeal to authority (the argument rests upon the credentials of a person, not the evidence).

Despite the fact that some primary sources can contain false information or lead readers to false conclusions based on the "facts" presented, they remain an invaluable resource regarding past events. Primary sources allow readers and researchers to come as close as possible to understanding the perceptions and context of events and thus to more fully appreciate how and why misconceptions occur.

Glossary

A

ABIOGENESIS: Also known as spontaneous generation; the incorrect theory that living things can be generated from nonliving things.

ABIOTIC: A term used to describe the portion of an ecosystem that is not living, such as water or soil.

ABSCESS: An abscess is a pus-filled sore, usually caused by a bacterial infection. It results from the body's defensive reaction to foreign material. Abscesses are often found in the soft tissue under the skin in areas such as the armpit or the groin. However, they may develop in any organ, and they are commonly found in the breast and gums. If they are located in deep organs such as the lung, liver, or brain, abscesses are far more serious and call for more specific treatment.

ACARACIDES: Chemicals that kill mites and ticks are acaracides.

ACQUIRED (ADAPTIVE) IMMUNITY: Immunity is the ability to resist infection and is subdivided into innate immunity, which an individual is born with, and acquired, or adaptive, immunity, which develops according to circumstances and is targeted to a specific pathogen. There are two types of acquired immunity, known as active and passive. Active immunity is either humoral, involving production of antibody molecules against a bacterium or virus, or cell-mediated, where T-cells are mobilized against infected cells. Infection and immunization can both induce acquired immunity. Passive immunity is induced by injection of the serum of a person who is already immune to a particular infection.

ACQUIRED IMMUNODEFICIENCY SYNDROME (AIDS): A disease of the immune system caused by the human immunodeficiency virus (HIV). It is characterized by the destruction of a particular type of white blood cell and increased susceptibility to infection and other diseases.

ACTIVE INFECTION: An active infection is one that is currently producing symptoms or in which the infective agent is multiplying rapidly. In contrast, a latent infection is one in which the infective agent is present, but not causing symptoms or damage to the body nor reproducing at a significant rate.

ADAPTIVE IMMUNITY: Adaptive immunity is another term for acquired immunity, referring to the resistance to infection that develops through life and is targeted to a specific pathogen. There are two types of adaptive immunity, known as active and passive. Active immunity is either humoral, involving production of antibody molecules against a bacterium or virus, or cell-mediated, in which T-cells are mobilized against infected cells. Infection and immunization can both induce acquired immunity.

ADHESION: Physical attraction between different types of molecules.

AEROBES: Aerobic microorganisms require the presence of oxygen for growth. Molecular oxygen functions in the respiratory pathway of the microbes to produce the energy necessary for life. Bacteria, yeasts, fungi, and algae are capable of aerobic growth.

AEROSOL: Particles of liquid or solid dispersed as a suspension in gas.

AGGREGATIONS: When blood clots (becomes solid, usually in response to injury), cells called platelets form clumps called aggregations. An instrument called an aggregometer measures the degree of platelet aggregation in blood.

AIDS (ACQUIRED IMMUNODEFICIENCY SYNDROME): A disease of the immune system caused by the human immunodeficiency virus (HIV). It is characterized by the destruction of a particular type of white blood cell and increased susceptibility to infection and other diseases.

AIRBORNE PRECAUTIONS: Airborne precautions are procedures that are designed to reduce the chance that certain disease-causing (pathogenic) microorganisms will be transmitted through the air.

AIRBORNE TRANSMISSION: Airborne transmission refers to the ability of a disease-causing (pathogenic) microorganism to be spread through the air by droplets expelled during sneezing or coughing.

ALLELE: Any of two or more alternative forms of a gene that occupy the same location on a chromosome.

ALLERGIES: An allergy is an excessive or hypersensitive response of the immune system to substances (allergens) in the environment. Instead of fighting off a disease-causing foreign substance, the immune system launches a complex series of actions against the particular irritating allergen. The immune response may be accompanied by a number of stressful symptoms, ranging from mild to life threatening. In rare cases, an allergic reaction leads to anaphylactic shock—a condition characterized by a sudden drop in blood pressure, difficulty in breathing, skin irritation, collapse, and possible death.

ALVEOLI: An alveolus (alveoli is plural) is a tiny air sac located within the lungs. The exchange of oxygen and carbon dioxide takes place within these sacs.

AMEBIC DYSENTERY: Amebic (or amoebic) dysentery, which is also referred to as amebiasis or amoebiasis, is an inflammation of the intestine caused by the parasite *Entamoeba histolytica*. The severe form of the malady is characterized by the formation of localized lesions (ulcers) in the intestine, especially in the region known as the colon; abscesses in the liver and the brain; vomiting; severe diarrhea with fluid loss leading to dehydration; and abdominal pain.

AMERICAN TYPE CULTURE COLLECTION: The American Type Culture Collection (ATCC) is a not-for-profit bioscience organization that maintains the world's largest and most diverse collection of microbiological life. Many laboratories and institutions maintain their own stockpile of microorganisms, usually those that are in frequent use in the facility. Some large culture collections are housed and maintained by universities or private enterprises, but none of these rivals the ATCC in terms of size.

AMPLIFICATION: A process by which something is made larger or the quantity increased.

ANADROMOUS: Fish that migrate from ocean (salt) water to fresh water, such as salmon, are termed anadromous.

ANAEROBIC BACTERIA: Bacteria that grow without oxygen, also called anaerobic bacteria or anaerobes. Anaerobic bacteria can infect deep wounds, deep tissues, and internal organs where there is little oxygen. These infections are characterized by abscess formation, foul-smelling pus, and tissue destruction.

ANTHRAX: Anthrax refers to a disease that is caused by the bacterium *Bacillus anthracis*. The bacterium can enter the body via a wound in the skin (cutaneous anthrax), via contaminated food or liquid (gastrointestinal anthrax), or can be inhaled (inhalation anthrax).

ANTIBACTERIAL: A substance that reduces or kills germs (bacteria and other microorganisms but not viruses). Also often a term used to describe a drug used to treat bacterial infections.

ANTIBIOTIC: A drug, such as penicillin, used to fight infections caused by bacteria. Antibiotics act only on bacteria and are not effective against viruses.

ANTIBIOTIC RESISTANCE: The ability of bacteria to resist the actions of antibiotic drugs.

ANTIBIOTIC SENSITIVITY: Antibiotic sensitivity refers to the susceptibility of a bacterium to an antibiotic. Each type of bacteria can be killed by some types of antibiotics and not be affected by other types. Different types of bacteria exhibit different patterns of antibiotic sensitivity.

ANTIBODIES: Antibodies, or Y-shaped immunoglobulins, are proteins found in the blood that help to fight against foreign substances called antigens. Antigens, which are usually proteins or polysaccharides, stimulate the immune system to produce antibodies. The antibodies inactivate the antigen and help to remove it from the body. While antigens can be the source of infections from pathogenic bacteria and viruses, organic molecules detrimental to the body from internal or environmental sources also act as antigens. Genetic engineering and the use of various mutational mechanisms allow the construction of a vast array of antibodies (each with a unique genetic sequence).

ANTIBODY RESPONSE: The specific immune response that utilizes B cells to kill certain kinds of antigens.

ANTIBODY-ANTIGEN BINDING: Antibodies are produced by the immune system in response to antigens (material perceived as foreign). The antibody response to a particular antigen is highly specific and often involves a physical association between the two molecules. Biochemical and molecular forces govern this association.

ANTIFUNGAL: Antifungals (also called antifungal drugs) are medicines used to fight fungal infections. They are of two kinds, systemic and topical. Systemic antifungal drugs are medicines taken by mouth or by injection to treat infections caused by a fungus. Topical antifungal drugs are medicines applied to the skin to treat skin infections caused by a fungus.

ANTIGEN: Antigens, which are usually proteins or polysaccharides, stimulate the immune system to produce antibodies. The antibodies inactivate the antigen and help to remove it from the body. While antigens can be the source of infections from pathogenic bacteria and viruses, organic molecules detrimental to the body from internal or environmental sources also act as antigens. Genetic engineering and the use of various mutational mechanisms allow the construction of a vast array of antibodies (each with a unique genetic sequence).

ANTIGENIC DRIFT: Antigenic drift describes the gradual accumulation of mutations in genes (e.g., in genes coding for surface proteins) over a period of time.

ANTIGENIC SHIFT: Antigenic shift describes an abrupt and major genetic change (e.g., in genes coding for surface proteins of a virus).

ANTIHELMINTHIC: Antihelminthic drugs are medicines that rid the body of parasitic worms.

ANTIMICROBIAL: An antimicrobial material slows the growth of bacteria or is able to kill bacteria. Antimicrobial materials include antibiotics (which can be used inside the body) and disinfectants (which can only be used outside the body).

ANTIRETROVIRAL (ARV) DRUGS: Antiretroviral (ARV) drugs prevent the reproduction of a type of virus called a retrovirus. The human immunodefiency virus (HIV), which causes acquired immune deficiency syndrome (AIDS, also cited as acquired immune deficiency syndrome), is a retrovirus. These ARV drugs are therefore used to treat HIV infections. These medicines cannot prevent or cure HIV infection, but they help to keep the virus in check.

ANTIRETROVIRAL (ARV) THERAPY: Treatment with antiretroviral (ARV) drugs prevents the reproduction of a type of virus called a retrovirus. The human immunodeficiency virus (HIV), which causes acquired immu-

nodeficiency syndrome (AIDS, also cited as acquired immune deficiency syndrome), is a retrovirus. ARV drugs are therefore used to treat HIV infections. These medicines cannot prevent or cure HIV infection, but they help to keep the virus in check.

ANTISENSE DRUG: An antisense drug binds to mRNA, thereby blocking gene activity. Some viruses have mRNA as their genetic material, so an antisense drug could inhibit their replication.

ANTISEPTIC: A substance that prevents or stops the growth and multiplication of microorganisms in or on living tissue.

ANTITOXIN: An antidote to a toxin that neutralizes its poisonous effects.

ANTIVIRAL DRUGS: Antiviral drugs are compounds that are used to prevent or treat viral infections, via the disruption of an infectious mechanism used by the virus, or to treat the symptoms of an infection.

ARBOVIRUS: An arbovirus is a virus that is typically spread by blood-sucking insects, most commonly mosquitoes. Over 100 types of arboviruses cause disease in humans. Yellow fever and dengue fever are two examples.

ARENAVIRUS: An arenavirus is a virus that belongs in a viral family known as Arenaviridae. The name arenavirus derives from the appearance of the spherical virus particles when cut into thin sections and viewed using a transmission electron microscope. The interior of the particles is grainy or sandy in appearance, due to the presence of ribosomes that have been acquired from the host cell. The Latin designation *arena* means "sandy."

ARTHROPOD: A member of the largest single animal phylum, consisting of organisms with segmented bodies, jointed legs or wings, and exoskeletons.

ARTHROPOD-BORNE DISEASE: A disease caused by one of a phylum of organisms characterized by exoskeletons and segmented bodies.

ARTHROPOD-BORNE VIRUS: A virus caused by one of a phylum of organisms characterized by exoskeletons and segmented bodies.

ASEPSIS: Asepsis means without germs, more specifically without microorganisms.

ASPIRATION: Aspiration is the drawing out of fluid from a part of the body; it can cause pneumonia when stomach contents are transferred to the lungs through vomiting.

ASSAY: A determination of an amount of a particular compound in a sample (e.g., to make chemical tests to determine the relative amount of a particular substance in a sample). A method used to quantify a biological compound.

ASYMPTOMATIC: A state in which an individual does not exhibit or experience symptoms of a disease.

ATAXIA: Ataxia is an unsteadiness in walking or standing that is associated with brain diseases such as kuru or Creutzfeldt-Jakob disease.

ATOPY: Atopy is an inherited tendency towards hypersensitivity towards immunoglobulin E, a key component of the immune system, which plays an important role in asthma, eczema, and hay fever.

ATROPHY: Decreasing in size or wasting away of a body part or tissue.

ATTENUATED: An attenuated bacterium or virus has been weakened and is often used as the basis of a vaccine against the specific disease caused by the bacterium or virus.

ATTENUATED STRAIN: A specific strain of bacteria that has been killed or weakened, often used as the basis of a vaccine against the specific disease caused by the bacterium.

AUTOCLAVE: An autoclave is a device that is designed to kill microorganisms on solid items and in liquids by exposure to steam at a high pressure.

AUTOIMMUNE DISEASE: A disease in which the body's defense system attacks its own tissues and organs.

AUTOINFECTION: Autoinfection is the reinfection of the body by a disease organism already in the body, such as eggs left by a parasitic worm.

B

B CELL: Also known as B lymphocyte; a kind of cell produced in bone marrow that secretes antibodies.

BABESIOSIS: An infection of the red blood cells caused by *Babesia microti*, a form of parasite (parasitic sporozoan).

BACILLUS ANTHRACIS: The bacterium that causes anthrax.

BACTEREMIA: Bacteremia occurs when bacteria enter the bloodstream. This condition may occur through a wound or infection or through a surgical procedure or injection. Bacteremia may cause no symptoms and resolve without treatment, or it may produce fever and other symptoms of infection. In some cases, bacteremia leads to septic shock, a potentially life-threatening condition.

BACTERIA: Single-celled microorganisms that live in soil, water, plants, and animals, and whose activities range from the development of disease to fermentation. They play a key role in the decay of organic matter and the cycling of nutrients. Bacteria exist in various shapes, including spherical, rod-shaped, and spiral. Some bacteria are agents of disease. Different types of bacteria cause many sexually transmitted diseases, including syphilis, gonorrhea, and chlamydia. Bacteria also cause diseases such as typhoid, dysentery, and tetanus. Bacterium is the singular form of bacteria.

BACTERIOCIDAL: Bacteriocidal is a term that refers to the treatment of a bacterium such that the organism is killed. A bacteriocidal treatment is always lethal and is also referred to as sterilization.

BACTERIOLOGICAL STRAIN: A bacterial subclass of a particular tribe and genus.

BACTERIOPHAGE: A bacteriophage is a virus that infects bacteria. When a bacteriophage that carries the diphtheria toxin gene infects diphtheria bacteria, the bacteria produce diphtheria toxin.

BACTERIOSTATIC: Bacteriostatic refers to a treatment that restricts the ability of the bacterium to grow.

BACTERIUM: Singular form of the term bacteria—single-celled microorganisms—bacterium refers to an individual microorganism.

BASIDIOSPORE: A fungal spore of Basidomycetes. Basidomycetes are classified under the Fungi kingdom as belonging to the phylum Mycota (i.e., Basidomycota or Basidiomycota), class Mycetes (i.e., Basidiomycetes). Fungi are frequently parasites that decompose organic material from their hosts, such as the parasites that grow on rotten wood, although some may cause serious plant diseases such as smuts (Ustomycetes) and rusts (Teliomycetes). Some live in a symbiotic relationship with plant roots (Mycorrhizae). A cell type termed basidium is responsible for sexual spore formation in Basidomycetes, through nuclear fusion followed by meiosis, thus forming haploid basidiospores.

BED NETS: A type of netting that provides protection from diseases caused by insects such as flies and mosquitoes. It is often used when sleeping to allow air to flow through its mesh structure while preventing insects from biting.

BIFURCATED NEEDLE: A bifurcated needle is a needle that has two prongs with a wire suspended between them. The wire is designed to hold a certain amount of vaccine. Development of the bifurcated needle was a major advance in vaccination against smallpox.

BIOFILM: A biofilm is a population of microorganisms that forms following the adhesion of bacteria, algae, yeast, or fungi to a surface. These surface growths can be found in natural settings such as on rocks in streams and in infections such as can occur on catheters. Microorganisms can colonize living and inert natural and synthetic surfaces.

BIOINFORMATICS: Bioinformatics, or computational biology, refers to the development of new database methods to store genomic information (information related to genes and the genetic sequence), computational software programs, and methods to extract, process, and evaluate this information. Bioinformatics also refers to the refinement of existing techniques to acquire the genomic data. Finding genes and determining their function, predicting the structure of proteins and sequence of ribonucleic acid (RNA) from the available sequence of deoxyribonucleic acid (DNA), and determining the evolutionary relationship of proteins and DNA sequences are aspects of bioinformatics.

BIOLOGICAL WARFARE: Biological warfare, as defined by The United Nations, is the use of any living organism (e.g., bacterium, virus) or an infective component (e.g., toxin), to cause disease or death in humans, animals, or plants. In contrast to bioterrorism, biological warfare is defined as the "state-sanctioned" use of biological weapons on an opposing military force or civilian population.

BIOLOGICAL WEAPON: A weapon that contains or disperses a biological toxin, disease-causing microorganism, or other biological agent intended to harm or kill plants, animals, or humans.

BIOMAGNIFICATION: The increasing concentration of compounds at a higher trophic level or the tendency of organisms to accumulate certain chemicals to a concentration larger than that occurring in their inorganic, non-living environment, such as soil or water, or, in the case of animals, larger than in their food.

BIOMODULATOR: A biomodulator, short for biologic response modulator, is an agent that modifies some characteristic of the immune system, which may help in the fight against infection.

BIOSAFETY LABORATORY: A laboratory that deals with all aspects of potentially infectious agents or biohazards.

BIOSAFETY LEVEL 4 FACILITY: A specialized biosafety laboratory that deals with dangerous or exotic infectious agents or biohazards that are considered high risks for spreading life-threatening diseases, either because the disease is spread through aerosols or because there is no therapy or vaccine to counter the disease.

BIOSHIELD PROJECT: A joint effort between the U.S. Department of Homeland Security and the Department of Health and Human Services, Project Bio-Shield is tasked to improve treatment of diseases caused by biological, chemical, and radiological weapons.

BIOSPHERE: The sum total of all life-forms on Earth and the interaction among those life-forms.

BIOTECHNOLOGY: Use of biological organisms, systems, or processes to make or modify products.

BIOWEAPON: A weapon that uses bacteria, viruses, or poisonous substances made by bacteria or viruses.

BLOODBORNE PATHOGENS: Disease-causing agents carried or transported in the blood. Bloodborne infections are those in which the infectious agent is transmitted from one person to another via contaminated blood.

BLOODBORNE ROUTE: Via the blood. For example, bloodborne pathogens are pathogens (disease-causing agents) carried or transported in the blood. Bloodborne infections are those in which the infectious agent is transmitted from one person to another via contaminated blood. Infections of the blood can occur as a result of the spread of an ongoing infection caused by bacteria such as *Yersinia pestis*, *Haemophilus influenzae*, or *Staphylococcus aureus*.

BOTULINUM TOXIN: Botulinum toxin is among the most poisonous substances known. The toxin, which can be ingested or inhaled, and which disrupts transmission of nerve impulses to muscles, is naturally produced by the bacterium *Clostridium botulinum*. Certain strains of *C. baratii* and *C. butyricum* can also be capable of producing the toxin.

BOTULISM: Botulism is an illness produced by a toxin that is released by the soil bacterium *Clostridium botulinum*. One type of toxin is also produced by *Clostridium baratii*. The toxins affect nerves and can produce paralysis. The paralysis can affect the functioning of organs and tissues that are vital to life.

BROAD-SPECTRUM: The term "broad-spectrum" refers to a series of objects or ideas with great variety between them. In medicine, the term is often applied to drugs, which act on a large number of different disease-causing agents.

BROAD-SPECTRUM ANTIBIOTICS: Broad-spectrum antibiotics are drugs that kill a wide range of bacteria rather than just those from a specific family. For example, Amoxicillin is a broad-spectrum antibiotic that is used against many common illnesses such as ear infections.

BRONCHIOLITIS: Bronciolitis is an inflammation (-itis) of the bronchioles, the small air passages in the lungs that enter the alveoli (air sacs).

BUBO: A swollen lymph gland, usually in the groin or armpit, characteristic of infection with bubonic plague.

BUSH MEAT: The meat of terrestrial wild and exotic animals, typically those that live in parts of Africa, Asia, and the Americas; also known as wild meat.

C

CADAVER: The body of a deceased human, especially one designated for scientific dissection or other research.

CAMPYLOBACTERIOSIS: Campylobacteriosis is a bacterial infection of the intestinal tract of humans. The infection, which typically results in diarrhea, is caused by members of the genus *Campylobacter*. In particular, *Campylobacter jejuni* is the most common cause of bacterial diarrhea in the United States, with more occurrences than salmonella (another prominent disease-causing bacteria associated with food poisoning). Worldwide, approximately 5 to 14% of all diarrhea may be the result of campylobacteriosis.

CAPSID: The protein shell surrounding a virus particle.

CARBOLIC ACID: An acidic compound that, when diluted with water, is used as an antiseptic and disinfectant.

CARCINOGEN: A carcinogen is any biological, chemical, or physical substance or agent that can cause cancer. There are over one hundred different types of cancer, which can be distinguished by the type of cell or organ that is affected, the treatment plan employed, and the cause of the cancer. Most of the carcinogens that are commonly discussed come from chemical sources artificially produced by humans. Some of the better-known carcinogens are the pesticide DDT (dichlorodiphenyltrichloroethane), asbestos, and the carcinogens produced when tobacco is smoked.

CASE FATALITY RATE: The rate of patients suffering disease or injury that die as a result of that disease or injury during a specific period of time.

CASE FATALITY RATIO: A ratio indicating the amount of persons who die as a result of a particular disease, usually expressed as a percentage or as the number of deaths per 1,000 cases.

CATALYST: Substance that speeds up a chemical process without actually changing the products of reaction.

CD4+ T CELLS: CD4 cells are a type of T cell found in the immune system that are characterized by the presence of a CD4 antigen protein on their surface. These are the cells most often destroyed as a result of HIV infection.

CELL CYCLE AND CELL DIVISION: The series of stages that a cell undergoes while progressing to division is known as cell cycle. In order for an organism to grow and develop, the organism's cells must be able to duplicate themselves. Three basic events must take place to achieve this duplication: the deoxyribonucleic acid (DNA), which makes up the individual chromosomes within the cell's nucleus must be duplicated; the two sets of DNA must be packaged up into two separate nuclei; and the cell's cytoplasm must divide itself to create two separate cells, each complete with its own nucleus. The two new cells—products of the single original cell—are known as daughter cells.

CELL MEMBRANE: The cell is bound by an outer membrane that, as described by a membrane model termed the fluid mosaic model, is comprised of a phospholipid lipid bilayer with proteins—molecules that also act as receptor sites—interspersed within the phospholipid bilayer. Varieties of channels exist within the membrane. In eukaryotes (cells with a true nucleus) there are a number of internal cellular membranes that can partition regions within the cells' interior. Some of these membranes ultimately become continuous with the nuclear membrane. Bacteria and viruses do not have inner membranes.

CENTERS FOR DISEASE CONTROL AND PREVENTION (CDC): The Centers for Disease Control and Prevention (CDC) is one of the primary public health institutions in the world. CDC is headquartered in Atlanta, Georgia, with facilities at nine other sites in the United States. The centers are the focus of U.S. government efforts to develop and implement prevention and control strategies for diseases, including those of microbiological origin.

CESTODE: A class of worms characterized by flat, segmented bodies, commonly known as tapeworms.

CHAGAS DISEASE: Chagas disease is a human infection that is caused by a microorganism that establishes a parasitic relationship with a human host as part of its life cycle. The disease is named for the Brazilian physician Carlos Chagas, who in 1909 described the involvement of the flagellated protozoan known as *Trypanosoma cruzi* in a prevalent disease in South America.

CHAIN OF TRANSMISSION: Chain of transmission refers to the route by which an infection is spread from its source to a susceptible host. An example of a chain of transmission is the spread of malaria from an infected animal to humans via mosquitoes.

CHANCRE: A sore that occurs in the first stage of syphilis at the place where the infection entered the body.

CHEMILUMINESCENT SIGNAL: A chemiluminescent signal is the production of light that results from a chemical reaction. A variety of tests to detect infectious organisms or target components of the organisms rely on the binding of a chemical-containing probe to the target and the subsequent development of light following the addition of a reactive compound.

CHEMOTHERAPY: Chemotherapy is the treatment of a disease, infection, or condition with chemicals that have a specific effect on its cause, such as a microorganism or cancer cell. The first modern therapeutic chemical was derived from a synthetic dye. The sulfonamide drugs developed in the 1930s, penicillin and other antibiotics of the 1940s, hormones in the 1950s, and more recent drugs that interfere with cancer cell metabolism and reproduction have all been part of the chemotherapeutic arsenal.

CHICKENPOX: Chickenpox (also called varicella disease and sometimes spelled chicken pox) is a common and extremely infectious childhood disease that can also affect adults. It produces an itchy, blistery rash that typically lasts about a week and is sometimes accompanied by a fever.

CHILDBED FEVER: A bacterial infection occurring in women following childbirth, causing fever and, in some cases, blood poisoning and possible death.

CHLORINATION: Chlorination refers to a chemical process that is used primarily to disinfect drinking water and spills of microorganisms. The active agent in chlorination is the element chlorine, or a derivative of chlorine (e.g., chlorine dioxide). Chlorination is a swift and economical means of destroying many, but not all, microorganisms that are a health-threat in fluids such as drinking water.

CHRONIC: Chronic infections persist for prolonged periods of time—months or even years—in the host. This lengthy persistence is due to a number of factors, which can include masking of the disease-causing agent (e.g., bacteria) from the immune system, invasion of host cells, and the establishment of an infection that is resistant to antibacterial agents.

CHRONIC FATIGUE SYNDROME: Chronic fatigue syndrome (CFS) is a condition that causes extreme tiredness. People with CFS have debilitating fatigue that lasts for six months or longer. They also have many other symptoms. Some of these symptoms are pain in the joints and muscles, headache, and sore throat. CFS appears to result from a combination of factors.

CILIA: Cilia are specialized arrangements of microtubules and have two general functions. They propel certain unicellular organisms, such as paramecium, through the water. In multicellular organisms, if cilia extend from stationary cells that are part of a tissue layer, they move fluid over the surface of the tissue.

CIRRHOSIS: Cirrhosis is a chronic, degenerative, irreversible liver disease in which normal liver cells are damaged and are then replaced by scar tissue. Cirrhosis changes the structure of the liver and the blood vessels that nourish it. The disease reduces the liver's ability to manufacture proteins and process hormones, nutrients, medications, and poisons.

CLINICAL TRIALS: According to the National Institutes of Health, a clinical trial is "a research study to answer specific questions about vaccines or new therapies or new ways of using known treatments." These studies allow researchers to determine whether new drugs or treatments are safe and effective. When conducted carefully, clinical trials can provide fast and safe answers to these questions.

CLOACA: The cavity into which the intestinal, genital, and urinary tracts open in vertebrates such as fish, reptiles, birds, and some primitive mammals.

CLUSTER: In epidemiology, cluster refers to a grouping of individuals contracting an infectious disease or foodborne illness very close in time or place.

COCCIDIUM: Any single-celled animal (protozoan) belonging to the sub-class Coccidia. Some coccidia species can infest the digestive tract, causing coccidiosis.

COHORT: A cohort is a group of people (or any species) sharing a common characteristic. Cohorts are identified and grouped in cohort studies to determine the frequency of diseases or the kinds of disease outcomes over time.

COHORTING: Cohorting is the practice of grouping persons with similar infections or symptoms together, in order to reduce transmission to others.

COLONIZATION: Colonization is the process of occupation and increase in number of microorganisms at a specific site.

COLONIZE: Colonize refers to the process in which a microorganism is able to persist and grow at a given location.

COMMUNITY-ACQUIRED INFECTION: Community-acquired infection is an infection that develops outside of a hospital, in the general community. It differs from hospital-acquired infections in that those who are infected are typically in better health than hospitalized people.

CONGENITAL: Existing at the time of birth.

CONJUNCTIVITIS: Conjunctivitis (also called pink eye) is an inflammation or redness of the lining of the white part of the eye and the underside of the eyelid (conjunctiva) that can be caused by infection, allergic reaction, or physical agents like infrared or ultraviolet light. Conjunctivitis is one of the most common eye infections in children and adults in the United States. Luckily, it is also one of the most treatable infections. Because it is so common in the United States and around the world, and is often not reported to health organizations, accurate statistics are not available for conjunctivitis.

CONTACT PRECAUTIONS: Contact precautions are actions developed to minimize the transfer of microorganisms directly by physical contact and indirectly by touching a contaminated surface.

CONTAGIOUS: A disease that is easily spread among a population, usually by casual person-to-person contact.

CONTAMINATED: The unwanted presence of a microorganism or compound in a particular environment. That environment can be in the laboratory setting, for example, in a medium being used for the growth of a species of bacteria during an experiment. Another environment can be the human body, where contamination by bacteria can produce an infection. Contamination by bacteria and viruses can occur on several levels and their presence can adversely influence the results of experiments. Outside the laboratory, bacteria and viruses can contaminate drinking water supplies, foodstuffs, and products, thus causing illness.

COWPOX: Cowpox refers to a disease that is caused by the cowpox or catpox virus. The virus is a member of the orthopoxvirus family. Other viruses in this family include the smallpox and vaccinia viruses. Cowpox is a rare disease and is mostly noteworthy as the basis of the formulation, over 200 years ago, of an injection by Edward Jenner that proved successful in curing smallpox.

CREPITANT: A crackling sound that accompanies breathing, a common symptom of pneumonia or other diseases of the lungs.

CREUTZFELDT-JAKOB DISEASE (CJD): Creutzfeldt-Jakob disease (CJD) is a transmissible, rapidly progressing, fatal neurodegenerative disorder related to bovine spongiform encephalopathy (BSE), commonly called mad cow disease.

CULL: A cull is the selection, often for destruction, of a part of an animal population. Often done just to reduce numbers, a widespread cull was carried out during the epidemic of bovine spongiform encephalopathy (BSE or mad cow disease) in the United Kingdom during the 1980s.

CULTURE: A culture is a single species of microorganism that is isolated and grown under controlled conditions. The German bacteriologist Robert Koch first developed culturing techniques in the late 1870s. Following Koch's initial discovery, medical scientists quickly sought to identify other pathogens. Today bacteria cultures are used as basic tools in microbiology and medicine.

CULTURE AND SENSITIVITY: Culture and sensitivity refer to laboratory tests that are used to identify the type of microorganism causing an infection and the compounds to which the identified organism is sensitive and resistant. In the case of bacteria, this approach permits the selection of antibiotics that will be most effective in dealing with the infection.

CUTANEOUS: Pertaining to the skin.

CYST: Refers to either a closed cavity or sac or the stage of life during which some parasites live inside an enclosed area. In a protozoan's life, it is a stage when it is covered by a tough outer shell and has become dormant.

CYTOKINE: Cytokines are a family of small proteins that mediate an organism's response to injury or infection. Cytokines operate by transmitting signals between cells in an organism. Minute quantities of cytokines are secreted, each by a single cell type, and regulate functions in other cells by binding with specific receptors. Their interactions with the receptors produce secondary signals that inhibit or enhance the action of certain genes within the cell. Unlike endocrine hormones, which can act throughout the body, most cytokines act locally near the cells that produced them.

CYTOTOXIC: A cytotoxic agent is one that kills cells. Cytotoxic drugs kill cancer cells but may also have application in killing bacteria.

D

DEBRIDEMENT: Debridement is the medical process of removing dead, damaged, or infected tissue from pressure ulcers, burns, and other wounds, in order to speed healing of the surrounding healthy tissue.

DEFINITIVE HOST: The organism in which a parasite reaches reproductive maturity.

DEGRADATION (CELLULAR): Degradation means breakdown and refers to the destruction of host cell components, such as DNA, by infective agents such as bacteria and viruses.

DEHYDRATION: Dehydration is the loss of water and salts essential for normal bodily function. It occurs when the body loses more fluid than it takes in. Water is very important to the human body because it makes up about 70% of the muscles, around 75% of the brain, and approximately 92% of the blood. A person who weights about 150 pounds (68 kilograms) will contain about 80 quarts (just over 75 liters) of water. About two cups of water are lost each day just from regular breathing. If the body sweats more and breathes more heavily than normal, the human body loses even more water. Dehydration occurs when that lost water is not replenished.

DEMENTIA: Dementia, which is from the Latin word *dement* meaning "away mind," is a progressive deterioration and eventual loss of mental ability that is severe enough to interfere with normal activities of daily living; lasts more than six months; has not been present since birth; and is not associated with a loss or alteration of consciousness. Dementia is a group of symptoms caused by gradual death of brain cells. Dementia is usually caused by degeneration in the cerebral cortex, the part of the brain responsible for thoughts, memories, actions, and personality. Death of brain cells in this region leads to the cognitive impairment that characterizes dementia.

DEMOGRAPHICS: The characteristics of human populations or specific parts of human populations, most often reported through statistics.

DEOXYRIBONUCLEIC ACID (DNA): Deoxyribonucleic acid (DNA) is a double-stranded, helical molecule that forms the molecular basis for heredity in most organisms.

DERMATOPHYTE: A dermatophyte is a parasitic fungus that feeds off keratin, a protein which is abundant in skin, nails, and hair and therefore often causes infection of these body parts.

DIAGNOSIS: Identification of a disease or disorder.

DIARRHEA: To most individuals, diarrhea means an increased frequency or decreased consistency of bowel movements; however, the medical definition is more exact than this explanation. In many developed countries, the average number of bowel movements is three per day. However, researchers have found that diarrhea, which is not a disease, best correlates with an increase in stool weight; a stool weight above 10.5 ounces (300 grams) per day generally indicates diarrhea. This is mainly due to excess water, which normally makes up 60 to 85% of fecal matter. In this way, true diarrhea is distinguished from diseases that cause only an increase in the number of bowel movements (hyperdefecation) or incontinence (involuntary loss of bowel contents). Diarrhea is also classified by physicians into acute, which lasts one to two weeks, and chronic, which continues for longer than four weeks. Viral and bacterial infections are the most common causes of acute diarrhea.

DIATOM: Algae are a diverse group of simple, nucleated, plant-like aquatic organisms that are primary producers. Primary producers are able to utilize photosynthesis to create organic molecules from sunlight, water, and carbon dioxide. Ecologically vital, algae account for roughly half of the photosynthetic production of organic material on Earth in both freshwater and marine environments. Algae exist either as single cells or as multicellular organizations. Diatoms are microscopic, single-celled algae that have intricate glass-like outer cell walls partially composed of silicon. Different species of diatom can be identified based upon the structure of these walls. Many diatom species are planktonic, suspended in the water column moving at the mercy of water currents. Others remain attached to submerged surfaces. One bucketful of water may contain millions of diatoms. Their abundance makes them important food sources in aquatic ecosystems.

DIMORPHIC: This refers to the occurrence of two different shapes or color forms within the species, usually occurring as sexual dimorphism between males and females.

DINOFLAGELLATE: Dinoflagellates are microorganisms that are regarded as algae. Their wide array of exotic shapes and, sometimes, armored appearance, is distinct from other algae. The closest microorganisms in appearance are the diatoms.

DIPHTHERIA: Diphtheria is a potentially fatal, contagious bacterial disease that usually involves the nose, throat, and air passages, but may also infect the skin. Its most striking feature is the formation of a grayish membrane covering the tonsils and upper part of the throat.

DISINFECTANT: Disinfection and the use of chemical disinfectants is one key strategy of infection control. Disinfectants reduce the number of living microorganisms, usually to a level that is considered to be safe for the particular environment. Typically, this entails the destruction of those microbes that are capable of causing disease.

DISSEMINATED: Disseminated refers to the previous distribution of a disease-causing microorganism over a larger area.

DISSEMINATION: The spreading of a disease in a population, or of disease organisms in the body, is dissemination. A disease that occurs over a large geographic area.

DISTAL: Distal comes from the same root word as "distant," and is the medical word for distant from some agreed-on point of reference. For example, the hand is at the distal end of the arm from the trunk.

DNA: Deoxyribonucleic acid, a double-stranded, helical molecule that is found in almost all living cells and that determines the characteristics of each organism.

DNA FINGERPRINTING: DNA fingerprinting is the term applied to a range of techniques that are used to show similarities and dissimilarities between the DNA present in different individuals (or organisms).

DNA PROBES: Substances (agents) that bind directly to a predefined specific sequence of nucleic acids in DNA.

DORMANT: Inactive, but still alive. A resting, non-active state.

DROPLET: A droplet is a small airborne drop or particle—less than 5 microns (a millionth of a meter) in diameter—of fluid, such as may be expelled by sneezing or coughing.

DROPLET TRANSMISSION: Droplet transmission is the spread of microorganisms from one space to another (including from person to person) via droplets that are larger than 5 microns in diameter. Drop-lets are typically expelled into the air by coughing and sneezing.

DRUG RESISTANCE: Drug resistance develops when an infective agent, such as a bacterium, fungus, or virus, develops a lack of sensitivity to a drug that would normally be able to control or even kill it. This tends to occur with overuse of anti-infective agents, which selects out populations of microbes most able to resist them, while killing off those organisms that are most sensitive. The next time the anti-infective agent is used, it will be less effective, leading to the eventual development of resistance.

DYSENTERY: Dysentery is an infectious disease that has ravaged armies, refugee camps, and prisoner-of-war camps throughout history. The disease is still a major problem in developing countries with primitive sanitary facilities.

DYSPLASIA: Abnormal changes in tissue or cell development.

E

ECTOPARASITES: Parasites that cling to the outside of their host, rather than their host's intestines. Common points of attachment are the gills, fins, or skin of fish.

ELBOW BUMP: The elbow bump is a personal greeting that can be used as an alternative to the handshake: the two people greeting each other bump elbows. It is recommended by the World Health Organization for use by researchers handling highly infectious organisms, such as Ebola virus.

ELECTROLYTES: Compounds that ionize in a solution; electrolytes dissolved in the blood play an important role in maintaining the proper functioning of the body.

ELECTRON: A fundamental particle of matter carrying a single unit of negative electrical charge.

EMBRYONATED: When an embryo has been implanted in a female animal, that animal is said to be embryonated.

EMERGING DISEASE: New infectious diseases such as SARS and West Nile virus, as well as previously known diseases such as malaria, tuberculosis, and bacterial pneumonias that are appearing in forms resistant to drug treatments are termed emerging infectious diseases.

ENCEPHALITIS: A type of acute brain inflammation, most often due to infection by a virus.

ENCEPHALOMYELITIS: Simultaneous inflammation of the brain and spinal cord is encephalomyelitis.

ENCEPHALOPATHY: Any abnormality in the structure or function of the brain.

ENCYSTED LARVAE: Encysted larvae are larvae that are not actively growing and dividing and are more resistant to environmental conditions.

ENDEMIC: Present in a particular area or among a particular group of people.

ENDOCYTOSIS: Endocytosis is a process by which host cells allow the entry of outside substances, including viruses, through their cell membranes.

ENTERIC: Involving the intestinal tract or relating to the intestines.

ENTEROBACTERIAL INFECTIONS: Enterobacterial infections are caused by a group of bacteria that dwell in the intestinal tract of humans and other warm-blooded animals. The bacteria are all Gram-negative and rod-shaped. As a group they are termed Enterobacteriaceae. A prominent member of this group is *Escherichia coli*. Other members are the various species in the genera *Salmonella*, *Shigella*, *Klebsiella*, *Enterobacter*, *Serratia*, *Proteus*, and *Yersinia*.

ENTEROPATHOGEN: An enteropathogen is a virus or pathogen that invades the large or small intestine, causing disease.

ENTEROTOXIN: Enterotoxin and exotoxin are two classes of toxin that are produced by bacteria.

ENTEROVIRUS: Enteroviruses are a group of viruses that contain ribonucleic acid as their genetic material. They are members of the picornavirus family. The various types of enteroviruses that infect humans are referred to as serotypes, in recognition of their different antigenic patterns. The different immune response is important, as infection with one type of enterovirus does not necessarily confer protection to infection by a different type of enterovirus. There are 64 different enterovirus serotypes. The serotypes include polio viruses, coxsackie A and B viruses, echo-viruses, and a large number of what are referred to as non-polio enteroviruses.

ENZYME: Enzymes are molecules that act as critical catalysts in biological systems. Catalysts are substances that increase the rate of chemical reactions without being consumed in the reaction. Without enzymes, many reactions would require higher levels of energy and higher temperatures than exist in biological systems. Enzymes are proteins that possess specific binding sites for other molecules (substrates).

A series of weak binding interactions allows enzymes to accelerate reaction rates. Enzyme kinetics is the study of enzymatic reactions and mechanisms. Enzyme inhibitor studies have allowed researchers to develop therapies for the treatment of diseases, including AIDS.

EPIDEMIC: *Epidemic*, from the Greek meaning prevalent among the people, is most commonly used to describe an outbreak of an illness or disease in which the number of individual cases significantly exceeds the usual or expected number of cases in any given population.

EPIDEMIOLOGIST: Epidemiologists study the various factors that influence the occurrence, distribution, prevention, and control of disease, injury, and other health-related events in a defined human population. By the application of various analytical techniques, including mathematical analysis of the data, the probable cause of an infectious outbreak can be pinpointed.

EPIDEMIOLOGY: Epidemiology is the study of the various factors that influence the occurrence, distribution, prevention, and control of disease, injury, and other health-related events in a defined human population. By the application of various analytical techniques, including mathematical analysis of the data, the probable cause of an infectious outbreak can be pinpointed.

EPIZOOTIC: The abnormally high occurrence of a specific disease in animals in a particular area, similar to a human epidemic.

EPSTEIN-BARR VIRUS (EBV): Epstein-Barr virus (EBV) is part of the family of human herpes viruses. Infectious mononucleosis (IM) is the most common disease manifestation of this virus, which, once established in the host, can never be completely eradicated. Very little can be done to treat EBV; most methods can only alleviate resultant symptoms.

ERADICATE: To get rid of; the permanent reduction to zero of global incidence of a particular infection.

ERADICATION: The process of destroying or eliminating a microorganism or disease.

ERYTHEMA: Erythema is skin redness due to excess blood in capillaries (small blood vessels) in the skin.

ESCHAR: Any scab or crust forming on the skin as a result of a burn or disease is an eschar. Scabs from cuts or scrapes are not eschars.

ETIOLOGY: The study of the cause or origin of a disease or disorder.

EX SITU: A Latin term meaning "from the place" or removed from its original place.

EXECUTIVE ORDER: Presidential orders that implement or interpret a federal statute, administrative policy, or treaty.

EXOTOXIN: A toxic protein produced during bacterial growth and metabolism and released into the environment.

EYE DROPS: Eye drops are saline-containing fluid that is added to the eye to cleanse the eye or is a solution used to administer antibiotics or other medication.

F

FASCIA: Fascia is a type of connective tissue made up of a network of fibers. It is best thought of as being the packing material of the body. Fascia surrounds muscles, bones, and joints and lies between the layers of skin. It functions to hold these structures together, protecting these structures and defining the shape of the body. When surrounding a muscle, fascia helps prevent a contracting muscle from catching or causing excessive friction on neighboring muscles.

FECAL-ORAL TRANSMISSION: The spread of disease through the transmission of minute particles of fecal material from one organism to the mouth of another organism. This can occur by drinking contaminated water, eating food that was exposed to animal or human feces (perhaps by watering plants with unclean water), or by the poor hygiene practices of those preparing food.

FIBROBLAST: A cell type that gives rise to connective tissue.

FILOVIRUS: A filovirus is any RNA virus that belongs to the family *Filoviridae*. Filoviruses infect primates. Marburg virus and Ebola virus are filoviruses.

FLEA: A flea is any parasitic insect of the order *Siphonaptera*. Fleas can infest many mammals, including humans, and can act as carriers (vectors) of disease.

FLORA: In microbiology, flora refers to the collective microorganisms that normally inhabit an organism or system. Human intestines, for example, contain bacteria that aid in digestion and are considered normal flora.

FOCI: In medicine, a focus is a primary center of some disease process (for example, a cluster of abnormal cells). Foci is plural for focus (more than one focus).

FOMITE: A fomite is an object or a surface to which infectious microorganisms such as bacteria or viruses can adhere and be transmitted. Papers, clothing, dishes, and other objects can all act as fomites. Transmission is often by touch.

FOOD PRESERVATION: The term food preservation refers to any one of a number of techniques used to prevent food from spoiling. It includes methods such as canning, pickling, drying and freeze-drying, irradiation, pasteurization, smoking, and the addition of chemical additives. Food preservation has become an increasingly important component of the food industry as fewer people eat foods produced on their own lands, and as consumers expect to be able to purchase and consume foods that are out of season.

FULMINANT: A fulminant infection is an infection that appears suddenly and whose symptoms are immediately severe.

G

GAMETOCYTE: A germ cell with the ability to divide for the purpose of producing gametes, either male gametes called spermatocytes or female gametes called oocytes.

GAMMA GLOBULIN: Gamma globulin is a term referring to a group of soluble proteins in the blood, most of which are antibodies that can mount a direct attack upon pathogens and can be used to treat various infections.

GANGRENE: Gangrene is the destruction of body tissue by a bacteria called *Clostridium perfringens* or a combination of streptococci and staphylococci bacteria. *C. perfringens* is widespread; it is found in soil and the intestinal tracts of humans and animals. It becomes dangerous only when its spores germinate, producing toxins and destructive enzymes, and germination occurs only in an anaerobic environment (one almost totally devoid of oxygen). While gangrene can develop in any part of the body, it is most common in fingers, toes, hands, feet, arms, and legs, the parts of the body most susceptible to restricted blood flow. Even a slight injury in such an area is at high risk of causing gangrene. Early treatment with antibiotics, such as penicillin, and surgery to remove the dead tissue will often reduce the need for amputation. If left untreated, gangrene results in amputation or death.

GASTROENTERITIS: Gastroenteritis is an inflammation of the stomach and the intestines. More commonly, gastroenteritis is called the stomach flu.

GENE: A gene is the fundamental physical and functional unit of heredity. Whether in a microorganism or in a human cell, a gene is an individual element of an organism's genome and determines a trait or characteristic by regulating biochemical structure or metabolic process.

GENE THERAPY: Gene therapy is the name applied to the treatment of inherited diseases by corrective genetic engineering of the dysfunctional genes. It is part of a broader field called genetic medicine, which involves the screening, diagnosis, prevention, and treatment of hereditary conditions in humans. The results of genetic screening can pinpoint a potential problem to which gene therapy can sometimes offer a solution. Genetic defects are significant in the total field of medicine, with up to 15 out of every 100 newborn infants having a hereditary disorder of greater or lesser severity. More than 2,000 genetically distinct inherited defects have been classified so far, including diabetes, cystic fibrosis, hemophilia, sickle-call anemia, phenylketonuria, Down syndrome, and cancer.

GENETIC ENGINEERING: Genetic engineering is the altering of the genetic material of living cells in order to make them capable of producing new substances or performing new functions. When the genetic material within the living cells (i.e., genes) is working properly, the human body can develop and function smoothly. However, should a single gene—even a tiny segment of a gene go awry—the effect can be dramatic: deformities, disease, and even death are possible.

GENOME: All of the genetic information for a cell or organism. The complete sequence of genes within a cell or virus.

GENOTYPE: The genetic information that a living thing inherits from its parents that affects its makeup, appearance, and function.

GEOGRAPHIC FOCALITY: The physical location of a disease pattern, epidemic, or outbreak; the characteristics of a location created by interconnections with other places.

GEOGRAPHIC INFORMATION SYSTEM (GIS): A system for archiving, retrieving, and manipulating data that has been stored and indexed according to the geographic coordinates of its elements. The system generally can utilize a variety of data types, such as imagery, maps, tables, etc.

GEOGRAPHIC MEDICINE: Geographic medicine, also called geomedicine, is the study of how human health is affected by climate and environment.

GERM THEORY OF DISEASE: The germ theory is a fundamental tenet of medicine that states that microorganisms, which are too small to be seen without the aid of a microscope, can invade the body and cause disease.

GLOBAL OUTBREAK ALERT AND RESPONSE NETWORK (GOARN): A collaboration of resources for the rapid identification, confirmation, and response to outbreaks of international importance.

GLOBALIZATION: The integration of national and local systems into a global economy through increased trade, manufacturing, communications, and migration.

GLOMERULONEPHRITIS: Glomerulonephritis is inflammation of the kidneys. Mostly it affects the glomeruli, the small capsules in the kidney where blood flowing through capillaries transfers body wastes to urine.

GRAM NEGATIVE BACTERIA: Gram-negative bacteria are bacteria whose cell walls are comprised of an inner and outer membrane that are separated from one another by a region called the periplasm. The periplasm also contains a thin but rigid layer called the peptidoglycan.

GRANULOCYTE: Any cell containing granules (small, grain-like objects) is a granulocyte. The term is often used to refer to a type of white blood cell (leukocyte).

GROUP A STREPTOCOCCUS (GAS): A type (specifically a serotype) of the streptococcus bacteria, based on the antigen contained in the cell wall.

H

HARM-REDUCTION STRATEGY: In public health, a harm-reduction strategy is a public-policy scheme for reducing the amount of harm caused by a substance such as alcohol or tobacco. The phrase may refer to any medical strategy directed at reducing the harm caused by a disease, substance, or toxic medication.

HELMINTH: A representative of various phyla of worm-like animals.

HELMINTHIC DISEASE: Helminths are parasitic worms such as hookworms or flatworms. Helminthic disease by such worms is infectious. A synonym for helminthic is verminous.

HELSINKI DECLARATION: A set of ethical principles governing medical and scientific experimentation on human subjects; it was drafted by the World Medical Association and originally adopted in 1964.

HEMAGGLUTININ: Often abbreviated as HA, hemagglutinin is a glycoprotein, a protein that contains a short chain of sugar as part of its structure.

HEMOLYSIS: The destruction of blood cells, an abnormal rate of which may lead to lowered levels of these cells. For example, Hemolytic anemia is caused by destruction of red blood cells at a rate faster than they can be produced.

HEMORRHAGE: Very severe, massive bleeding that is difficult to control.

HEMORRHAGIC FEVER: A hemorrhagic fever is caused by viral infection and features a high fever and copious (high volume of) bleeding. The bleeding is caused by the formation of tiny blood clots throughout the bloodstream. These blood clots—also called microthrombi—deplete platelets and fibrinogen in the bloodstream. When bleeding begins, the factors needed for the clotting of the blood are scarce. Thus, uncontrolled bleeding (hemorrhage) ensues.

HEPA FILTER: A HEPA (high efficiency particulate air) filter is a filter that is designed to nearly totally remove airborne particles that are 0.3 microns (millionth of a meter) in diameter or larger. Such small particles can penetrate deeply into the lungs if inhaled.

HEPADNAVIRUSES: Hepadnaviridae is a family of hepadnaviruses comprised by two genera, *Avihepadnavirus* and *Orthohepadnavirus*. Hepadnaviruses have partially double-stranded DNA and they replicate their genome in the host cells using an enzyme called reverse transcriptase. Because of this, they are also termed retroviruses. The viruses invade liver cells (hepatocytes) of vertebrates. When hepadna retroviruses invade a cell, a complete viral double-stranded (ds) DNA is made before it randomly inserts in one of the host's chromosomes. Once part of the chromosomal DNA, the viral DNA is then transcribed into an intermediate messenger RNA (mRNA) in the hosts' nucleus. The viral mRNA then leaves the nucleus and undergoes reverse transcription, which is mediated by the viral reverse transcriptase.

HEPATITIS AND HEPATITIS VIRUSES: Hepatitis is an inflammation of the liver, a potentially life-threatening disease most frequently caused by viral infections but which may also result from liver damage caused by toxic substances such as alcohol and certain drugs. There are six major types of hepatitis viruses: hepatitis A (HAV), hepatitis B (HBV), hepatitis C (HCV), hepatitis D (HDV), hepatitis E (HEV), and hepatitis G (HGV).

HERD IMMUNITY: Herd immunity is a resistance to disease that occurs in a population when a proportion of them have been immunized against it. The theory is that it is less likely that an infectious disease will spread in a group where some individuals are unlikely to contract it.

HERPESVIRUS: Herpesvirus is a family of viruses, many of which cause disease in humans. The *herpes simplex*-1 and *herpes simplex*-2 viruses cause infection in the mouth or on the genitals. Other common types of herpesvirus include chickenpox, Epstien-Barr virus, and cytomegalovirus. Herpesvirus is notable for its ability to remain latent, or inactive, in nerve cells near the area of infection, and to reactivate long after the initial infection. *Herpes simplex*-1 and -2, along with chickenpox, cause familiar skin sores. Epstein-Barr virus causes mononucleosis. Cytomegalovirus also causes a like-like infection, but it can be dangerous to the elderly, infants, and those with weakened immune systems.

HETEROPHILE ANTIBODY: A heterophile antibody is an antibody that is found in the blood of someone with infectious mononucleosis, also known as glandular fever.

HIGH-LEVEL DISINFECTION: High-level disinfection is a process that uses a chemical solution to kill all bacteria, viruses, and other disease-causing agents except for bacterial endospores and prions. High-level disinfection should be distinguished from sterilization, which removes endospores (a bacterial structure that is resistant to radiation, drying, lack of food, and other things that would be lethal to the bacteria) and prions (misshapen proteins that can cause disease) as well.

HIGHLY ACTIVE ANTIRETROVIRAL THERAPY (HAART): Highly active antiretroviral therapy (HAART) is the name given to the combination of drugs given to people with human immunodeficiency virus (HIV) infection to slow or stop the progression of their condition to AIDS (acquired human immunodeficiency syndrome). HIV is a retrovirus and the various components of HAART block its replication by different mechanisms.

HISTAMINE: Histamine is a hormone that is chemically similar to the hormones serotonine, epinephrine, and norepinephrine. A hormone is generally defined as a chemical produced by a certain cell or tissue that causes a specific biological change or activity to occur in another cell or tissue located elsewhere in the body. Specifically, histamine plays a role in localized immune responses and in allergic reactions.

HISTOCOMPATIBILITY: The histocompatibility molecules (proteins) on the cell surfaces of one individual of a species are unique. Thus, if the cell is transplanted into another person, the cell will be recognized by the immune system as being foreign. The histocompatibility molecules act as antigens in the recipient and so can also be called histocompatibility antigens or transplantation antigens. This is the basis of the rejection of transplanted material.

HISTOPATHOLOGY: Histopathology is the study of diseased tissues. A synonym for histopathology is pathologic histology.

HIV (HUMAN IMMUNODEFICIENCY VIRUS): The virus that causes AIDS (acquired immunodeficiency syndrome).

HOMOZYGOUS: A condition in which two alleles for a given gene are the same.

HORIZONTAL GENE TRANSFER: Horizontal gene transfer is a major mechanism by which antibiotic resistance genes get passed between bacteria. It accounts for many hospital-acquired infections.

HORIZONTAL TRANSMISSION: Horizontal transmission refers to the transmission of a disease-causing microorganism from one person to another, unrelated person by direct or indirect contact.

HOST: An organism that serves as the habitat for a parasite or possibly for a symbiont. A host may provide nutrition to the parasite or symbiont, or it may simply provide a place in which to live.

HOST FOCALITY: Host focality refers to the tendency of some animal hosts, such as rodents carrying hantavirus and other viruses, to exist in groups in specific geographical locations and act as a local reservoir of infection.

HUMAN GROWTH HORMONE: Human growth hormone is a protein that is made and released from the pituitary gland, which increases growth and manufacture of new cells.

HUMAN IMMUNODEFICIENCY VIRUS (HIV): The human immunodeficiency virus (HIV) belongs to a class of viruses known as the retroviruses. These viruses are known as RNA viruses because they have RNA (ribonucleic acid) as their basic genetic material instead of DNA (deoxyribonucleic acid).

HUMAN T-CELL LEUKEMIA VIRUS: Two types of human T-cell leukemia virus (HTLV) are known. They are also known as human T-cell lymphotrophic viruses. HTLV-I often is carried by a person with no obvious symptoms. However, HTLV-I is capable of causing a number of maladies. These include abnormalities of the T cells and B cells, a chronic infection

of the myelin covering of nerves that causes a degeneration of the nervous system, sores on the skin, and an inflammation of the inside of the eye. HTLV-II infection usually does not produce any symptoms. However, in some people a cancer of the blood known as hairy cell leukemia can develop.

HYBRIDIZATION: A process of combining two or more different molecules or organisms to create a new molecule or organism (oftentimes called a hybrid organism).

HYGIENE: Hygiene refers to the health practices that minimize the spread of infectious microorganisms between people or between other living things and people. Inanimate objects and surfaces such as contaminated cutlery or a cutting board may be a secondary part of this process.

HYPERENDEMIC: A disease that is endemic (commonly present) in all age groups of a population is hyperendemic. A related term is holoendemic, meaning a disease that is present more in children than in adults.

HYPERINFECTION: A hyperinfection is an infection that is caused by a very high number of disease-causing microorganisms. The infection results from an abnormality in the immune system that allows the infecting cells to grow and divide more easily than would normally be the case.

I

IATROGENIC: Any infection, injury, or other disease condition caused by medical treatment is iatrogenic (pronounced eye-at-roh-GEN-ik).

IMMUNITY HUMORAL REGULATION: One way in which the immune system responds to pathogens is by producing soluble proteins called antibodies. This is known as the humoral response and involves the activation of a special set of cells known as the B lymphocytes, because they originate in the bone marrow. The humoral immune response helps in the control and removal of pathogens such as bacteria, viruses, fungi, and parasites before they enter host cells. The antibodies produced by the B cells are the mediators of this response.

IMMIGRATION: The relocation of people to a different region or country from their native lands; also refers to the movement of organisms into an area in which they were previously absent.

IMMUNE GLOBULIN: Globulins are a type of protein found in blood. The immune globulins (also called immunoglobulins) are Y-shaped globulins that act as antibodies, attaching themselves to invasive cells or materials in the body so that they can be identified and attacked by the immune system. There are five immune globulins, designated IgM, IgG, IgA, IgD, and IgE.

IMMUNE RESPONSE: The body's production of antibodies or some types of white blood cells in response to foreign substances.

IMMUNE SYNAPSE: Before they can help other immune cells respond to a foreign protein or pathogenic organism, helper T cells must first become activated. This process occurs when an antigen-presenting cell submits a fragment of a foreign protein, bound to a Class II MHC molecule (virus-derived fragments are bound to Class I MHC molecules), to the helper T cell. Antigen-presenting cells are derived from bone marrow, and include both dendritic cells and Langerhans cells, as well as other specialized cells. Because T cell responses depend upon direct contact with their target cells, their antigen receptors, unlike antibodies made by B cells, exist bound to the membrane only. In the intercellular gap between the T cell and the antigen-presenting cell, a special pattern of various receptors and complementary ligands forms that is several microns in size.

IMMUNE SYSTEM: The body's natural defense system that guards against foreign invaders and that includes lymphocytes and antibodies.

IMMUNO-BASED TEST: An immuno-based test is a medical technology that tests for the presence of a disease by looking for a reaction between disease organisms that may be present in a tissue or fluid sample and antibodies contained in the test kit.

IMMUNOCOMPROMISED: A reduction of the ability of the immune system to recognize and respond to the presence of foreign material.

IMMUNODEFICIENCY: In immunodeficiency disorders, part of the body's immune system is missing or defective, thus impairing the body's ability to fight infections. As a result, the person with an immunodeficiency disorder will have frequent infections that are generally more severe and last longer than usual.

IMMUNOGENICITY: Immunogenicity is the capacity of a host to produce an immune response to protect itself against infectious disease.

IMMUNOLOGY: Immunology is the study of how the body responds to foreign substances and fights off infection and other disease. Immunologists study the

molecules, cells, and organs of the human body that participate in this response.

IMMUNOSUPPRESSION: A reduction of the ability of the immune system to recognize and respond to the presence of foreign material.

IMPETIGO: Impetigo refers to a very localized bacterial infection of the skin. It tends to afflict primarily children, but can occur in people of any age. Impetigo caused by the bacteria *Staphylococcus aureus* (or staph) affects children of all ages, while impetigo caused by the bacteria called group A streptococci (Streptoccus pyogenes or strep) is most common in children ages two to five years.

IMPORTED CASE OF DISEASE: Imported cases of disease happen when an infected person who is not yet showing symptoms travels from his home country to another country and develops symptoms of his disease there.

IN SITU: A Latin term meaning "in place" or in the body or natural system.

INACTIVATED VACCINE: An inactivated vaccine is a vaccine that is made from disease-causing microorganisms that have been killed or made incapable of causing the infection. The immune system can still respond to the presence of the microorganisms.

INACTIVATED VIRUS: An inactivated virus is incapable of causing disease but still stimulates the immune system to respond by forming antibodies.

INCIDENCE: The number of new cases of a disease or injury that occur in a population during a specified period of time.

INCUBATION PERIOD: Incubation period refers to the time between exposure to a disease-causing virus or bacteria and the appearance of symptoms of the infection. Depending on the microorganism, the incubation time can range from a few hours (for example, food poisoning due to *Salmonella*) to a decade or more (for example, acquired immunodeficiency syndrome, or AIDS).

INFECTION CONTROL: Infection control refers to policies and procedures used to minimize the risk of spreading infections, especially in hospitals and health care facilities.

INFECTION CONTROL PROFESSIONAL (ICP): Infection control professionals are a group of nurses, doctors, laboratory workers, microbiologists, public health officials, and others who have specialized training in the prevention and control of infectious disease. Infection control professionals develop methods to control infection and instruct others in their use. These methods include proper handwashing; correct wearing of protective masks, eye-guards, gloves, and other specialized clothing; vaccination; monitoring for infection; and investigating ways to treat and prevent infection. Courses and certifications are available for those wishing to become infection control professionals.

INFORMED CONSENT: An ethical and informational process in which a person learns about a procedure or clinical trial, including potential risks or benefits, before deciding to voluntarily participate in a study or undergo a particular procedure.

INNATE IMMUNITY: Innate immunity is the resistance against disease that an individual is born with, as distinct from acquired immunity, which develops with exposure to infectious agents.

INOCULUM: An inoculum is a substance such as virus, bacterial toxin, or a viral or bacterial component that is added to the body to stimulate the immune system, which then provides protection from an infection by the particular microorganism.

INPATIENT: A patient who is admitted to a hospital or clinic for treatment, typically requiring the patient to stay overnight.

INSECTICIDE: A chemical substance used to kill insects.

INTERMEDIATE HOST: An organism infected by a parasite while the parasite is in a developmental form, not sexually mature.

INTERMEDIATE-LEVEL DISINFECTION: Intermediate-level disinfection is a form of disinfection that kills bacteria, most viruses, and mycobacteria.

INTERNATIONAL HEALTH REGULATIONS: International regulations introduced by the World Health Organization (WHO) that aim to control, monitor, prevent, protect against, and respond to the spread of disease across national borders while avoiding unnecessary interference with international movement and trade.

INTERTRIGO: Intertrigo, sometimes called eczema intertrigo, is a skin rash, often occurring in obese persons on parts of the body symmetrically opposite each other. It is caused by irritation of skin trapped under hanging folds of flesh such as pendulous breasts.

INTRAVENOUS: In the vein. For example, the insertion of a hypodermic needle into a vein to instill a fluid, withdraw or transfuse blood, or start an intravenous feeding.

IONIZING RADIATION: Any electromagnetic or particulate radiation capable of direct or indirect ion production in its passage through matter. In general use: Radiation that can cause tissue damage or death.

IRRADIATION: A method of preservation that treats food with low doses of radiation to deactivate enzymes and to kill microorganisms and insects.

ISOLATION: Isolation, within the health community, refers to the precautions that are taken in the hospital to prevent the spread of an infectious agent from an infected or colonized patient to susceptible persons. Isolation practices are designed to minimize the transmission of infection.

ISOLATION AND QUARANTINE: Public health authorities rely on isolation and quarantine as two important tools among the many they use to fight disease outbreaks. Isolation is the practice of keeping a disease victim away from other people, sometimes by treating them in their homes or by the use of elaborate isolation systems in hospitals. Quarantine separates people who have been exposed to a disease but have not yet developed symptoms from the general population. Both isolation and quarantine can be entered voluntarily by patients when public health authorities request it, or it can be compelled by state governments or by the federal Centers for Disease Control and Prevention.

J

JAUNDICE: Jaundice is a condition in which a person's skin and the whites of the eyes are discolored a shade of yellow due to an increased level of bile pigments in the blood as a result of liver disease. Jaundice is sometimes called icterus, from a Greek word for the condition.

K

KERITITIS: Keratitis, sometimes called corneal ulcers, is an inflammation of the cornea, the transparent membrane that covers the colored part of the eye (iris) and pupil of the eye.

KOCH'S POSTULATES: Koch's postulates are a series of conditions that must be met for a microorganism to be considered the cause of a disease. German microbiologist Robert Koch (1843–1910) proposed the postulates in 1890.

KOPLIK'S SPOTS: Koplik's spots, named after American pediatrician Henry Koplik (1858-1927) and also called Koplik's sign, are red spots with a small blue-white speck in the center found on the tongue and the insides of the cheeks during the early stages of measles.

L

LARVAE: Immature forms (wormlike in insects; fishlike in amphibians) of an organism capable of surviving on its own. Larvae do not resemble the parent and must go through metamorphosis, or change, to reach the adult stage.

LATENT: A condition that is potential or dormant, not yet manifest or active, is latent.

LATENT INFECTION: An infection already established in the body but not yet causing symptoms, or having ceased to cause symptoms after an active period, is a latent infection.

LATENT VIRUS: Latent viruses are those viruses that can incorporate their genetic material into the genetic material of the infected host cell. Because the viral genetic material can then be replicated along with the host material, the virus becomes effectively "silent" with respect to detection by the host. Latent viruses usually contain the information necessary to reverse the latent state. The viral genetic material can leave the host genome to begin the manufacture of new virus particles.

LEGIONNAIRES' DISEASE: Legionnaires' disease is a type of pneumonia caused by *Legionella* bacteria. The bacterial species responsible for Legionnaires' disease is *L. pneumophila*. Major symptoms include fever, chills, muscle aches, and a cough that is initially nonproductive. Definitive diagnosis relies on specific laboratory tests for the bacteria, bacterial antigens, or antibodies produced by the body's immune system. As with other types of pneumonia, Legionnaires' disease poses the greatest threat to people who are elderly, ill, or immunocompromised.

LENS: An almost clear, biconvex structure in the eye that, along with the cornea, helps to focus light onto the retina. It can become infected, causing inflammation, for example, when contact lenses are improperly used.

LEPTOSPIRE: Also called a leptospira, a leptospire is any bacterial species of the genus *Leptospira*. Infection with leptospires causes leptospirosis.

LESION: The tissue disruption or the loss of function caused by a particular disease process.

LIPOPOLYSACCHARIDE (LPS): Lipopolysaccharide (LPS) is a molecule that is a constituent of the outer membrane of Gram-negative bacteria. The molecule can also be referred to as endotoxin. LPS can help protect the bacterium from host defenses and can contribute to illness in the host.

LIVE VACCINE: A live vaccine uses a virus or bacteria that has been weakened (attenuated) to cause an immune response in the body without causing disease. Live vaccines are preferred to killed vaccines, which use a dead virus or bacteria, because they cause a stronger and longer-lasting immune response.

LOW-LEVEL DISINFECTION: Low-level disinfection is a form of disinfection that is capable of killing some viruses and some bacteria.

LYMPHADENOPATHY: Any disease of the lymph nodes (gland-like bodies that filter the clear intercellular fluid called lymph to remove impurities) is lymphadenopathy.

LYMPHATIC SYSTEM: The lymphatic system is the body's network of organs, ducts, and tissues that filters harmful substances out of the fluid that surrounds body tissues. Lymphatic organs include the bone marrow, thymus, spleen, appendix, tonsils, adenoids, lymph nodes, and Peyer's patches (in the small intestine). The thymus and bone marrow are called primary lymphatic organs, because lymphocytes are produced in them. The other lymphatic organs are called secondary lymphatic organs. The lymphatic system is a complex network of thin vessels, capillaries, valves, ducts, nodes, and organs that runs throughout the body, helping protect and maintain the internal fluids system of the entire body by both producing and filtering lymph and by producing various blood cells. The three main purposes of the lymphatic system are to drain fluid back into the bloodstream from the tissues, to filter lymph, and to fight infections.

LYMPHOCYTE: A type of white blood cell; includes B and T lymphocytes. A type of white blood cell that functions as part of the lymphatic and immune systems by stimulating antibody formation to attack specific invading substances.

M

M PROTEIN: M protein is an antibody found in unusually large amounts in the blood or urine of patients with multiple myeloma, a form of cancer that arises in the white blood cells that produce antibodies.

MACAQUE: A macaque is any short-tailed monkey of the genus *Macaca*. Macaques, including rhesus monkeys, are often used as subjects in medical research because they are relatively affordable and resemble humans in many ways.

MACULOPAPULAR: A macule is any discolored skin spot that is flush or level with the surrounding skin surface: a papule is a small, solid bump on the skin. A maculopapular skin disturbance is one that combines macules and papules.

MAJOR HISTOCOMPATIBILITY COMPLEX (MHC): The proteins that protrude from the surface of a cell that identify the cell as "self." In humans, the proteins coded by the genes of the major histocompatibility complex (MHC) include human leukocyte antigens (HLA), as well as other proteins. HLA proteins are present on the surface of most of the body's cells and are important in helping the immune system distinguish "self" from "non-self" molecules, cells, and other objects.

MALAISE: Malaise is a general or nonspecific feeling of unease or discomfort, often the first sign of disease infection.

MALIGNANT: A general term for cells that can dislodge from the original tumor, then invade and destroy other tissues and organs.

MATERIEL: A French-derived word for equipment, supplies, or hardware.

MEASLES: Measles is an infectious disease caused by a virus of the paramyxovirus group. It infects only humans, and the infection results in life-long immunity to the disease. It is one of several exanthematous (rash producing) diseases of childhood, the others being rubella (German measles), chickenpox, and the now rare scarlet fever. The disease is particularly common in both preschool and young school children.

MENINGITIS: Meningitis is an inflammation of the meninges—the three layers of protective membranes that line the spinal cord and the brain. Meningitis can occur when there is an infection near the brain or spinal cord, such as a respiratory infection in the sinuses, the mastoids, or the cavities around the ear. Disease organisms can also travel to the meninges through the bloodstream. The first signs may be a severe headache and neck stiffness followed by fever, vomiting, a rash, and, then, convulsions leading to loss of consciousness. Meningitis generally involves two types: non-bacterial meningitis, which is often called aseptic meningitis, and bacterial meningitis, which is referred to as purulent meningitis.

MENINGITIS BELT: The Meningitis Belt is an area of Africa south of the Sahara Desert, stretching from the Atlantic to the Pacific coast, where meningococcal meningitis is common.

MEROZOITE: The motile, infective stage of malaria, responsible for disease symptoms.

MESSENGER RIBONUCLEIC ACID (MRNA): A molecule of RNA that carries the genetic information for producing one or more proteins; mRNA is produced by copying one strand of DNA, but in eukaryotes it is able to move from the nucleus to the cytoplasm (where protein synthesis takes place).

MICROBICIDE: A microbicide is a compound that kills microorganisms such as bacteria, fungi, and protozoa.

MICROFILIAE: Live offspring produced by adult nematodes within the host's body.

MICROORGANISM: Microorganisms are minute organisms. With only a single currently known exception (i.e., *Epulopiscium fishelsonia*, a bacterium that is billions of times larger than the bacteria in the human intestine and is large enough to view without a microscope), microorganisms are minute organisms that require microscopic magnification to view. To be seen, they must be magnified by an optical or electron microscope. The most common types of microorganisms are viruses, bacteria, blue-green bacteria, some algae, some fungi, yeasts, and protozoans.

MIGRATION: In medicine, migration is the movement of a disease symptom from one part of the body to another, apparently without cause.

MIMICKED: In biology, mimicry is the imitation of another organism, often for evolutionary advantage. A disease that resembles another (for whatever reason) is sometimes said to have mimicked the other. Pathomimicry is the faking of symptoms by a patient, also called malingering.

MINIMAL INHIBITORY CONCENTRATION (MIC): The minimal inhibitory concentration (MIC) refers to the lowest level of an antibiotic that prevents growth of the particular type of bacteria in a liquid food source after a certain amount of time. Growth is detected by clouding of the food source. The MIC is the lowest concentration of the antibiotic at which the no cloudiness occurs.

MITE: A mite is a tiny arthropod (insect-like creature) of the order *Acarina*. Mites may inhabit the surface of the body without causing harm, or may cause various skin ailments by burrowing under the skin. The droppings of mites living in house dust are a common source of allergic reactions.

MMR VACCINE: MMR (measles, mumps, rubella) vaccine is a vaccine that is given to protect someone from measles, mumps, and rubella. The vaccine is made up of viruses that cause the three diseases. The viruses are incapable of causing the diseases but can still stimulate the immune system.

MONO SPOT TEST: The mononucleosis (mono) spot test is a blood test used to check for infection with the Epstein-Barr virus, which causes mononucleosis.

MONOCLONAL ANTIBODIES: Antibodies produced from a single cell line that are used in medical testing and, increasingly, in the treatment of some cancers.

MONONUCLEAR LEUKOCYTE: A mononuclear leukocyte is a type of white blood cell active in the immune system.

MONOVALENT VACCINE: A monovalent vaccine is one that is active against just one strain of a virus, such as the one that is in common use against the poliovirus.

MORBIDITY: The term "morbidity" comes from the Latin word *morbus*, which means sick. In medicine it refers not just to the state of being ill, but also to the severity of the illness. A serious disease is said to have a high morbidity.

MORPHOLOGY: The study of form and structure of animals and plants. The outward physical form possessed by an organism.

MORTALITY: Mortality is the condition of being susceptible to death. The term mortality comes from the Latin word *mors*, which means death. Mortality can also refer to the rate of deaths caused by an illness or injury, i.e., rabies has a high mortality rate.

MOSQUITO COILS: Mosquito coils are spirals of inflammable paste that, when burned, steadily release insect repellent into the air. They are often used in Asia, where many coils release octachlorodipropyl ether, which can cause lung cancer.

MOSQUITO NETTING: Fine meshes or nets hung around occupied spaces, especially beds, to keep out disease-carrying mosquitoes. Mosquito netting is a cost-effective way of preventing malaria.

MRSA: Methicillin-resistant *Staphylococcus aureus* are bacteria resistant to most penicillin-type antibiotics, including methicillin.

MULTIBACILLARY: The more severe form of leprosy (Hansen's disease) is called multibacillary leprosy. It is defined as the presence of more than 5 skin lesions on the patient with a positive skin-smear test. The less severe form of leprosy is called paucibacillary leprosy.

MULTI-DRUG RESISTANCE: Multi-drug resistance is a phenomenon that occurs when an infective agent loses its sensitivity against two or more of the drugs that are used against it.

MULTI-DRUG THERAPY: Multi-drug therapy is the use of a combination of drugs against infection, each of which attacks the infective agent in a different way. This strategy can help overcome resistance to anti-infective drugs.

MUTABLE VIRUS: A mutable virus is one whose DNA changes rapidly so that drugs and vaccines against it may not be effective.

MUTATION: A mutation is a change in an organism's DNA that occurs over time and may render it less sensitive to the drugs that are used against it.

MYALGIA: Muscular aches and pain.

MYCOBACTERIA: *Mycobacteria* is a genus of bacteria that contains the bacteria causing leprosy and tuberculosis. The bacteria have unusual cell walls that are harder to dissolve than the cell walls of other bacteria.

MYCOTIC: Mycotic means having to do with or caused by a fungus. Any medical condition caused by a fungus is a mycotic condition, also called a mycosis.

MYCOTIC DISEASE: Mycotic disease is a disease caused by fungal infection.

N

NATIONAL ELECTRONIC TELECOMMUNICATIONS SYSTEM FOR SURVEILLANCE (NETSS): A computerized public health surveillance information system that provides the Centers for Disease Control and Prevention (CDC) with weekly data regarding cases of nationally notifiable diseases.

NECROPSY: A necropsy is a medical examination of a dead body: also called an autopsy.

NECROTIC: Necrotic tissue is dead tissue in an otherwise living body. Tissue death is called necrosis.

NEEDLESTICK INJURY: Any accidental breakage or puncture of the skin by an unsterilized medical needle (syringe) is a needlestick injury. Health-care providers are at particular risk for needlestick injuries (which may transmit disease) because of the large number of needles they handle.

NEGLECTED TROPICAL DISEASE: Many tropical diseases are considered to be neglected because, despite their prevalence in less-developed areas, new vaccines and treatments are not being developed for them.

Malaria was once considered to be a neglected tropical disease, but recently a great deal of research and money have been devoted to its treatment and cure.

NEMATODES: Also known as roundworms; a type of helminth characterized by long, cylindrical bodies.

NEURAMINIDASE: Also abbreviated (NA), neuraminidase is a glycoprotein, a protein that contains a short chain of sugar as part of its structure.

NEUROTOXIN: A poison that interferes with nerve function, usually by affecting the flow of ions through the cell membrane.

NEUTROPHIL: An immune cell that releases a bacteria-killing chemical; neutrophils are prominent in the inflammatory response. A type of white blood cell that phagocytizes foreign microorganisms. It also releases lysozyme.

NOBEL PEACE PRIZE: An annual prize bequeathed by Swedish inventor Alfred Nobel (1833–1896) and awarded by the Norwegian Nobel Committee to an individual or organization that has "done the most or the best work for fraternity between the nations, for the abolition or reduction of standing armies and for the holding and promotion of peace congresses."

NODULE: A nodule is a small, roundish lump on the surface of the skin or of an internal organ.

NON-GOVERNMENTAL ORGANIZATION (NGO): A voluntary organization that is not part of any government; often organized to address a specific issue or perform a humanitarian function.

NORMAL FLORA: The bacteria that normally inhabit some part of the body, such as the mouth or intestines, are normal flora. Normal flora are essential to health.

NOROVIRUS: Norovirus is a type of virus that contains ribonucleic acid as the genetic material and causes an intestinal infection known as gastroenteritis. A well-known example is Norwalk-like virus.

NOSOCOMIAL INFECTION: A nosocomial infection is an infection that is acquired in a hospital. More precisely, the Centers for Disease Control in Atlanta, Georgia, defines a nosocomial infection as a localized infection or an infection that is widely spread throughout the body that results from an adverse reaction to an infectious microorganism or toxin that was not present at the time of admission to the hospital.

NOTIFIABLE DISEASES: Diseases that the law requires must be reported to health officials when diagnosed, including active tuberculosis and several sexually transmitted diseases; also called reportable diseases.

NUCLEOTIDE: The basic unit of a nucleic acid. It consists of a simple sugar, a phosphate group, and a nitrogen–containing base.

NUCLEOTIDE SEQUENCE: A particular ordering of the chain structure of nucleic acid that provides the necessary information for a specific amino acid.

NUCLEUS, CELL: Membrane–enclosed structure within a cell that contains the cell's genetic material and controls its growth and reproduction. (Plural: nuclei.)

NUTRITIONAL SUPPLEMENTS: Nutritional supplements are substances necessary to health, such as calcium or protein, that are taken in concentrated form to compensate for dietary insufficiency, poor absorption, unusually high demand for that nutrient, or other reasons.

NYMPH: In aquatic insects, the larval stage.

O

ONCOGENIC VIRUS: An oncogenic virus is a virus that is capable of changing the cells it infects so that the cells begin to grow and divide uncontrollably.

OOCYST: An oocyst is a spore phase of certain infectious organisms that can survive for a long time outside the organism and so continue to cause infection and resist treatment.

OOPHORITIS: Oophoritis is an inflammation of the ovary, which happens in certain sexually transmitted diseases.

OPPORTUNISTIC INFECTION: An opportunistic infection is so named because it occurs in people whose immune systems are diminished or not functioning normally; such infections are opportunistic insofar as the infectious agents take advantage of their hosts' compromised immune systems and invade to cause disease.

OPTIC SOLUTION: Any liquid solution of a medication that can be applied directly to the eye is an optic solution.

ORAL REHYDRATION THERAPY: Patients who have lost excessive water from their tissues are said to be dehydrated. Restoring body water levels by giving the patient fluids through the mouth (orally) is oral rehydration therapy. Often, a special mixture of water, glucose, and electrolytes called oral rehydration solution is given.

ORCHITIS: Orchitis is inflammation of one or both testicles. Swelling and pain are typical symptoms. Orchitis may be caused by various sexually transmitted diseases or escape of sperm cells into the tissues of the testicle.

OUTBREAK: The appearance of new cases of a disease in numbers greater than the established incidence rate, or the appearance of even one case of an emergent or rare disease in an area.

OUTPATIENT: A person who receives health care services without being admitted to a hospital or clinic for an overnight stay.

OVA: Mature female sex cells produced in the ovaries. (Singular: ovum.)

OVIPOSITION: Ovum is Latin for "egg." To oviposition is to position or lay eggs, especially when done by an insect.

P

PANCREATITIS: Pancreatitis is an inflammation of the pancreas, an organ that is important in digestion. Pancreatitis can be acute (beginning suddenly, usually with the patient recovering fully) or chronic (progressing slowly with continued, permanent injury to the pancreas).

PANDEMIC: Pandemic, which means all the people, describes an epidemic that occurs in more than one country or population simultaneously.

PAPULAR: A papule is a small, solid bump on the skin; papular means pertaining to or resembling a papule.

PAPULE: A papule is a small, solid bump on the skin.

PARAMYXOVIRUS: Paramyxovirus is a type of virus that contains ribonucleic acid as the genetic material and has proteins on its surface that clump red blood cells and assist in the release of newly made viruses from the infected cells. Measles virus and mumps virus are two types of paramyxoviruses.

PARASITE: An organism that lives in or on a host organism and that gets its nourishment from that host. The parasite usually gains all the benefits of this relationship, while the host may suffer from various diseases and discomforts, or show no signs of the infection. The life cycle of a typical parasite usually includes several developmental stages and morphological changes as the parasite lives and moves through the environment and one or more hosts. Parasites that remain on a host's body surface to feed are called ectoparasites, while those that live inside a host's body are called endoparasites. Parasitism is a highly successful biological adaptation. There are more known parasitic species than nonparasitic ones, and parasites affect just about every form of life, including most all animals, plants, and even bacteria.

PAROTITIS: Parotitis is inflammation of the parotid gland. There are two parotid glands, one on each side of the jaw, at the back. Their function is to secret saliva into the mouth.

PAROXYSM: In medicine, a paroxysm may be a fit, convulsion, or seizure. It may also be a sudden worsening or recurrence of disease symptoms.

PASTEURIZATION: Pasteurization is a process where fluids such as wine and milk are heated for a predetermined time at a temperature that is below the boiling point of the liquid. The treatment kills any microorganisms that are in the fluid but does not alter the taste, appearance, or nutritive value of the fluid.

PATHOGEN: A disease-causing agent, such as a bacteria, virus, fungus, etc.

PATHOGENIC: Something causing or capable of causing disease.

PATHOGENS: Agents or microorganisms causing or capable of causing disease.

PAUCIBACILLARY: Paucibacillary refers to an infectious condition, such as a certain form of leprosy, characterized by few, rather than many, bacilli, which are a rod-shaped type of bacterium.

PCR (POLYMERASE CHAIN REACTION): The polymerase chain reaction, or PCR, refers to a widely used technique in molecular biology involving the amplification of specific sequences of genomic DNA.

PERSISTENCE: Persistence is the length of time a disease remains in a patient. Disease persistence can vary from a few days to life-long.

PESTICIDE: Substances used to reduce the abundance of pests, any living thing that causes injury or disease to crops.

PHAGOCYTOSIS: The process by which certain cells engulf and digest microorganisms and consume debris and foreign bodies in the blood.

PHENOTYPE: The visible characteristics or physical shape produced by a living thing's genotype.

PLAGUE: A contagious disease that spreads rapidly through a population and results in a high rate of death.

PLASMID: A circular piece of DNA that exists outside of the bacterial chromosome and copies itself independently. Scientists often use bacterial plasmids in genetic engineering to carry genes into other organisms.

PLEURAL CAVITY: The lungs are surrounded by two membranous coverings, the pleura. One of the pleura is attached to the lung, the other to the ribcage. The space between the two pleura, the pleural cavity, is normally filled with a clear lubricating fluid called pleural fluid.

PNEUMONIA: Pneumonia is inflammation of the lung accompanied by filling of some air sacs with fluid (consolidation). It can be caused by a number of infectious agents, including bacteria, viruses, and fungi.

POSTEXPOSURE PROPHYLAXIS: Postexposure prophylaxis is treatment with drugs immediately after exposure to an infectious microorganism. The aim of this approach is to prevent an infection from becoming established.

POSTHERPETIC NEURALGIA: Neuralgia is pain arising in a nerve that is not the result of any injury. Postherpetic neuralgia is neuralgia experienced after infection with a herpesvirus, namely *Herpes simplex* or *Herpes zoster.*

POTABLE: Water that is clean enough to drink safely is potable water.

PREVALENCE: The actual number of cases of disease (or injury) that exist in a population.

PRIMARY HOST: The primary host is an organism that provides food and shelter for a parasite while allowing it to become sexually mature, while a secondary host is one occupied by a parasite during the larval or asexual stages of its life cycle.

PRIONS: Prions are proteins that are infectious. Indeed, the name prion is derived from "proteinaceous infectious particles." The discovery of prions and confirmation of their infectious nature overturned a central dogma that infections were caused only by intact organisms, particularly microorganisms such as bacteria, fungi, parasites, or viruses. Since prions lack genetic material, the prevailing attitude was that a protein could not cause disease.

PRODROMAL SYMPTOMS: Prodromal symptoms are the earliest symptoms of a disease.

PRODROME: A prodrome of a disease is a symptom indicating the disease's onset; it may also be called a prodroma. For example, painful swallowing is often a prodrome of infection with a cold virus.

PROPHYLAXIS: Pre-exposure treatments (e.g., immunization) that prevents or reduces severity of disease or symptoms upon exposure to the causative agent.

PROSTRATION: A condition marked by nausea, disorientation, dizziness, and weakness caused by dehydration and prolonged exposure to high temperatures; also called heat exhaustion or hyperthermia.

PROTOZOA: Single-celled animal-like microscopic organisms that live by taking in food rather than making it by photosynthesis and must live in the presence of water. (Singular: protozoan.) Protozoa are a diverse group of single-celled organisms, with more than 50,000 different types represented. The vast majority are microscopic, many measuring less than 5 one-thousandth of an inch (0.005 millimeters), but some, such as the freshwater Spirostomun, may reach 0.17 inches (3 millimeters) in length, large enough to enable it to be seen with the naked eye.

PRURITIS: Pruritis is the medical term for itchiness.

PRURULENT: Containing, discharging, or producing pus.

PUERPERAL: An interval of time around childbirth, from the onset of labor through the immediate recovery period after delivery.

PUERPERAL FEVER: Puerperal fever is a bacterial infection present in the blood (septicemia) that follows childbirth. The Latin word *puer* meaning boy or child, is the root of this term. Puerperal fever was much more common before the advent of modern aseptic practices, but infections still occur. Louis Pasteur showed that puerperal fever is most often caused by *Streptococcus* bacteria, which is now treated with antibiotics.

PULMONARY: Having to do with the lungs or respiratory system. The pulmonary circulatory system delivers deoxygenated blood from the right ventricle of the heart to the lungs, and returns oxygenated blood from the lungs to the left atrium of the heart. At its most minute level, the alveolar capillary bed, the pulmonary circulatory system is the principle point of gas exchange between blood and air that moves in and out of the lungs during respiration.

PURULENT: Any part of the body that contains or releases pus is said to be purulent. Pus is a fluid produced by inflamed, infected tissues and is made up of white blood cells, fragments of dead cells, and a liquid containing various proteins.

PUSTULES: A pustule is a reservoir of pus visible just beneath the skin. It is usually sore to the touch and surrounded by inflamed tissue.

PYELONEPHRITIS: Inflammation caused by bacterial infection of the kidney and associated blood vessels is termed pyelonephritis.

PYROGENIC: A substance that causes fever is pyrogenic. The word "pyrogenic" comes from the Greek word *pyr* meaning fire.

Q

QUANTITATED: An act of determining the quantity of something, such as the number or concentration of bacteria in an infectious disease.

QUARANTINE: Quarantine is the practice of separating people who have been exposed to an infectious agent but have not yet developed symptoms from the general population. This can be done voluntarily or involuntarily by the authority of states and the federal Centers for Disease Control and Prevention.

R

RALES: French term for a rattling sound in the throat or chest.

RASH: A rash is a change in appearance or texture of the skin. A rash is the popular term for a group of spots or red, inflamed skin that is usually a symptom of an underlying condition or disorder. Often temporary, a rash is only rarely a sign of a serious problem.

REASSORTMENT: A condition resulting when two or more different types of viruses exchange genetic material to form a new, genetically different virus.

RECEPTOR: Protein molecules on a cell's surface that acts as a "signal receiver" and allow communication between cells.

RECOMBINANT DNA: DNA that is cut using specific enzymes so that a gene or DNA sequence can be inserted.

RECOMBINATION: Recombination is a process during which genetic material is shuffled during reproduction to form new combinations. This mixing is important from an evolutionary standpoint because it allows the expression of different traits between generations. The process involves a physical exchange of

nucleotides between duplicate strands of deoxyribonucleic acid (DNA).

RED TIDE: Red tides are a marine phenomenon in which water is stained a red, brown, or yellowish color because of the temporary abundance of a particular species of pigmented dinoflagellate (these events are known as "blooms"). Also called phytoplankton, or planktonic algae, these single-celled organisms of the class Dinophyceae move using a tail-like structure called a flagellum. They also photosynthesize, and it is their photosynthetic pigments that can tint the water during blooms. Dinoflagellates are common and widespread. Under appropriate environmental conditions, various species can grow very rapidly, causing red tides. Red tides occur in all marine regions with a temperate or warmer climate.

RE-EMERGING INFECTIOUS DISEASE: Re-emerging infectious diseases are illnesses such as malaria, diphtheria, tuberculosis, and polio that were once nearly absent from the world but are starting to cause greater numbers of infections once again. These illnesses are reappearing for many reasons. Malaria and other mosquito-borne illnesses increase when mosquito-control measures decrease. Other diseases are spreading because people have stopped being vaccinated, as happened with diphtheria after the collapse of the Soviet Union. A few diseases are re-emerging because drugs to treat them have become less available or drug-resistant strains have developed.

REHYDRATION: Dehydration is excessive loss of water from the body; rehydration is the restoration of water after dehydration.

REITER'S SYNDROME: Reiter's syndrome (also called Reiter syndrome, Reiter disease, or reactive arthritis), named after German doctor Hans Reiter (1881-1969), is a form of arthritis (joint inflammation) that appears in response to bacterial infection in some other part of the body.

RELAPSE: Relapse is a return of symptoms after the patient has apparently recovered from a disease.

REPLICATE: To replicate is to duplicate something or make a copy of it. All reproduction of living things depends on the replication of DNA molecules or, in a few cases, RNA molecules. Replication may be used to refer to the reproduction of entire viruses and other microorganisms.

REPLICATION: A process of reproducing, duplicating, copying, or repeating something, such as the duplication of DNA or the recreation of characteristics of an infectious disease in a laboratory setting.

REPORTABLE DISEASE: By law, occurrences of some diseases must be reported to government authorities when observed by health-care professionals. Such diseases are called reportable diseases or notifiable diseases. Cholera and yellow fever are examples of reportable diseases.

RESERVOIR: The animal or organism in which the virus or parasite normally resides.

RESISTANCE: Immunity developed within a species (especially bacteria) via evolution to an antibiotic or other drug. For example, in bacteria, the acquisition of genetic mutations that render the bacteria invulnerable to the action of antibiotics.

RESISTANT BACTERIA: Resistant bacteria are microbes that have lost their sensitivity to one or more antibiotic drugs through mutation.

RESISTANT ORGANISM: An organism that has developed the ability to counter something trying to harm it. Within infectious diseases, the organism, such as a bacterium, has developed a resistance to drugs, such as antibiotics.

RESPIRATOR: A respirator is any device that assists a patient in breathing or takes over breathing entirely for them.

RESTRICTION ENZYME: A special type of protein that can recognize and cut DNA at certain sequences of bases to help scientists separate out a specific gene. Restriction enzymes recognize certain sequences of DNA and cleave the DNA at those sites. The enzymes are used to generate fragments of DNA that can be subsequently joined together to create new stretches of DNA.

RETROVIRUS: Retroviruses are viruses in which the genetic material consists of ribonucleic acid (RNA) instead of the usual deoxyribonucleic acid (DNA). Retroviruses produce an enzyme known as reverse transcriptase that can transform RNA into DNA, which can then be permanently integrated into the DNA of the infected host cells.

REVERSE TRANSCRIPTASE: An enzyme that makes it possible for a retrovirus to produce DNA (deoxyribonucleic acid) from RNA (ribonucleic acid).

RHINITIS: An inflammation of the mucous lining of the nose. A nonspecific term that covers infections, allergies, and other disorders whose common feature is the location of their symptoms. These symptoms include infected or irritated mucous membranes, producing a discharge, congestion, and swelling of the tissues of the nasal passages. The most widespread form of infectious rhinitis is the common cold.

RIBONUCLEIC ACID (RNA): Any of a group of nucleic acids that carry out several important tasks in the synthesis of proteins. Unlike DNA (deoxyribonucleic acid), it has only a single strand. Nucleic acids are complex molecules that contain a cell's genetic information and the instructions for carrying out cellular processes. In eukaryotic cells, the two nucleic acids, ribonucleic acid (RNA) and deoxyribonucleic acid (DNA), work together to direct protein synthesis. Although it is DNA that contains the instructions for directing the synthesis of specific structural and enzymatic proteins, several types of RNA actually carry out the processes required to produce these proteins. These include messenger RNA (mRNA), ribosomal RNA (rRNA), and transfer RNA (tRNA). Further processing of the various RNAs is carried out by another type of RNA called small nuclear RNA (snRNA). The structure of RNA is very similar to that of DNA, however, instead of the base thymine, RNA contains the base uricil in its place.

RING VACCINATION: Ring vaccination is the vaccination of all susceptible people in an area surrounding a case of an infectious disease. Since vaccination makes people immune to the disease, the hope is that the disease will not spread from the known case to other people. Ring vaccination was used in eliminating the smallpox virus.

RNA VIRUS: An RNA virus is one whose genetic material consists of either single- or double-stranded ribonucleic acid (RNA) rather than deoxyribonucleic acid (DNA).

ROUNDWORM: Also known as nematodes; a type of helminth characterized by long, cylindrical bodies. Roundworm infections are diseases of the digestive tract and other organ systems that are caused by roundworms. Roundworm infections are widespread throughout the world, and humans acquire most types of roundworm infection from contaminated food or by touching the mouth with unwashed hands that have come into contact with the parasite larva. The severity of infection varies considerably from person to person. Children are more likely to have heavy infestations and are also more likely to suffer from malabsorption and malnutrition than adults.

ROUS SARCOMA VIRUS: Rous sarcoma virus, named after American doctor Francis Peyton Rous (1879-1970), is a virus that can cause cancer in some birds, including chickens. It was the first virus known to be able to cause cancer.

RUMINANTS: Cud-chewing animals with a four-chambered stomachs and even-toed hooves.

S

SANITATION: Sanitation is the use of hygienic recycling and disposal measures that prevent disease and promote health through sewage disposal, solid waste disposal, waste material recycling, and food processing and preparation.

SCHISTOSOMES: Blood flukes that infect an estimated 200 million people.

SEIZURE: A seizure is a sudden disruption of the brain's normal electrical activity accompanied by altered consciousness and/or other neurological and behavioral abnormalities. Epilepsy is a condition characterized by recurrent seizures that may include repetitive muscle jerking called convulsions. Seizures are traditionally divided into two major categories: generalized seizures and focal seizures. Within each major category, however, there are many different types of seizures. Generalized seizures come about due to abnormal neuronal activity on both sides of the brain, while focal seizures, also named partial seizures, occur in only one part of the brain.

SELECTION: Process which favors one feature of organisms in a population over another feature found in the population. This occurs through differential reproduction—those with the favored feature produce more offspring than those with the other feature, such that they become a greater percentage of the population in the next generation.

SELECTION PRESSURE: Selection pressure refers to factors that influence the evolution of an organism. An example is the overuse of antibiotics, which provides a selection pressure for the development of antibiotic resistance in bacteria.

SELECTIVE PRESSURE: Selective pressure refers to the tendency of an organism that has a certain characteristic to be eliminated from an environment or to increase in numbers. An example is the increased prevalence of bacteria that are resistant to multiple kinds of antibiotics.

SENTINEL: A sentinel is a guard or watcher; in medicine, a sentinel node is a lymph node near the breast in which cancer cells from a breast tumor are likely to be found at an early stage of the cancer's spreading (metastasization).

SENTINEL SURVEILLANCE: Sentinel surveillance is a method in epidemiology where a subset of the population is surveyed for the presence of communicable diseases. Also, a sentinel is an animal used to indicate the presence of disease within an area.

SEPSIS: Sepsis refers to a bacterial infection in the bloodstream or body tissues. This is a very broad term covering the presence of many types of microscopic disease-causing organisms. Sepsis is also called bacteremia. Closely related terms include septicemia and septic syndrome. According to the Society of Critical Care Medicine, severe sepsis affects about 750,000 people in the United States each year. However, it is predicted to rapidly rise to one million people by 2010 due to the aging U.S. population. Over the decade of the 1990s, the incident rate of sepsis increased over 91%.

SEPTIC: The term "septic" refers to the state of being infected with bacteria, particularly in the bloodstream.

SEPTICEMIA: Prolonged fever, chills, anorexia, and anemia in conjunction with tissue lesions.

SEQUENCING: Finding the order of chemical bases in a section of DNA.

SEROCONVERSION: The development in the blood of antibodies to an infectious organism or agent. Typically, seroconversion is associated with infections caused by bacteria, viruses, and protozoans. But seroconversion also occurs after the deliberate inoculation with an antigen in the process of vaccination. In the case of infections, the development of detectable levels of antibodies can occur quickly, in the case of an active infection, or can be prolonged, in the case of a latent infection. Seroconversion typically heralds the development of the symptoms of the particular infection.

SEROTYPES: Serotypes or serovars are classes of microorganisms based on the types of molecules (antigens) that they present on their surfaces. Even a single species may have thousands of serotypes, which may have medically quite distinct behaviors.

SEXUALLY TRANSMITTED DISEASE (STD): Sexually transmitted diseases (STDs) vary in their susceptibility to treatment, their signs and symptoms, and the consequences if they are left untreated. Some are caused by bacteria. These usually can be treated and cured. Others are caused by viruses and can typically be treated but not cured. More than 15 million new cases of STDs are diagnosed annually in the United States.

SHED: To shed is to cast off or release. In medicine, the release of eggs or live organisms from an individual infected with parasites is often referred to as shedding.

SHOCK: Shock is a medical emergency in which the organs and tissues of the body are not receiving an adequate flow of blood. This condition deprives the organs and tissues of oxygen (carried in the blood) and allows the buildup of waste products. Shock can result in serious damage or even death.

SOCIOECONOMIC: Concerning both social and economic factors.

SOUTHERN BLOT ANALYSIS: Southern blot refers to an electrophoresis technique in which pieces of deoxyribonucleic acid (DNA) that have resulted from enzyme digestion are separated from one another on the basis of size, followed by the transfer of the DNA fragments to a flexible membrane. The membrane can then be exposed to various probes to identify target regions of the genetic material.

SPECIAL PATHOGENS BRANCH: A group within the U.S. Centers for Disease Control and Prevention (CDC) whose goal is to study highly infectious viruses that produce diseases within humans.

SPIROCHETE: A bacterium shaped like a spiral. Spiral-shaped bacteria, which live in contaminated water, sewage, soil, and decaying organic matter, as well as inside humans and animals.

SPONGIFORM: Spongiform is the clinical name for the appearance of brain tissue affected by prion diseases, such as Creutzfeld-Jakob disease or bovine spongiform encephalopathy (mad cow disease). The disease process leads to the formation of tiny holes in brain tissue, giving it a spongy appearance.

SPONTANEOUS GENERATION: Also known as abiogenesis; the incorrect and discarded assumption that living things can be generated from nonliving things.

SPORE: A dormant form assumed by some bacteria, such as anthrax, that enables the bacterium to survive high temperatures, dryness, and lack of nourishment for long periods of time. Under proper conditions, the spore may revert to the actively multiplying form of the bacteria.

SPOROZOAN: The fifth Phylum of the Protist Kingdom, known as Apicomplexa, comprises several species of obligate intracellular protozoan parasites classified as Sporozoa or Sporozoans, because they form reproductive cells known as spores. Many sporozoans are parasitic and pathogenic species, such as *Plasmodium falciparum, P. malariae, P. vivax, Toxoplasma gondii, Pneumocysts carinii, Cryptosporidum parvum* and *Cryptosporidum muris.* The Sporozoa reproduction cycle has both asexual and sexual phases. The asexual phase is termed schizogony (from the Greek, meaning generation through division), in which merozoites (daughter cells) are produced through multiple nuclear fissions. The sexual phase is known as sporogony (i.e., generation of spores) and is followed by gametogony or the production of sexually reproductive cells termed gamonts.

SPOROZOITE: Developmental stage of a protozoan (e.g., a malaria protozoan) during which it is transferred from vector (with malaria, a mosquito) to a human host.

STAINING: Staining refers to the use of chemicals to identify target components of microorganisms.

STANDARD PRECAUTIONS: Standard precautions are the safety measures taken to prevent the transmission of disease-causing bacteria. These include proper handwashing; wearing gloves, goggles, and other protective clothing; proper handling of needles; and sterilization of equipment.

STERILIZATION: Sterilization is a term that refers to the complete killing or elimination of living organisms in the sample being treated. Sterilization is absolute. After the treatment the sample is either devoid of life or the possibility of life (as from the subsequent germination and growth of bacterial spores) or it is not considered sterile.

STRAIN: A subclass or a specific genetic variation of an organism.

STREP THROAT: Streptococcal sore throat, or strep throat as it is more commonly called, is an infection caused by group A *Streptococcus* bacteria. The main target of the infection is the mucous membranes lining the pharynx. Sometimes the tonsils are also infected (tonsillitis). If left untreated, the infection can develop into rheumatic fever or other serious conditions.

STREPTOCOCCUS: A genus of bacteria that includes species such as *Streptococci pyogenes,* a species of bacteria that causes strep throat.

SUPERINFECTION: When a new infection occurs in a patient who already has some other infection, it is called a superinfection. For example, a bacterial infection appearing in a person who already had viral pneumonia would be a superinfection.

SURVEILLANCE: The systematic analysis, collection, evaluation, interpretation, and dissemination of data. In public health, it assists in the identification of health threats and the planning, implementation, and evaluation of responses to those threats.

SYLVATIC: Sylvatic means pertaining to the woods and refers to diseases such as plague that are spread by animals such as ground squirrels and other wild rodents.

SYSTEMIC: Any medical condition that affects the whole body (i.e., the whole system) is systemic.

T

T CELL: Immune-system white blood cells that enable antibody production, suppress antibody production, or kill other cells. When a vertebrate encounters substances that are capable of causing it harm, a protective system known as the immune system comes into play. This system is a network of many different organs that work together to recognize foreign substances and destroy them. The immune system can respond to the presence of a disease-causing agent (pathogen) in two ways. In cell-mediated immunity, immune cells known as the T cells produce special chemicals that can specifically isolate the pathogen and destroy it. The other branch of immunity is called humoral immunity, in which immune cells called B cells can produce soluble proteins (antibodies) that can accurately target and kill the pathogen.

TAPEWORM: Tapeworms are parasitic flatworms of class *Cestoidea*, phylum *Platyhelminthes*, that live inside the intestine. Tapeworms have no digestive system, but absorb predigested nutrients directly from their surroundings.

T-CELL VACCINE: A T-cell vaccine is one that relies on eliciting cellular immunity, rather than humoral antibody-based immunity, against infection. T cell vaccines are being developed against the human immunodeficiency virus (HIV) and hepatitis C.

TICK: A tick is any blood-sucking parasitic insect of suborder *Ixodides*, superfamily *Ixodoidea*. Ticks can transmit a number of diseases, including Lyme disease and Rocky Mountain spotted fever.

TOGAVIRUS: Togaviruses are a type of virus. Rubella is caused by a type of togavirus.

TOPICAL: Any medication that is applied directly to a particular part of the body's surface is termed topical; for example, a topical ointment.

TOXIC: Something that is poisonous and that can cause illness or death.

TOXIN: A poison that is produced by a living organism.

TOXOID: A toxoid is a bacterial toxin that has been altered chemically to make it incapable of causing damage, but is still capable of stimulating an immune response. Toxoids are used to stimulate antibody production, which is protective in the event of exposure to the active toxin.

TRANSFUSION-TRANSMISSIBLE INFECTIONS: Any infection that can be transmitted to a person by a blood transfusion (addition of stored whole blood or blood fractions to a person's own blood) is a transfusion-transmissible infection. Some diseases that can be transmitted in this way are AIDS, hepatitis B, hepatitis C, syphilis, malaria, and Chagas disease.

TRANSMISSION: Microorganisms that cause disease in humans and other species are known as pathogens. The transmission of pathogens to a human or other host can occur in a number of ways, depending upon the microorganism.

TREMATODES: Trematodes, also called flukes, are a type of parasitic flatworm. In humans, flukes can infest the liver, lung, and other tissues.

TRICLOSAN: A chemical that kills bacteria. Most antibacterial soaps use this chemical.

TRISMUS: Trismus is the medical term for lockjaw, a condition often associated with tetanus, infection by the *Clostridium tetani* bacillus. In trismus or lockjaw, the major muscles of the jaw contract involuntarily.

TROPHOZOITE: The amoeboid, vegetative stage of the malaria protozoa.

TYPHUS: A disease caused by various species of *Rickettsia*, characterized by fever, rash, and delirium. Insects such as lice and chiggers transmit typhus. Two forms of typhus, epidemic typhus and scrub typhus, are fatal if untreated.

U

UNIVERSAL PRECAUTION: Universal precaution refers to an infection control strategy in which all human blood and other material is assumed to be potentially infectious, specifically with organisms such as human immunodeficiency virus (HIV) and hepatitis B virus. The precautions are aimed at preventing contact with blood or the other materials.

V

VACCINATION: Vaccination is the inoculation, or use of vaccines, to prevent specific diseases within humans and animals by producing immunity to such diseases. It is the introduction of weakened or dead viruses or microorganisms into the body to create immunity by the production of specific antibodies.

VACCINE: A substance that is introduced to stimulate antibody production and thus provide immunity to a particular disease.

VACCINIA VIRUS: The vaccinia virus is a usually harmless virus that is closely related to the virus that causes smallpox, a dangerous disease. Infection with the vaccinia virus confers immunity against smallpox, so vaccinia virus has been used as a vaccine against smallpox.

VARICELLA ZOSTER IMMUNE GLOBULIN (VZIG): Varicella zoster immune globulin is a preparation that can give people temporary protection against chickenpox after exposure to the Varicella virus. It is used for children and adults who are at risk of complications of the disease or who are susceptible to infection because they have weakened immunity.

VARICELLA ZOSTER VIRUS (VZV): Varicella zoster virus is a member of the alpha herpes virus group and is the cause of both chickenpox (also known as varicella) and shingles (herpes zoster).

VARIOLA VIRUS: Variola virus (or variola major virus) is the virus that causes smallpox. The virus is one of the members of the poxvirus group (Family Poxviridae). The virus particle is brick shaped and contains a double strand of deoxyribonucleic acid. The variola virus is among the most dangerous of all the potential biological weapons.

VARIOLATION: Variolation was the pre-modern practice of deliberately infecting a person with smallpox in order to make them immune to a more serious form of the disease. It was dangerous, but did confer immunity on survivors.

VECTOR: Any agent that carries and transmits parasites and diseases. Also, an organism or chemical used to transport a gene into a new host cell.

VECTOR-BORNE DISEASE: A vector-borne disease is one in which the pathogenic microorganism is transmitted from an infected individual to another individual by an arthropod or other agent, sometimes with other animals serving as intermediary hosts. The transmission depends upon the attributes and requirements of at least three different living organisms: the pathologic agent, either a virus, protozoa, bacteria, or helminth (worm); the vector, commonly arthropods such as ticks or mosquitoes; and the human host.

VENEREAL DISEASE: Venereal diseases are diseases that are transmitted by sexual contact. They are named after Venus, the Roman goddess of female sexuality.

VESICLE: A membrane-bound sphere that contains a variety of substances in cells.

VIRAL SHEDDING: Viral shedding refers to the movement of the herpes virus from the nerves to the surface of the skin. During shedding, the virus can be passed on through skin-to-skin contact.

VIRION: A virion is a mature virus particle, consisting of a core of ribonucleic acid (RNA) or deoxyribonucleic acid (DNA) surrounded by a protein coat. This is the form in which a virus exists outside of its host cell.

VIRULENCE: Virulence is the ability of a disease organism to cause disease: a more virulent organism is more infective and liable to produce more serious disease.

VIRUS: Viruses are essentially nonliving repositories of nucleic acid that require the presence of a living prokaryotic or eukaryotic cell for the replication of the nucleic acid. There are a number of different viruses that challenge the human immune system and that may produce disease in humans. A virus is a small, infectious agent that consists of a core of genetic material—either deoxyribonucleic acid (DNA) or ribonucleic acid (RNA)—surrounded by a shell of protein. Very simple microorganisms, viruses are much smaller than bacteria that enter and multiply within cells. Viruses often exchange or transfer their genetic material (DNA or RNA) to cells and can cause diseases such as chickenpox, hepatitis, measles, and mumps.

VISCERAL: Visceral means pertaining to the viscera. The viscera are the large organs contained in the main cavities of the body, especially the thorax and abdomen, for example, the lungs, stomach, intestines, kidneys, or liver.

W

WATER-BORNE DISEASE: Water-borne disease refers to diseases that are caused by exposure to contaminated water. The exposure can occur by drinking the water or having the water come in contact with the body. Examples of water-borne diseases are cholera and typhoid fever.

WAVELENGTH: A distance of one cycle of a wave; for instance, the distance between the peaks on adjoining waves that have the same phase.

WEAPONIZATION: The use of any bacterium, virus, or other disease-causing organism as a weapon of war. Among other terms, it is also called germ warfare, biological weaponry, and biological warfare.

WEIL'S DISEASE: Weil's disease, named after German doctor Adolf Weil (1848-1916), is a severe form of leptospirosis or seven-day fever, a disease caused by infection with the corkscrew-shaped bacillus *Leptospira interrogans.*

WILD VIRUS: Wild- or wild-type virus is a genetic description referring to the original form of a virus, first observed in nature. It may remain the most common form in existence but mutated forms develop over time and sometimes become the new wild type virus.

Z

ZOONOTIC: A zoonotic disease is a disease that can be transmitted between animals and humans. Examples of zoonotic diseases are anthrax, plague, and Q-fever.

Chronology

c.2500 The characteristic symptoms of malaria are first described in Chinese medical writings.

c.1000 Hindu physicians exhibit broad clinical knowledge of tuberculosis. In India, the Laws of Manu consider it to be an unclean, incurable disease and an impediment to marriage.

c.430 Plague of Athens caused by unknown infectious agent. One third of the population (increased by those fleeing the Spartan army) die.

c.400 Hippocrates (460–370 BC), Greek physician, and his disciples found their medical practice based on reason and experiment. They attribute disease to natural causes and use diet and medication to restore the body's balance of humors.

c.400 Hippocratic texts recommend irrigation with fresh water as a treatment for septic wounds.

c.300 A medical school is set up in Alexandria where the first accurate anatomical observations using dissection are made. The principal exponents of the school are Greek physician Herophilus (c.335–c.280 BC) and Greek physician Erasistratus (c.304–c.250 BC).

c.300 Herophilus, Greek anatomist, establishes himself as the first systemic anatomist and the first to perform human dissections.

91 Greek scientific medicine takes hold in Rome when the physician Asclepiades (c.130–40 BC) of Bithynia settles in the West.

c.30 Aulus Cornelius Celsus, Roman encyclopedist, writes his influential book *De Re Medicina*. This work *On Medicine* contains descriptions of many conditions and operations, and is probably drawn mostly from the collection of writings of the school of Hippocrates. It is rediscovered during the fifteenth century and becomes highly influential. (See 1426)

c.75 Dioscorides, Greek physician, writes the first systematic pharmocopoeia. His *De Materia Medica* in five volumes provides accurate botanical and pharmacological information. It is preserved by the Arabs and, when translated into Latin and printed in 1478, becomes a standard botanical reference.

150 Cladius Galen says that pus formation is required for wound healing. This proves to be incorrect and hinders the treatment of wounds for centuries.

c.160 Bubonic plague (termed "barbarian boils") sweeps China.

c.160 Galen (c.130-c.200), Greek physician, in his *De Usu Partium* describes the pineal gland as a secretory organ that is important to thinking. He names it the pineal because it resembles a pine cone.

c.166 Plague in Rome (possibly smallpox or bubonic plague) eventually kills millions throughout the weakening Roman empire.

167 Stabiae, a popular health resort for tuberculosis sufferers, is established near Naples,

Italy. It is believed that the fumes from nearby Mt. Vesuvius are beneficial for lung ulcers.

170   Galen, the Greek physician, first describes gonorrhea.

c.200 Galen describes internal inflammations as caused by personal factors.

c.370 Basil of Caesarea (330–379) founds and organizes a large hospital at Caesarea (near Palestine).

c.400 Fabiola, a Christian noblewoman, founds the first nosocomium or hospital in Western Europe. After establishing the first hospital in Rome, she founds a hospice for pilgrims in Porto, Italy.

430   Earliest recorded plague in Europe is an epidemic that breaks out in Athens, Greece.

c.500 During this century, the "plague of Justinian" kills about one million people.

529   Benedict of Nursia founds the monastery at Monte Cassino in central Italy. It becomes, if not an actual medical school, at least an important center of scholarship in which medicine played a great part. It also acquires great fame throughout the West and its medical teachings are spread by the Benedictines to their monasteries scattered all over Europe.

610   In China, Ch'ao Yuan-fang writes a treatise on the causes and symptoms of diseases. Medical knowledge spreads from China to Japan via the Korean peninsula.

644   Rotharus, King of Lombardy also called Rothari, issues his edict ordering the segregation of all lepers.

c.700 Benedictus Crispus, archbishop of Milan from 681 to about 730, writes his *Commentarium Medicinale*, an elementary practical manual in verse. It describes the use of medicinal plants for curing illnesses.

c.850 Christian physician Sabur ibn Sahl of Jundishapur compiles a twenty-two volume work on antidotes that dominates Islamic pharmacopeia for the next 400 years.

c.850 Islamic philosopher al-Kindi (813–873) writes his *De Medicinarum Compositarum Gradibus*, which attempts to base dosages of medicine on mathematical measurements.

c.875 Bertharius, the abbot of Montcasino from 857 to 884, writes two treatises, *De Innu-meris Remediorum Utilitatibus* and *De Innumeris Morbis* that give insight into the kind of medicine practiced in the monasteries.

896   Abu Bakr al-Razi (also known as Rhazes (c.845-c.930), Persian physician and alchemist, distinguishes between the specific characteristics of measles and smallpox. He is also believed to be the first to classify all substances into the great classification of animal, vegetable, and mineral. (See 918)

c.900 First medical books written in Anglo-Saxon appear. *Lacnunga* and the *Leech Book of Bald* appear and have some botanical sections.

c.955 Jewish "prince of medicine," Isaac Israeli, dies. He writes classic works on fever and uroscopy, as well as a *Guide of the Physicians*.

c.980 Abu Al–Qasim Al–Zahravi (Abucasis) creates a system and method of human dissection along with the first formal specific surgical techniques.

c.1000 Ibn Sina, or Avicenna, publishes *Al-Quanun*, or Canon of Medicine, where he held that medicines could be discovered and tried by experiment or by reasoning.

1137   St. Bartholomew's hospital is founded in London.

1140   Bologna, Italy, begins to develop as a major European medical center. In the next century, the Italian physician Taddeo Alderotti (c.1233–1303) opens a school of medicine there.

1200   Physicians in Italy begin to write case-histories that describe symptoms and observable pathology of diseases.

c.1267 Roger Bacon (1214–1292), English philosopher and scientist, asserts that natural phenomena should be studied empirically.

1302   First formally recorded post-mortem or judicial autopsy is performed in Bologna, Italy, by Italian physician Bartolomeo da Varignana. A postmortem is ordered by the court in a case of suspected poisoning.

1333   Public botanical garden is established in Venice, Italy, to grow herbs that have medical uses.

1345   First apothecary shop or drug store opens in London, England.

1348 The beginning of a three-year epidemic caused by *Yersinia pestis* kills almost one-third of the population of urban Europe. In the aftermath of the epidemic, measures are introduced by the Italian government to improve public sanitation, marking the origin of public health.

1374 As the plague spreads, the Republic of Ragusa places the first quarantines on crews of ships thought to be infected.

1388 Richard II (1367–1400), king of England, establishes the first sanitary laws in England.

1489 Typhus is first brought to Europe by soldiers who had been fighting in Cyprus.

1491 First anatomical book to contain printed illustrations is German physician Johannes de Ketham's *Fasciculus Medicinae.*

1492 Venereal diseases, smallpox, and influenza are brought by the Columbus expedition (and subsequent European explorers) to the New World. Millions of native peoples eventually die from these diseases because of a lack of prior exposure to stimulate immunity. In some regions, whole villages succumb, and across broader regions up to 95% of the native population dies.

1525 Gonzalo Hernandez de Oviedo y Valdes (1478–1557) of Spain publishes the first systematic description of the medicinal plants of Central America.

1525 Paracelsus (1493–1541), Swiss physician and alchemist, begins the use of mineral substances as medicines.

1527 Paracelsus (1493–1541), Swiss physician and alchemist, publicly burns the writings of Galen at Basel. He rejects the traditional medical methods as irrational, and he founds iatrochemistry, asserting that the body is linked in some way to the laws of chemistry.

1528 The Italian physician Fracastorius describes an epidemic of typhus among French troops invading Naples.

1530 Girolamo Fracastoro (1478–1553), Italian physician and poet, writes his poem called "Syphilis" (*Syphilis sive Morbus Gallici*), which gives the definitive name to the sexually transmitted disease that is spreading throughout Europe.

1536 Paracelsus (1493–1541), Swiss physician and alchemist, publishes his surgical treatise, *Chirurgia Magna.*

1543 Andreas Vesalius (1514–1564), Dutch anatomist, publishes his *De Corporis Humani Corporis Fabrica*, the first accurate book on human anatomy. Its illustrations are of the highest level of both realism and art, and the result revolutionizes biology.

1546 Girolamo Fracastoro (1478–1553), Italian physician, writes his *De Contagione et Contagiosis Morbis*, which contains new ideas on the transmission of contagious diseases and is considered as the scientific beginning of that study.

1563 Epidemic cholera is described by Garcia del Huerto, working in Goa, India.

1567 A book on miner's tuberculosis by Swiss physician and alchemist Paracelsus (1493–1541) is posthumously published.

1602 Felix Platter (1536–1614), Swiss anatomist, publishes his *Praxis Medica*, which is the first modern attempt at the classification of diseases.

1621 Johannes Baptista van Helmont (1577–1635), Dutch physician and alchemist, writes his *Ortus Medicinae* in which he becomes one of the founders of modern pathology. He studies the anatomical changes that occur in disease.

1624 Adriaan van den Spigelius (1578–1625), Dutch anatomist, publishes the first account of malaria.

1640 Juan del Vigo introduces cinchona into Spain. Native to the Andes, the bark of this tree is processed to obtain quinine, used in the treatment of malaria.

1642 First treatise on the use of cinchona bark (quinine powder) for treating malaria is written by Spanish physician Pedro Barba (1608–1671).

1648 René Descartes (1596–1650), French philosopher and mathematician, writes *De Homine*, the first European textbook on physiology. He considers the body to be a material machine and offers his mechanist theory of life.

1648 Willem Piso (1611–1678), Dutch physician and botanist (also called Le Pois), points out the effectiveness of ipecac against dysentery in his book *De Medicina Brasiliensi.* He is among the first to become acquainted with tropical diseases, and he distinguishes between yaws and syphilis.

1660   The Royal Society of London is founded in England with Henry Oldenburg (c.1618–1677) Secretary and Robert Hooke (1635–1702) Curator of Experiments. Two years later (1662), King Charles II (1630–1685) grants it a royal charter, and it becomes known as the "Royal Society of London for the Promotion of Natural Knowledge."

1665   Bubonic plague epidemic in London kills 75,000 people. It is during this scourge that English scientist and mathematician Isaac Newton (1642–1727) leaves school in London and stays at his mother' farm in the country. There he formulates his laws of motion.

1665   First drawing of the cell is made by Robert Hooke (1635–1703), English physicist. While observing a sliver of cork under a microscope, Hooke notices it is composed of a pattern of tiny rectangular holes he calls "cells" because each looks like a small, empty room. Although he does not observe living cells, the name is retained.

1665   Robert Hooke (1635–1703), English physicist, publishes his landmark book on microscopy called *Micrographia.* Containing some of the most beautiful drawings of microscopic observations ever made, his book led to many discoveries in related fields.

1666   Robert Boyle (1627–1691), English physicist and chemist, publishes *The Origine of Formes and Qualities* in which he begins to explain all chemical reactions and physical properties through the existence of small, indivisible particles or atoms.

1668   Francesco Redi (1626–1697), Italian physician, conducts experiments to disprove spontaneous generation and shows that maggots are not born spontaneously, but come from eggs laid by flies. He publishes his *Esperienze Intorno all Generazione degli Insetti.*

1671   Michael Ettmüller (1644–1683), German physician, attributes the contagiousness of tuberculosis to sputum.

1672   French physician Le Gras introduces ipecac into Europe as he brings it to Paris this year. The root of the Brazilian plant ipeca-cuanha is used to cure dysentery. (See 1625)

1674   Antoni van Leeuwenhoek (1632–1723), Dutch biologist and microscopist, observes "animacules" in lake water viewed through a ground glass lens. This observation of what will eventually be known as bacteria represents the start of the formal study of microbiology.

1675   John Josselyn, English botanist, publishes an account of the plants and animals he encounters while living in America and indicates that tuberculosis existed among the Native Americans before the coming of the Europeans.

1677   Antoni van Leeuwenhoek (1632–1723), Dutch biologist and microscopist, discovers spermatozoa and describes them in a letter he publishes in *Philosophical Transactions* in 1679. In the same year, Johan Ham also sees them microscopically, but the semen he observes comes from a patient suffering from gonorrhea, and Ham concludes that spermatozoa are a consequence of the disease.

1700   Bernardino Ramazzini (1633–1714), Italian physician, publishes the first systematic treatment on occupational diseases. His book, *De Morbis Artificum,* opens up an entirely new department of modern medicine—diseases of trade or occupation and industrial hygiene.

1721   The word "antiseptic" first appears in print.

1730   George Martine performs the first tracheostomy on a patient with diphtheria.

1735   Botulism first described.

1748   John Fothergill describes diphtheria in "Account of the Putrid Sore Throat."

1762   Marcus Anton von Plenciz, Sr. (1705–1786), Austrian physician, expresses the idea that all infectious diseases are caused by living organisms and that there is a specific organism for each disease.

1767   William Heberden demonstrates that chicken-pox is not a mild form of smallpox, but a different disease.

1780   George Adams (1750–1795), English engineer, devises the first microtome. This mechanical instrument cuts thin slices for examination under a microscope, thus replacing the imprecise procedure of cutting by hand-held razor.

1789   Polio is first described by Michael Underwood in England.

1796   Edward Jenner (1749 1823) uses cowpox virus to develop a smallpox vaccine. By modern standards, this was human experimentation as Jenner injected healthy eight-year-old James Phillips with cowpox and then after a period of months with smallpox.

1798   Government legislation is passed to establish hospitals in the United States devoted to the care of ill mariners. This initiative leads to the establishment of a Hygenic Laboratory that eventually grows to become the National Institutes of Health.

1800   Marie-François-Xavier Bichat publishes his first major work, *Treatise on Tissues,* which establishes histology as a new scientific discipline. Bichat distinguishes 21 kinds of tissue and relates particular diseases to particular tissues.

1801   A hospital is established in London, England, to treat the victims of typhus.

1802   John Dalton introduces modern atomic theory into the science of chemistry.

1814   The Royal Hospital for Diseases of the Chest is founded in London, England, in an attempt to keep consumptive patients (people with tuberculosis) segregated.

1816   The stethoscope, which is an important tool for diagnosing pneumonia, is introduced by Rene LaËnnec.

1817   Start of first cholera pandemic, which spreads from Bengal to China in the east and to Eygpt in the west.

1818   William Charles Wells suggests the theory of natural selection in an essay dealing with human color variations. He notes that dark-skinned people seem more resistant to tropical diseases than lighter-skinned people. Wells also calls attention to selection carried out by animal breeders. Jerome Lawrence, James Cowles Prichard, and others make similar suggestions, but do not develop their ideas into a coherent and convincing theory of evolution.

1818   Xavier Bichat (1771–1802), French physician, publishes his first major work, *Trait, des membranes en general,* in which he propounds the notion of tissues. This work also founds histology, distinguishing 21 kinds of tissue and relating disease to them.

1820   First United States *Pharmacopoeia* is published.

1824   Start of second cholera pandemic, which penetrates as far as Russia and also reaches England, North America, the Caribbean, and Latin America.

1826   Pierre Bretonneau (1778–1862), French physician, describes and names diptheria in his specification of diseases.

1829   Salicin, the precursor of aspirin, is purified from the bark of the willow tree.

1831   Charles Robert Darwin (1809–1882) begins his historic voyage on the H.M.S. *Beagle* (1831–1836). His observations during the voyage lead to his theory of evolution by means of natural selection.

1835   Jacob Bigelow (1787–1879), American physician, publishes his book *On Self-Limited Diseases* in which he states the commonsense idea that some diseases will simply run their course and subside without the benefit of any treatment from a physician.

1836   Theodor Schwann carries out experiments that refute the theory of the spontaneous generation. He also demonstrates that alcoholic fermentation depends on the action of living yeast cells. The same conclusion is reached independently by Charles Caignard de la Tour.

1837   Pierre-Françs-Olive Rayer (1793–1867), French physician, is the first to describe the disease glanders as found in man and to prove that it is not a form of tuberculosis.

1838   Angelo Dubini (1813–1902), Italian physician, discovers *Ankylostoma duodenale,* the cause of hookworm disease, in the intestinal tract.

1838   Matthias Jakob Schleiden notes that the nucleus first described by Robert Brown is a characteristic of all plant cells. Schleiden describes plants as a community of cells and cell products. He helps establish cell theory and stimulates Theodor Schwann's recognition that animals are also composed of cells and cell products.

1839 Third cholera pandemic begins with entry of British troops in Afghanistan and travels to Persia, Central Asia, Europe, and the Americas.

1841 Friedrich Gustav Jacob Henle (1809–1885), German pathologist and anatomist, publishes his *Allegemeine Anatomie*, which becomes the first systematic textbook of histology (the study of minute tissue structure and includes the first statement of the germ theory of communicable disease).

1842 Edwin Chadwick, a pioneer in sanitary reform, reports that deaths from typhus in 1838 and 1839 in England exceeded those from smallpox.

1842 Oliver Wendell Holmes recommends that surgeons wash their hands using calcium chloride to prevent spread of infection from corpses to patients.

1843 First outbreak of polio in the United States occurs.

1843 Gabriel Andral (1797–1876), French physician, is the first to urge that blood be examined in cases of disease.

1846 American Medical Association establishes a code of ethics for physicians which declares their obligation to treat victims of epidemic diseases even at a risk to their own lives. (See 1912)

1847 A series of yellow fever epidemics sweeps the American Southern states. The epidemics recur for more than thirty years.

1847 The first sexually transmitted disease clinic is opened at the London Docks Hospital.

1849 John Snow (1813–1858), English physician, first states the theory that cholera is a water-borne disease. During a cholera epidemic in London in 1854, Snow breaks the handle of the Broad Street Pump, thereby shutting down the main source of disease transmission during the outbreak.

1849 John Snow publishes the groundbreaking paper "On the Transmission of Cholera."

1855 Third, or Modern, pandemic of plague probably begins in Yunan province, China.

1857 Louis Pasteur demonstrates that lactic acid fermentation is caused by a living organism. Between 1857 and 1880, he performs a series of experiments that refute the doctrine of spontaneous generation. He also introduces vaccines for fowl cholera, anthrax, and rabies, based on attenuated strains of viruses and bacteria.

1858 Rudolf Ludwig Carl Virchow publishes his landmark paper "Cellular Pathology" and establishes the field of cellular pathology. Virchow asserts that all cells arise from pre-existing cells (*Omnis cellula e cellula*). He argues that the cell is the ultimate locus of all disease.

1859 Charles Robert Darwin publishes his landmark book *On the Origin of Species by Means of Natural Selection*.

1861 Carl Gegenbaur confirms Theodor Schwann's suggestion that all vertebrate eggs are single cells.

1862 First demonstration of pasteurization.

1864 Fourth cholera pandemic starts and revisits locations of previous pandemics.

1865 An epidemic of rinderpest kills 500,000 cattle in Great Britain. Government inquiries into the outbreak pave the way for the development of contemporary theories of epidemiology and the germ theory of disease.

1865 French physiologist Claude Bernard publishes *Introduction to the Study of Human Experimentation*, which advocates "Never perform an experiment which might be harmful to the patient even if advantageous to science...."

1866 The Austrian botanist and monk Johann Gregor Mendel (1822–1884) discovers the laws of heredity and writes the first of a series of papers on heredity (1866–1869). The papers formulate the laws of hybridization. Mendel's work is disregarded until 1900, when Hugo de Vries rediscovers it. Unbeknownst to both Darwin and Mendel, Mendelian laws provide the scientific framework for the concepts of gradual evolution and continuous variation.

1867 Joseph Lister publishes a study that implicates microorganisms with infection. Based on this, his use of early disinfectants during surgery markedly reduces post-operative infections and death.

1867 Robert Koch establishes the role of bacteria in anthrax, providing the final piece of evidence in support of the germ theory of disease. Koch goes on to formulate postulates that, when fulfilled, confirm bacteria or viruses as the cause of an infection.

1868 Carl August Wunderlich (1815–1877), German physician, publishes his major work on the relation of animal heat or fever to disease. He is the first to recognize that fever is not itself a disease, but is rather a symptom.

1869 Johann Friedrich Miescher discovers nuclein, a new chemical isolated from the nuclei of pus cells. Two years later, he isolates nuclein from salmon sperm. This material comes to be known as nucleic acid.

1871 Ferdinand Julius Cohn coins the term bacterium.

1871 First U.S. city to use a filter on its public water supply is Poughkeepsie, New York. The evidence mounts that much disease is spread by contaminated drinking water.

1873 Franz Anton Schneider describes cell division in detail. His drawings include both the nucleus and chromosomal strands.

1875 Ferdinand Cohn publishes a classification of bacteria in which the genus name *Bacillus* is used for the first time.

1875 Koch's postulates used for the first time to demonstrate that anthrax is caused by *Bacillus anthracis*, validating the germ theory of disease.

1877 Louis Pasteur (1822–1895), French chemist, first distinguishes between aerobic and anaerobic bacteria.

1877 Paul Erlich recognizes the existence of the mast cells of the immune system.

1877 Robert Koch describes new techniques for fixing, staining, and photographing bacteria.

1877 Wilhelm Friedrich Kühne proposes the term enzyme (meaning "in yeast"). Kühne establishes the critical distinction between enzymes, or "ferments," and the microorganisms that produce them.

1878 Joseph Lister publishes a paper describing the role of a bacterium he names *Bacterium lactis* in the souring of milk.

1878 Robert Koch (1843–1910), German bacteriologist, publishes his landmark findings on the etiology or cause of infectious disease. Koch' postulates state that the causative microorganism must be located in a diseased animal, and that after it is cultured or grown, it must then be capable of causing disease in a healthy animal. Finally, the newly-infected animal must yield the same bacteria as those found in the original animal.

1878 Thomas Burrill demonstrates that a plant disease (pear blight) is caused by a bacterium (*Micrococcus amylophorous*).

1879 Albert Nisser (1855–1916) identifies the bacterium *Neiserria gonorrhoeoe* as the cause of gonorrhea.

1880 C. L. Alphonse Laveran isolates malarial parasites in erythrocytes of infected people and demonstrates that the organism can replicate in the cells.

1880 The first issue of the journal *Science* is published by the American Association for the Advancement of Science.

1881 Fifth cholera pandemic begins and is widespread in China and Japan in the Far East, as well as Germany and Russia in Europe, although the disease does not spread in North America.

1881 *Streptococcus pneumoniae*, a major cause of bacterial pneumonia, is discovered independently by Louis Pasteur and George Sternberg.

1882 Angelina Fannie and Walter Hesse in Koch's laboratory develop agar as a solid grow medium for microorganisms. Agar replaces gelatin as the solid growth medium of choice in microbiology.

1882 Friedrich August Johannes Loffler (1852–1915), German bacteriologist, and F. Schulze discover the bacterium causing glanders, a contagious and destructive disease of animals, especially horses, that can be transmitted to humans.

1883 Edwin Theodore Klebs and Frederich Loeffler independently discover *Corynebacterium diphtheriae*, the bacterium that causes diphtheria.

1883 Robert Koch discovers *V. cholerae* as the causative agent of cholera in Egypt.

1883   Surgical gowns and headgear begin to be used by surgeons.

1884   Elie Metchnikoff discovers the antibacterial activity of white blood cells, which he calls "phagocytes," and formulates the theory of phagocytosis. He also develops the cellular theory of vaccination.

1884   Hans Christian J. Gram develops the Gram stain, a method of categorizing bacteria into one of two groups (gram-positive and gram-negative) based upon the chemical reaction of the bacteria cell walls to a staining procedure.

1884   Louis Pasteur and coworkers publish a paper entitled *A New Communication on Rabies.* Pasteur proves that the causal agent of rabies can be attenuated and the weakened virus can be used as a vaccine to prevent the disease. This work serves as the basis of future work on virus attenuation, vaccine development, and the concept that variation is an inherent characteristic of viruses.

1885   Francis Galton devises a new statistical tool, the correlation table.

1885   French chemist Louis Pasteur (1822–1895) inoculates a boy, Joseph Meister, against rabies. Meister had been bitten by a dog infected with rabies, and the treatment saved his life. This is the first time Pasteur uses an attenuated (weakened) germ on a human being.

1885   Russian hematologist Antonin Filatov makes the first formal description of mononucleosis.

1885   Theodor Escherich identifies a bacterium inhabiting the human intestinal tract that he names *Bacterium coli* and shows that the bacterium causes infant diarrhea and gastroenteritis. The bacterium is subsequently named *Escherichia coli.*

1886   Camillo Golgi describes two forms of malaria, with fever occurring every two and every three days, respectively.

1887   Julius Richard Petri develops a culture dish that has a lid to exclude airborne contaminants. The innovation is subsequently termed the Petri dish.

1888   Francis Galton publishes *Natural Inheritance,* considered a landmark in the establishment of biometry and statistical studies of variation. Galton also proposes the Law of Ancestral Inheritance, a statistical description of the relative contributions to heredity made by previous generations.

1888   Martinus Beijerinck uses a growth medium enriched with certain nutrients to isolate the bacteria *Rhizobium,* demonstrating that nutritionally-tailored growth media are useful in bacterial isolation.

1888   The diphtheria toxin is discovered by Emile Roux and Alexandre Yersin.

1888   The Institute Pasteur is formed in France.

1890   Emil Adolf von Behring (1854–1917), German bacteriologist, uses his new discovery of antitoxins to develop an antitoxin for diphtheria—a disease that usually brought death to the children it attacked.

1891   First child is treated with the diphtheria antitoxin.

1891   Paul Ehrlich (1854–1915), German bacteriologist, discovers that methyl blue dye immobilizes malaria bacterium and begins searching for other, more potent microbial dyes. (See 1904)

1891   Paul Ehrlich proposes that antibodies are responsible for immunity.

1891   Prussian State dictates that even jailed prisoners must give consent prior to treatment (for tuberculosis).

1891   Robert Koch proposes the concept of delayed type hypersensitivity.

1892   Dmitri Ivanowski demonstrates that filterable material causes tobacco mosaic disease. The infectious agent is subsequently showed to be the tobacco mosaic virus. Ivanowski's discovery heralds the field of virology.

1892   First vaccine for diphtheria becomes available.

1892   Albert Neisser, the discoverer of gonorrhea bacteria, injects human subjects with syphilis, prompting debate and leading to regulations on human experimentation.

1892   Richard Pfeiffer discovers *Haemophilius influenzae,* a cause of both pneumonia and influenza.

1894   Alexandre Yersin isolates *Yersinia (Pasteurella) pestis,* the bacterium responsible for bubonic plague.

1894   Wilhelm Konrad Roentgen discovers x-rays.

1895   Heinrich Dreser, working for the Bayer Company in Germany, produces a drug he thought to be as effective an analgesic as morphine, but without its harmful side effects. Bayer begins mass production of diacetylmorphine, and in 1898, markets the new drug under the brand name "heroin" as a cough sedative.

1896 Edmund Beecher Wilson, American zoologist, publishes the first edition of his highly influential treatise *The Cell in Development and Heredity*. Wilson calls attention to the relationship between chromosomes and sex determination.

1896 William Joseph Dibdin (1850–1925), English engineer, and his colleague Schweder improve the sewage disposal systems in England with the introduction of a bacterial system of water purification. These improvements greatly reduce the number of water-borne diseases like cholera and typhoid fever.

1897 American physician William Welch describes and names *Plasmodium falciparum,* a protozoan parasite and cause of malaria.

1898 First state-run sanatorium for tuberculosis in the United States opens in Massachusetts.

1898 Friedrich Loeffler and Paul Frosch publish their *Report on Foot-and-Mouth Disease.* They prove that this animal disease is caused by a filterable virus and suggest that similar agents might cause other diseases.

1898 Martinus Wilhelm Beijerinck (1851–1931), Dutch botanist, discovers and names the causative agent of the tobacco mosaic disease. He describes it as a new type of microscopically-visible organism which eventually comes to be known as a virus.

1898 The First International Congress of Genetics is held in London.

1898 The transmission of plague by flea-infested rodents is shown by French bacteriologist Paul-Louis Simond (1858–1947).

1899 A meeting to organize the Society of American Bacteriologists is held at Yale University. The society will later become the American Society for Microbiology.

1899 George Henry Falkiner Nuttall (1862–1937), American biologist, first summarizes the role of insects, arachnids, and myriapods as transmitters of bacterial and parasitic diseases.

1899 Start of the sixth cholera pandemic, which affects the Far East, apart from sporadic outbreaks in parts of Euorpe.

1900 Karl Landsteiner discovers the blood-agglutination phenomenon and the four major blood types in humans.

1900 Pandemic plague becomes widely disseminated throughout the world, reaching Europe, North and South America, India, the Middle East, Africa, and Australia.

1900 Paul Erlich proposes the theory concerning the formation of antibodies by the immune system.

1900 Walter Reed (1851–1902), American surgeon, discovers that the yellow fever virus is transmitted to humans by a mosquito. This is the first demonstration of a viral cause of a human disease.

1901 Joseph Everett Dutton (1874-1905), English physician, and his colleague J. L. Todd discover the parasite *Trypanosoma gambiense* that is responsible for the African sleeping sickness disease.

1902 Ronald Ross (1857–1932), a British officer with the Indian Medical Service, receives the Nobel Prize for identifying mosquitoes as the transmitter of malaria.

1904 Paul Ehrlich (1854–1915), German bacteriologist, discovers a microbial dye called trypan red that helps destroy the trypanosomes that cause such diseases as sleeping sickness. This is the first such active agent against trypanosomes (parasitic protozoa).

1905 Fritz Richard Schaudinn (1871–1906), German zoologist, discovers *Treponema pallidum*, the organism or parasite causing syphilis. His discovery of this almost invisible parasite is due to his consummate technique and staining methods.

1905 Jules-Jean-Baptiste-Vincent Bordet (1870–1961), Belgian bacteriologist, and his colleague, Octave Gengou, discover the bacillus of whooping cough (*B. pertussis*). Bordet goes on to discover a method of immunization against this dreaded childhood disease.

1906 Charles Nicolle of the Pasteur Institute in Paris shows a link between typhus and lice.

1906 Pure Food and Drugs Act passed in the United States, beginning the organization that would become the FDA (Food and Drug Administration).

1906   Viennese physician Clemens von Pirquet (1874–1929) coins the term allergy to describe the immune reaction to certain compounds.

1907   Alphonse Laveran, a French army surgeon stationed in Algeria, identifies malaria parasites (protozoa) in blood.

1907   Charles Franklin Craig (1872–1950), American physician, and Percy Moreau Ashburn (1872–1940), American surgeon, work in the Phillipines and are the first to prove that dengue fever (also called "breakbone fever") is caused by a virus. (See 1925)

1907   Clemens Peter Pirquet von Cesenatico (1874–1929), Austrian physician, first introduces the cutaneous or skin reaction test for the diagnosis of tuberculosis.

1907   William Bateson urges biologists to adopt the term "genetics" to indicate the importance of the new science of heredity.

1909   Sigurd Orla-Jensen proposes that the physiological reactions of bacteria are primarily important in their classification.

1909   Thomas Hunt Morgan selects the fruit fly *Drosophila* as a model system for the study of genetics. Morgan and his coworkers confirm the chromosome theory of heredity and realize the significance of the fact that certain genes tend to be transmitted together. Morgan postulates the mechanism of "crossing over." His associate, Alfred Henry Sturtevant demonstrates the relationship between crossing over and the rearrangement of genes in 1913.

1909   Walter Reed General Hospital opens in Washington, D.C.

1909   Wilhelm Ludwig Johannsen argues the necessity of distinguishing between the appearance of an organism and its genetic constitution. He invents the terms "gene" (carrier of heredity), "genotype" (an organism's genetic constitution), and "phenotype" (the appearance of the actual organism).

1910   Howard Taylor Ricketts, discoverer of the *Rickettsia* genus of bacteria, dies of the *Rickettsia*-caused disease typhus while investigating an outbreak in Mexico City.

1910   Paul Ehrlich (1854–1915), German bacteriologist, announces his discovery of an effective treatment for syphilis. He names this new drug Salvarsan, and it is now called arsphenamine. His discovery marks the first chemotherapeutic agent for a bacterial disease.

1911   The first known retrovirus, Rous sarcoma virus, is discovered by Peyton Rous, who also showed that the virus could induce cancer.

1912   The United States Public Health Service is established.

1913   Shick designs a skin test which determines immunity to diphtheria.

1914   Frederick William Twort (1877–1950), English bacteriologist, and Felix H. D'Herelle (1873–1949), Canadian-Russian physician, independently discover bacteriophage, viruses which destroy bacteria.

1915   A typhus epidemic in Serbia causes 150,000 deaths.

1915   Stanislaus Prowazek dies of typhus when investigating an outbreak in a Russian prisoner of war camp, having identified *R. prowazekii*, the causative agent.

1915   U.S. Public Health Office allows induction of pellagra in Mississippi prisoners.

1916   Felix Hubert D'Herelle carries out further studies of the agent that destroys bacterial colonies and gives it the name "bacteriophage" (bacteria eating agent). D'Herelle and others unsuccessfully attempted to use bacteriophages as bactericidal therapeutic agents.

1917   D'Arcy Wentworth Thompson publishes *On Growth and Form*, which suggests that the evolution of one species into another occurs as a series of transformations involving the entire organism, rather than a succession of minor changes in parts of the body.

1918   Global influenza pandemic kills more people than numbers of soldiers who died fighting during World War I (1914–1918). By the end of 1918, more than 25 million people die from virulent strain of Spanish influenza.

1918   Thomas Hunt Morgan and coworkers publish *The Physical Basis of Heredity*, a survey of the remarkable development of the new science of genetics.

1919   James Brown uses blood agar to study the destruction of blood cells by the bacterium *Streptococcus*. He observes three reactions that he designates alpha, beta, and gamma.

1919   The Health Organization of the League of Nations was established for the prevention and control of disease around the world.

1920   Data on diphtheria is gathered for the first time in the United States, showing around 13,000 deaths per year.

1920   Sprunt and Evans coined the term infectious mononucleosis, as they described the abnormal mononuclear leukocytes observed in patients with the condition.

1921   Otto Loewi (1873–1961), German-American physiologist, discovers that acetylcholine functions as a neurotransmitter. It is the first such brain chemical to be so identified.

1922   John Stephens describes *P. ovale*.

1924   Albert Jan Kluyver publishes *Unity and Diversity in the Metabolism of Microorganisms*. He demonstrates that different microorganisms have common metabolic pathways of oxidation, fermentation, and synthesis of certain compounds. Kluyver also states that life on Earth depends on microbial activity.

1924   The last urban epidemic of plague in the United States begins in Los Angeles.

1926   James B. Sumner publishes a report on the isolation of the enzyme urease and his proof that the enzyme is a protein. This idea is controversial until 1930 when John Howard Northrop confirms Sumner's ideas by crystallizing pepsin. Sumner, Northrop, and Wendell Meredith Stanley ultimately share the Nobel Prize for chemistry in 1946.

1927   Thomas Rivers publishes a paper that differentiates bacteria from viruses, establishing virology as a field of study that is distinct from bacteriology.

1928   Fred Griffith discovers that certain strains of pneumococci could undergo some kind of transmutation of type. After injecting mice with living R type pneumococci and heat-killed S type, Griffith is able to isolate living virulent bacteria from the infected mice. Griffith suggests that some unknown

"principle" had transformed the harmless R strain of the pneumococcus to the virulent S strain.

1928   Philip and Cecil Drinker of Harvard School of Public Health introduce the "iron lung" for treatment of paralytic polio.

1928   Scottish biochemist Alexander Fleming (1881–1955) discovers penicillin. In his published report (1929), Fleming observes that the mold *Penicillium notatum* inhibits the growth of some bacteria. This is the first anti-bacterial, and it opens a new era of "wonder drugs."

1929   Alexander Fleming publishes account of bacteriolytic power of penicillin.

1929   Francis O. Holmes introduces the technique of "local lesion" as a means of measuring the concentration of tobacco mosaic virus. The method becomes extremely important in virus purification.

1929   Willard Myron Allen, American physician, and George Washington Corner, American anatomist, discover progesterone. They demonstrate that it is necessary for the maintenance of pregnancy.

1930   Max Theiler demonstrates the advantages of using mice as experimental animals for research on animal viruses. Theiler uses mice in his studies of the yellow fever virus.

1930   Ronald A. Fisher publishes *Genetical Theory of Natural Selection*, a formal analysis of the mathematics of selection.

1930   United States Food, Drug, and Insecticide Administration is renamed Food and Drug Administration (FDA).

1932   At Tuskegee, Alabama, African-American sharecroppers become unknowing and unwilling subjects of experimentation on the untreated natural course of syphilis. Even after penicillin came into use in the 1940's, the men remained untreated.

1932   William J. Elford and Christopher H. Andrewes develop methods of estimating the sizes of viruses by using a series of membranes as filters. Later studies prove that the viral sizes obtained by this method were comparable to those obtained by electron microscopy.

1933   "Regulation on New Therapy and Experimentation" decreed in Germany.

1934   Discovery of chloroquine is announced by Hans Andersag at Bayer, in Germany

1934   J.B.S. Haldane presents the first calculations of the spontaneous mutation frequency of a human gene.

1934   John Marrack begins a series of studies that leads to the formation of the hypothesis governing the association between an antigen and the corresponding antibody.

1935   Wendall Meredith Stanley (1904–1971), American biochemist, discovers that viruses are partly protein-based. By purifying and crystallizing viruses, he enables scientists to identify the precise molecular structure and propagation modes of several viruses.

1936   George P. Berry and Helen M. Dedrick report that the Shope virus could be "transformed" into myxomatosis/Sanarelli virus. This virological curiosity was variously referred to as "transformation," "recombination," and "multiplicity of reactivation." Subsequent research suggests that it is the first example of genetic interaction between animal viruses, but some scientists warn that the phenomenon might indicate the danger of reactivation of virus particles in vaccines and in cancer research.

1937   American researcher H. R. Cox cultures *Rickettsiae* in the yolks of fertilized hens' eggs, opening the door to research into a vaccine.

1938   Emory L. Ellis and Max Delbrück perform studies on phage replication that mark the beginning of modern phage work. They introduce the "one-step growth" experiment, which demonstrates that after bacteriophages attack bacteria, replication of the virus occurs within the bacterial host during a "latent period," after which viral progeny are released in a "burst."

1939   Ernest Chain and H. W. Florey refine the purification of penicillin, allowing the mass production of the antibiotic.

1939   Paul Müller in Switzerland discovers the insecticidal properties of DDT.

1939   Richard E. Shope reports that the swine influenza virus survived between epidemics in an intermediate host. This discovery is an important step in revealing the role of intermediate hosts in perpetuating specific diseases.

1941   George W. Beadle and Edward L. Tatum publish their classic study on the biochemical genetics entitled Genetic Control of Biochemical Reactions in Neurospora. Beadle and Tatum irradiate red bread mold *Neurospora* and prove that genes produce their effects by regulating particular enzymes. This work leads to the one-gene-one enzyme theory.

1941   Norman M. Gregg of Australia discovers that rubella during pregnancy can cause congenital abnormalities. Children of mothers who had rubella (German measles) during their pregnancy are found to suffer from blindness, deafness, and heart disease.

1941   The term "antibiotic" is coined by Selman Waksman.

1942   Jules Freund and Katherine McDermott identify adjuvants (e.g., paraffin oil) that act to boost antibody production.

1942   Luria and Max Delbrück demonstrate statistically that inheritance of genetic characteristics in bacteria follows the principles of genetic inheritance proposed by Charles Darwin. For their work, the two (along with Alfred Day Hershey) are awarded the 1969 Nobel Prize in Medicine or Physiology.

1942   Neil Hamilton Fairley, the Australian physician, wins a Fellowship of the Royal Society for work on anemia caused by the rupture of red blood cells in malaria.

1943   At University of Cincinnati Hospital experiments are performed using mentally disabled patients.

1943   Penicillin starts to become available as a therapy for Allied troops.

1944   Oswald T. Avery, Colin M. MacLeod, and Maclyn McCarty publish a landmark paper on the pneumococcus transforming principle. The paper is entitled *Studies on the chemical nature of the substance inducing transformation of pneumococcal types*. Avery suggests that the transforming principle seems to be deoxyribonucleic acid (DNA), but contemporary ideas about the structure of nucleic acids suggest that

DNA does not possess the biological specificity of the hypothetical genetic material.

1944 Selman Waksman introduces streptomycin.

1944 To combat battle fatigue during World War II (1939–1945), nearly 200 million amphetamine tablets are issued to American soldiers stationed in Great Britain during the war.

1944 The United States Public Health Service Act is passed.

1944 University of Chicago Medical School professor Dr. Alf Alving conducts malaria experiments on more than 400 Illinois prisoners.

1945 Joshua Lederberg and Edward L. Tatum demonstrate genetic recombination in bacteria.

1946 Felix Bloch and Edward Mills Purcell develop nuclear magnetic resonance (NMR) as viable tool for observation and analysis.

1946 Hermann J. Muller is awarded the Nobel Prize in Medicine or Physiology for his contributions to radiation genetics.

1946 Max Delbrück and W. T. Bailey, Jr. publish a paper entitled *Induced Mutations in Bacterial Viruses*. Despite some confusion about the nature of the phenomenon in question, this paper establishes the fact that genetic recombinations occur during mixed infections with bacterial viruses. Alfred Hershey and R. Rotman make the discovery of genetic recombination in bacteriophage simultaneously and independently. Hershey and his colleagues prove that this phenomenon can be used for genetic analyses. They construct a genetic map of phage particles and show that phage genes can be arranged in a linear fashion.

1946 Nazi physicians and scientists tried by international court at Nuremberg.

1947 Four years after the mass-production and use of penicillin, microbial resistance is detected.

1947 Nuremberg Code issued regarding voluntary consent of human subjects.

1948 Barbara McClintock publishes her research on transposable regulatory elements ("jumping genes") in maize. Her work was not appreciated until similar phenomena were discovered in bacteria and fruit flies in the 1960s

and 1970s. McClintock was awarded the Nobel Prize in physiology or medicine in 1983.

1948 Chloramphenicol and tetracycline are shown to be effective treatments for typhus.

1948 James V. Neel reports evidence that the sickle-cell disease is inherited as a simple Mendelian autosomal recessive trait.

1948 World Health Organization (WHO) is formed. The WHO subsequently becomes the principle international organization managing public health related issues on a global scale. Headquartered in Geneva, the WHO becomes, by 2002, an organization of more than 190 member countries. The organization contributes to international public health in areas including disease prevention and control, promotion of good health, addressing disease outbreaks, initiatives to eliminate diseases (e.g., vaccination programs), and development of treatment and prevention standards.

1949 John F. Endes, Thomas H. Weller, and Frederick C. Robbins publish "Cultivation of Polio Viruses in Cultures of Human Embryonic Tissues." The report by Enders and coworkers is a landmark in establishing techniques for the cultivation of poliovirus in cultures on non-neural tissue and for further virus research. The technique leads to the polio vaccine and other advances in virology.

1949 Macfarlane Burnet and his colleagues begin studies that lead to the immunological tolerance hypothesis and the clonal selection theory. Burnet receives the 1960 Nobel Prize in Physiology or Medicine for this research.

1950 Dr. Joseph Stokes of the University of Pennsylvania infects 200 women prisoners with viral hepatitis.

1950 Robert Hungate develops the roll-tube culture technique, which is the first technique that allows anaerobic bacteria to be grown in culture.

1951 Esther M. Lederberg discovers a lysogenic strain of *Escherichia coli* K12 and isolates a new bacteriophage, called lambda.

1951 Rosalind Franklin obtains sharp x-ray diffraction photographs of deoxyribonucleic acid (DNA).

1951　The eradication of malaria from the United States is announced.

1951　University of Pennsylvania under contract with U.S. Army conducts psychopharmacological experiments on hundreds of Pennsylvania prisoners.

1952　Alfred Hershey and Martha Chase publish their landmark paper "Independent Functions of Viral Protein and Nucleic Acid in Growth of Bacteriophage." The famous "blender experiment" suggests that DNA is the genetic material.

1952　James T. Park and Jack L. Strominger demonstrate that penicillin blocks the synthesis of the peptidoglycan of bacteria. This represents the first demonstration of the action of a natural antibiotic.

1952　Karl Maramorosch demonstrate that some viruses could multiply in both plants and insects. This work leads to new questions about the origins of viruses.

1952　Joshua Lederberg and Esther Lederberg develop the replica plating method that allows for the rapid screening of large numbers of genetic markers. They use the technique to demonstrate that resistance to antibacterial agents such as antibiotics and viruses is not induced by the presence of the antibacterial agent.

1952　Polio peaks in the United States, with 57,268 cases recorded.

1952　Renato Dulbecco develops a practical method for studying animal viruses in cell cultures. His so-called plaque method is comparable to that used in studies of bacterial viruses, and the method proves to be important in genetic studies of viruses. These methods are described in his paper *Production of Plaques in Monolayer Tissue Cultures by Single Particles of an Animal Virus*.

1952　Rosalind Franklin completes a series of x-ray crystallography studies of two forms of DNA. Her colleague, Maurice Wilkins, gives information about her work to James Watson.

1952　Selman Abraham Waksman, Russian-American microbiologist, is awarded the Nobel Prize for Physiology or Medicine for his discovery of streptomycin, the first antibiotic effective against tuberculosis.

1952　William G. Gochenour of the United States demonstrates that pretibial fever (also called Fort Bragg Fever) is not caused by a virus but rather is an infection caused by a microorganism called *Leptospira*.

1952　William Hayes isolates a strain of *E. coli* that produces recombinants thousands of times more frequently than previously observed. The new strain of K12 is named Hfr (high-frequency recombination) by Hayes.

1953　James D. Watson and Francis H. C. Crick publish two landmark papers in the journal *Nature*: "Molecular structure of nucleic acids: a structure for deoxyribonucleic acid," and "Genetical implications of the structure of deoxyribonucleic acid." Watson and Crick propose a double helical model for DNA and call attention to the genetic implications of their model. Their model is based, in part, on the x-ray crystallographic work of Rosalind Franklin and the biochemical work of Erwin Chargaff. Their model explains how the genetic material is transmitted.

1953　Jonas Salk begins testing a polio vaccine comprised of a mixture of killed viruses.

1954　John Enders, Thomas Weller and Frederick Robbins of Harvard School of Public Health receive the Nobel Prize for Physiology or Medicine for their work on poliovirus

1954　John Franklin Enders (1897-1985), American micrologist, and Thomas Peebles, American pediatrician, develop the first vaccine for measles. A truly practical and successful vaccine requires more time. (See 1963)

1954　Jonas Edward Salk, American virologist, produces the first successful anti-poliomyelitis vaccine, which prevents paralytic polio. It is soon (1955) followed by the Polish-American virologist, Albert Bruce Sabin's (1906-1993) development of the first oral vaccine. (See 1959)

1954　Thomas Weller isolated the varicella zoster virus from chickenpox lesions.

1955　Fred L. Schaffer and Carlton E. Schwerdt report on their successful crystallization of the polio virus. Their achievement is the first successful crystallization of an animal virus.

1955 Jonas Salk's inactivated polio vaccine is approved for use.

1955 National Institutes of Health organizes a Division of Biologics Control within FDA, following death from faulty polio vaccine.

1956 Alfred Gierer and Gerhard Schramm demonstrate that naked RNA from tobacco mosaic virus is infectious. Subsequently, infectious RNA preparations are obtained for certain animal viruses.

1956 Niels Kai Jerne, Danish physician, proposes the clonal selection theory of antibody selection to explain how white blood cells are able to produce a large range of antibodies.

1956 Researchers start hepatitis experiments on mentally disabled children at The Willowbrook State School.

1957 Alick Isaacs (1921-1967), Scottish virologist, demonstrates that antibodies act only against bacteria. This means that antibodies are not one of the body's natural forms of defense against viruses. This knowledge leads eventually to the discovery of interferon this same year by Isaacs and his colleague, Jean Lindenmann of Switzerland. They find that the generation of a small amount of protein is the body's first line of defense against a virus. (See c.1968)

1957 Alick Isaacs and Jean Lindenmann publish their pioneering report on the drug interferon, a protein produced by interaction between a virus and an infected cell that can interfere with the multiplication of viruses.

1957 François Jacob and Elie L. Wollman demonstrate that the single linkage group of *Escherichia coli* is circular and suggest that the different linkage groups found in different Hfr strains result from the insertion at different points of a factor in the circular linkage group that determines the rupture of the circle.

1957 The World Health Organization advances the oral polio vaccine developed by Albert Sabin (1906-1993) as a safer alternative to the Salk vaccine.

1958 George W. Beadle, Edward L. Tatum, and Joshua Lederberg were awarded the Nobel Prize in physiology or medicine. Beadle and Tatum were honored for the work in

Neurospora that led to the one gene-one enzyme theory. Lederberg was honored for discoveries concerning genetic recombination and the organization of the genetic material of bacteria.

1958 Matthew Meselson and Frank W. Stahl publish their landmark paper "The replication of DNA in *Escherichia coli*," which demonstrated that the replication of DNA follow the semiconservative model.

1959 Albert Bruce Sabin (1906-1993), Polish-American virologist, announces successful results from testing live attenuated polio vaccine. His vaccine eventually is preferred over the Salk vaccine, since it can be administered orally and offers protection with a single dose.

1959 English biochemist Rodney Porter begins studies that lead to the discovery of the structure of antibodies. Porter receives the 1972 Nobel Prize in Physiology or Medicine for this research.

1959 Robert L. Sinsheimer reports that bacteriophage ØX174, which infects *Escherichia coli*, contains a single-stranded DNA molecule, rather than the expected double-stranded DNA. This provides the first example of a single-stranded DNA genome.

1959 Sydney Brenner and Robert W. Horne publish a paper entitled *A Negative Staining Method for High Resolution Electron Microscopy of Viruses*. The two researchers develop a method for studying the architecture of viruses at the molecular level using the electron microscope.

1961 Francis Crick, Sydney Brenner, and others propose that a molecule called transfer RNA uses a three base code in the manufacture of proteins.

1961 French pathologist Jacques Miller discovers the role of the thymus in cellular immunity.

1961 Marshall Warren Nirenberg synthesizes a polypeptide using an artificial messenger RNA (a synthetic RNA containing only the base uracil) in a cell-free protein-synthesizing system. The resulting polypeptide only contains the amino acid phenylalanine, indicating that UUU was the codon for phenylalanine. This important step in deciphering the genetic code is described in the landmark paper by Nirenberg and J. Heinrich Matthaei, *The Dependence of Cell-Free Synthesis in E. coli upon Naturally Occurring or Synthetic Polyribonucleotides.* This work establishes the messenger concept and a system that could be used to work out the relationship between the sequence of nucleotides in the genetic material and amino acids in the gene product.

1961   Noel Warner establishes the physiological distinction between the cellular and humoral immune responses.

1962   James D. Watson, Francis Crick, and Maurice Wilkins are awarded the Nobel Prize in physiology or medicine for their work in elucidating the structure of DNA.

1962   United States Congress passes Kefauver-Harris Drug Amendments that shift the burden of proof of clinical safety to drug manufacturers. For the first time, drug manufacturers had to prove their products were safe and effective before they could be sold.

1963   Albert Sabin's live polio vaccine is approved for use.

1964   Michael Epstein and Yvonne Barr discover the Epstein-Barr virus that is the cause of mononucleosis.

1964   Retrovir is developed as a cancer treatment. While not useful for cancer, the drug subsequently becomes the first drug approved for the treatment of AIDS.

1964   World Medical Association adopts Helsinki Declaration.

1965   Anthrax vaccine adsorbed (AVA), is approved for use in the United States.

1965   François Jacob, André Lwoff, and Jacques Monod are awarded the Nobel Prize in physiology or medicine for their discoveries concerning genetic control of enzymes and virus synthesis.

1966   Bruce Ames develops a test to screen for compounds that cause mutations, including those that are cancer causing. The so-called Ames test utilizes the bacterium *Salmonella typhimurium.*

1966   Daniel Carleton Gajdusek, American pediatrician, transfers for the first time a viral disease of the central nervous system from humans to another species. The viral disease kuru is found in New Guinea and is spread by the ritual eating of the deceased's brains.

1966   FDA and National Academy of Sciences begin investigation of effectiveness of drugs previously approved because they were thought safe.

1966   Marshall Nirenberg and Har Gobind Khorana lead teams that decipher the genetic code. All of the 64 possible triplet combinations of the four bases (the codons) and their associated amino acids are determined and described.

1966   Merck, Sharp, and Dohme Laboratories began research into a varicella-zoster vaccine.

1966   *New England Journal of Medicine* article exposes unethical Tuskegee syphilis study.

1966   NIH Office for Protection of Research Subjects ("OPRR") created.

1966   Paul D. Parman and Harry M. Myer, Jr., develop a live-virus rubella vaccine.

1967   A hemorrhagic fever outbreak in Marburg, Germany occurs. The virus responsible is subsequently named the marburg virus, and the disease called marburg hemorrhagic fever.

1967   British physician M. H. Pappworth publishes "Human Guinea Pigs," advising "No doctor has the right to choose martyrs for science or for the general good."

1968   FDA administratively moves to Public Health Service.

1968   Mark Steven Ptashne and Walter Gilbert independently identify the bacteriophage genes that are the repressors of the lac operon.

1968   Robert W. Holley, Har Gobind Khorana, and Marshall W. Nirenberg are awarded the Nobel Prize in physiology or medicine for their interpretation of the genetic code and its function in protein synthesis.

1968   Werner Arber discovers that bacteria defend themselves against viruses by producing DNA-cutting enzymes. These enzymes quickly become important tools for molecular biologists.

1969   By Executive Order, the United States renounces first-use of biological weapons and restricts future weapons research programs to issues concerning defensive responses (e.g., immunization, detection, etc.).

1969   Jonathan R. Beckwith, American molecular biologist, and colleagues isolate a single gene.

1969   Max Delbrück, Alfred D. Hershey, and Salvador E. Luria are awarded the Nobel Prize in physiology or medicine for their discoveries concerning the replication mechanism and the genetic structure of viruses.

1969   United States Surgeon General William Stewart announces: "The time has come to close the book on infectious diseases."

1970   First outbreak of drug-resistant tuberculosis recorded in the United States.

1970   Howard Martin Temin and David Baltimore independently discover reverse transcriptase in viruses. Reverse transcriptase is an enzyme that catalyzes the transcription of RNA into DNA.

1972   Biological and Toxin Weapons Convention first signed. BWC prohibits the offensive weaponization of biological agents (e.g., anthrax spores). The BWC also prohibits the transformation of biological agents with established legitimate and sanctioned purposes into agents of a nature and quality that could be used to effectively induce illness or death.

1972   Introduction of amoxcillin, a drug related to penicillin, which is a treatment of choice for bacterial pneumonia.

1972   Mishiaka Takahashi isolated the varicella virus from a 3-year-old patient and named it Oka, after the patient's name. The isolated virus was later used by Merck to develop a vaccine.

1972   Paul Berg and Herbert Boyer produce the first recombinant DNA molecules.

1972   Recombinant technology emerges as one of the most powerful techniques of molecular biology. Scientists are able to splice together pieces of DNA to form recombinant genes. As the potential uses, therapeutic and industrial, became increasingly clear, scientists and venture capitalists establish biotechnology companies.

1973   Concerns about the possible hazards posed by recombinant DNA technologies, especially work with tumor viruses, leads to the establishment of a meeting at Asilomar, California. The proceedings of this meeting are subsequently published by the Cold Spring Harbor Laboratory as a book entitled *Biohazards in Biological Research*.

1973   Herbert Wayne Boyer and Stanley H. Cohen create recombinant genes by cutting DNA molecules with restriction enzymes. These experiments mark the beginning of genetic engineering.

1974   National Research Act establishes "The Common Rule" for protection of human subjects.

1974   Peter Doherty and Rolf Zinkernagl discover the basis of immune determination of self and non-self.

1975   César Milstein and George Kohler create monoclonal antibodies.

1975   David Baltimore, Renato Dulbecco, and Howard Temin share the Nobel Prize in physiology or medicine for their discoveries concerning the interaction between tumor viruses and the genetic material of the cell and the discovery of reverse transcriptase.

1975   HHS promulgates Title 45 of Federal Regulations titled "Protection of Human Subjects," requiring appointment and utilization of Institutional Review Board (IRB).

1976   First outbreak of Ebola virus observed in Zaire, resulting in more than 300 cases with a 90% death rate.

1976   Swine flu breaks identified in soldiers stationed in New Jersey. Virus identified as H1N1 virus causes concern due to its similarities to H1N1 responsible for Spanish Flu pandemic. President Gerald Ford calls for emergency vaccination program. More than 20 deaths result from Guillain-Barre syndrome related to the vaccine.

1977   Carl R. Woese and George E. Fox publish an account of the discovery of a third major branch of living beings, the Archaea. Woese suggests that an rRNA database could be used to generate phylogenetic trees.

1977   Earliest known AIDS (acquired immunodeficiency syndrome) victims in the United States are two homosexual men in New York who are diagnosed as suffering from Kaposi's sarcoma.

1977   Frederick Sanger develops the chain termination (dideoxy) method for sequencing DNA, and uses the method to sequence the genome of a microorganism.

1977   The first known human fatality from H5N1 avian flu occurs in Hong Kong.

1977   The last reported smallpox case is recorded. Ultimately, the World Health Organization (WHO) declares the disease eradicated.

1979   National Commission issues Belmont Report.

1979   The last case of wild poliovirus infection is recorded in the United States.

1980   Congress passes the Bayh-Dole Act, the Act is amended by the Technology Transfer Act in 1986.

1980   In *Diamond v. Chakrabarty* the U.S. Supreme Court rules that a genetically modified bacterium can be patented.

1980   Researchers successfully introduce a human gene, which codes for the protein interferon, into a bacterium.

1980   The FDA promulgates 21 CFR 50.44 prohibiting use of prisoners as subjects in clinical trials.

1981   AIDS (acquired immunodeficiency syndrome) is officially recognized by the U.S. Center for Disease Control, and the first clinical description of this disease is made. It soon becomes recognized that AIDS is an infectious disease caused by a virus that spreads virtually exclusively by infected blood or body fluids.

1981   First disease-causing human retrovirus, human T-cell leukemia virus, discovered.

1981   The first cases of AIDS are reported among previously healthy young men in Los Angeles, California, and New York presenting with *Pneumocystis carinii* pneumonia and Kaposi's sarcoma.

1982   The U.S. Food and Drug Administration approves the first genetically engineered drug, a form of human insulin produced by bacteria.

1983   *Escherichia coli* O157:H7 is identified as a human pathogen.

1983   Luc Montainer and Robert Gallo discover the human immunodeficiency virus that causes acquired immunodeficiency syndrome.

1984   Niels Kai Jerne, Danish-English immunologist, Georges J. F. Kohler, German immunologist, and Cesar Milstein, Argentinian immunologist, are awarded the Nobel Prize for Physiology or Medicine for theories concerning the specificity in development and control of the immune system and the discovery of the principle for production of monoclonal antibodies.

1984   WHO begins a program to control trypanosomiasis.

1985   Alec Jeffreys develops "genetic fingerprinting," a method of using DNA polymorphisms (unique sequences of DNA) to identify individuals. The method, which has been used in paternity, immigration, and murder cases, is generally referred to as "DNA fingerprinting."

1985   First vaccine for *H. influenzae* type B is licensed for use.

1985   Japanese molecular biologist Susuma Tonegawa discovers the genes that code for immunoglobulins. He receives the 1986 Nobel Prize in Physiology or Medicine for this discovery.

1985   Kary Mullis, who was working at Cetus Corporation, develops the polymerase chain reaction (PCR), a new method of amplifying DNA. This technique quickly becomes one of the most powerful tools of molecular biology. Cetus patents PCR and sells the patent to Hoffman-LaRoche, Inc. in 1991.

1986   Congress passes the National Childhood Vaccine Injury Act, requiring patient information on vaccines and reporting of adverse events after vaccination.

1986   First genetically-engineered vaccine approved for human use is the hepatitis B vaccine. The U.S. Food and Drug Administration gives its approval.

1986   First license to market a living organism that was produced by genetic engineering is granted by the U.S. Department of Agriculture. It allows Biologics Corporation to sell a virus that is used as a vaccine against a herpes disease in pigs.

1986   International Committee on the Taxonomy of Viruses officially names the AIDS virus as HIV (human immunosufficiency virus).

1987 An illness outbreak in Prince Edward Island, Canada, which sickens over 100 people and kills three, leads to the first isolation and identification of domoic acid.

1987 Maynard Olson creates and names yeast artificial chromosomes (YACs), which provided a technique to clone long segments of DNA.

1987 The U.S. Congress charters a Department of Energy advisory committee, the Health and Environmental Research Advisory Committee (HERAC), which recommends a 15-year, multidisciplinary, scientific, and technological undertaking to map and sequence the human genome. DOE designates multidisciplinary human genome centers. National Institute of General Medical Sciences at the National Institutes of Health (NIH NIGMS) began funding genome projects.

1988 First report of vancomycin-resistant enterococci, a type of Streptococcus that is resistant to almost all antiobitics.

1988 The Human Genome Organization (HUGO) is established by scientists in order to coordinate international efforts to sequence the human genome. The Human Genome Project officially adopts the goal of determining the entire sequence of DNA comprising the human chromosomes.

1988 The World Health Organization (WHO) and its partners announce the Global Polio Eradication Initiative.

1989 Ebola-Reston virus is the source of an outbreak at an animal facility in Virginia. The outbreak becomes the basis for the best-selling book "The Hot Zone."

1989 Sidney Altman and Thomas R. Cech are awarded the Nobel Prize in chemistry for their discovery of ribozymes (RNA molecules with catalytic activity). Cech proves that RNA could function as a biocatalyst as well as an information carrier.

1990 Only 24 cases of diphtheria reported in the United States during preceding ten-year period.

1991 Cholera returns to the Western Hemisphere when an outbreak in Peru spreads to other Latin American countries.

1991 World Health Organization announces CIOMS Guidelines (the International Ethical Guidelines for Biomedical Research Involving Human Subjects).

1992 Craig Venter establishes The Institute for Genomic Research (TIGR) in Rockville, Maryland. TIGR later sequences the genome of *Haemophilus influenzae* and many other bacterial genomes.

1993 An international research team, led by Daniel Cohen, of the Center for the Study of Human Polymorphisms in Paris, produces a rough map of all 23 pairs of human chromosomes.

1993 Beginning in April, a five-week contamination of the drinking water supply of Milwaukee, Wisconsin, by *Cryptosporidium parvum* sickens 400,000 people and kills an estimated 104 people.

1993 Hanta virus emerged in the United States in a 1993 outbreak on a "Four Corners" (the juncture of Utah, Colorado, New Mexico, Arizona) area Native American Reservation. The resulting Hanta pulmonary syndrome (HPS) had a 43% mortality rate.

1993 Outbreaks in Moscow and St. Petersburg mark the return of epidemic diphtheria to the Western world.

1994 AZT (zidovudine) approved by the FDA for use in reducing maternal-fetal HIV transmission.

1994 DOE announces the establishment of the Microbial Genome Project as a spin off of the Human Genome Project.

1994 Ebola-Ivory Coast virus discovered.

1994 Geneticists determine that DNA repair enzymes perform several vital functions, including preserving genetic information and protecting the cell from cancer.

1994 The WHO declares the Americas free of polio.

1994 The WHO reports the start of epidemics of plague in Malawi, Mozambique, and India after 15 years absence.

1995 Edward B. Lewis, Christiane Nüsslein-Volhard, and Eric F. Wieschaus, developmental biologists, shared the Nobel Prize in physiology or medicine to cover discrimination based on genetic information related to illness, disease, or other conditions.

1995 Peter Funch and Reinhardt Moberg Kristensen create a new phylum, Cycliophora, for a novel invertebrate called *Symbion pandora*, which is found living in the mouths of Norwegian lobsters.

1995 Public awareness of potential use of chemical or biological weapons by a terrorist group increases following an Aum Shinrikyo, a Japanese cult, attack, which releases sarin gas in a Tokyo subway, killing a dozen people and sending thousands to the hospital.

1995 The U.S. FDA approved the varicella-zoster vaccine developed by Merck for vaccinations of persons 12 months of age and older.

1995 The Programme Against African Trypanosomiasis (PAAT) is created.

1995 The sequence of *Mycoplasma genitalium* is completed. *M. genitalium*, regarded as the smallest known bacterium, is considered a model of the minimum number of genes needed for independent existence.

1996 FDA approves the antidepressant buproprion (Zyban) and a nicotine nasal spray for the treatment of nicotine dependence.

1996 H5N1 avian flu virus is identified in Guangdong, China.

1996 International participants in the genome project meet in Bermuda and agree to formalize the conditions of data access. The agreement, known as the "Bermuda Principles," calls for the release of sequence data into public databases within 24 hours.

1996 Researchers C. Cheng and L. Olson demonstrate that the spinal cord can be regenerated in adult rats. Experimenting on rats with severed spinal cords, Cheng and Olson use peripheral nerves to connect white matter and gray matter.

1996 Researchers find that abuse and violence can alter a child's brain chemistry, placing him or her at risk for various problems, including drug abuse, cognitive disabilities, and mental illness, later in life.

1996 Scientists discover a link between autoptosis (cellular suicide, a natural process whereby the body eliminates useless cells) gone awry and several neurodegenerative conditions, including Alzheimer's disease.

1996 Scientists report further evidence that individuals with two mutant copies of the CC-CLR-5 gene are generally resistant to HIV infection.

1996 The Health Care Portability and Accountability Act incorporates provisions to prohibit the use of genetic information in certain health-insurance eligibility decisions. The Department of Health and Human Services was charged with the enforcement of health-information privacy provisions.

1996 U.S. Comprehensive Methamphetamine Control Act increases penalties for the manufacture, distribution, and possession of methamphetamines, as well as the reagents and chemicals needed to make it.

1996 William R. Bishai and co-workers report that SigF, a gene in the tuberculosis bacterium, enables the bacterium to enter a dormant stage.

1997 FDA reports and investigates correlation of heart valve disease in patients using phen-fen drug combination for weight loss. Similar reports were reported for patients using only dexfenluramine or fenfluramine. The FDA noted that the combination phen-fen treatment had not received FDA approval.

1997 Institute of Medicine (IOM), a branch of the National Academy of Sciences, publishes the report, *Marijuana: Assessing the Science Base*, which concludes that cannabinoids show significant promise as analgesics, appetite stimulants, and anti-emetics, and that further research into producing these medicines is warranted.

1997 Mickey Selzer, neurologist at the University of Pennsylvania, and co-workers, find that in lampreys, which have a remarkable ability to regenerate a severed spinal cord, neurofilament messenger RNA effects the regeneration process by literally pushing the growing axons and moving them forward.

1997 The DNA sequence of *Escherichia coli* is completed.

1997 While performing a cloning experiment, Christof Niehrs, a researcher at the German Center for Cancer Research, identifies a protein responsible for the creation of the head in a frog embryo.

1997 William Jacobs and Barry Bloom create a biological entity that combines the characteristics of a bacterial virus and a plasmid (a

DNA structure that functions and replicates independently of the chromosomes). This entity is capable of triggering mutations in *Mycobacterium tuberculosis.*

1997 Outbreaks of highly pathogenic H5N1 influenza are reported in poultry at farms and live animal markets in Hong Kong.

1998 A live, orally-administered rotavirus vaccine is approved for use in the United States. Use was discontinued in 1999 due to complications in some vaccinated children.

1998 Craig Venter forms a company (later named Celera), and predicts that the company would decode the entire human genome within three years. Celera plans to use a "whole genome shotgun" method, which would assemble the genome without using maps. Venter says that his company would not follow the Bermuda principles concerning data release.

1998 U.S. Department of Energy (Office of Science) funds bacterial artificial chromosome and sequencing projects.

1998 Scientists find that an adult human's brain can, with certain stimuli, replace cells. This discovery heralds potential breakthroughs in neurology.

1998 Sibutramine (Meridia), introduced as a weight-loss drug. Sibutramine inhibits the reuptake of the brain chemicals norepinephrine, dopamine, and serotonin, but does not promote monoamine release like the amphetamines.

1998 The World Health Organization reports a resurgence in tuberculosis cases worldwide; TB is killing more people than at any other point in history. Recommends Directly Observed Therapy (DOT) treatment, which is 95% effective in curing patients, even in developing nations.

1999 Pharmaceutical research in Japan leads to the discovery of donepezil (Aricept), the first drug intended to help ward off memory loss in Alzheimer's disease and other age-related dementias.

1999 Scientists announce the complete sequencing of the DNA making up human chromosome 22. The first complete human chromosome sequence is published in December 1999.

1999 The National Institutes of Health and the Office for Protection from Research Risks (OPRR) require researchers conducting or overseeing human subjects to ethics training.

1999 The public genome project responds to Craig Venter's challenge with plans to produce a draft genome sequence by 2000. Most of the sequencing is done in five centers, known as the "G5": the Whitehead Institute for Biomedical Research in Cambridge, MA; the Sanger Centre near Cambridge, UK; Baylor College of Medicine in Houston, TX; Washington University in St. Louis, MO; the DOE's Joint Genome Institute (JGI) in Walnut Creek, CA.

2000 On June 26, 2000, leaders of the public genome project and Celera announce the completion of a working draft of the entire human genome sequence. Ari Patrinos of the DOE helps mediate disputes between the two groups so that a fairly amicable joint announcement could be presented at the White House in Washington, D.C.

2000 Office for Protection from Research Risks (OPRR) becomes part of the Department of Health and Human Services, Office of Human Research Protection (OHRP).

2000 The federal government approves irradiation of raw meat, the only technology known to kill *E. coli* O157 bacteria while preserving the integrity of the meat.

2000 The first volume of *Annual Review of Genomics and Human Genetics* is published. Genomics is defined as the new science dealing with the identification and characterization of genes and their arrangement in chromosomes and human genetics as the science devoted to understanding the origin and expression of human individual uniqueness.

2000 The municipal water supply of Walkerton, Ontario, Canada, is contaminated in the summertime by a strain of the bacterium *Escherichia coli* O157:H7, sickening 2,000 people and killing 7.

2000 The WHO declares the Western Pacific region, including China, free of polio.

2001 *American Journal of Psychiatry* publishes studies providing evidence that methamphetamine can cause brain damage that results in slower motor and cognitive functioning—even in users who take the drug for less than a year.

2001 In February, the complete draft sequence of the human genome is published. The public sequence data is published in the British journal *Nature* and the Celera sequence is published in the American journal *Science*. Increased knowledge of the human genome allows greater specificity in pharmacological research and drug interaction studies.

2001 Microbiologists reveal that bacteria possess an internal protein structure similar to that of human cells.

2001 President George W. Bush announces the United States will allow and support limited forms of stem cell research.

2001 Researchers at Eli Lilly in Minneapolis sequence the genome of *Streptoccocus pneumoniae*.

2001 Scientists from the Whitehead Institute announce test results that show patterns of errors in cloned animals that might explain why such animals die early and exhibit a number of developmental problems. The report stimulates new debate on ethical issues related to cloning.

2001 Study entitled *Global Illicit Drug Trends* conducted by the United Nations Office for Drug Control and Crime Prevention (ODCCP), estimates that 14 million people use cocaine worldwide. Although cocaine use leveled off, the United States still maintains the highest levels of cocaine abuse.

2001 Terrorists attack United States on September 11, 2001, and kill thousands by crashing airplanes into buildings.

2001 Letters containing a powdered form of *Bacillus anthracis*, the bacteria that causes anthrax, are mailed to government representatives, members of the news media, and others in the United States. More than 20 cases and five deaths eventually result. As of August 2007, the case remains open and unsolved.

2001 The Chemical and Biological Incident Response Force (CBIRF) sends a 100-member initial response team into the Dirksen Senate Office Building in Washington alongside Environmental Protection Agency

(EPA) specialists to detect and remove anthrax. A similar mission was undertaken at the Longworth House Office Building in October, during which time samples were collected from more than 200 office spaces.

2001 The Pan African Trypanosomiasis and Tsetse Eradication campaign (PATTEC) begins operation.

2001 U.S. military endorses the situational temporary usefulness of caffeine, recommending it as a safe and effective stimulant for its soldiers in good health.

2002 A company called DrinkSafe Technology announces the invention of a coaster that can be used to test whether a drink has been drugged by changing color when a drop of the tampered drink is placed on it.

2002 Following September 11, 2001, terrorist attacks on the United States, the Public Health Security and Bioterrorism Preparedness and Response Act of 2002 is passed in an effort to improve the ability to prevent and respond to public health emergencies.

2002 In June 2002, traces of biological and chemical weapon agents are found in Uzbekistan on a military base used by U.S. troops fighting in Afghanistan. Early analysis dates and attributes the source of the contamination to former Soviet Union biological and chemical weapons programs that utilized the base.

2002 In the aftermath of the September 11, 2001, terrorist attacks on the United States, by the first few months of 2002 the United States government dramatically increases funding to stockpile drugs and other agents that could be used to counter a bioterrorist attack.

2002 Scientists found that stockpiled smallpox vaccine doses can be effective if diluted to one-tenth their original concentration, greatly enhancing the number of doses available to respond to an emergency.

2002 Severe acute respiratory syndrome (SARS) virus is found in patients in China, Hong Kong, and other Asian countries. The newly discovered coronavirus is not identified until early 2003. The spread of the virus reaches epidemic proportions in Asia and expands to the rest of the world.

2002 The Best Pharmaceuticals for Children Act passed in an effort to improve safety and efficacy of patented and off-patent medicines for children.

2002   The Defense Advanced Research Projects Agency (DARPA) initiates the Biosensor Technologies program in 2002 to develop fast, sensitive, automatic technologies for the detection and identification of biological warfare agents.

2002   The Pathogen Genomic Sequencing program is initiated by the Defense Advanced Research Project Agency (DARPA) to focus on characterizing the genetic components of pathogens in order to develop novel diagnostics, treatments, and therapies for the diseases they cause.

2002   The planned destruction of stocks of smallpox causing Variola virus at the two remaining depositories in the U.S. and Russia is delayed over fears that large scale production of vaccine might be needed in the event of a bioterrorist action.

2002   The WHO declares the 51 countries of its European region free of polio.

2003   Almost 500,000 civic and health care workers at strategic hospitals, governmental facilities, and research centers across the United States are slated to receive smallpox immunizations as part of a strategic plan for ready response to a biological attack using the smallpox virus.

2003   An international research team funded by NINR found that filters made from old cotton saris cut the number of cholera cases in rural Bangladesh villages almost in half. Other inexpensive cloth should work just as well in other parts of the world where cholera is endemic. Cholera is a waterborne disease that causes severe diarrhea and vomiting, killing thousands of people around the world every year. This simple preventive measure has the potential to make a significant impact on a global health problem.

2003   By early May, WHO officials have confirmed reports of more than 3,000 cases of SARS from 18 different countries with 111 deaths attributed to the disease. United States health officials reported 193 cases with no deaths. Significantly, all but 20 of the U.S. cases are linked to travel to infected areas, and the other 20 cases are accounted

for by secondary transmission from infected patients to family members and health care workers. Health authorities assert that the emergent virus responsible for SARS will remain endemic (part of the natural array of viruses) in many regions of China well after the current outbreak is resolved.

2003   Canadian scientists at the British Columbia Cancer Agency in Vancouver announce the sequence of the genome of the coronavirus most likely to be the cause of SARS. Within days, scientists at the Centers for Disease Control (CDC) in Atlanta, Georgia, offer a genomic map that confirms more than 99% of the Canadian findings.

2003   Differences in outbreaks in Hong Kong between 1997 and 2003 cause investigators to conclude that the H5N1 virus has mutated.

2003   Following approximately five deaths by heart attack correlated to individuals receiving the new smallpox vaccine, U.S. health officials at the Centers for Disease Control (CDC) announce a suspension of administration of the new smallpox vaccine to patients with a history of heart disease until the matter can be fully investigated.

2003   Preliminary trials for a malaria vaccine are scheduled to begin in malaria-endemic African areas, where approximately 3,000 children die from the disease every day.

2003   SARS cases in Hanoi reach 22, as a simultaneous outbreak of the same disease occurs in Hong Kong. The World Health Organization issues a global alert about a new infectious disease of unknown origin in both Vietnam and Hong Kong.

2003   SARS is added to the list of quarantinable diseases in the United States.

2003   Studies indicate that women with a history of some sexually transmitted diseases, including the human papillomavirus, are at increased risk for developing cervical cancer.

2003   Studies show no correlation between immunization schedules and sudden infant death syndrome (SIDS) occurrences.

2003   The first case of an unusually severe pneumonia occurs in Hanoi, Vietnam, and is identified two days later as severe acute respiratory syndrome (SARS) by Italian physician and epidemiologist Carlo

Urbani, who formally identifies SARS as a unique disease and names it. Urbani later dies of SARS.

2003   The first case of bovine spongiform encephalopathy (BSE, mad cow disease) in the United States is found in a cow in Washington state. Investigations later reveal that the cow was imported from a Canadian herd, which included North America's first "home-grown" case of BSE six months earlier.

2003   The World Health Organization (WHO) takes the unusual step of issuing a travel warning that describes SARS as a worldwide health threat. WHO officials announced that SARS cases, and potential cases, had been tracked from China to Singapore, Thailand, Vietnam, Indonesia, Philippines, and Canada.

2003   United States invades Iraq and finds chemical, biological, and nuclear weapons programs, but no actual weapons.

2003   WHO Global Influenza Surveillance Network intensifies work on development of a H5N1 vaccine for humans.

2004   A 35-year-old television producer in the Guangdong province of China is the first person to become ill with SARS since the end of the May 2003, the initial outbreak of the newly-identified disease. Within two weeks, three other persons are suspected of having SARS in the region, and teams from the World Health Organization return to investigate possible human-to-human, animal-to-human, and environmental sources of transmission of the disease.

2004   Chinese health officials in the Guangdong province of China launch a mass slaughter of civet cats, a cousin of the mongoose considered a delicacy and thought to be a vector of SARS, in an attempt to control the spread of the disease.

2004   On December 26, the most powerful earthquake in more than 40 years occurred underwater off the Indonesian island of Sumatra. The tsunami produced a disaster of unprecedented proportion in the modern era. The International Red Cross puts the death toll at over 150,000 lives.

2004   Project BioShield Act of 2004 authorizes U.S. government agencies expedite procedures related to rapid distribution of treatments as countermeasures to chemical, biological, and nuclear attack.

2005   A massive 7.6-magnitude earthquake leaves more than 3 million homeless and without food and basic medical supplies in the Kashmir mountains between India and Pakistan; 80,000 people die.

2005   H5N1 virus, responsible for avian flu moves from Asia to Europe. The World Health Organization attempts to coordinate multinational disaster and containment plans. Some nations begin to stockpile antiviral drugs.

2005   Hurricane Katrina slams into the U.S. Gulf Coast, causing levee breaks and massive flooding to New Orleans. Damage is extensive across the coasts of Louisiana, Mississippi, and Alabama. Federal Emergency Management Agency (FEMA) is widely criticized for a lack of coordination in relief efforts. Three other major hurricanes make landfall in the United States within a two-year period, stressing relief and medical supply efforts. Long-term health studies begin of populations in devastated areas.

2005   The WHO reports outbreaks of plague in the Democratic Republic of Congo.

2005   U.S. FDA Drug Safety Board is founded.

2005   United States president George W. Bush addresses the issue of HIV/AIDS in black women in the United States, acknowledging it as a public health crisis.

2006   European Union bans the importation of avian feathers (non-treated feathers) from countries neighboring or close to Turkey.

2006   Mad cow disease confirmed in an Alabama cow as third reported case in the United States.

2006   More than a dozen people are diagnosed with avian flu in Turkey, but U.N. health experts assure the public that human-to-human transmission is still rare and only suspected in a few cases in Asia.

2006   Researchers begin human trials for vaginal microbicide gels.

2007   Texas governor Rick Perry adds the HPV vaccine to the list of required vaccines for school-age girls.

2007 Four people are hospitalized with botulism poisoning in the United States after more than 90 potentially contaminated meat products, including canned chili, were removed from grocery shelves across the country.

2007 The Centers for Disease Control and Prevention (CDC) issues a rare order for isolation when a New Jersey man infected with a resistant strain of tuberculosis flies on multiple trans-Atlantic commercial flights.

African Sleeping Sickness (Trypanosomiasis)

■ Introduction

Trypanosomiasis (tri-PAN-o-SO-my-a-sis), which is also known as African sleeping sickness because of the semiconscious stupor and excessive sleep that can occur in someone who is infected, is an infection passed to humans through the bite of the tsetse fly. Thus, it is a vector-borne disease. The fly bite transfers either *Trypanosoma brucei rhodesiense*, which causes a version of the disease called East African trypanosomiasis, or *T. brucei gambiense*, which causes West African trypanosomiasis. If left untreated, trypanosomiasis is ultimately fatal.

Trypanosomiasis is common in Africa. In the 1960s the disease was almost eradicated, but interruptions in the delivery of public health to affected regions due to government indifference and warfare caused a re-emergence of the disease, now resulting in tens of thousands of cases every year. The World Health Organization (WHO) estimates that in 2005 there were 50,000–70,000 new cases. This is a drop from higher numbers reported during the 1990s. An ongoing effort involving WHO, Médecines Sans Frontières (Doctors Without Borders), and several pharmaceutical companies is again attempting to bring trypanosomiasis under control.

■ Disease History, Characteristics, and Transmission

Trypanosomiasis has been known for centuries. It was first described in the fourteenth century in the land-locked region of northwestern Africa that today is known as Mali. The involvement of the trypanosomes and the tsetse fly were discovered by Sir David Bruce in 1902-1903. A few years later, a massive epidemic that affected millions of Africans and killed 500,000 people called attention to the seriousness of the disease. Shortly afterward, the association between trypanosomiasis and the tsetse fly was established.

T. brucei rhodesiense and *T. brucei gambiense* are protozoa. Protozoans are single-celled organisms that are more complex in structure than bacteria and viruses; the organisms are considered to be animals. The protozoa responsible for sleeping sickness are native to Africa. The few cases of trypanosomiasis that occur outside of Africa each year generally result from travelers who acquire the protozoa in Africa, then leave and subsequently develop the disease in another country.

The two protozoans have a complex life cycle. In the animal host, the organisms that are injected by a tsetse fly progressively change their shape to what is described as the stumpy form. This form is able to infect a tsetse fly when it takes a blood meal from an animal. While inside the gut of the fly, the protozoans change again into a form that is able to migrate to the salivary glands of the fly. Finally, another change in the organism occurs; the protozoan is now capable of infecting another animal when the tsetse fly seeks a blood meal. This animal-to-human cycle can continue until the chain of transmission (also called the cycle of infection) is interrupted, usually by an organized effort by agencies such as WHO.

T. brucei rhodesiense is naturally carried by antelopes. The antelopes are not harmed by the protozoan and serve as the natural reservoir of the *T. brucei rhodesiense*. Tsetse flies who obtain a blood meal from an antelope can acquire the protozoan, which they can transfer to humans or cows. The resulting infection is lethal in cattle. People who are most likely to become infected are those who come into contact with cattle or antelopes. Thus, those who raise cattle, or the game wardens and visitors to East African game reserves and other rural areas are at risk.

T. brucei gambiense does not infect antelope or cattle. It resides in creatures that live in the tropical rain forests found in Central and West Africa. The disease caused by this protozoan in humans produces more severe symptoms and more often results in death. Fortunately, because of its isolated distribution, fewer people contract this form of trypanosomiasis.

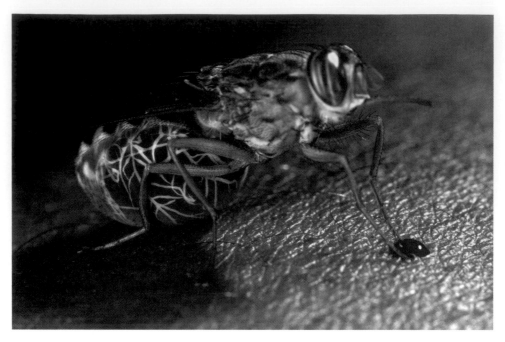

Glossina morsitans morsitans is a species of tsetse fly that can transmit the trypanosome parasite responsible for trypanosomiasis, also called African sleeping sickness. © *Robert Patrick/Corbis Sygma.*

The infection due to *T. brucei rhodesiense* progresses more swiftly than the longer-lasting infection that is caused by *T. brucei gambiense*. Both infections inevitably lead to death if they are not treated.

Sleeping sickness is a complex disease, with interactions between humans, the tsetse fly vector, and the animal host. This can complicate efforts to control the disease.

Typically, the first indication of both types of trypanosomiasis is the development of redness, pain, and swelling at the site of the fly bite several days after having been bitten. The sore is also referred to as a chancre. Some people also develop a rash. Both forms of the disease then progress in two stages. The first stage begins two to three weeks following the bite and the entry of the protozoans into the bloodstream. The symptoms of this stage develop as the trypanosome is carried throughout the body in the bloodstream. The lymphatic system, which is an important part of the immune system, can also become infected. Because at this stage the disease affects the whole body, it is termed the systemic phase. A hallmark of the illness at this point is an extreme fluctuation of body temperature. A person's temperature will cycle from normal to very high and back again, which is a consequence of the immune system's reaction to the protozoan. Additionally, a person may experience a feeling of extreme itchiness and develop a headache. Some people become mentally disoriented. If left untreated, a person can lapse into a coma and die.

West African trypanosomiasis also produces marked swelling of lymph nodes, especially those located behind the ear and at the base of the neck, and swelling of both the spleen and the liver. East African trypanosomiasis can cause the heart to become inflamed and to malfunction.

Some of the symptoms of trypanosomiasis that can occur during the first stage of the illness are a result of the immune reaction to the infection. The immune response remains strong, since invading trypanosomes can shift the composition of their outer surface. As the immune system hones in on one surface configuration, that configuration can rapidly change. This trait is known as antigenic variation. The trypanosomes are capable of expressing thousands of different surface profiles during the years that an infection can last. A consequence of the heightened immune response due to the changing surface of the protozoan is the cycling fever, as well as organ damage and weakened blood vessels; the latter aid in the spread of the organism throughout the body.

The second stage of trypanosomiasis involves the nervous system. As the brain becomes affected, a person can experience difficulties in speaking, mental disorientation, and periods of near-unconsciousness or sleep during the daytime (hence the term sleeping sickness). During the night, insomnia robs a person of sleep. Other symptoms can develop that mimic those of Parkinson's disease; these include difficulty in movement, with difficulty in walking that can require a shuffling motion to avoid falling down, involuntary movement or trembling of arms and legs, and a tightening of muscles. With more time, a person can lapse into a coma and die.

Trypanosomiasis can also be transferred from a pregnant woman to her baby prior to birth or via transfusion with infected blood or a contaminated organ that is transplanted. However, these routes of infection are rare.

■ Scope and Distribution

Trypanosomiasis is prevalent in regions of Africa. East African trypanosomiasis is found in Uganda, Tanzania, Kenya, Malawi, Zaire, Ethiopia, Botswana, and Zimbabwe. West African trypanosomiasis is prevalent in Western and Central Africa.

According to the WHO, in 2002 trypanosomiasis was constantly present in 11 countries and almost as prevalent in a further 12 countries. As of 2007, epidemics are occurring in the Democratic Republic of Congo, Angola, and Sudan.

Spread of the disease to humans occurs only in Africa, since the tsetse fly is only found on the African continent. On the rare occasions that trypanosomiasis occurs elsewhere in the world, it is usually the result of travel by someone who became infected while in Africa. As of February 2006, the United States Centers for Disease Control and Prevention (CDC) has records of only 36 cases of the disease in the United States, and all involved people who contracted the disease in Africa.

A version of trypanosomiasis called Chagas disease, which is caused by *Trypanosoma cruzi*, occurs in South America and sometimes in Central and North America.

The WHO estimates that there are 50,000 or more cases of East and West African trypanosomias every year. However, since the majority of cases occur in regions of Africa where organized medical care and reporting is scant, the actual number of cases is likely much higher. The CDC estimates that there are over 100,000 new cases every year.

■ Treatment and Prevention

The diagnosis of trypanosomiasis involves examination of the fluid from either the site of the tsetse fly bite or from a swollen lymph node or blood, to detect the presence of infecting protozoa. As well, fluid can be injected into rats, which can develop an infection. Blood recovered from the rats after several weeks will contain the protozoa.

Medications are available to treat trypanosomiasis. A drug called pentamidine is used for the early stage of *T. brucei gambiense* infections, and the drug suramin is used for the early stage of infections caused by *T. brucie rhodesiense*. More advanced stages of both forms of the disease are treated using a drug called melarsoprol. Those who do not respond to melarsoprol can be given another drug called eflornithine. Unfortunately, the drugs can have undesirable side effects. For example, suramin, eflornithine, and pentamidine can cause a fatal reaction in the kidney or liver, or inflammation in the brain. These drugs must be used with care and their effects monitored; they

WORDS TO KNOW

CHAIN OF TRANSMISSION: Chain of transmission refers to the route by which an infection is spread from its source to susceptible host. An example of a chain of transmission is the spread of malaria from an infected animal to humans via mosquitoes.

EPIDEMIC: From the Greek *epidemic*, meaning "prevalent among the people," is most commonly used to describe an outbreak of an illness or disease in which the number of individual cases significantly exceeds the usual or expected number of cases in any given population.

PROTOZOA: Single-celled animal-like microscopic organisms that live by taking in food rather than making it by photosynthesis and must live in the presence of water. (Singular: protozoan.) Protozoa are a diverse group of single-celled organisms, with more than 50,000 different types represented. The vast majority are microscopic, many measuring less than 5 one-thousandth of an inch (or 0.005 millimeters), but some, such as the freshwater Spirostomun, may reach 0.17 inches (3 millimeters) in length, large enough to enable it to be seen with the naked eye.

RE-EMERGING INFECTIOUS DISEASE: Re-emerging infectious diseases are illnesses such as malaria, diphtheria, tuberculosis, and polio that were once nearly absent from the world but are starting to cause greater numbers of infections once again. These illnesses are reappearing for many reasons. Malaria and other mosquito-borne illnesses increase when mosquito-control measures decrease. Other diseases are spreading because people have stopped being vaccinated, as happened with diphtheria after the collapse of the Soviet Union. A few diseases are reemerging because drugs to treat them have become less available or drug-resistant strains have developed.

RESERVOIR: The animal or organism in which the virus or parasite normally resides.

VECTOR: Any agent, living or otherwise, that carries and transmits parasites and diseases. Also, an organism or chemical used to transport a gene into a new host cell.

are usually only used in a hospital setting. While these drugs can be effective, the CDC does not recommend any particular medication.

Trypanosomiasis cannot clear up on its own. Hospitalization and treatment is necessary. Those who recover from the infection should be monitored for several years afterward to ensure that the infection does not recur.

As of 2007, there is no vaccine for either form of trypanosomiasis. Prevention of the disease consists of avoiding contact with the tsetse fly. For example, contact with bushes should be minimized, as the flies often rest there. Bushes and other shrubbery that are near rivers or waterholes are prime spots for tsetse flies, and so should be avoided. This habitat tends to be rural, so people who spend time traveling or staying in rural areas of regions where trypanosomiasis is prevalent are at risk and should be appropriately cautious.

Clothing can be protective. The clothing should be fairly thick, as the tsetse fly can bite through light fabric. Also, because the fly is attracted to bright colors, clothing should be bland; khaki- or olive-colored clothing is recommended. The clothing should fit tightly at the wrists and ankles to make it harder for flies to enter. Riding in the back of open-air vehicles is unwise; tsetse flies are also attracted to dust. Another wise precaution, which has also proven useful in reducing the incidence of malaria, is the use of protective netting over a bed.

■ Impacts and Issues

The resurgence of trypanosomiasis during the 1970s highlights the vigilance that is necessary to control infectious diseases and prevent their re-emergence. The loss of control over trypanosomiasis was due to the interruptions in the monitoring of disease outbreaks, the displacement of people due to regional conflicts, and environmental changes. These problems are ongoing. In particular, the documented warming of the atmosphere will make Africa even more hospitable to the spread of the territory of the tsetse fly, which could increase the geographical distribution of trypanosomiasis.

Trypanosomiasis is a major health concern in approximately 20 countries in Africa. The WHO estimates that over 66 million people are at risk of developing the disease. However, fewer than 4 million people are being monitored and only about 40,000 people are treated every year. The proportion of people being monitored or treated is smaller than other tropical diseases, even though trypanosomiasis can increase to epidemic proportions and the death rate for those who are not treated is 100%.

Epidemics disrupt families as well as national economies, as large numbers of people become unable to work or care for themselves. According to WHO estimates, in 2004 the number of healthy years of life lost due to premature death and disability caused by trypanosomia-

sis was 1.5 million. Since many regions are still agricultural, the rural-based disease affects those who are most important to the economy. Of the 48,000 deaths that occurred in 2004, 31,000 were males, who are often the working family members. Epidemics can decimate the population of a region.

Taking care of those diagnosed with trypanosomiasis is a daunting task for the poor nations, since two-thirds of people diagnosed with the disease already have the advanced stage of the infection, in which the nervous system has been affected. The only treatment that is effective once the central nervous system has been affected—the drug melarsoprol—contains arsenic, and so the treatment itself can sometimes be fatal. Compounding the problem, some strains of the trypanosomes that are resistant to drugs used to treat the disease at an earlier stage have been detected. It seems a matter of time before these resistant strains become more common, as the resistance gives them a selective advantage over nonresistant trypanosomes.

Treatment can also be hampered by the cost of the drugs. An example is eflornithine. Originally developed as an anticancer compound, the drug has been promising against *T. brucei gambiense*. However, it costs between 300 and 500 U.S. dollars per patient, which makes it unaffordable for mass use by a poor nation.

The WHO is actively involved in programs intended to monitor and treat trypanosomiasis. As one example, since 1975, WHO, the United Nations Children's Fund (UNICEF), the World Bank, and the United Nations Development Program (UNDP) have collaborated on The Special Program for Research and Training in Tropical Diseases. The aim of the program is to develop means of combating infectious diseases, including trypanosomiasis, in a way that is effective and affordable to poorer countries that otherwise are unable to meet the economic and logistical burdens of treatment.

In addition, the WHO Communicable Disease Surveillance and Response unit works with countries experiencing epidemics to set up national programs to control the disease. This can be challenging, since governments can treat trypanosomiasis as a low priority issue until an epidemic strikes. By acting earlier and with a more coordinated national effort, however, epidemics might well be avoided.

■ Primary Source Connection

With international cooperation among African countries and international health authorities, intensive insecticide spraying, and efficient drug delivery to treat the disease in its early stages, trypanosomiasis was nearly eradicated from Africa in the mid-1960s. By the late 1980s, major epidemics in east and central Africa heralded a dramatic re-emergence of the disease. In the article for the magazine *Foreign Policy*, author Peter Hotez discusses re-emerging diseases, including those that could re-emerge

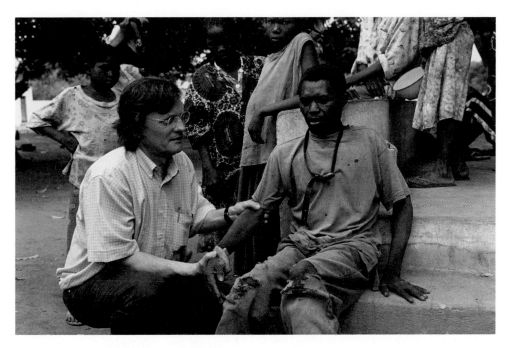

Jean Jannin (left), who led the World Health Organization (WHO) campaign to fight sleeping sickness, examines a man exhibiting signs of trypanosomiasis in Chad in 2002. Although sleeping sickness is estimated to be carried by about 500,000 people, it is not yet considered a top priority even though it is a fatal disease if left untreated. © *Patrick Robert/Corbis.*

deliberately through acts of bioterrorism, along with the political, social, and natural causes that allow diseases to re-emerge. Peter Hotez is professor and chair of microbiology and tropical medicine at The George Washington University and a senior fellow at the Sabin Vaccine Institute.

Dark Winters Ahead

During the 1990s, the eruption of military conflicts posed one of the strongest stimuli for the reemergence of infectious diseases in poor nations. The civil wars in Angola, Rwanda, and Sudan produced devastating outbreaks of African sleeping sickness, cholera, and polio, even though experts had assumed that these infections had been eliminated a decade or so earlier.

New links between political turmoil and public health crises are forcing the traditional foreign-policy community to consider the latest trends in global disease. Enter *Emerging Infectious Diseases*, a seven-year-old bimonthly journal published by the Centers for Disease Control and Prevention (CDC) in Atlanta. The journal provides a valuable service by studying infectious agents like the West Nile or Ebola viruses, which have the potential to emerge because of new human or animal migrations or environmental changes. A recent article by Scott Dowell, the acting associate director for global health at the CDC's National Center for Infectious Diseases, examines the seasonal aspects of infectious disease, offering insights

that could prove useful to global public health initiatives as well as antibioterrorism efforts around the world.

In an article titled "Seasonal Variation in Host Susceptibility and Cycles of Certain Infectious Diseases," Dowell explains how human viral epidemics seem to depend on the calendar, suddenly appearing and disappearing with the seasons. A good example is the regular January arrival of influenza in the United States. Similarly, rotavirus gastroenteritis appears in the southwestern United States and then slowly migrates to northeastern cities like Boston and Washington, D.C., striking young children during the winter months. Some 200 years ago, these same cities faced predictable and devastating summer epidemics of yellow fever introduced by cargo ships carrying infected mosquitoes from the West Indies.

Dowell argues that this seasonal variation of infection might not depend solely on the weather, as is commonly thought. He notes that the same viral infection—such as influenza—can appear on both sides of the equator during January, despite it being winter in the North and summer in the South. Because some aspects of human physiology (including sensitivity to light and certain immunities) also vary with the calendar, Dowell maintains, the regular arrival of certain epidemic infections might be explained by seasonal changes in human susceptibility to microbial invasion.

On this particular point, Dowell's hypothesis is less convincing since it diminishes the crucial role of the infectious agent itself in producing a clinical infection. Indeed, infectious pathogens have coevolved with humans in an intricate and remarkable dance that has taken millions of years. Recognizing the tentative nature of his hypothesis, Dowell calls for fellow researchers to review past clinical trials for further evidence.

Nevertheless, Dowell's larger emphasis on the seasonal nature of infection has important implications for the implementation of public health efforts. For instance, when national immunization days are held in polio- and measles-endemic regions of the developing world, they are best conducted well before the seasonal onset of these infections, thus allowing sufficient time for a child's immune system to respond to the vaccine. The same time-urgency applies to so-called days of tranquility, when vaccinations help to implement effective cease-fires in war-torn areas of Central Asia and sub-Saharan Africa.

Dowell's insights can also help those who seek to mitigate the potential impact of bioterrorism attacks. U.S. civil defense officials are concerned by the similarity between the early symptoms produced by biological warfare agents—such as bacterial agents of tularemia and Q fever—with the symptoms produced by influenza. In the initial stages of infection, all three will produce fever, chills, headaches, muscle pains, and appetite loss. The similarity may delay the detection of biological attacks during the winter, when public health officials might erroneously attribute an increase in complaints of such symptoms to a common flu outbreak.

Responding to such concerns, the CDC has initiated a national system of Centers for Public Health Preparedness to ensure that local health workers can respond to a bioterrorism attack. Similarly, the U.S. Defense Department's Advanced Research Projects Agency is developing new technologies aimed at differentiating infectious agents used as biological weapons from common seasonal viruses. However, such efforts are far from sufficient. A January 2001 CDC report concluded that the nation's public health infrastructure is not prepared to detect a bioterrorist event. In June 2001, the Center for Strategic and International Studies and the Johns Hopkins University Center for Civilian Biodefense Studies simulated a bioterrorist attack in a war game exercise known as "Dark Winter." Their conclusion: A smallpox attack on the United States would produce massive civilian casualties and rapid breakdown of the country's essential institutions. Unfortunately, the United States remains years away from replenishing key vaccine stockpiles and even further from having improved detection technologies in place.

Peter Hotez

HOTEZ, PETER. "DARK WINTERS AHEAD." *FOREIGN POLICY* (NOVEMBER-DECEMBER 2001): 84.

SEE ALSO *Chagas Disease; Médecins Sans Frontières (Doctors Without Borders); Mosquito-borne Diseases; Re-emerging Infectious Diseases.*

BIBLIOGRAPHY

Books

Hoppe, Kirk. *Lords of the Fly: Sleeping Sickness Control in British East Africa, 1900-1960*. Westport, Conn.: Praeger, 2003.

Kruel, Donald. *Trypanosomiasis*. London: Chelsea House, 2007.

Tyler, Kevin M., and Michael A. Miles. *American Trypanosomiasis*. New York: Springer, 2006.

Brian Hoyle

AIDS (Acquired Immunodeficiency Syndrome)

■ Introduction

First reported in the United States in 1981, acquired immunodeficiency syndrome (AIDS, also cited as acquired immune deficiency syndrome) has since become a major worldwide pandemic. Medical research has demonstrated that AIDS is caused by HIV (the human immunodeficiency virus), a retrovirus, so named because its genes are coded in ribonucleic acid (RNA) instead of the more common deoxyribonucleic acid (DNA). Essentially, the virus causes disease by killing or damaging cells of the human immune system. HIV gradually destroys a person's ability to battle infections and certain types of cancer. This loss of immune system functioning causes victims to be vulnerable to often-deadly opportunistic infections, which are caused by pathogens (disease-causing organisms) that are usually harmless to healthy people.

Because the spread of the AIDS epidemic in the United States has been extensively tracked and analyzed, the most reliable information regarding its transmission, treatment, and prevention comes from United States-based research. However, it should be understood that the vast majority of people infected with HIV now live outside of the United States. While modes of transmission of HIV have been determined to be the same across the world, risk patterns among different peoples have varied according to cultural influences. For example, outside of Western Europe and North America, homosexual activity has been comparatively more circumscribed and suppressed; hence the major pattern of sexual transmission of HIV occurs among heterosexuals in non-Westernized countries. Although the HIV epidemic acquired its original momentum in the United States, the future focuses of the pandemic lie outside of the United States, mainly in the developing countries of Africa and Asia.

■ Disease History, Characteristics, and Transmission

The most common way to transmit HIV is by having unprotected sex with an infected partner. The virus can enter the body through the mucous membranes of the vagina, vulva, penis, rectum, or mouth during sexual activity.

HIV is transmitted by the exchange of bodily fluids such as blood, semen, and saliva. Therefore certain behaviors put people at risk for contracting HIV, including sharing drug syringes, anal, vaginal or oral sexual contact with an infected person without using a condom, and having sexual contact with someone with unknown HIV status.

Contact with Infected Blood

It is possible to contract HIV through contact with infected blood. This risk has given rise to extensive screening of donated blood for evidence of HIV infection, and also heat-treatment techniques to destroy HIV in blood products used in medical practice. Prior to these measures, HIV was transmitted through transfusions of contaminated blood or blood products such as serum, platelets, and clotting factors. Screening for HIV and heat treatment has practically eliminated the risk of getting HIV from such transfusions.

Contaminated Needles

One of the primary means of spreading infection with HIV is the sharing of syringes contaminated with very small quantities of blood among injection drug users from someone that has been infected with the virus.

There have also been rare cases of health care workers that have been infected by accidental punctures with needles or other medical instruments that have been contaminated by contact with patients, or, conversely, patients that have been infected by contaminated needles used by health care workers. In the health care setting,

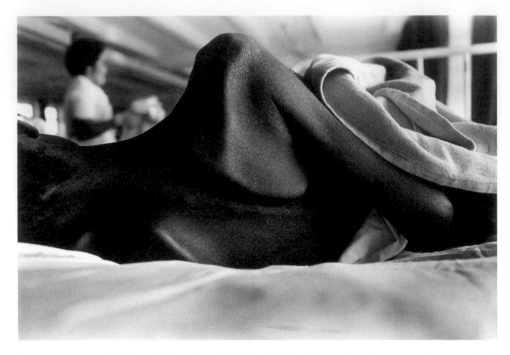

A young woman suffers from AIDS at a hospital in South Africa. Because there is a strong stigma associated with the disease in her community, she has been ostracized by family and abandoned in the hospital. South Africa has the highest number of people living with HIV of any nation in the world, estimated at six million people.   © Gideon Mendel/Corbis.

workers have been infected with HIV after being stuck with needles containing HIV-infected blood or, less frequently, after infected blood gets into a worker's open cut or a mucous membrane (for example, the eyes or inside of the nose). According to the CDC, there has been only one instance of patients being infected by a health care worker in the United States; this involved HIV transmission from one infected dentist to six patients. Investigations have been completed involving more than 22,000 patients of 63 HIV-infected physicians, surgeons, and dentists, and no other cases of this type of transmission have been identified in the United States.

Mother-to-child Transmission

Women can transmit HIV to their babies during pregnancy or birth. About one-quarter to one-third of HIV-positive pregnant women will pass the virus on to their babies. HIV can also be transmitted from infected mothers to babies through breast milk. Available drug treatment for the mother during pregnancy can significantly reduce the probability of such infection. Cesarean section delivery can further reduce mother-to-newborn infection rates to just one percent. Drug treatment and cesarean delivery has nearly eradicated mother-to-baby transmission of HIV in the United States. Use of these measures has increased worldwide. A study in Uganda sponsored by the U.S. National Institute of Allergy and Infectious Diseases (NIAID) and confirmed by inde-

pendent research has established the safety and effectiveness of an affordable drug treatment with nevirapine (NVP) for preventing mother-to-newborn transmission of HIV. A single oral dose of this antiretroviral drug given to an HIV-infected woman in labor and another to her baby within three days of birth reduces the transmission rate of HIV by 50%.

Saliva and Other Bodily Fluids

Researchers have detected HIV in the saliva of infected people. Nevertheless, no evidence has yet been produced that the virus is transmitted by contact with saliva. Laboratory studies indicate that saliva has natural properties that limit the infectivity of HIV, and the concentration of virus in saliva has been found to be very low. Studies of HIV-positive individuals have found no evidence that the virus can be spread through saliva by kissing. Because of the potential for contact with blood during open-mouth kissing, the CDC recommends against engaging in this activity with a person known to be infected with HIV. However, the risk of acquiring HIV during open-mouth kissing is considered to be very low. CDC has investigated only one case of HIV infection that may be attributed to contact with blood during open-mouth kissing. Nevertheless, the mucous membrane of the mouth can be infected by HIV, and there have been documented instances of HIV transmission through oral sex.

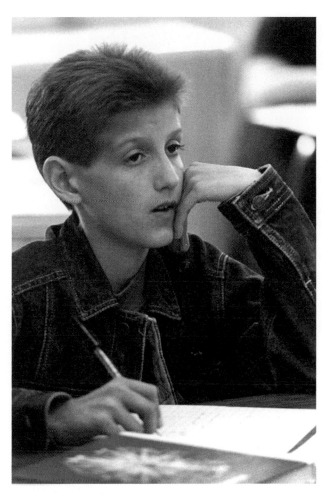

Ryan White, 15, won a legal battle allowing him access to a public education despite having contracted AIDS. © *UPI/Corbis-Bettmann.*

Researchers have found no evidence that HIV is spread through sweat, tears, urine, or feces that is not contaminated with blood.

Biting

In 1997, the CDC published findings from a state health department investigation of an incident that suggested blood-to-blood transmission of HIV by a human bite. There have been other reports in the medical literature in which HIV appeared to have been transmitted by a bite. Severe trauma with extensive tissue tearing and damage and presence of blood were reported in each of these instances. Biting is not a common way of transmitting HIV. In fact, there are numerous reports of bites that did not result in HIV infection.

Casual Contact and Environmental Transmission

Extensive studies of families of HIV-infected people have shown conclusively that HIV is not spread through casual contact such as the sharing of food utensils, towels and bedding, swimming pools, telephones, or toilet seats. HIV is not spread by biting insects such as mosquitoes or bedbugs.

From the beginning of the AIDS epidemic, some people feared that HIV might be transmitted in other common ways, but no scientific evidence to support these fears has been found. If HIV were being transmitted through other routes (such as through air, water, or by insects), the pattern of reported AIDS cases would be much different from what has been observed. For example, if mosquitoes could transmit HIV infection, many more young children and adolescents would have been diagnosed with AIDS. All reported cases suggesting new or potentially unknown routes of transmission are thoroughly investigated by state and local health departments with the assistance, guidance, and laboratory support from the CDC. No additional routes of transmission have been recorded, despite a national sentinel system (an early warning system using animals or population data to detect the presence of disease) designed to detect just such an occurrence.

Households

Although HIV has been transmitted between family members in a household setting, such transmission is very rare. These transmissions are argued to have resulted from contact between skin or mucous membranes and infected blood. To prevent even such rare occurrences, precautions should be taken in all settings including the home to prevent exposures to the blood of persons who are HIV infected, at risk for HIV infection, or whose infection and risk status are unknown. CDC guidelines stipulate that 1) gloves should be worn during contact with blood or other body fluids that could possibly contain visible blood, such as urine, feces, or vomit; 2) cuts, sores, or breaks on both the care giver's and the patient's exposed skin should be covered with bandages; 3) hands and other parts of the body should be washed immediately after contact with blood or other body fluids, and surfaces soiled with blood should be disinfected appropriately; 4) practices that increase the likelihood of blood contact, such as sharing of razors and toothbrushes should be avoided; needles and other sharp instruments should be used only when medically necessary and handled according to recommendations for health-care settings.

Businesses and Other Settings   There is no known risk of HIV transmission to co-workers, clients, or consumers from contact in industries such as food-service establishments. Food-service workers known to be infected with HIV need not be restricted from work unless they have other infections or illnesses (such as diarrhea or hepatitis A) for which any food-service worker, regardless of HIV infection status, should be restricted. The CDC recommends that all food-service workers follow

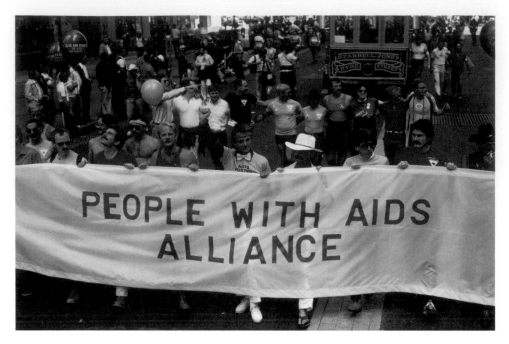

Activists from the People with AIDS Alliance participate in the Gay Freedom Day Parade in San Francisco, California, in June 1983. © *Roger Ressmeyer/Corbis.*

recommended standards and practices of good personal hygiene and food sanitation.

In 1985, CDC issued routine precautions that all personal-service workers (such as hairdressers, barbers, cosmetologists, and massage therapists) should follow, even though there is no evidence of transmission from a personal-service worker to a client or vice versa. Instruments that penetrate the skin (such as tattooing and acupuncture needles, ear piercing devices) should be used once and disposed of or thoroughly cleaned and sterilized. Instruments not intended to penetrate the skin, but which may become contaminated with blood (for example, razors) should be used for only one client and disposed of or thoroughly cleaned and disinfected after each use. Personal-service workers can use the same cleaning procedures that are recommended for health care institutions.

The CDC reports no instances of HIV transmission through tattooing or body piercing, although hepatitis B virus has been transmitted during some of these practices. One case of HIV transmission from acupuncture has been documented. Body piercing (other than ear piercing) is relatively new in the United States, and the medical complications for body piercing appear to be greater than for tattoos. Healing of piercings generally will take weeks, and sometimes even months, and the pierced tissue could conceivably be abraded (torn or cut) or inflamed even after healing. Therefore, a theoretical HIV transmission risk does exist if the unhealed or abraded tissues come into contact with an infected person's blood or other infectious body fluid. Additionally,

HIV could be transmitted if instruments contaminated with blood are not sterilized or disinfected between clients.

Sexually Transmitted Infections

Sexually transmitted infections (STI) such as syphilis, genital herpes, chlamydia, gonorrhea, or bacterial vaginosis appear to increase susceptibility to infection with HIV during sex with infected partners.

In the United States, condoms are regulated by the Food and Drug Administration (FDA) and condom manufacturers are required to test each latex condom for defects such as holes prior to packaging. The proper and consistent use of latex or polyurethane condoms when engaging in vaginal, anal, or oral sexual intercourse can greatly reduce the risk of acquiring or transmitting sexually transmitted diseases, including HIV infection.

Only latex or polyurethane condoms provide a highly effective mechanical barrier to HIV. In laboratories, viruses occasionally have been shown to pass through natural membrane ("skin" or lambskin) condoms, which may contain natural pores and are therefore not recommended for disease prevention, although they are documented to be effective for contraception. For condoms to provide maximum protection, they must be used consistently and correctly. Numerous studies among sexually active people have demonstrated that a properly used latex condom provides a high degree of protection against a variety of sexually transmitted diseases, including HIV infection.

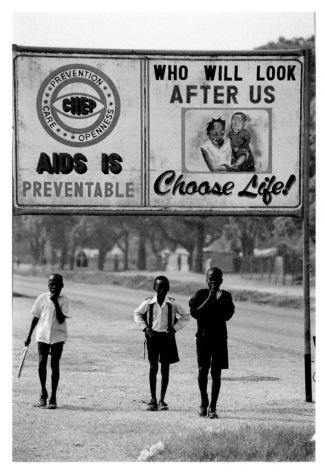

Boys in Kitwe, Zambia, play below a road sign designed to raise public awareness of AIDS prevention and the growing number of children orphaned due to the disease in Africa. © Louise Gubb/ Corbis Saba.

Early Signs and Symptoms of HIV Infection

Most people show no early symptoms when initially infected with HIV. In a minority of cases, people may have a flulike illness within a month or two after exposure that could include fever, headache, fatigue, and swollen lymph nodes in the neck and groin. These symptoms usually disappear within a week to a month and are often attributed to some other viral infection. During this early period, people are very contagious, and HIV is present in large quantities in genital fluids.

Long-lasting, debilitating symptoms may not appear for 10 or more years after infection with HIV in adults, or within 2 years in children born with HIV infection. This latent period without symptoms varies greatly by individual, ranging from a few months to more than a decade. However, even during the asymptomatic (without symptoms) period, the virus is actively multiplying and destroying immune system cells, or can be dormant (inactive) within infected cells. The most readily apparent laboratory sign of HIV infection is a gradual decline in the blood concentration of CD4 positive T (CD4+) cells, which are cells the immune system's most important infection fighters. HIV slowly disables or destroys these cells without causing symptoms.

As the immune system deteriorates, various complications appear. The first persistent symptoms experienced by many persons with HIV include enlarged lymph nodes for more than three months, fatigue, weight loss, frequent fevers and sweats, persistent or frequent yeast infections (oral or vaginal), persistent skin rashes or flaky skin, pelvic inflammatory disease in women that does not respond to treatment, and short-term memory loss. Some people develop frequent and severe herpes infections that cause mouth, genital, or anal sores, or a resurgence of the dormant virus that causes chickenpox known as shingles. Children may fail to thrive and grow.

Acquired Immunodeficiency Syndrome (AIDS)

Usually after a long assault on the immune system, victims reach the most advanced stage of HIV infection, which is known as AIDS. The CDC, the agency responsible for tracking the AIDS epidemic in the United States, has developed official criteria that define AIDS. The CDC's definition of AIDS includes all HIV-infected people who have fewer than 200 CD4+ T cells per cubic millimeter of blood. (Healthy adults usually have CD4+ T-cell counts of 1,000 or more.) In addition, the definition includes 26 clinical conditions, mainly opportunistic infections that affect people with advanced HIV disease. In people with AIDS, these infections are generally severe and can be fatal because the immune system is so ravaged by HIV that the body loses its ability to fight off certain bacteria, viruses, fungi, parasites, and other microbes.

Common symptoms of opportunistic infections in both adults and children with AIDS include persistent coughing and shortness of breath, seizures, lack of coordination, difficult or painful swallowing, confusion or forgetfulness, severe and persistent diarrhea, fever, vision loss, nausea, abdominal cramps, vomiting, weight loss, extreme fatigue, and severe headaches. In addition, children may also have severe forms of the common childhood bacterial infections, such as conjunctivitis (pink eye), otitis media (ear infection), and tonsillitis.

In addition to opportunistic infections, people with AIDS are also prone to various cancers that are associated with persistent exposure to certain viruses such as Kaposi's sarcoma and cervical cancer, or cancers of the immune system known as lymphomas. These cancers are usually more aggressive and difficult to treat in people with AIDS.

As HIV infection progresses and the number of CD4+ T cells declines, people with CD4+ T cells above 200 may experience some of the early symptoms of HIV disease. Conversely, others with their CD4+ T-cell count below 200 may have no symptoms. Victims

WORDS TO KNOW

ANTIBODY: Antibodies, or Y-shaped immunoglobulins, are proteins found in the blood that help to fight against foreign substances called antigens. Antigens, which are usually proteins or polysaccharides, stimulate the immune system to produce antibodies. The antibodies inactivate the antigen and help to remove it from the body. While antigens can be the source of infections from pathogenic bacteria and viruses, organic molecules detrimental to the body from internal or environmental sources also act as antigens. Genetic engineering and the use of various mutational mechanisms allow the construction of a vast array of antibodies (each with a unique genetic sequence).

ASYMPTOMATIC: A state in which an individual does not exhibit or experience symptoms of a disease.

CD4+ T CELLS: CD4 cells are a type of T cell found in the immune system, which are characterized by the presence of a CD4 antigen protein on their surface. These are the cells most often destroyed as a result of HIV infection.

HIGHLY ACTIVE ANTIRETROVIRAL THERAPY (HAART): Highly active antiretroviral therapy (HAART) is the name given to the combination of drugs given to people with human immunodeficiency virus (HIV) infection to slow or stop the progression of their condition to AIDS (acquired human immunodeficiency syndrome). HIV is a retrovirus and the various components of HAART block its replication by different mechanisms.

LATENT INFECTION: An infection already established in the body but not yet causing symptoms, or having ceased to cause symptoms after an active period, is a latent infection.

OPPORTUNISTIC INFECTION: An opportunistic infection is so named because it occurs in people whose immune systems are diminished or are not functioning normally; such infections are opportunistic insofar as the infectious agents take advantage of their hosts' compromised immune systems and invade to cause disease.

PANDEMIC: Pandemic, which means all the people, describes an epidemic that occurs in more than one country or population simultaneously.

REPLICATE: To replicate is to duplicate something or make a copy of it. All reproduction of living things depends on the replication of DNA molecules or, in a few cases, RNA molecules. Replication may be used to refer to the reproduction of entire viruses and other microorganisms.

RETROVIRUS: Retroviruses are viruses in which the genetic material consists of ribonucleic acid (RNA) instead of the usual deoxyribonucleic acid (DNA). Retroviruses produce an enzyme known as reverse transcriptase that can transform RNA into DNA, which can then be permanently integrated into the DNA of the infected host cells.

SEXUALLY TRANSMITTED DISEASE (STD): Sexually transmitted diseases (STDs) vary in their susceptibility to treatment, their signs and symptoms, and the consequences if they are left untreated. Some are caused by bacteria. These usually can be treated and cured. Others are caused by viruses and can typically be treated but not cured. More than 15 million new cases of STD are diagnosed annually in the United States.

SENTINEL: Sentinel surveillance is a method in epidemiology where a subset of the population is surveyed for the presence of communicable diseases. Also, a sentinel is an animal used to indicate the presence of a disease within an area.

STRAIN: A subclass or a specific genetic variation of an organism.

---

frequently become so debilitated by the symptoms of AIDS that they are unable to work or do household chores. Other persons with AIDS may experience intermittent phases of life-threatening illness followed by periods during which they appear to be reasonably healthy.

A few people known to have been infected with HIV ten or more years ago have not developed symptoms of AIDS. Scientists are trying to ascertain what factors may account for this lack of progression to AIDS, such as whether their immune systems have particular characteristics, whether they were infected with a less aggressive strain of the virus or whether their genes may protect them from the effects of HIV. Researchers hope that understanding the body's natural method of controlling infection may produce ideas for protective HIV vaccines that can prevent the disease from progressing in the general population.

Diagnosis

Because early HIV infection often causes no symptoms, health care providers can usually diagnose it by testing blood for the presence of antibodies (disease-fighting proteins) to HIV. HIV antibodies generally do not reach noticeable levels in standard blood tests in the blood for one to three months or more following infection. In order to determine whether a person has been recently infected, health care providers can screen for the presence of HIV genetic material. Such direct screening of HIV is extremely critical in order to prevent transmission of HIV from recently infected individuals. Such individuals can discuss with health care providers when they should start treatment to help combat HIV and prevent the emergence of opportunistic infections. Early testing also alerts people to avoid high-risk behaviors that could transmit the virus to others. Health care providers often provide counseling to individuals who test HIV positive. People can be tested anonymously at many sites if they are concerned about confidentiality.

The diagnosis of HIV infection is established by using two different types of antibody tests: ELISA and Western Blot. Individuals who are highly likely to be infected with HIV, but have received negative results for both tests may request additional tests or may be told to repeat antibody testing at a later date, when antibodies are more likely to have developed.

Babies born to HIV infected mothers may or may not be infected with the virus, but all carry their mothers' antibodies to HIV for several months. If these babies lack symptoms, a doctor cannot make a definitive diagnosis of HIV infection using standard antibody tests. New technologies have been developed to more accurately determine HIV infection in infants between ages 3–15 months. Researchers are evaluating a number of blood tests to determine which ones can best diagnose HIV infection in infants younger than three months.

■ Scope and Distribution

Since 1981, more than 900,000 cases of AIDS have been reported in the United States. At least as many Americans may be infected with HIV, 25% of whom are not yet aware of their infection. AIDS has been spreading most rapidly among non-Caucasian populations and is one of the foremost killers of adult African-American males between the ages 25–44. The CDC has produced statistics showing that AIDS affects nearly seven times more African-Americans and three times more Hispanics than whites in the United States.

Worldwide, the AIDS epidemic has killed more than 25 million people since 1981, and an estimated 40 million people are living with AIDS today. Young people, under 25 years old, now account for more than half of all new HIV infections.

IN CONTEXT: CULTURAL CONNECTIONS

Following the discovery of AIDS, scientists attempted to identify the virus that causes the disease. In 1983–84, two scientists and their teams reported isolating HIV, the virus that causes AIDS. One was French immunologist Luc Montagnier (1932–), working at the Pasteur Institute in Paris, and the other was American immunologist Robert Gallo (1937–) at the National Cancer Institute in Bethesda, Maryland. Both identified HIV as the cause of AIDS and showed the pathogen to be a retrovirus, meaning that its genetic material is RNA, instead of DNA. Following the discovery, a dispute ensued over who made the initial discovery, but today Gallo and Montagnier are credited as co-discoverers.

■ Treatment and Prevention

When AIDS first appeared in the United States, there were no medicines that were effective against HIV and few treatments existed for the associated opportunistic diseases. Within a relatively short time after the discovery of HIV, researchers began to develop drugs to fight both HIV infection and its associated infections and cancers.

The first group of drugs used to treat HIV infection, called nucleoside reverse transcriptase (RT) inhibitors, interrupts an early stage of the virus as it replicates (duplicates). These drugs slow the spread of HIV in the body and delay the start of opportunistic infections. This class of drugs, called nucleoside analogs, includes AZT (azidothymidine), ddC (zalcitabine), ddI (dideoxyinosine), d4T (stavudine), 3TC (lamivudine), abacavir, tenofovir, and emtricitabine.

Physicians can also prescribe non-nucleoside reverse transcriptase inhibitors (NNRTIs) to treat HIV infection, such as delavridine, nevirapine, and efravirenz, often in combination with other antiretroviral drugs.

A second class of drugs for treating HIV infection called protease inhibitors was later approved. Protease inhibitors interrupt the virus from replicating itself at a later step in its life cycle. They include ritonavir, saquinivir, indinavir, amprenivir, nelfinavir, lopinavir, atazanavir, and fosamprenavir.

A third new class of drugs known as HIV fusion inhibitors includes enfuvirtide, the first approved fusion inhibitor, which works by interfering with HIV-1's ability to enter into cells by blocking the merging of the virus with the cell membranes. This inhibition blocks HIV's ability to enter and infect the human immune cells. Enfuvirtide is designed for use in combination with other anti-HIV treatments. It reduces the level of HIV infection in the blood and may be active against HIV that has become resistant to current antiviral treatment schedules.

IN CONTEXT: TRENDS AND STATISTICS

The list below reflects data on the percentage (%) of all deaths in children under 5 years of age due to HIV/AIDS as reported by World Health Organization in February 2007.

Data is shown for countries reporting approximately that 4% or more of children under 5 years of age die from AIDS/HIV

- Burkina Faso: 4.00%
- Chad: 4.06%
- Trinidad and Tobago: 4.69%
- Ukraine: 4.95%
- Nigeria: 4.96%
- Rwanda: 4.99%
- Bahamas: 5.34%
- Côte d'Ivoire: 5.59%
- Ghana: 5.74%
- Togo: 5.78%
- Jamaica: 6.09%
- Thailand: 6.18%
- Eritrea: 6.21%
- Honduras: 6.28%
- Cameroon: 7.24%
- Equatorial Guinea: 7.39%
- Uganda: 7.67%
- Guyana: 7.68%
- Burundi: 8.00%
- Haiti: 8.28%
- United Republic of Tanzania: 9.29%
- Congo: 9.33%
- Gabon: 10.10%
- Central African Republic: 12.40%
- Mozambique: 12.94%
- Malawi: 14.04%
- Kenya: 14.57%
- Zambia: 16.12%
- Zimbabwe: 40.59%
- Swaziland: 47.00%
- Namibia: 52.96%
- Botswana: 53.85%
- Lesotho: 56.19%
- South Africa: 57.08%

SOURCE: *World Health Organization*

Because HIV can become resistant to any of these drugs, health care providers must use a combination treatment to effectively suppress the virus. When multiple drugs (three or more) are used in combination, it is referred to as highly active antiretroviral therapy, or HAART, and can be used by people who are newly infected with HIV as well as people with AIDS. Researchers have credited HAART as being a major factor in significantly reducing the number of deaths from AIDS

in the U.S. While HAART is not a cure for AIDS, it has greatly improved the health of many people with AIDS and reduces the amount of virus circulating in the blood to nearly undetectable levels. Researchers, however, have shown that HIV remains present in some places in the body, such as the lymph nodes, brain, testes, and retina of the eye, even in people who have been treated.

Opportunistic Infections A number of available drugs help treat the opportunistic infections of AIDS. These drugs include foscarnet and ganciclovir to treat CMV (cytomegalovirus) eye infections, fluconazole to treat yeast and other fungal infections, and TMP/SMX (trimethoprim/sulfamethoxazole) or pentamidine to treat a pneumonia known as PCP (*Pneumocystis carinii* pneumonia) that is sometimes associated with AIDS.

Cancers Health care providers use radiation, chemotherapy, or injections of alpha interferon, a genetically engineered protein that occurs naturally in the human body, to treat Kaposi's sarcoma or other cancers associated with HIV infection.

Prevention

In the absence of a vaccine for HIV, the only means to prevent infection by the virus is to avoid behaviors that put people at risk of infection, such as sharing needles and having unprotected sex. Because many people infected with HIV have no symptoms, there is no way of knowing with certainty whether a sexual partner is infected unless he or she has repeatedly tested negative for the virus and has not engaged in any risky behavior. Abstaining from having sex offers the most protection from AIDS. Using male latex condoms or female polyurethane condoms have been shown in prospective studies to offer partial protection during oral, anal, or vaginal sex. Only water-based lubricants should be used with male latex condoms.

Although some laboratory evidence shows that spermicides can kill HIV, researchers have not found that these products can prevent the transmission of HIV during sex.

Ongoing Research

Research is ongoing in all areas of HIV infection, including developing and testing preventive HIV vaccines and new treatments for HIV infection and AIDS-associated opportunistic infections. Researchers also are trying to determine exactly how HIV damages the immune system. Recently, an electron micrograph was taken of HIV binding to a cell wall and is being examined for precise information about how the virus infects healthy cells. Such research is identifying new and more effective targets for drugs and vaccines. Investigators also continue to trace how the disease progresses in different people.

Current research also includes testing chemical barriers, such as topical microbicides (germ-killing compounds) that people can use in the vagina or in the rectum during sex to help prevent HIV transmission. Scientists are also examining

IN CONTEXT: ANTIRETROVIRAL THERAPY COVERAGE

The list below reflects selected data on antiretroviral therapy coverage from countries selected across the spectrum of data (ranked lowest to highest in terms of percentage of those estimated to need antiretroviral therapy who have actual access to the treatment) as reported by the World Health Organization in February 2007.

Selected non-reporting countries, or countries for which data was otherwise not available, included the Republic of Korea, Singapore, Afghanistan, and Iraq.

- Sudan: 1% of persons estimated to need ARV therapy have access to the treatment (data reported: Dec 2005)
- Nepal: 1% (Dec 2005)
- Bangladesh: 1% (Dec 2005)
- Somalia: 1% (Dec 2005)
- Guinea-Bissau: 1% (Dec 2005)
- Pakistan: 2% (Dec 2005)
- Sierra Leone: 2% (Dec 2005)
- Central African Republic: 3% (Dec 2005)
- Philippines: 5% (Dec 2005)
- Russian Federation: 5% (Dec 2005)
- Belarus: 5% (Dec 2005)
- Nigeria: 6% (Dec 2005)
- Angola: 6% (Dec 2005)
- Sri Lanka: 6% (Dec 2005)
- Ukraine: 6 % (Dec 2005)
- India: 7% (Dec 2005)
- United Republic of Tanzania: 7 % (Dec 2005)
- Ghana: 7% (Dec 2005)
- Ethiopia: 7% (Dec 2005)
- Myanmar: 7% (Dec 2005)
- Zimbabwe: 8% (Dec 2005)
- Mozambique: 9% (Dec 2005)
- Gambia: 9% (Dec 2005)

- Turkey: 9% (Dec 2005)
- Iran (Islamic Republic of): 9% (Dec 2005)
- Egypt: 12% (Dec 2005)
- Viet Nam: 12% (Dec 2005)
- South Africa: 21% (Dec 2005)
- Kenya: 24% (Dec 2005)
- China: 25% (Dec 2005)
- Swaziland: 31% (Dec 2005)
- Tunisia: 34% (Dec 2005)
- Cambodia: 36% (Dec 2005)
- Rwanda: 39% (Dec 2005)
- Guatemala: 43% (Dec 2005)
- Colombia: 44% (Dec 2005)
- Senegal: 47% (Dec 2005)
- Guyana: 50% (Dec 2005)
- Uganda: 51% (Dec 2005)
- Mexico: 71% (Dec 2005)
- Canada: 75% (Dec 2005)
- Israel: 75% (Dec 2005)
- Italy: 75% (Dec 2005)
- New Zealand: 75% (Dec 2005)
- United Kingdom: 75% (Dec 2005)
- United States of America: 75% (Dec 2005)
- Costa Rica: 80% (Dec 2005)
- Argentina: 81% (Dec 2005)
- Brazil: 83% (Dec 2005)
- Venezuela (Bolivarian Republic of): 84% (Dec 2005)
- Botswana: 85% (Dec 2005)
- Cuba: 100% (Dec 2005)

SOURCE: *World Health Organization, Progress on global access to HIV antiretroviral therapy. A report on "3 by 5" and beyond. Geneva, World Health Organization and Joint United Nations Programme on HIV/AIDS, March 2006.*

the effectiveness of other ways of preventing HIV transmission, such controlling other sexually transmitted infections like chlamydia that have a role in making HIV easier to contract.

■ Impacts and Issues

As the AIDS pandemic nears its 30th year, the number of people infected with HIV continues to climb steadily. Approximately two thirds of infected persons live in Africa, where the epidemic grew exponentially during the decade of the 1990s, and one fifth are in Asia, where the epidemic has been growing most rapidly in recent years. By the end of 2006, more than 40 million people worldwide were living with HIV infection. Worldwide funding from public and private sources to combat the epidemic has similarly risen dramatically, in an increasingly urgent effort to reverse the growth trajectory of the epidemic. Recent estimates of worldwide HIV infections and deaths have been revised downward, but these downward revisions do not reflect the uncertainty and unreliability of global HIV statistics outside of the major industrial nations.

Analysis of the reliable data has shown that the primary modes of HIV transmission have not changed significantly over time from those outlined above: unprotected heterosexual intercourse, unprotected anal sex between men, injection-drug use, unsafe medical injections and blood transfusions, and transmission from mother to child during pregnancy, labor and delivery, or breast-feeding. Direct blood contact, such as the sharing of drug-injection equipment, is by far the most efficient means of transmitting the virus. However the specific features of the epidemic vary among regions and within countries. Globally, in the *World Health Report 2004*, the World Health Organization (WHO) states that "unprotected sexual intercourse between men and women is the

IN CONTEXT: DISEASE IN DEVELOPING NATIONS

The World Health Organization (WHO) states that "in the developing world, 6 million people infected with HIV need access to antiretroviral (ARV) therapy. Only 300,000 have such access. To address the HIV/AIDS crisis, the World Health Organization, with the Joint United Nations Programme on AIDS (UNAIDS) and other partners, has committed itself to having 3 million people living with HIV/AIDS in developing countries on ARV treatment by the end of 2005."

SOURCE: *World Health Organization*

predominant mode of transmission of the virus." This report also states that "In sub-Saharan Africa and the Caribbean, women are at least as likely as men to become infected." In India, a large proportion of infected persons are prostitutes and long-haul truck drivers. In areas of China, India, Thailand, and Vietnam, HIV transmission is being fueled primarily by injection-drug use. In other parts of Southeast Asia, Cambodia, Myanmar, Thailand, and Vietnam, men having sex with prostitutes are a major factor.

The most recent statistics underline global disparities in AIDS deaths. Absent treatment with antiretroviral drugs, it usually takes about 10 years for HIV infection to progress to AIDS. More than two million people in sub-Saharan Africa died of AIDS in 2006 (accounting for three-quarters of the worldwide total). By comparison, in Western Europe, where drug treatment is widely available, only a few thousand people died of AIDS. In the most recent year of statistics, more than 12 million children in sub-Saharan Africa were orphaned by AIDS. Because the rapid growth of the epidemic is more recent in Asia, the number of deaths from AIDS has been comparatively lower than in Africa, given the number of infected people and a similar lack of drug treatment. Still, tens of thousands of people have died in Thailand and China each year in the past several years and death rates are increasing as asymptomatic infections acquired in the past decade progress to full-blown AIDS. Sub-Saharan Africa continues to have the most mother-to-child transmission of the virus, where more than a half-million children died of AIDS in 2005.

Increasingly the mantra of the international community is access for all to effective antiretroviral therapy. Only two approaches to containing the epidemic have been effective: preventing new HIV infections and providing antiretroviral treatment to victims of HIV. As there is no AIDS vaccine, prevention efforts focus on education about sexual and other practices, behavioral change, and outreach to marginalized groups of people, including injection-drug users and sex workers and their clients. Many infected people do not realize that they are

infected; others may not seek available care because of the stigma of being HIV positive. Cambodia and Thailand are cited as examples of nations that have prevention programs promoting increased condom use by prostitutes and their clients that have been demonstrably effective.

Even if ambitious WHO goals for increasing access to antiretroviral treatment are successful, and despite substantial progress toward these goals, less than 10 percent of the people globally that need treatment for HIV infection are receiving it. A few countries such as Botswana, Senegal, and Uganda in Africa, and Brazil in South America are doing better. Brazil has a universal program for the distributing antiretroviral medications. Botswana, with one of the highest HIV infection rates in the world, has a program of routine HIV testing and is also successfully expanding access to drug treatment.

In summary, there is some evidence that the global HIV epidemic is starting to slow slightly, both in the rate of new infections and in the AIDS death rate. Behavioral change based on detailed knowledge of the means of viral transmission has been successful in saving millions of lives, and access to modern drug therapy has and can save millions more. Although the ultimate eradication of HIV infection remains a cherished goal of the worldwide medical research community, efforts to change behavior and expand access to currently available treatments will save untold millions of lives until the enigma of HIV infection is finally solved.

■ Primary Source Connection

In the commentary that follows, Nicholas D. Kristof describes the failures of political and health policies during the first quarter century of the AIDS pandemic in the context of family impacts in Swaziland. At the time of publication, Nicholas D. Kristof served as a columnist for the *The New York Times* since November 2001. In 1990, Kristof shared a Pulitzer Prize for coverage of China's Tiananmen Square uprising and democracy movement. In 2006, Mr. Kristof won a second Pulitzer for commentary.

At 12, a Mother of Two

MHLATUZE, Swaziland. We're now marking the 25th anniversary of the detection of AIDS, and it has been a sad chapter in the history of humanity. It's been a quarter-century of self-delusion, dithering and failure at every level.

In America, we may think of AIDS as something that is behind us, but this year it will kill almost three million people worldwide. And a new victim is still being infected every eight seconds.

Southern Africa is becoming the land of orphans, kids like Nomzamo Ngubeni, a fifth grader who is now the head of her household.

Nomzamo is 12, a soft-spoken schoolgirl with close-cropped hair here in central Swaziland, the country with the highest HIV infection rate in the world. Two out of five adults here have the virus, and very few get the antiretroviral medicines that can save their lives.

Although Nomzamo probably does not have the virus (although it's hard to be sure because she's never been tested for it), her life is entirely framed by the epidemic. Her parents both died of AIDS, so she and her two younger sisters moved in with an aunt—only to find that the aunt was dying of AIDS as well.

Nomzamo nursed the aunt for months and buried her last year. So at the age of 11, she found herself in charge of the family and its thatch-roofed hut, which has no electricity or running water. She is now both mother and father to her little sisters, Nokwanda, 9, and Temhlanga, 7.

She wakes them up in the morning to go to school, and forces them to take their baths and do their homework. She washes their clothes and cuts their hair. She consoles them when they miss their parents. When they misbehave, she beats them. She fetches water and firewood, and in the evenings she cooks for them—if there is food.

"If there is no food, then we just go to sleep with nothing," Nomzamo explains. "The kids don't cry. They just go to sleep."

If all of this seems too much for a 12-year-old, it is. The stress is wearing her down and causing her to do poorly in school.

Like many households in southern Africa, this family no longer has any able-bodied person to till the ground, so the family's land lies fallow. These sisters get one good meal each day—at school, supplied by the World Food Program—and they beg or borrow the rest.

There are indeed some heroes in the AIDS saga, including American nuns, the Missionaries of the Sacred Heart, known as the Cabrini Sisters (www.cabrinifoundation.org). Nuns like Sister Barbara Staley, originally from Pennsylvania, live in this remote pocket of Swaziland and look after the flotsam of the AIDS crisis. With help from CARE, the sisters shelter and school many of the orphans; they pay the fees that allow Nomzamo and her sisters to attend the public school.

But mostly the last quarter-century of AIDS has been a shameful period of neglect. In the U.S., President Ronald Reagan didn't let the word "AIDS" slip past his lips in public until 1987. And nobody behaved more immorally than the moralizers, people like Patrick Buchanan, who declared in 1983: "The poor homosexuals—they have declared war against nature, and now nature is exacting an awful retribution." The Rev. Jerry Falwell put it this way: "AIDS is the wrath of a just God against homosexuals."

In retrospect, the gross immorality of the 1980's wasn't committed in San Francisco bathhouses, but in the corridors of power by self-righteous political and religious leaders whose indifference to the suffering of gays allowed the epidemic to spread.

Misgovernance has been even worse in Africa. South Africa's president, Thabo Mbeki, refused for years to address AIDS seriously and is probably responsible for more deaths of blacks than any of his white racist predecessors. And here in Swaziland, the playboy king sets a horrendous example of sexual excess by publicly reviewing tens of thousands of bare-breasted teenage virgins so he can choose new wives for his harem.

There are some signs that leaders around the world have finally been waking up to the challenge of AIDS in the last few years. Some countries, like Kenya, Zimbabwe and China, may have turned the corner. President Bush has vastly increased the funds for AIDS in Africa.

But the bottom line remains that for the last 25 years, we've faced an enormous public health challenge—one expected to be comparable to the mortality an earlier generation faced from World War II. And in that test, we have disgraced ourselves.

And that is one reason why, in this forgotten part of Swaziland, a 12-year-old looks old beyond her years.

Nicholas D. Kristof

KRISTOF, NICHOLAS D. "AT 12, A MOTHER OF TWO." *THE NEW YORK TIMES.* MAY 28, 2006.

SEE ALSO *AIDS: Origin of the Modern Pandemic; Bloodborne Pathogens; Epidemiology; Opportunistic Infection; Public Health and Infectious Disease; Sexually Transmitted Diseases.*

BIBLIOGRAPHY

Books

Johanson, Paula. *HIV and AIDS (Coping in a Changing World).* New York: Rosen, 2007.

World Health Organization. *Preventing HIV/AIDS in Young People.* Geneva: WHO, 2006.

Periodicals

Steinbrook R. Global Health: The AIDS Epidemic in 2004. New England Journal of Medicine 2004; 351:115–117, Jul 8, 2004.

Steinbrook R. HIV in India—The Challenges Ahead. New England Journal of Medicine 2007; 356: 1197–1201, Mar 22, 2007.

Steinbrook R. HIV in India—A Complex Epidemic. New England Journal of Medicine 2007; 356: 1089–1093, Mar 15, 2007.

Web Sites

AIDSinfo. <http://aidsinfo.nih.gov> (accessed April 9, 2007).

NIH Vaccine Research Center. "Become an HIV Vaccine Study Volunteer." <http://www.niaid.nih.gov/vrc/clintrials/clin_steps.htm%20%20%20> (accessed April 9, 2007).

Kenneth T. LaPensee

AIDS: Origin of the Modern Pandemic

■ Introduction

The world has reached the twenty-fifth year of the modern AIDS pandemic, which has been acknowledged by the United Nations (UN) to be among the deadliest epidemics in human history. AIDS has killed 25 million people and infected an estimated additional 40 million people since 1981, many of whom will die of the disease without effective treatment.

■ History and Policy Response

Little is yet known about the incidence and prevalence of AIDS prior to the first reported cases in the United States in the early 1980s. In the 1970s, the HIV virus was unknown and, given its latency period with which clinicians are now familiar, transmission was not associated with signs or symptoms significant enough to be noticed. A small number of case reports of AIDS and medical archaeological studies have uncovered human infections with HIV prior to 1970. Scientists have pieced together evidence suggesting that AIDS originated in Africa, but the precise location of the pandemic's origin remains unknown. AIDS is thought to have begun in the primordial forests of West Africa when a virus harbored in the blood of a monkey or a chimpanzee made the genetic leap to humans, possibly after a hunter was

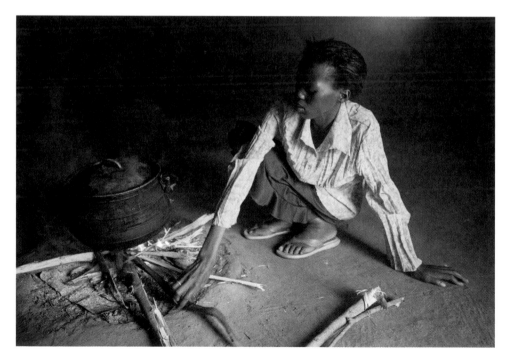

An African woman weakened by AIDS struggles to summon the energy to cook a meal for her family. When AIDS was first identified in homosexual males in the United States, the disease was already spreading among heterosexual Africans in Uganda and was known simply as "slim." © Gideon Mendel/Corbis.

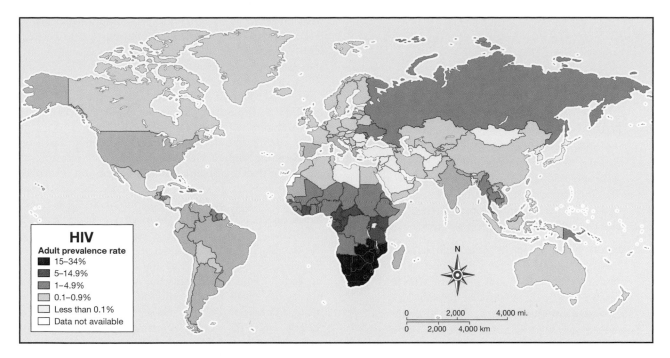

Map showing HIV prevalence rates in adults (15–49) in 2005. *© Copyright World Health Organization (WHO). Reproduced by permission.*

infected by a bite. HIV was discovered by researchers in a blood sample collected in 1959 from a man in Kinshasa, Congo. Further genetic analysis of the man's blood indicated that the HIV infection was caused by a single virus in the late 1940s or early 1950s. Thus, it appears that the earliest human infections went unnoticed on a continent where people routinely die from tropical diseases with unusual manifestations.

Analyses of medical records in African countries have shown that there had been striking increases in opportunistic infections now known to be AIDS-related during the late 1970s and early 1980s. These included "slim" disease in Zaire (late 1970s) and in Uganda and Tanzania (early 1980s); esophageal candidiasis in Rwanda (from 1983); aggressive Kaposi's sarcoma in Zaire (early 1980s) and in Zambia and Uganda (1982 and 1983); and crypotococcal meningitis in Zaire (late 1970s to early 1980s). Research suggests that although isolated cases of AIDS may have occurred in Africa earlier, it was probably rare until the late 1970s and early 1980s. Studies further suggest that demographic groups and the routes of disease transmission have been largely similar in Africa and Western nations, implicating sexual activity among young and middle-aged people, blood transfusions, vertical transmission from mother to infant, and frequent exposure to unsterilized needles as the most likely means of transmitting AIDS.

Thus, available data suggest that the modern AIDS pandemic started in the mid- to late-1970s. By 1980, HIV had spread to North America, South America, Europe, and Australia. During this early stage of the

epidemic, the transmission of the virus was unhindered by awareness of the disease or any preventive action, and approximately 100,000–300,000 persons are estimated to have contracted the infection.

In March 1981, however, a few cases of an aggressive form of Kaposi's sarcoma (KS) were documented among young gay men in New York. This development caused concern because KS was known as a rare, relatively benign cancer that tended to occur in elderly people with immune system impairment. Simultaneously, there was an increase in California and New York in the incidence of *Pneumocystis carinii* pneumonia (PCP), an unusual lung infection. The Centers for Disease Control and Prevention (CDC) noticed this increase in April in the course of monitoring prescriptions that were dispensed for rare drugs and detected a spike in requests for pentamine to treat PCP. In June 1981, the CDC published a report outlining the occurrence of five cases of PCP without identifiable cause in Los Angeles. This report marks the beginning of a more general awareness of AIDS, and, shortly thereafter, the CDC formed a task force to investigate a syndrome that they called Kaposi's sarcoma and Opportunistic Infections (KSOI).

Speculation among scientists soon centered on whether this apparently new disease was a consequence of the widespread recreational use of amyl nitrate for sexual stimulation among gay men, or the possibility of immune system overload in this population due to exposure to repeated sexually transmitted infections such as cytomegalovirus (CMV). CDC officials issued statements indicating that the disease appeared to be limited

WORDS TO KNOW

ANTIRETROVIRAL DRUGS: Antiretroviral (ARV) drugs prevent the reproduction of a type of virus called a retrovirus. The human immunodefiency virus (HIV), which causes acquired immune deficiency syndrome (AIDS, also cited as acquired immune deficiency syndrome), is a retrovirus. These ARV drugs are therefore used to treat HIV infections. These medicines cannot prevent or cure HIV infection, but they help to keep the virus in check.

IMMUNODEFICIENCY: In immunodeficiency disorders, part of the body's immune system is missing or defective, thus impairing the body's ability to fight infections. As a result, the person with an immunodeficiency disorder will have frequent infections that are generally more severe and last longer than usual.

LATENT INFECTION: An infection already established in the body but not yet causing symptoms, or having ceased to cause symptoms after an active period, is a latent infection.

OPPORTUNISTIC INFECTION: An opportunistic infection is so named because it occurs in people whose immune systems are diminished or are not functioning normally; such infections are opportunistic insofar as the infectious agents take advantage of their hosts' compromised immune systems and invade to cause disease.

PANDEMIC: Pandemic, which means all the people, describes an epidemic that occurs in more than one country or population simultaneously.

to gay men and that there was no apparent risk of spreading the disease through contagion.

By 1982, however, AIDS was reported among injection drug users, and disease patterns among a group of gay men in California appeared to support the notion that the disease was sexually transmitted. Later in the year, cases appeared among citizens of Haiti and among persons with hemophilia, a blood disorder that is treated with infusions of blood clotting factors. After the spreading disease shed its exclusive association with gay men, the CDC characterized the disease as acquired immunodeficiency syndrome (AIDS, also cited as acquired immune deficiency syndrome). This terminology for the ailment was chosen because the immune system impairment that was its hallmark was acquired rather

than inherited as in other known immunodeficiencies. AIDS was labeled a syndrome because it was associated with a group of diseases rather than a single disease. By the end of 1982, cases of AIDS began to appear in European countries, and a wasting syndrome dubbed "slim" was reported in Uganda, which was soon linked to AIDS. By the end of the year, over 600 cases had been reported in the United States.

In 1983, physicians diagnosed the first cases of AIDS among women with no other apparent risk factors, indicating that the disease could be transmitted by heterosexual contact. In view of the evidence that AIDS was an infection that could be transmitted via blood and blood products, the CDC mounted a concerted effort to discover an infectious agent responsible for causing the disease. In May, doctors at the Institute Pasteur in France reported the isolation of a new virus, which they suggested might be the cause of AIDS. Although scant notice was taken of this announcement when it was made, a sample of the virus was sent to the CDC. Several months later, the virus was named lymphadenopathy-associated virus or LAV, and a sample of LAV was sent to the National Cancer Institute (NCI). In the meantime, public anxiety over the means of AIDS transmission, viewed by some people as potentially spread through casual contact due to its incidence among children, continued to grow, giving rise to increasingly numerous panic-driven and sometimes cruel interactions involving people either with AIDS or seen as at risk for AIDS. These incidents included evictions of persons with AIDS from housing; families and loved ones abandoning their relatives or partners with AIDS; and use of surgical masks during police work with individuals suspected of having AIDS. The CDC soon issued information that confirmed that there was no evidence for casual transmission and explained the possibility of bloodborne transmission of infection of AIDS from mothers to children.

By 1984, it became clear that the AIDS epidemic had been established in central Africa among populations that were not at risk from homosexuality, drug use, blood transfusion, or hemophilia. In Africa, cases often had an aggressive and often fatal form of Kaposi's sarcoma, which had up to this point been endemic to the region, but had been easily treatable. The main risk factor in Africa for AIDS appeared to be heterosexual contact. American and European scientists began to focus on the African epidemic, particularly because it appeared more likely to spread throughout the world due to its predominantly heterosexual mode of transmission than the epidemic in America and Europe.

The Institute Pasteur continued to claim that LAV was the cause of AIDS, but a related virus called human t-cell leukemia virus III (HTLV-III) was discovered by a research team in San Francisco. Investigators began to suspect that these viruses were identical. By the end of

1984, the CDC had reported nearly 8,000 AIDS cases and 3,500 deaths from the disease.

In 1985, the U.S. Food and Drug Administration confirmed that LAV and HTLV-III were identical, and that the virus was indeed the cause of AIDS. The FDA additionally ordered testing of the national blood supply and required that anyone testing positive for the virus would not be allowed to donate blood. Now that the cause of AIDS could be detected, public bewilderment over AIDS transmission gave way to concern over the dissemination and use of information about HTLV-III/LAV infection. The gay community voiced fears of stigmatization of persons found to carry the virus, believing the information would be misused by employers and insurance companies to exclude infected individuals. Incidents of cruelty and prejudice directed toward AIDS victims and perceived risk groups continued to mount, though Haitians were removed from the list of high-risk groups in view of new understanding of heterosexual and injection drug transmission risks. The year 1985 ended with more than 20,000 reported U.S. AIDS cases, with over 15,000 cases reported in other nations.

The International Committee on the Taxonomy of Viruses ruled in May 1986 that the LAV and HTLV-III virus names should be dropped in favor of Human Immunodeficiency Virus (HIV). During that year, the Director of the WHO announced that some 10 million people worldwide could already have been infected with HIV by June 1986. The true scope and devastation of the disease had begun to be apparent to the scientific community.

■ Impacts and Issues

As of early 2007, officials at UNAIDS, a United Nations organization tasked with uniting efforts to treat and eliminate HIV, estimated that another 50 million people could die from AIDS in India and China alone by the year 2025. In Africa, where research indicates that the epidemic likely began, AIDS will have killed 100 million people by that time if trends continue. Although antiretroviral medications have begun to lower expected death rates, AIDS could still kill 40 million additional Africans by 2025. To date, all vaccine development programs have failed. Prevention programs focused on changing sexual and drug-use behaviors have had mixed success across regions and across cultural and political divides.

■ Primary Source Connection

The primary source "Many Blood Banks Deny Request of Hemophiliacs" demonstrates the confusion and fears surrounding the earliest days of the AIDS epidemic in the United States, when the cause of the disease was known, but erroneously linked only to specific groups.

IN CONTEXT: THE FIRST REPORTS OF AIDS

Within an eight-month period in 1980–1981, five young men were hospitalized in the Los Angeles area with a rare, severe form of pneumonia caused by the pathogen (disease-causing microorganism) *Pneumocystis carinii*. In reporting the outbreak to the Centers for Disease Control and Prevention (CDC), physician Michael S. Gottlieb and his colleagues first documented in medical literature the disease that was to become known as AIDS. The report jarred physicians in New York and San Francisco, who noticed a handful of similar cases occurring at about the same time. In another unusual occurrence, eight young men in the New York area with Kaposi's sarcoma had recently died. Kaposi's sarcoma is a form of skin cancer that was usually seen mainly in elderly persons. Suspecting a new or emerging disease among young men, the Centers for Disease Control and Prevention (CDC) formed a task force to investigate the outbreaks. Gottlieb was an assistant professor of medicine at the University of California at Los Angeles (UCLA) in 1981 when he submitted the featured report as its lead author. In 1985, Gottlieb co-founded the American Foundation for AIDS Research.

IN CONTEXT: REAL TIME DELAYS IN RECOGNIZING GLOBAL LINKS

In initial reports to the CDC, all of the young men with both *Pneumocystis* pneumonia and Kaposi's sarcoma were actively homosexual, and early on, the task force considered the disease likely to be confined to the community of homosexual males. By the end of 1981, it became clear that that the newly recognized disease affected other population groups, as the first cases of *Pneumocystis* pneumonia were reported in drug users who injected their drugs. It also became clear that the disease was not confined to the United States when similar cases were found within a year in the United Kingdom, Haiti, and in Uganda, where the disease was already known as "slim."

The author/creator, The Associated Press, is a worldwide and multiple Pulitzer Prize winning news agency based in New York.

Editor's note: As set forth in the introduction, the perspective of time and accumulation of subsequent information can often make assertions contained in primary sources—even if based upon the best information available at the time written—subsequently misleading or wrong. Readers should be mindful that primary

IN CONTEXT: SCIENTIFIC, POLITICAL, AND ETHICAL ISSUES

The advent of AIDS (Acquired Immunity Deficiency Syndrome) in early 1981 stunned the scientific community, as many researchers at that time viewed the world to be on the brink of eliminating infectious disease. Victims of AIDS most often die from opportunistic infections that take hold of the body because the immune system is severely impaired. AIDS is caused by the Human Immune Deficiency Virus (HIV). HIV belongs to a class of viruses known as retroviruses. These viruses are known as RNA viruses, because they have RNA (ribonucleic acid) as their basic genetic material instead of DNA (deoxyribonucleic acid).

Following its discovery and spread in Western nations, the urgency of combating AIDS significantly altered the distribution of research funding in the biomedical sciences—including increased funding for research on retroviruses. Whether such shifts in funding were insufficient (i.e., more research money should have been spent sooner) or to the overall detriment of world health—because it sometime shifted money from research on diseases that kill more people worldwide—is often a contentious scientific, political, and ethical issue.

researchers say it may be transmitted through sexual contact or blood.

The hemophilia foundation recommended Monday that blood banks ask male donors if they are homosexual and then ban all blood donations from homosexual men. It also said blood collection should be halted in areas heavily populated by homosexual men.

Associated Press

"AROUND THE NATION; MANY BLOOD BANKS DENY REQUEST OF HEMOPHILIACS;" *NEW YORK TIMES.* JANUARY 21, 1983.

SEE ALSO *AIDS (Acquired Immunodeficiency Syndrome); Antiviral Drugs; Bloodborne Pathogens; Developing Nations and Drug Delivery; Epidemiology; Opportunistic Infection; Public Health and Infectious Disease; Sexually Transmitted Diseases.*

BIBLIOGRAPHY

Books

Mayer, Kenneth H., and H.F. Pizer. *The AIDS Pandemic: Impact on Science and Society.* San Diego: Academic Press, 2004.

Periodicals

Hymes, K.B., J.B. Greene, A. Marcus, et al. "Kaposi's Sarcoma in Homosexual Men: A Report of Eight Cases." *Lancet* 2 (1981): 598–600.

Gottlieb, M.S., et.al. "*Pneumocystis* Pneumonia—Los Angeles" Morbidity and Mortality Weekly Report (June 5, 1981): (30) 21, 1–3. Available online at <http://www.cdc.gov/mmwr/preview/ mmwrhtml/june_5.htm> (accessed April 21, 2007).

Web Sites

Kaiser Family Foundation. "The Global HIV-AIDS Timeline." <http://www.kff.org/hivaids/ timeline/hivtimeline.cfm> (accessed February 19, 2007).

Centers for Disease Control and Prevention. "Milestones in the U.S. HIV Epidemic." <http:// www.thebody.com/cdc/pdfs/timeline.pdf> (accessed March 25, 2007).

Kenneth T.LaPensee

sources often contain information later proven to be false, or contain viewpoints and terms unacceptable to future generations. It is important to view primary sources within the historical and social context existing at the time of creation.

Many Blood Banks Deny Request of Hemophiliacs

Many of the nation's blood banks say they will not heed the advice of the National Hemophilia Foundation that male donors be asked whether they are homosexuals. The question is part of a effort to screen possible carriers of a disease that cripples the body's immune system.

The disease, Acquired Immunodeficiency Syndrome, or AIDS, is most common among homosexual and bisexual men. The cause of the disease is not known, but some

Airborne Precautions

■ Introduction

Airborne precautions are procedures that are designed to reduce the chance that certain disease-causing (pathogenic) microorganisms will be transmitted through the air.

The precautions relate to airborne, microbe-containing droplets that are less than five microns in diameter (a micron is 10^{-6} meters). Such droplets can remain suspended in the air for a long time and so can be transported a considerable distance (such as from room to room) in even a gentle current of air. As well, particles of this size can be inhaled deeply into the lung, where the chance of establishing an infection can be increased.

Airborne precautions that involve the treatment of the air and ventilation systems are necessary for patients who have tuberculosis, and often for those with herpes zoster (shingles), varicella (chickenpox), and rubeola (measles). As of 2007, the precautions also apply to severe acute respiratory syndrome (SARS), as the mechanisms of spread of the virus are still being investigated. Other diseases do not require these mandated precautions.

■ History and Scientific Foundations

It has been known for over a century that some bacteria and viruses can be dispersed into the air, and that they can cause infection if they are inhaled or enter a wound. Indeed, the physical isolation of a operating theater from the rest of a hospital and the wearing of a face mask by health care providers is designed in part to limit the airborne spread of microbes.

In the United States, regulated airborne precautions were instituted by the Centers for Disease Control and Prevention (CDC). The latest guidelines were issued in 1996. The CDC also formulated separate guidelines that were specific for patients with tuberculosis.

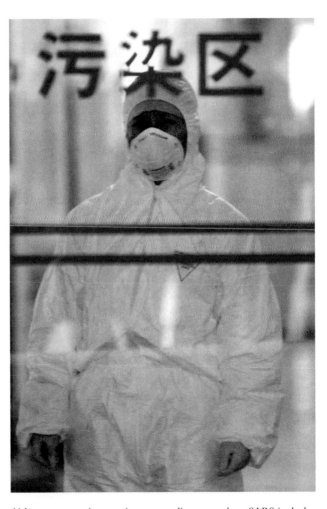

Airborne precautions against severe diseases such as SARS include high-filtration N95 masks, suits to prevent respiratory droplets from contacting the body, and negative-pressure ventilation in isolation areas, as illustrated by this medical worker standing inside an isolated area for SARS patients at a hospital in Guangdong, China, in 2004. © Wilson Wen/epa/Corbis.

WORDS TO KNOW

COHORT: A cohort is a group of people (or any species) sharing a common characteristic. Cohorts are identified and grouped in cohort studies to determine the frequency of diseases or the kinds of disease outcomes over time.

CONTACT PRECAUTIONS: Contact precautions are actions developed to minimize the person-to-person transfer of microorganisms by direct physical contact and indirectly by inhalation or touching a contaminated surface.

HEPA FILTER: A HEPA (high efficiency particulate air) filter is a filter that is designed to nearly totally remove airborne particles that are 0.3 microns (millionth of a meter) in diameter or larger. Such small particles can penetrate deeply into the lungs if inhaled.

■ Applications and Research

The airborne precautions pertain to patient placement in the hospital, transport of the patient from one area of the hospital to another, and the protective breathing gear worn by health care providers when around the patient.

According to the precautions, the affected patients must be housed in a room that has what is termed a negative air pressure relative to the surrounding spaces. Negative air pressure means that the number of air molecules in the room is less than the number of air molecules in the areas adjacent to the room. The result is that air will move into but not out of the room, reducing the chance that airborne microbes in the patient's room will disperse more widely. The air pressure of the room is monitored, the air in the room must be completely changed 6 to 12 times every hour, and the exhausted air is passed through a special type of air filter called a high-efficiency particulate (HEPA) filter that traps extremely small particles. The filter ensures that the exhausted air is not contaminated with the pathogenic microbes. The filter is changed at regular intervals and disposed of in a certain way to make sure that the trapped microbes do not pose a further hazard.

The room should also be separated from adjacent rooms and hallways by a door, which is left closed when not in use.

Ideally, the room should be just for the affected patient. If this is not possible, then more than one patient can be housed in the same room (this is called cohorting). These cohorts should have the same infection that is caused by the same microorganism (there are exceptions for tuberculosis). However, the patients should not have any other infections. If these precautions cannot be met, then another strategy should not be undertaken without the advice of infection control experts.

The precaution concerning respiratory protection is specific. When entering the affected patient's room, health care providers must wear an N-95 respirator, which is a mask certified by CDC's National Institute for Occupational Safety and Health (NIOSH). The mask is equipped with a filter that can trap over 95% of particles that are 0.3 microns or greater in diameter in an aerosol that is free of oil (oil can affect droplet size and is not the sort of aerosol encountered in hospitals).

Anyone who is susceptible to rubeola or chickenpox should not enter the room of a patient with these diseases without an N-95 mask. A person who has a compromised immune system should not have close contact with a person whose illness requires airborne precautions. This applies to other patients as well as visitors and health care personnel.

Airborne precautions also pertain to the movement of patients within the hospital. This movement should only be done when absolutely necessary. During transport, a surgical mask is placed over the patient's nose and mouth to minimize the dispersal of droplets.

■ Impacts and Issues

Airborne precautions reduce the spread of certain infections. But this safeguard comes with a price tag. Equipping hospital rooms to be negative pressure rooms, installing and maintaining HEPA filters, and equipping staff with respirators is expensive. Furthermore, the requirements to frequently document compliance with the precautions is an added burden to hospital caretakers.

One recent example highlighting airborne precautions concerns a type of recently emergent *Mycobacterium tuberculosis* that is extremely resistant to antibiotics. According to the World Health Organization (WHO), the extreme drug-resistant tuberculosis (XDR-TB) is virtually untreatable using the present arsenal of drugs. Strains of XDR-TB have been noted in individuals mainly in South Africa, but also in Russia, North America, South America, and Asia. According to WHO, people infected with the human immunodeficiency virus (HIV) are particularly susceptible to XDR-TB. As of 2007, prevention and containment through the use of airborne precautions constitute the main line of defense against XDR-TB.

SEE ALSO *Anthrax; Bioterrorism; Contact Precautions; Droplet Precautions; Standard Precautions.*

BIBLIOGRAPHY

Books

Lawrence, Jean and Dee May. *Infection Control in the Community.* New York: Churchill Livingstone, 2003.

Tierno, Philip M. *The Secret Life of Germs: What They Are, Why We Need Them, and How We Can Protect Ourselves Against Them.* New York: Atria, 2004.

Periodicals

Booth, Timothy F., et al. "Detection of Airborne Severe Acute Respiratory Syndrome (SARS) Cornonavirus and Environmental Contamination in SARS Outbreak Units." *Journal of Infectious Diseases* 191 (2005): 1472–1477.

Yu, Ignatius T.S., Tze Wai Wong, Yuk Lan Chiu, Nelson Lee, Yuguo Li. "Temproal-spation Analysis of Severe Acute Respiratory Syndrome among Hospital Inpatients." *Clinical Infectious Diseases* 40 (2005): 1237–1243.

Brian Hoyle

IN CONTEXT: AVAILABILITY OF HOSPITAL BEDS

Airborne precautions pertain to patient placement in the hospital, transport of the patient from one area of the hospital to another, and the protective gear worn by health care providers when around the patient.

But how available are the hospital beds?

The list below reflects selected data from the World Health Organization that demonstrates the wide disparity in results reported by WHO as of February 2007. Data was not available for all countries, including a lack of data for: Angola, Botswana, Burkina Faso, Central African Republic, Chad, Ethiopia, Ghana, Kenya, Mali, Niger, Rwanda, Senegal, Togo, Uganda, and South Africa.

Country; Hospital beds (per 10,000 people); (Year data gathered).

- Nepal 1.5 beds (2001)
- Bangladesh 3.4 beds (2001)
- Afghanistan 3.9 beds (2001)
- Somalia 4.2 beds (1997)
- Guatemala 5 beds (2003)
- Cambodia 5.72 beds (2004)
- India 6.9 beds (1998)
- Sudan 7.1 beds (2003)
- Haiti 8 beds (2000)
- Mexico 10 beds (2003)
- Philippines 11.45 beds (2002)
- Iran (Islamic Republic of) 16.3 beds (2001)
- Egypt 21.7 beds (2003)
- Thailand 22.3 beds (1999)
- Maldives 22.6 beds (2003)
- Viet Nam 22.8 beds (2003)
- China 23.11 beds (2004)
- Sweden 30 beds (2004)
- United States 33 beds (2003)
- Ireland 35 beds (2004)
- Canada 36 beds (2003)
- United Kingdom 40 beds (2003)
- Italy 41 beds (2003)
- Cuba 49 beds (2004)
- Switzerland 59 beds (2003)
- France 76 beds (2003)
- Russian Federation 99 beds (2004)
- Belarus 107 beds (2004)
- Japan 129.37 beds (2001)
- Monaco 196 beds (1995)

SOURCE: *WHOSIS (WHO Statistical Information System), World Health Organization, Regional Office websites and publications.*

Alveolar Echinococcosis

■ Introduction

Alveolar echinococcosis (al-VEE-oh-ler ee-keye-ni-kah-KOH-sis) is an infection caused by the tapeworm *Echinococcus multilocularis*. The infection is rare in humans, although is serious when it occurs as, if not treated, the infection is nearly always lethal. Tumorlike formations—due to the growth of the larval form of the tapeworm—occur most commonly in the liver, but can also be present in the brain, lungs, and elsewhere in the body.

■ Disease History, Characteristics, and Transmission

E. multilocularis has a life cycle that consists of an egg phase and a larval phase. The eggs are excreted in the feces of the infected animal. If the feces are eaten by another animal, the eggs can germinate to form the larva, which matures in the intestine. As part of the maturation process, eggs are produced, which are shed in the feces. The cycle can then repeat in another animal.

Humans acquire the infection by ingesting the eggs. This usually occurs in one of two ways. First, food that is contaminated with fox or coyote feces is eaten. This can happen when, for example, a person hiking in the woods eats herbs or berries collected along the route. Second and more commonly, eggs that have stuck to the fur of family pets as they have been shed by the animal (or picked up as the dog or cat has rubbed against vegetation) transfer to the hands of the owner when the animal is petted or groomed, and are accidentally ingested when the hands are put into the mouth.

As the larvae of the tapeworm grow, they aggregate (come together) to create tumorlike formations. These typically occur in the liver, but can spread elsewhere. The symptoms, which develop slowly over years, include abdominal pain, a feeling of weakness, and loss of weight. The symptoms can be mistaken for the slow growth of a liver tumor or the type of progressive liver damage that can result from the chronic over-consumption of alcohol.

■ Scope and Distribution

Alveolar echinococcosis is widespread in animal populations in northern latitudes including Europe, China, Russia, Asia, Japan, and North America (primarily in the north-central area of the United States from Montana to Ohio, Alaska, and most of Canada). In these

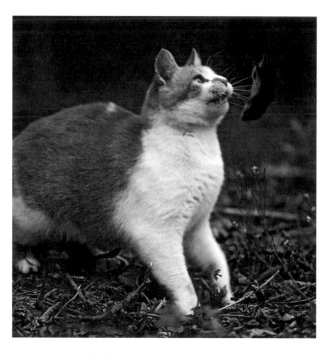

As the habitats of wildlife and domestic animals converge, domestic cats and dogs can become a source of alveolar echinococcosis disease in humans. Dogs and cats can become infected with *Echinococcus multilocularis* tapeworm larvae found in wild rodents, which in turn get the tapeworm larvae from wildlife such as coyotes. *James L. Amos/Photo Researchers, Inc.*

regions, the tapeworm is present in over 50% of the fox and coyote populations. Human cases have rarely been reported in North America; in the twentieth century only two cases are known to have occurred: one in the state of Minnesota and the other in the western Canadian province of Manitoba.

In addition to foxes and coyotes, *E. mulitlocularis* can be found in the intestinal tract of dogs and cats. The animals can also become infected when they eat rodents, voles, or field mice that are infected with the tapeworm larvae.

Because the infection occurs most often in wild foxes, people who are most at risk are those who spend much of their time outdoors. These include park rangers, trappers, and hunters. Urban and rural veterinarians also run a risk of contact because they handle animals that may carry the tapeworm eggs. There is no evidence of racial or gender association with the infection. The higher tendency of men to be infected could reflect the traditional dominance of men in occupations like logging and in pursuits like hunting.

The distribution of the infection may be spreading as the territory of wild foxes contracts and they come into closer contact with humans. This is partially due to the expansion of urban areas; the availability of food attracts foxes that had not previously inhabited these areas.

■ Treatment and Prevention

As of 2007, there is no cure for alveolar echinococcosis. The most common treatment involves surgery to remove the tumorlike larval mass, followed by drug therapy to attempt to prevent the germination of eggs that may still be present in the individual. Drug therapy, typically with the anti-fungal compound benzimidazole, can be long and expensive.

The best prevention is to lessen the chances of contacting *E. multilocularis*. Avoiding contact with living or dead wild animals unless protective gloves are worn is a sensible precaution. Keeping domestic pets close to home and away from contact with wild animals is another wise move. Washing hands after handling pets is another preventative step, but one that is difficult for most people to consistently follow.

■ Impacts and Issues

The main impact on human health of alveolar echinococcosis is the high death rate of the infection if it is not treated. The odds of survival for five years if the infection is untreated is only 40% versus almost 90% if treatment is provided.

Even with treatment, persons treated for alveolar echinococcosis often face a diminished quality of life.

WORDS TO KNOW

LARVA: Immature form (wormlike in insects; fishlike in amphibians) of an organism capable of surviving on its own. A larva does not resemble the parent and must go through metamorphosis, or change, to reach its adult stage. The initial stage of a mosquito after it hatches from its egg.

PARASITE: An organism that lives in or on a host organism and that gets its nourishment from that host. The parasite usually gains all the benefits of this relationship, while the host may suffer from various diseases and discomforts, or show no signs of the infection. The life cycle of a typical parasite usually includes several developmental stages and morphological changes as the parasite lives and moves through the environment and one or more hosts. Parasites that remain on a host's body surface to feed are called ectoparasites, while those that live inside a host's body are called endoparasites. Parasitism is a highly successful biological adaptation. There are more known parasitic species than nonparasitic ones, and parasites affect just about every form of life, including most all animals, plants, and even bacteria.

Furthermore, treatment comes with a high price tag; up to $300,000 per person.

The infection is an example of how political or economic decisions can influence a disease. The clearing of forests to provide more farmland or timber can cause rodent populations to become more concentrated in urban areas, increasing the chances for the spread of *E. multilocularis*.

SEE ALSO *Tapeworm Infections; Vector-borne Disease; Zoonoses.*

BIBLIOGRAPHY

Books

Black, Jacquelyn G. *Microbiology: Principles and Explorations.* New York: John Wiley & Sons, 2004.

Pelton, Robert Young. *Robert Young Pelton's The World's Most Dangerous Places.* 5th ed. New York: Collins, 2003.

Wobeser, Gary A. *Essentials of Disease in Wild Animals.* Boston: Blackwell Publishing Professional, 2005.

IN CONTEXT: PERSONAL RESPONSIBILITY AND PREVENTION

The Centers for Disease Control and Prevention recommends that people who live in an area where *E. multilocularis* is often found in rodents and wild canines, take the following precautions to avoid infection:

- Don't touch a fox, coyote, or other wild canine, dead or alive, unless you are wearing gloves. Hunters and trappers should use plastic gloves to avoid exposure.
- Don't keep wild animals, especially wild canines, as pets or encourage them to come close to your home.
- Don't allow your cats and dogs to wander freely or to capture and eat rodents.
- If you think that your pet may have eaten rodents, consult your veterinarian about the possible need for preventive treatments.
- After handling pets, always wash your hands with soap and warm water.
- Fence in gardens to keep out wild animals.
- Do not collect or eat wild fruits or vegetables picked directly from the ground. All wild-picked foods should be washed carefully or cooked before eating.

SOURCE: *Centers for Disease Control and Prevention (CDC)*

Periodicals

Sréter, Tamás, Zoltáa Széll, Zsuzsa Egyed, István Varga. "Echinococcus Multilocularis: An Emerging Pathogen in Hungary and Central Eastern Europe?" *Emerging Infectious Diseases.* 9 (2003): 384–386.

Brian Hoyle

Amebiasis

■ Introduction

Amebiasis (am-e-BI-a-sis) is an infection that is caused by a one-celled parasite called *Entamoeba histolytica*. The infection, which produces an inflammation of the cells lining the intestinal tract, is also referred to as amebic (or amoebic) dysentery.

Amebiasis often results in relatively mild illness, producing diarrhea and abdominal pain. However, the infection can be quite severe, with inflammation being so extensive that the intestinal wall in the colon can become perforated, and damage can occur to both the liver and the brain. As well, diarrhea can be copious and often accompanied by vomiting, which can lead to dehydration if fluids are not replaced.

■ Disease History, Characteristics, and Transmission

E. histolytica can occur in two forms. One form is known as a cyst. This form is very tough, and can survive harsh conditions of temperature and lack of moisture that would kill the other, growing form of the organism called the trophozoite. This hardiness makes a cyst similar to a bacterial spore. The parasite is excreted in feces as a cyst. It can survive for a long time until it finds itself in a more favorable environment, such as the intestinal tract of another person. There, the cyst can resume growth. The trophozoite is the form that causes amebiasis. Some trophozoites will form cysts and can be excreted, beginning another cycle of infection.

The cysts can also invade the walls of the intestine, where they can germinate into the trophozoite forms. Then, ulcers and diarrhea can be produced. Or, much more seriously, the cysts may enter the bloodstream and can be carried all over the body. Damage to tissues such as the brain and liver can result.

When symptoms develop, they tend to begin about 2 to 4 weeks after the parasite has entered the body, although some people develop symptoms in only a few days.

Amebiasis has been known since the early years of the twentieth century. Despite this, the diagnosis of amebiasis has not changed in over a century, still relying on the visual detection of the cyst in feces from the person suspected of having the infection. This can be a tedious and lengthy process, often requiring days of examination. Complicating diagnosis, the cysts of *E. histolytica* resemble that of other amoeba called *Entamoeba coli* and *Entamoeba dispar*, which are normal and harmless residents of the intestinal tract of warm-blooded animals, including humans. Indeed, *E. histolytica* and *E. dipar* are

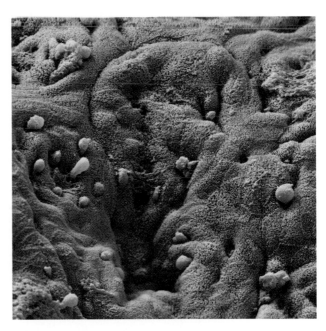

Entamoeba histolytica, a species of parasitic protozoa, cause entamoebiasis and amebic dysentery. Humans are infected most often through food or water contaminated with human fecal material. *Eye of Science/Photo Researchers, Inc.*

WORDS TO KNOW

DYSENTERY: Dysentery is an infectious disease that has ravaged armies, refugee camps, and prisoner-of-war camps throughout history. The disease still is a major problem in developing countries with primitive sanitary facilities.

TROPHOZOITE: The amoeboid, vegetative stage of the malaria protozoa.

virtually identical in appearance. This means that many cases of amebiasis are likely diagnosed incorrectly.

Scope and Distribution

Some people who are infected carry *E. histolytica* in their intestinal tract without displaying symptoms. Since the parasite can be excreted along with feces, a person can unknowingly pass the parasite to someone else by handling food with unwashed hands after going to the bathroom, by person-to-person contact (including sexual intercourse), or by contaminating drinking water with feces. This route of transmission can persist for years after a person has been exposed to the parasite. The persons who subsequently become infected might become ill.

Amebiasis affects about 50 million people worldwide each year, making it one of the two most common causes of intestinal inflammation; the other is caused by *Shigella*. Approximately 100,000 people die of the infection each year. Those most often affected are in poorer health; thus, amebiasis tends to be more common in developing countries, where sanitation is inadequate and where people live in crowded conditions, making the spread of the parasite much easier. However, anyone is susceptible; several hundred cases are reported each year in the United States, for example. In developed countries, those who become infected tend to be pregnant women, the young and the elderly, and those whose immune systems have become compromised due to malnourishment or disease (such as acquired immunodeficiency syndrome [AIDS]).

Treatment and Prevention

Amebiasis is treatable using a combination of drug therapies. Some drugs generically called amebicides kill the organisms that are growing in the intestinal tract, while other drugs can lessen the chance that the infection will spread to tissues such as the liver.

Impacts and Issues

Persons who travel to high-risk countries such as parts of Africa, India, Latin America, and Southeast Asia, where the infection is commonly prevalent in some regions (such an infection is described as being endemic) should take precautions against contracting amebiasis. Precautions include drinking bottled water or boiling drinking water for at least one minute, peeling the skins off fresh fruits and vegetables before eating them, and proper handwashing using soap.

An important issue concerning amebiasis is that the parasite can be excreted in the feces of someone who has no symptoms of the infection. In fact, this is true for the majority of people; estimates are that only one in ten people who are infected actually become sick. While this is a small percent, the fact that millions of people become infected each year still means that a great many people become ill, with many more remaining capable of spreading the infection to others.

Research is ongoing to find more definitive ways of treating amebiasis, and in preventing the infection in the first place. As of 2007, there is no vaccine for the infection. A blood test is available that can detect the presence of the parasite. However, because the test detects the presence of antibodies—molecules produced by the immune system that are targeted against the particular invading organism—the test only reveals if someone has ever had an infection, not necessarily an ongoing infection.

The World Health Organization (WHO) recommends that if the presence of amoeba in the feces is confirmed microscopically but the person is not experiencing any symptoms, then it should not be assumed that the person has amebiasis.

On a larger scale, the WHO is building an international network, now totaling over 100 organizations, that together aim to reduce worldwide deaths from diseases such as amebiasis. The group, called the International Network to Promote Household Water Treatment and Safe Storage, plans to implement sustainable and affordable methods of purifying drinking water supplies in communities without access to sanitation or treated water, or with water that is improved but from unsafe sources. Although large waterborne outbreaks of amebiasis are uncommon, water treatment and sanitation measures are complimentary and are developed together when possible.

In the era of molecular biology, procedures have been developed that can detect the genetic material of *E. histolytica* in feces. However, the test is relatively expensive and requires specialized equipment and training that may not be part of a clinic, especially in an underdeveloped region.

SEE ALSO *Giardiasis; Parasitic Diseases; Sanitation.*

BIBLIOGRAPHY

Books

Guerrant, Richard I., David H. Walker, and Peter F. Weller. *Tropical Infectious Diseases: Principles, Pathogens & Practice.* Oxford: Churchill Livingstone, 2005.

Web Sites

Centers for Disease Control and Prevention. "Amebiasis." <http://www.cdc.gov/ncidod/dpd/parasites/ amebiasis/factsht_amebiasis.htm> (accessed March 15, 2007).

Brian Hoyle

AVOIDING INFECTION WITH *E. HISTOLYTICA*

To avoid infection with *E. histolytica*, The Centers for Disease Control and Prevention (CDC) recommends that a person traveling to a country that has poor sanitary conditions should observe the following with regard to eating and drinking:

- Drink only bottled or boiled (for 1 minute) water or carbonated (bubbly) drinks in cans or bottles. Do not drink fountain drinks or any drinks with ice cubes. Another way to make water safe is by filtering it through an "absolute 1 micron or less" filter and dissolving iodine tablets in the filtered water. "Absolute 1 micron" filters can be found in camping/outdoor supply stores.
- Do not eat fresh fruit or vegetables that you did not peel yourself.
- Do not eat or drink milk, cheese, or dairy products that may not have been pasteurized.
- Do not eat or drink anything sold by street vendors.

SOURCE: *Centers for Disease Control and Prevention (CDC)*

IN CONTEXT: IMPROVED WATER ACCESS

The list below reflects data from the World Health Organization indicating countries recently reporting access to improved water sources for less than 50% of the population (with the year of the report indicated):

- Afghanistan 13% of the population (year reported: 2002)
- Somalia 29% (2002)
- Cambodia 34% (2002)
- Chad 34% (2002)
- Papua New Guinea 39% (2002)
- Mozambique 42% (2002)
- Lao People's Democratic Republic 43% (2002)
- Equatorial Guinea 44% (2002)
- Madagascar 45% (2002)
- Congo 46% (2002)
- Democratic Republic of the Congo 46% (2002)
- Niger 46% (2002)
- Mali 48% (2002)

SOURCE: *World Health Organization (WHO)*

Angiostrongyliasis

■ Introduction

Angiostrongyliasis (ann-gee-o-stronge-uh-luss) is an infection caused by the internal parasites *Angiostrongylus cantonensis* and *Angiostrongylus costaricensis*. These worms are transmitted as eggs or larvae from rats to other animals such as snails, slugs, and some crustaceans. Humans become infected when they ingest immature parasites, usually after eating undercooked or raw mollusks, crustaceans, and especially snails. Angiostrongyliasis infection often has no symptoms, or mild symptoms, although some cases result in the development of meningitis. Infection disappears as the worms die in the body.

The majority of outbreaks of angiostrongyliasis occur in Southeast Asia and the Pacific Islands, although cases have been reported in other countries. The first appearance of the parasites in humans was noted in 1944 and since then, there have been numerous reported infections.

■ Disease History, Characteristics, and Transmission

Angiostrongyliasis is caused by the ingestion of one of two parasites, *Angiostrongylus cantonensis* or *Angiostrongylus costaricensis*. Both are parasites of rats and are

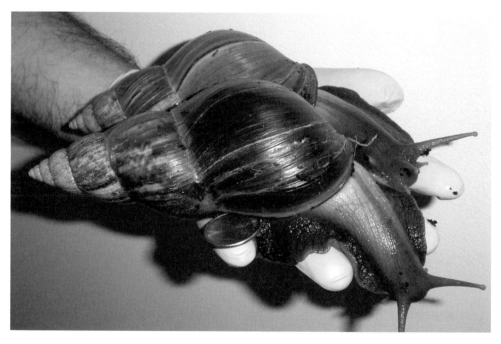

African snails, which can reach a length of 8 in (20 cm), can carry the *Angiostrongylus cantonensis* parasite that causes meningitis in humans. When administrators at an Illinois school realized that these giant snails could pose a health risk for the 28 fourth graders caring for them in 2004, they asked students to return them to school, where they were seized by the U.S. Department of Agriculture. *AP Images.*

transmitted to snails and slugs when they eat rat feces. Crustaceans such as prawns can also carry the parasite. Transmission to humans occurs when humans eat undercooked or raw intermittent hosts containing the parasite. Most humans become infected after eating in restaurants that do not cook the animals properly, or when they accidentally ingest a snail or slug attached to a salad item that has not been washed properly.

Infection by *A. cantonensis*, which travels to the brain or lungs and eventually dies there, usually results in mild symptoms, or no symptoms, although eosinophilic meningitis can develop. Meningitis is usually accompanied by headaches, a stiff neck, fever, nausea, and vomiting. Infection by *A. costaricensis*, which travels to the digestive tract and dies there, can result in abdominal pain as the dying parasites cause inflammatory pain in the abdomen.

■ Scope and Distribution

The *Angiostrongylus* parasites were first discovered in rats in China in 1933 and in humans in Taiwan in 1944. Infection of rats first spread throughout the Indo-pacific basin and through Madagascar, Cuba, Egypt, Puerto Rico, and New Orleans. Following the end of World War II in 1945, infected rats spread to Micronesia, Australia, and Polynesia. During the 1950s, infected rats were reported in the Philippines, Saipan, New Caledonia, Rarotonga, and Tahiti; during the 1960s, infected rats had spread to Thailand, Cambodia, Java, Sarawak, Guam, and Hawaii.

During 2000, students from Chicago traveling through Jamaica became infected with eosinophilic meningitis. The cause of infection was pinpointed to a salad that was eaten by all the students and that most likely contained secretions from infected slugs or snails.

In August 2006, a number of cases of angiostrongyliasis infection were reported in Beijing, China. Over the course of two months, an outbreak occurred during which the number of infected people rose to 132. The cause of this outbreak was linked to a restaurant chain that served Amazonian snails, known hosts of the parasites. These snails were most likely undercooked, causing the parasite to infect humans.

■ Treatment and Prevention

Angiostrongyliasis parasites die within weeks to months. Sometimes the body reacts to the dying parasites, which causes mild symptoms such as abdominal pain. Infected humans usually recover fully without treatment, although treatment may be administered to treat symptoms. Eosinophilic meningitis can also develop and is characterized by neck pain, headaches, and nausea. Although there is no specific treatment for angiostron-

WORDS TO KNOW

HELMINTHIC DISEASE: Helminths are parasitic worms such as hookworms or flatworms. Helminthic disease is infectious by such worms. A synonym for helminthic is verminous.

PARASITE: An organism that lives in or on a host organism and that gets its nourishment from that host. The parasite usually gains all the benefits of this relationship, while the host may suffer from various diseases and discomforts, or show no signs of the infection. The life cycle of a typical parasite usually includes several developmental stages and morphological changes as the parasite lives and moves through the environment and one or more hosts. Parasites that remain on a host's body surface to feed are called ectoparasites, while those that live inside a host's body are called endoparasites. Parasitism is a highly successful biological adaptation. There are more known parasitic species than nonparasitic ones, and parasites affect just about every form of life, including most all animals, plants, and even bacteria.

gyliasis, analgesics, corticosteroids, and certain anti-helminthic drugs may be administered.

Infections can be prevented by cooking snails, crustaceans, and slugs thoroughly so that the parasite is killed. In addition, careful washing of salad items will prevent infected snails and slugs from being present in salads and potentially being ingested. Although some cases have been attributed to the ingestion of mucus and secretions, some scientists insist that it is still unknown whether transmission can occur following ingestion of mucus from infected snails and slugs. Ingestion of mucus may occur when people who collect snails touch their mouths or nasal passages. Infection can also be prevented by wearing gloves while collecting snails.

■ Impacts and Issues

The main mode of transmission of the parasites that cause angiostrongyliasis is through poor preparation of food. Therefore, infection is more likely to occur in countries with soft regulations on food preparation. People traveling through countries in which rats are infected by the parasites need to be aware of the risks

IN CONTEXT: HAVE CASES OCCURRED IN THE CONTINENTAL UNITED STATES?

The Centers for Disease Control and Prevention (CDC) states that "In 1993, a boy got infected by swallowing a raw snail 'on a dare.' The type of snail he swallowed isn't known. He became ill a few weeks later, with muscle aches, headache, stiff neck, a slight fever, and vomiting. Although he had eosinophilic meningitis, his symptoms went away in about 2 weeks, without treatment of the infection."

The CDC specifically recommends that to avoid infection: "Don't eat raw or undercooked snails or slugs. If you handle snails or slugs, wear gloves and wash your hands. Always remember to thoroughly wash fresh produce."

SOURCE: *Centers for Disease Control and Prevention (CDC)*

abundant. In the islands of French Polynesia, most infections occur in adults.

In the United States, Giant African land snails are illegal to import as pets. They are considered an invasive species capable of supporting the emergence of angiostrongyliasis in the United States, as well as an agricultural pest. In 2004, authorities seized the snails in over 100 U.S. exotic pet shops and among private owners. Additionally, several schools that kept Giant African land snails as projects turned them over to public health authorities.

SEE ALSO *Food-borne Disease and Food Safety; Parasitic Diseases.*

BIBLIOGRAPHY

Books

Mandell, G.L., J.E. Bennett, and R. Dolin. *Principles and Practice of Infectious Diseases*, Vol. 2. Philadelphia, Penn: Elsevier, 2005.

Web Sites

Centers for Disease Control and Prevention (CDC). "Angiostrongyliasis." Sep. 27, 2004 <http://www.dpd.cdc.gov/DPDx/HTML/ImageLibrary/Angiostrongyliasis_il.asp?body=A-F/Angiostrongyliasis/body_Angiostrongyliasis_il2.htm> (accessed Jan. 25, 2007).

Centers for Disease Control and Prevention (CDC). "Fact Sheet: *Angiostrongylus cantonensis* Infection." May 13, 2004 <http://www.cdc.gov/ncidod/dpd/parasites/angiostrongylus/factsht_angiostrongylus.htm> (accessed Jan. 25, 2007).

International Society for Infectious Diseases. "Angiostrongylus Meningitis—China (04)." Oct. 1, 2006 <http://www.promedmail.org/pls/promed/f?p=2400:1202:1604187183216986886::NO::F2400_P1202_CHECK_DISPLAY,F2400_P1202_PUB_MAIL_ID:X,34650> (accessed Jan. 25, 2007).

associated with eating food in these countries. Reducing the rodent population in endemic countries also reduces the available population for the initial reservoir of the parasite, and thus, minimizes the opportunity for infection.

The type of snails eaten and the methods used to cook these snails also impact infection. Therefore, restaurants that sell certain snails could potentially contribute towards spreading the infection. Furthermore, as the proper cooking of snails can render the parasites harmless, thorough cooking of snails would prevent infection.

Giant African land snails are frequent hosts of the angiostrongyliasis parasite. In Taiwan, angiostrongyliasis occurs most often among children who play with (and sometimes eat) the giant African land snail during the rainy months of June to October when they are most

Animal Importation

■ Introduction

The prevention of zoonotic diseases (those capable of transmission from animal to human populations) is the primary focus of animal importation regimes. Every nation (as well as supranational bodies such as the European Union) has established protocols concerning the admission of foreign animals into domestic jurisdictions. In the United States, various governmental departments and agencies assume concurrent jurisdiction for the development, promulgation (publishing), and enforcement of animal importation standards. The primary American bodies that direct these initiatives are the Centers for Disease Control (CDC), specifically the National Center for Zoonotic, Vector-Borne, and Enteric Diseases, and the United States Department of Agriculture (USDA).

■ History and Scientific Foundations

The organized transport of livestock and other domesticated animals has played an important role in human

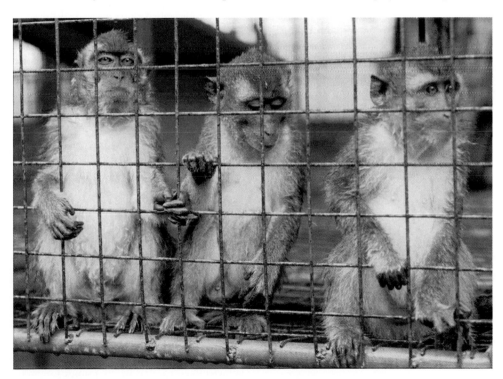

Three Philippine macaque monkeys are shown as they wait to be fed at a breeding farm south of Manila. More than 600 monkeys at the farm were ordered to be destroyed in 1979 following the discovery of an Ebola virus strain in two of them. The infected monkeys were shipped to the United States for scientific research. *AP Images.*

WORDS TO KNOW

EPIZOOTIC: The abnormally high occurrence of a specific disease in animals in a particular area, similar to a human epidemic.

PRIONS: Prions are proteins that are infectious. Indeed, the name prion is derived from "proteinaceous infectious particles." The discovery of prions and confirmation of their infectious nature overturned a central dogma that infections were caused by intact organisms, particularly microorganisms such as bacteria, fungi, parasites, or viruses. Since prions lack genetic material, the prevailing attitude was that a protein could not cause disease.

QUARANTINE: Quarantine is the practice of separating people who have been exposed to an infectious agent but have not yet developed symptoms from the general population. This can be done voluntarily or involuntarily by the authority of states and the federal Centers for Disease Control and Prevention.

STRAIN: A subclass or a specific genetic variation of an organism.

ZOONOSES: Zoonoses are diseases of microbiological origin that can be transmitted from animals to people. The causes of the diseases can be bacteria, viruses, parasites, and fungi.

food production since prehistoric times. The empires of Mesopotamia, Greece, and Rome employed successively more sophisticated methods to move desired animals more efficiently between various geographic regions.

The first Industrial Revolution (c.1780–1830) precipitated a European population surge that generated a corresponding demand for increased food production. After 1820, Britain was the world leader in the importation of cattle, securing both dairy and beef breeds from various parts of Europe to bolster its domestic stock. This burgeoning industry was essentially unregulated; any sickness or disease noted in an imported cattle herd or among domestic livestock that had contact with imported animals was regarded as a local phenomenon; contaminated beef was usually disguised by vendors and sold in the normal course of business.

In this *laissez-faire* industrial environment, the first great cattle epidemics swept both Britain and Europe after 1839. Foot and mouth disease (*aphthovirus*), bovine pleuro-pneumonia, and sheep pox were the most common of the epizootic outbreaks that posed significant challenges to veterinary medicine. The prominent British practitioner John Gamgee (1828-1886) was the first expert to propose the comprehensive government regulation of animals entering Britain to prevent "contagionism," his rudimentary appreciation of the viral properties of these newly identified animal plagues.

Rinderpest (*Morbillivirus*), a highly infectious and fatal bovine virus, became the impetus to European government regulation of imported cattle. In 1865, rinderpest caused the deaths of over 400,000 cattle in Britain alone and an estimated one million more livestock across continental Europe. Britain established the world's first state veterinary service that year. Rinderpest is transmitted between animals through direct physical contact and has remained a potent agricultural industry threat across modern Africa, where war and political unrest have often prevented effective regulation of cattle imports.

■ Applications and Research

There are three distinct but interrelated elements of the public interest that are addressed through governmental animal import controls: public health and disease prevention, the security of national food supplies, and enhanced scientific research capabilities.

Many types of imported livestock are intended for both breeding and direct food production. Cattle are the most prominent example of a dual-purpose animal. As all cattle breeds are susceptible to a myriad of highly contagious diseases, both zoonotic and bovine-specific, national import regulation is designed to anticipate such risks through mandatory inspections and reporting provisions.

The most prominent threat to the international animal importation regulatory framework was the discovery of bovine spongiform encephalopathy (BSE) in Britain in 1986. Also known as "mad cow disease," BSE is a progressive and fatal neurological condition that ultimately destroys the function of an animal's central nervous system. BSE is highly contagious, although the incubation period of the disease is in excess of five years. The precise cause of BSE remains unknown, although there is a scientifically validated relationship between the disease and the presence in a subject animal of infectious proteins known as prions. The disease is most likely transmitted through either direct animal-to-animal contact or through the ingestion of feed prepared from the bone marrow of infected animals. Creutzfeldt-Jakob Disease (CJD) is a condition similar to BSE that occurs in humans; a variant of CJD is capable of being transmitted to humans through the consumption of BSE-contaminated beef.

The danger of BSE to both livestock and humans is so sufficiently grave that when a single cow was determined to be afflicted with BSE in Washington State in 2003, the Canada-United States border was closed to all cattle imports between each nation for 15 months. As BSE has no known treatment or cure except to slaughter and incinerate the affected animal, national border authorities inevitably err on the side of caution when BSE is suspected.

Scientific research involving animal experiments engages additional animal importation issues. The scientific community places a premium upon the ability to use monkeys and other non-human primates for research purposes, given the physiological similarities between these animals and humans. Primates also represent a significant risk to the human population as disease carriers.

The Ebola and Marburg viruses are the most prominent component of the Filoviridae family. African and Southeast Asian primates are known carriers of the various forms of these viruses. The strain that causes Ebola Hemorrhagic Fever (EHF) is a remarkably virulent virus that is transmitted by direct contact with a contaminated person or through the exchange of bodily fluids. EHF will trigger an often fatal attack upon the contaminated person's internal organs. The four most prolific outbreaks of Ebola occurred in the African nations of Zaire, Sudan, Gabon, and Cote d'Ivoire between 1976 and 1997, killing hundreds of people; in each instance the EHF mortality rates exceeded 60%. A typical victim will die within 21 days of contracting this disease.

It was for these reasons that the identification of a new Ebola strain at a primate research facility in Reston, Virginia in 1989 attracted significant international attention and touched off a fresh consideration of American research animal importation controls. The Reston animals were monkeys imported from the Philippines. Twenty-one of the animals were determined to have contracted this Ebola strain (later referenced as Ebola-R). Four human handlers became ill from exposure to Ebola-R, but each subsequently recovered. As the epidemiology and pathology of all Ebola variants remains poorly understood, strict importation rules, including express CDC permission for non-human primates, remain in force in the United States. The primary risk concerning a recurrence of Ebola-R in the United States or elsewhere is that this strain may mutate at a future time into a variant that is deadly to the human population.

■ Impacts and Issues

The transport of pets across national borders is the third significant aspect of animal import regulation. Dogs and cats form the vast majority of such animals. The number of pet dogs owned worldwide is difficult to estimate; the two largest domestic dog populations are located in the United States (60 million dogs) and Brazil (30 million dogs) respectively. The sheer number of household pets and the corresponding ability of a large number of animal-borne zoonotic diseases to move quickly through a given population to infect both pets and humans has led to rigorous pet importation controls being enacted in most countries.

Exotic or unconventional pets, including large members of the cat family and various reptiles, are governed by species-specific regulations throughout the world. As an example, a turtle with a shell measuring less than 4 in (10 cm) in length may not be imported into the United States without the advance permission of the CDC, due to a heightened risk to humans that Salmonellosis, a bacterial disease caused by contact with the bacterium *Salmonella*, may be contracted through the handling of these creatures.

Dogs and cats are subject to similar entry and quarantine regulations in most Western nations. In the United States, a pet cat or dog entering the country must be both quarantined and be proven free of any contagious disease. The standard requirement is a certificate from a licensed veterinarian confirming that the animal is free of rabies or any other infectious disease. The USDA possesses the discretion to quarantine any pet entering the United States, but, as a general rule, once rabies certification is available the animal will not be quarantined. These regulations apply equally to animals imported as pets or for breeding purposes. The most common of the zoonotic diseases sought to be contained through import control are rabies (Lyssavirus, transmitted through the bite of an infected animal), ringworm (*Tinea*, a fungal skin disease), and roundworm (*Trinchinella spiralis*, a parasitic worm that attacks a mammal's gastrointestinal tract).

SEE ALSO *Ebola; Emerging Infectious Diseases; Globalization and Infectious Disease; Zoonoses.*

BIBLIOGRAPHY

Books

Swabe, Joanna. *Animals, Disease, and Human Society: Human-Animal Relations and the Rise of Veterinary Medicine.* London: Routledge, 1999.

Periodicals

Gips, Michael A. "Open Border, Insert Foot and Mouth." *Security Management* 45, 6 (2001): 14.

Grischow, Jeff D. "K.R.S. Morris and Tsetse Eradication in the Gold Coast, 1928-51." *Africa* 76, 3 (2006): 381-409.

Peters, C.J., and J.W. Leduc. "An Introduction to Ebola: The Virus and the Disease." *Journal of Infectious Diseases* Supp.1 (1999): 179-187.

Web Sites

Centers for Disease Control and Prevention. "Frequently Asked Questions about Animal Importation." <http://www.cdc.gov/ncidod/dq/faq_animal_importation.htm> (accessed June 8, 2007).

Bryan Davies

Anisakiasis

■ Introduction

Anisakiasis is an infection in humans caused by ingesting the larvae of nematodes (parasitic roundworms with long, cylindrical bodies) in raw or undercooked saltwater fish. When the larvae infect humans, the anisakiasis infection causes discomfort to the stomach and intestinal areas. According to the U.S. Food and Drug Administration's Center for Food Safety and Applied Nutrition, *Anisakis simplex* (herring worm) and *Pseudoterranova (Phocanema, Terranova) decipiens* (cod or seal worm) are linked to human infections in North America.

Before ingestion into the human body, anisakiads travel through a complex life cycle involving the ingestion by various marine and anadromous fish (those that breed by returning from the sea to the water bodies where they were born) and crustaceans.

Usually, marine life infected with *Anisakidae* larvae are only found in seawater because larvae need to grow within waters of higher salinity. It is also uncommon in areas where cetaceans (large ocean mammals like whales) are not found, such as waters in the southern North Sea.

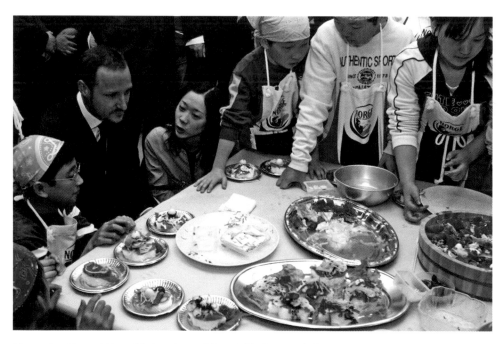

Norwegian Crown Prince Haakon (second from left) observes sixth graders preparing sushi using Norwegian salmon during a 2005 goodwill tour in Tokyo, Japan. People in countries such as Norway and Japan, where raw fish is often consumed, have the greatest incidence of contracting illnesses such as Anisakiasis that result from ingesting parasite-laden fish. *AP Images.*

Disease History, Characteristics, and Transmission

Human anisakiasis was first reported in Japan during the middle part of the twentieth century. *Anisakis simplex* and *Pseudoterranova decipiens* is found frequently inside saltwater fish. *P. decipiens* is found typically in temperate and arctic environments.

The characteristics of anisakids include a long, cylindrical body shape (what is called vermiform, or worm-like). It does not contain segments. The posterior part narrows to a cavity (pseudocoel), with the anus somewhat off-centered. The mouth is encircled by projections, which are used for sensing and feeding.

Transmission of the adult *Anisakis simplex* and *Pseudoterranova decipiens* begins in the stomach of marine mammals, specifically in the mucosa (mucous membranes). The eggs of female anisakids are expelled as feces of infected mammals. The eggs develop into embryos in seawater, where first-stage larvae are formed. The larvae then molt and become second-stage larvae. Upon hatching, free-swimming larvae are ingested by crustaceans, turning into mature, third-stage larvae.

Infected crustaceans are eaten by fish and squid, who become intermediate hosts. Inside fish, anisakids are coil-shaped. When uncoiled, their average length is 0.8 inches (2 centimeters). When these fish and squid die, the larvae move into muscle tissues. Anisakids transfer between fish when larger fish eat smaller ones. During these times, larvae are infective to humans and marine mammals. Sometimes, larvae are ingested by humans when infected seafood is eaten raw, is undercooked, or improperly prepared. After humans ingest third-stage larvae, the larvae attach themselves to, or burrow into, stomach or intestine tissues.

When third-stage larvae are digested by marine mammals, the larvae molt two times and develop into adult worms. These parasites are longer than two centimeters when uncoiled, with a thicker and sturdier body than when inside fish. The adult worms produce eggs that are expelled by marine mammals.

Scope and Distribution

Anisakiasis is found worldwide. However, it is more common in areas where raw fish is eaten such as Scandinavian countries, the Netherlands, Japan, and along the Pacific Ocean coast of South American countries. As of 2007, according to the FDA, Japan has the highest incidence of infection. The incidence of anisakiasis in the United States is unknown, but is thought to be fewer than 400 cases per year. Fish and marine mammals most affected include cod, crabs, cuttlefish, halibut, herring, mackerel, porpoises, rockfish, salmon, seals, sea lions, squid, tuna, and whales.

WORDS TO KNOW

ANADROMOUS: Fish that migrate from ocean (salt) water to fresh water, such as salmon, are termed anadromous.

INTERMEDIATE HOST: An organism infected by a parasite while the parasite is in a developmental form, not sexually mature.

NEMATODES: Also known as roundworms; a type of helminth characterized by long, cylindrical bodies.

PARASITE: An organism that lives in or on a host organism and that gets its nourishment from that host. The parasite usually gains all the benefits of this relationship, while the host may suffer from various diseases and discomforts, or show no signs of the infection. The life cycle of a typical parasite usually includes several developmental stages and morphological changes as the parasite lives and moves through the environment and one or more hosts. Parasites that remain on a host's body surface to feed are called ectoparasites, while those that live inside a host's body are called endoparasites. Parasitism is a highly successful biological adaptation. There are more known parasitic species than nonparasitic ones, and parasites affect just about every form of life, including most all animals, plants, and even bacteria.

Treatment and Prevention

Diagnosis cannot be accomplished from stool specimens. Instead, it is made by x-ray images and medical examinations of the patient's stomach and intestines using a flexible endoscope. In addition, microscopic examination of tissue can be made in which larvae are removed through biopsy or during surgery. *Anisakis simplex* and *Pseudoterranova decipiens* cannot survive in human hosts. They eventually die while inside the inflamed tissue.

In some case, invasive treatments may be attempted. Endoscopy may be used for the removal of larvae, especially in emergency cases involving obstruction or rupture of the bowel. Also, nasogastric suction (suction through a tube inserted through the nose and into the stomach) may be used, followed by drugs that target parasitic worms. If such action fails, worms can be removed surgically.

Surgical procedures sometimes may be avoided by drug treatments, including albendazole (marketed under

Albenza®, Eskazole®, and Zentel® brands). As of March 2007, albendazole has not been approved by the U.S. Federal Drug Administration (FDA) for treatment of the infection in the United States.

Anisakiasis infection can be prevented by heating seafood to a temperature higher than 122°F (50°C), or freezing it to at least −4°F (−20°C) for at least 24 hours. Such actions kill the larvae. If fish or shellfish is to be consumed raw or semi-raw, the FDA recommends that the food be blast frozen to −31°F (−35°C) or below for 15 hours, or regularly frozen to −4°F (−20°C) for seven days.

■ Impacts and Issues

When anisakid worms can infect humans, within several hours of ingestion they can produce severe sickness that affects the stomach and intestines. Sometimes the larvae are vomited or coughed up. Symptoms include vomiting, diarrhea, nausea, and severe abdominal pain that may resemble appendicitis, so cases are often misdiagnosed. With the increasing popularity of raw seafood dishes, government and medical organizations have made efforts to educate physicians to consider the possibility of anisakiasis in patients with these symptoms.

If larvae pass into the bowel, major symptoms may occur within one to two weeks due to tissue inflammation. They can also produce a minor chronic disease that causes stomach or intestinal irritation, which may last between weeks and years. These symptoms resemble stomach ulcers and tumors, or irritable bowel syndrome.

Fish and shellfish are important foods to maintain a healthy lifestyle. They are high in protein and other essential nutrients. However, the growing international popularity of eating such raw seafood dishes as sushi, sashimi, ceviche, and pickled herring, has produced an increase in the number of cases of anisakiasis, a trend that health authorities expect to continue upward.

SEE ALSO *Cancer and Infectious Disease; Food-borne Disease and Food Safety; Helminth Disease; Host and Vector; Parasitic Diseases; Tropical Infectious Diseases.*

BIBLIOGRAPHY

Books

Adley, Catherine C., ed. *Food-borne Pathogens: Methods and Protocols.* Totowa, NJ: Humana Press, 2006.

Guerrant, Richard L., David H. Walker, and Peter F. Weller. *Tropical Infectious Diseases: Principles, Pathogens, and Practice.* Philadelphia, PA: Elsevier Churchill Livingstone, 2006.

Parker, James N., and Philip M. Parker, eds. *The Official Patient's Sourcebook on Anisakiasis: A Revised and Updated Directory for the Internet Age.* San Diego, CA: Icon Health Publications, 2002.

Web Sites

Center for Food Safety and Applied Nutrition, Federal Food and Drug Administration. "*Anisakis simplex* and related worms." <http://www.cfsan.fda.gov/~mow/chap25.html> (accessed March 1, 2007).

Centers for Disease Control and Prevention. "Anisakiasis." <http://www.dpd.cdc.gov/dpdx/HTML/Anisakiasis.htm> (accessed March 1, 2007).

ProMED Mail, International Society for Infectious Diseases. "Anisakiasis—Israel: suspected." <http://www.promedmail.org/pls/promed/f?p=2400:1202:16245428003054921509::NO::F2400_P1202_CHECK_DISPLAY,F2400_P1202_PUB_MAIL_ID:X,23022> (accessed March 1, 2007).

Anthrax

■ Introduction

Anthrax is an infection caused by the bacterium *Bacillus anthracis*. Its name comes from the black spots that can appear on the body in the cutaneous (skin) form of the disease; to suggest the color of the spots, doctors used the Greek word for coal, "anthrax." Anthrax is usually transmitted through hardy spores that can survive in soil for decades. Anthrax exists naturally in many parts of the world as an infection of herbivores (plant-eating animals), such as cattle and sheep. Because its spores are small enough to become airborne, anthrax can be contracted by humans as a lung infection. In this form it is fatal in at least 95% of cases that do not receive immediate antibiotic treatment. Because

of the high fatality rate of the inhaled form of the disease, anthrax has been developed as a biological weapon by several major nations, including Japan, Russia, the United Kingdom, and the United States. No nation is known today to retain stocks of weaponized anthrax, but there is concern that terrorists might use anthrax as a weapon.

■ Disease History, Characteristics, and Transmission

History

Anthrax is a naturally occurring disease afflicting livestock and occasionally, through contact with livestock,

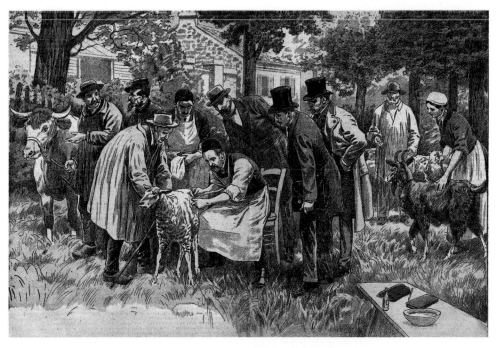

In this illustration, French microbiologist Louis Pasteur (1822–1895) is shown vaccinating sheep and other animals against anthrax. *© Stefano Bianchetti/Corbis.*

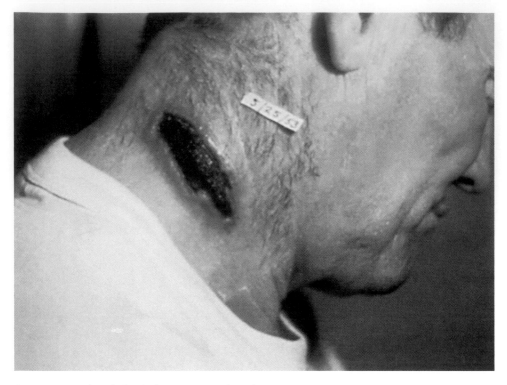

A cutaneous anthrax lesion is shown on a man's neck. © *CDC/PHIL/Corbis.*

humans. Records show that in Europe in the 1600s, a cattle disease that was almost certainly anthrax, called the Black Bane, killed about 60,000 cattle. Until the development of antibiotics and an effective veterinary vaccine for anthrax in the mid-twentieth century, anthrax was

WORDS TO KNOW

CUTANEOUS: Pertaining to the skin.

ENTERIC: Involving the intestinal tract or relating to the intestines.

HYPERENDEMIC: A disease that is endemic (commonly present) in all age groups of a population is hyperendemic. A related term is holoendemic, meaning a disease that is present more in children than in adults.

SPORE: A dormant form assumed by some bacteria, such as anthrax, that enable the bacterium to survive high temperatures, dryness, and lack of nourishment for long periods of time. Under proper conditions, the spore may revert to the actively multiplying form of the bacteria.

one of the most common causes of death for cattle, goats, horses, pigs, and sheep.

In 1876, the German physician Robert Koch (1843–1910) showed that a bacterium was responsible for the disease, making anthrax one of the first diseases to be identified as having a bacterial cause. Koch, who was awarded a Nobel Prize in Medicine in 1905, also discovered the bacterial causes of tuberculosis and cholera. Cattle were first successfully inoculated against anthrax in 1880 by the French biologist Louis Pasteur (1822–1895).

The use of anthrax in modern warfare began in 1915 during World War I, when a German-American agent working for the Imperial German Government set up a secret laboratory in Washington, D.C., to produce anthrax bacteria. These were then used to infect cattle and draft animals being shipped to the Allied armies in Europe. Several hundred Allied military personnel were infected by the anthrax-ridden cattle.

During World War II (1939–1945), anthrax was developed as a major weapon by several countries. A biological warfare unit, Unit 731, was formed in the Japanese Imperial Army, which carried out experiments on thousands of Chinese prisoners of war in the 1930s. In one facility, about 4,000 prisoners were killed by biological agents, mostly anthrax. By 1945, Japan had prepared about 880 lb (400 kg) of powdered anthrax spores for use in fragmentation bombs intended to spread the spores in the air to be inhaled. Japan

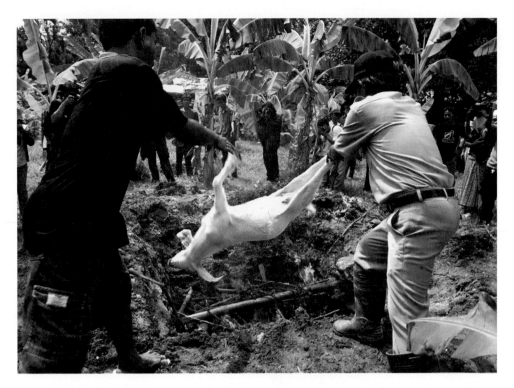

An Indonesian official (right) from the animal husbandry department gets help from a resident with burning goats suspected of being infected by anthrax disease in October 2004. The infected animals were destroyed after six people died of anthrax disease after consuming mutton from a sick goat. © *Dadang Tri/ Reuters/Corbis.*

surrendered before using anthrax bombs, but historians estimate that Japan may have killed over a half a million Chinese civilians using other forms of biological warfare. All members of Unit 731 were granted amnesty by the United States after the war in exchange for full disclosure of their wartime activities.

Japan was not the only country to place anthrax in bombs during World War II. In the United States, a major offensive biowar program was established at the Army's Camp Detrick, Maryland, in 1942. Anthrax and a number of other agents were developed as weapons there, and a plant for producing biological weapons was constructed near Terre Haute, Indiana. Thousands of anthrax bombs were produced, but none were used during the war. The British government, which was cooperating with the United States and Canada in developing anthrax as a weapon, contaminated the Scottish island of Gruinard with anthrax spores in 1942. Due to the long-lived nature of the spores, the island was off-limits for 48 years afterward, when it was finally decontaminated. The difficulty of decontaminating Gruinard shows how a large-scale attack with anthrax spores might render large areas of land uninhabitable. Decontamination of the small island involved soaking it in 308 tons (280 metric tons) of formaldehyde diluted in seawater and the removal of tons of topsoil in sealed containers.

The Soviet Union also instituted a biological warfare program during World War II, focusing on anthrax and other agents. The Soviet program continued for decades after the war, as did the U.S. program. In 1979, one of the worst anthrax outbreaks of the twentieth century occurred in the Ural Mountains in western Russia. The official toll was 96 people infected, resulting in 66 deaths, but the actual toll was probably higher. The Soviet government claimed that the outbreak was natural, but the United States and others accused the Soviets of violating the 1972 Biological and Toxic Weapons Convention. This treaty had been designed to ban the manufacture and stockpiling of biological and poison-gas weapons. In

IN CONTEXT: CULTURAL CONNECTIONS

The description of the sooty "morain" in the Book of *Exodus* is reminiscent of anthrax, and the disease is probably the "burning wind of plague" in Homer's *Iliad*. The mass death of horses and cattle (the primary targets of anthrax infection, along with sheep) during the Eurasian campaign of the Huns in 80 AD was also likely due to anthrax.

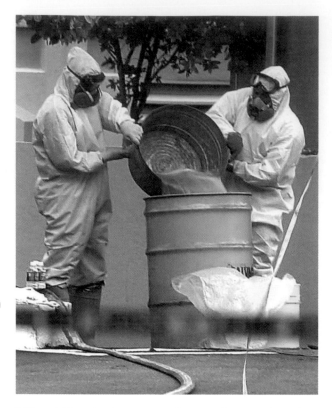

FBI special investigation team members wear hazmat suits as they work to decontaminate the American Media Inc. office in Florida in 2001. The publishing facility became a bio-hazard crime scene following the death of a worker from exposure to anthrax. *AP Images.*

the early 1990s, after the breakup of the Soviet Union, Russian and American scientists were able to study the 1979 outbreak in detail. They concluded that it was caused by an accidental release of anthrax spores from a military facility on the outskirts of the city Sverdlovsk (now called Yekaterinburg). All the cases in cattle and humans occurred in narrow oval pattern downwind of the facility.

In response to a 1969 decision by President Richard Nixon (1913–1994), the U.S. army destroyed all its anti-personnel biological warfare stocks, including anthrax, in 1971 and 1972.

The potential of even a small quantity of anthrax to disrupt a society and drain its resources was shown in 2001, when attacks were carried out through the U.S. mail using anthrax spores. The attacks began on September 18, a week after the attacks on the World Trade Center and Pentagon. Letters containing anthrax spores in powder form were mailed from a public mailbox in Princeton, New Jersey, and received by several TV networks, the newspaper the *New York Post,* and the offices of two senators, Tom Daschle (D-SD) and Patrick Leahy (D-VT). Five people were killed by the anthrax and seventeen others were made ill. (Neither of the senators

was infected.) As of early 2007, no group or individual had claimed responsibility for the attacks, and the case remained unsolved.

Early news reports characterized the 2001 anthrax powder as weapons-grade, but, in 2006, the U.S. Federal Bureau of Investigation (FBI) confirmed that the powder did not have any of the special technical features (such as a coating on the spores to keep them from sticking together) that would identify it as coming from a military facility.

Anthrax, like other biological weapons, has little value as a battlefield weapon. It has several disadvantages for combat use:

1. No disease acts quickly enough to be decisive in combat.

2. Wind and other factors make it difficult to deliver spores or viruses in a controlled way to enemy troops.

3. Soldiers are the best-defended of any target group, often being equipped with protective clothing, filter masks, and immunizations.

Biological weapons, whether employed by nation-states or smaller organizations, are therefore primarily a terror threat to civilian populations. The U.S. National Academy of Sciences estimated in 2003 that 2.2 lb (1 kg) of anthrax spores sprayed aerially over a large city could kill over 100,000 people. Anthrax spores could also render hundreds of square miles uninhabitable for a many decades by lodging in the soil, causing immense economic damage.

Characteristics

Anthrax bacteria in their vegetative form are shaped like rods about 1 millionth of a meter (1 μm) wide and 6 μm long. The vegetative form multiplies inside a host animal. When conditions are not right for anthrax to grow and multiply—namely, when temperature, acidity, humidity, and nutrient levels are outside the favorable range—some of the vegetative anthrax bacteria sporulate, that is, take on a spore form. A spore is an extremely small, one-celled reproductive unit that is usually able to survive extreme environmental conditions. Unlike a seed, a spore does not store a significant amount of nutrients. Anthrax spores can survive in soil or as a dry powder for many years and are the most common source of anthrax infection.

Once in the body, anthrax spores germinate and multiply. Toxins released by the bacteria cause the immune system to break down. In the final phase of infection, the bacteria build rapidly in the blood, doubling in number every 0.75–2 hours. At death, there may be more than 10^8 (100,000,000) anthrax bacteria per milliliter of blood. (A milliliter is about the size of a small drop.) Toxins from the bacteria break down the blood vessels, causing death by internal bleeding.

After death, the bacteria continue to multiply in the carcass. Large numbers of spores are shed to the surrounding soil. The anthrax life cycle is continued when other creatures either eat the flesh of the dead animal or ingest enough of the spores.

There are three basic types of anthrax infection: pulmonary, cutaneous, and gastrointestinal (also called enteric, meaning of the intestines) anthrax. Pulmonary or lung infection with anthrax is caused by inhalation of spores; cutaneous or skin infection is caused by entry of spores or bacteria into cuts or sores; and gastrointestinal infection is caused by eating anthrax-contaminated meat.

Transmission

Anthrax is usually contracted either by taking spores or bacteria into the body through a lesion (cut or open sore), through the bite of a fly, by eating the flesh of an anthrax-infected animal, or by inhaling spores. Direct transmission of anthrax between humans is extremely rare.

Humans are moderately resistant to anthrax. The infectious dose for inhalation anthrax, measured by spore count, is probably between 2,500 and 760,000 spores, the range recorded for non-human primates. The U.S. Department of Defense estimates that 8,000–10,000 spores is the anthrax LD50 for humans; LD50 stands for "lethal dose 50," the amount of an agent that will be fatal in about 50% of cases. Scientists have shown that in contaminated industrial settings, people can inhale over 1,000 anthrax spores per day without contracting the disease. When anthrax is developed as a weapon, it is meant to be delivered in extremely large quantities. For example, 220 lb (100 kg) of spores, often cited as a working figure in discussions of possible large-scale military use, contain about 10^{13} (10,000,000,000,000 or ten trillion) LD50 doses—about 1,500 times the population of the world. However, most of the spores distributed by a weapon would not end up being inhaled.

■ Scope and Distribution

As a naturally occurring disease, anthrax mostly afflicts cattle. In humans, it is relatively rare. Persons in agricultural settings in poor nations, who are likelier to contract the disease from livestock, account for the great majority of human anthrax cases worldwide. Natural anthrax remains hyperendemic or epidemic in about 14 countries today, including Burma (also known as Myanmar), Chad, Niger, Turkey, and Zambia. It is endemic in China, India, Indonesia, much of Latin America and Africa, and sporadic in most of the rest of the world, including Australia, the United States, and Europe. (A sporadic disease occurs only occasionally; an endemic disease coexists normally with its host population; a hyperendemic disease co-exists with its host population at a high rate; and an epidemic disease is one that episodically occurs at a high rate.) Human case rates are

highest today in central and southern Asia, the Middle East, and Africa.

The human anthrax rate normally depends on the livestock anthrax rate in a given area. There is about one human cutaneous anthrax case for every 10 anthrax-infected livestock carcasses processed and one enteric case for every 100–200 cutaneous cases. Inhalation anthrax is relatively rare.

■ Treatment and Prevention

Prevention of anthrax is based on breaking the cycle of infection, which primarily means controlling its appearance in livestock. The World Health Organization (WHO) of the United Nations is trying to set up a global network of anthrax experts and diagnostic laboratories to better monitor and respond to anthrax outbreaks worldwide. WHO says that the following steps must be rigorously implemented when dealing with anthrax-infected livestock:

1. Correct disposal of carcasses of animals with anthrax. This means deep burial, heat treatment, or incineration without a post-mortem (to avoid releasing spores).

2. Disinfection and disposal of all contaminated materials. This includes the processing of possibly infected animal hides before export, the incineration or burial of dung, the chemical sterilization of tools, and the thorough washing of hands.

3. Vaccination of susceptible animals and humans in at-risk occupations, such as those processing meat, hides, and wool.

Vaccination is not universal for livestock because of its expense. It is not universal for humans because of the expense and the risk of presently available anthrax vaccines. The only anthrax vaccine that is approved by the government for use in the United States—trade name Biothrax, first licensed in 1970—involves giving the subject six injections over 18 months. This vaccine is mandatory for some categories of U.S. military personnel and civilian defense contractors. However, because the potency of the vaccine varies greatly, some scientists argue that many military personnel have suffered health damage from the vaccine.

For persons in contact with human anthrax patients, prophylactic (preventative) antibiotics are given. Treatment of anthrax infection is with large doses of antibiotics, both swallowed (oral) and injected directly into the bloodstream (intravenous). Especially for inhalation anthrax, treatment must begin soon after infection—generally within a day and before symptoms are seen.

■ Impacts and Issues

In countries where anthrax is naturally present, it exacts a steady human and economic toll. Persons contracting the disease may die or live with a decreased quality of life. Animals that contract the disease must be destroyed, and their carcasses are economically worthless.

The mere threat of the use of anthrax as a weapon has caused the U.S. government to undertake extraordinary preventive efforts in addition to its military vaccination program. In 2004, as part of a $5.6 billion program called

Project BioShield, intended to protect the public from biological threats, the federal government ordered 75 million doses ($877 million worth) of a new anthrax vaccine from a private company, VaxGen Inc., to be stockpiled in case of an anthrax attack on the United States. The new vaccine was to have required no more than three separate injections. The U.S. Department of Health and Human Services (HHS) has also stockpiled over a billion antibiotic tablets, enough to treat 20 million people for two months. The new anthrax vaccine was to be delivered in 2006, but the program was delayed. In December 2006, HHS cancelled its contract with VaxGen because the company was not able to start human clinical trials of its new vaccine on time. This leaves Project Bioshield without a plan for producing an emergency stock of anthrax vaccine for public use.

SEE ALSO *Biological Weapons Convention; Bioterrorism; Koch's Postulates; War and Infectious Disease; Zoonoses.*

BIBLIOGRAPHY

Books

Sarasin, Philipp, and Giselle Weiss. *Anthrax: Bioterror as Fact and Fantasy.* Cambridge, MA: Harvard University Press, 2006.

Periodicals

Broad, William J. "Anthrax Not Weapons Grade, Official Says." *New York Times* (September 26, 2006).

Enserink, Martin, and Jocelyn Kaiser. "Accidental Anthrax Shipment Spurs Debate Over Safety." *Nature* 304 (2004): 1726–1727.

Hilts, Philip J. "'79 Anthrax Traced to Soviet Military." *New York Times* (November 18, 1994).

Lipton, Eric. "Bid to Stockpile Bioterror Drugs Stymied by Setbacks." *New York Times* (September 18, 2006).

Rosovitz, M.J., and Stephen H. Leppla. "Virus Deals Anthrax a Killer Blow." *Nature* 418 (2002): 825–826.

Web Sites

British Broadcasting Corporation. "Britain's 'Anthrax Island.'" July 25, 2001. <http://news.bbc.co.uk/2/low/uk_news/scotland/1457035.stm> (accessed January 30, 2007).

World Health Organization. "Guidelines for the Surveillance and Control of Anthrax in Humans and Animals." <http://www.who.int/csr/resources/publications/anthrax/WHO_EMC_ZDI_98_6/en/> (accessed January 30, 2007).

World Health Organization. "World Anthrax Data Site." September 30, 2003. <http://www.vetmed.lsu.edu/whocc/mp_world.htm> (accessed January 30, 2007).

Antibacterial Drugs

■ Introduction

Antibacterial drugs stop bacterial infections in two ways: they prevent bacteria from dividing and increasing in number, or they kill the bacteria. The former drugs, which prevent bacteria from increasing in number but do not kill the bacteria, are termed bacteriostatic drugs. The latter, which kill the infectious bacteria, are known as bactericidal drugs. Both types of drugs can stop an infection.

The terms antibacterial drugs and antibiotics are often used interchangeably. Though the most common antibacterial drugs are the many types of antibiotics, other compounds can also be considered antibacterial. One example is alcohol, which kills bacteria by dissolving the cell membrane. Another example is carbolic acid, which was famously used by Joseph Lister (1827–1912) in the mid-nineteenth century as a spray to prevent bacterial contamination of wounds during operations. Antibacterial agents such as alcohol and carbolic acid are more accurately considered disinfectants, chemicals that kill or inactivate bacteria on surfaces and instruments, rather than antibiotics, which are generally taken internally and can create resistant strains of bacteria.

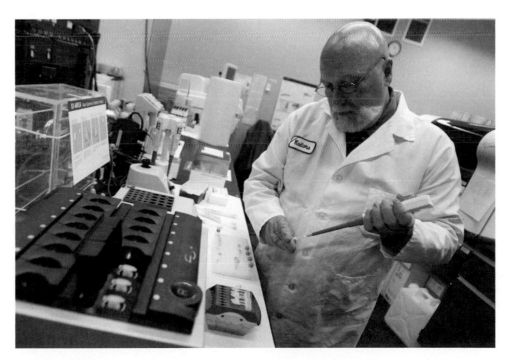

A technician loads patient samples with PCR reagents into a thermocycler, which heats and cools the samples and amplifies the DNA. Using fluorescence, the instrument then detects the resistant organism in the sample. The results are sent to a computer. *© Jerry McCrea/Star Ledger/Corbis.*

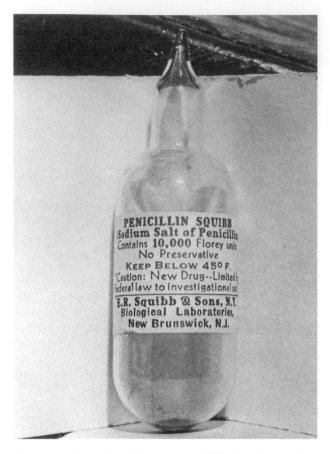

An early container of penicillin is shown c.1943 when the new drug was in short supply and mainly restricted to treating wounded soldiers in World War II.   © *Bettmann/Corbis.*

■ History and Scientific Foundations

The use of antibacterial drugs is ancient. Thousands of years ago, although the scientific basis of infection and its treatment was unknown, infections were sometimes successfully treated with molds and plants. Centuries later, the production of antibiotics by some species of molds and plants was discovered. One argument against the large-scale deforestation of regions, such as the Amazon basin, is that there are likely still many antibiotic-producing molds and plants yet to be discovered.

The antibiotic era began in the first decade of the twentieth century, when Paul Ehrlich (1854–1915) discovered a compound that proved to be an effective treatment for syphilis. In 1928, Sir Alexander Fleming (1881–1955) discovered the antibiotic penicillin. With recognition of the compound's prowess in killing a wide variety of bacteria, interest in antibiotics soared. In 1941, Selman Waksman (1888–1973) coined the term antibiotic. In the ensuing decades, much work focused on the discovery of new antibiotics from natural sources,

the laboratory alteration of existing compounds to increase their potency (and, later, to combat the problem of antibiotic resistance), and the synthesis of entirely new antibiotics.

Antibiotics kill bacteria in a variety of ways. Some alter the structure of the bacteria so that the bacteria become structurally weakened and unable to withstand physical stresses, such as pressure, with the result that the bacteria explode. Other antibiotics halt the production of various proteins in a number of ways: inhibiting the decoding of the genes specifying the proteins (transcriptional inhibition); blocking the production of the proteins following the production of the genetic message, messenger ribonucleic acid (mRNA, in a process termed translational inhibition); blocking the movement of the manufactured protein to its final location in the bacterium; or blocking the import of compounds that are crucial to the continued survival of the bacterium.

Some antibiotics—described as broad-spectrum—are effective against many different bacteria. Other antibiotics—described as narrow-spectrum—are very specific in their action and, as a result, affect fewer bacteria.

Penicillin is the classic example of a class of antibiotics known as beta-lactam antibiotics. The term beta-lactam refers to the ring structure that is the backbone of these antibiotics. Other classes of antibiotics, which are based on the structure and/or the mechanism of action of the antibiotic, are tetracyclines, rifamycins, quinolones, aminoglycosides, and sulphonamides.

Beta-lactam antibiotics kill bacteria by altering the construction of a portion of the bacterial membrane called the peptidoglycan. This component is a thin layer located between the inner and outer membranes of Gram-negative bacteria (an example is *Escherichia coli*) and a much thicker layer in Gram-positive bacteria (an example is *Bacillus anthracis*, the bacterium that causes anthrax). The peptidoglycan is a tennis racket-like mesh of sugar molecules and other compounds that is very strong when intact. This network has to expand to accommodate the growth of the bacteria. This is done by introducing breaks in the peptidoglycan so that newly made material can be inserted and incorporated into the existing network, cross-linking the newly inserted material with the older material. Beta-lactam antibiotics disrupt the final cross-linking step by inhibiting the activity of enzymes called penicillin-binding proteins, which are the enzymes that catalyze the cross-linkage. Other enzymes called autolysins also are released. The autolysins degrade the exposed peptidoglycan at the sites that are defectively cross-linked. The result is the weakening of the peptidoglycan layer, which causes the bacterium to essentially self-destruct.

Another class of antibiotics with a mode of action similar to the beta-lactam antibiotics are the cephalosporins. There have been various versions, or generations, of cephalosporins that have improved the ability

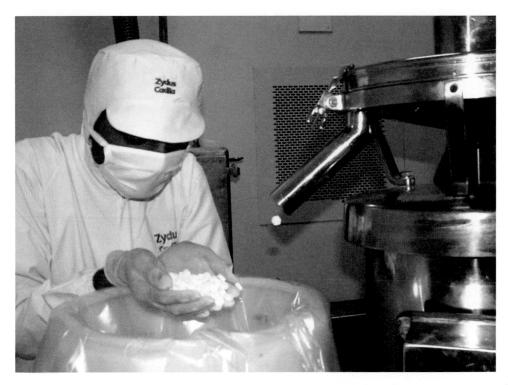

A technician from an Indian pharmaceutical company works to produce ciprofloxacin, which is used to combat anthrax. Production of the pills at this facility increased to 100,000 per hour as worldwide demand for the drug skyrocketed after anthrax spores were mailed to several locations in the United States in 2001. *AP Images.*

of these antibiotics to withstand enzyme breakdown. The latest cephalosporins are the fourth generation of these antibiotics.

Aminoglycoside antibiotics bind to certain regions of the cellular structure called ribosomes. Ribosomes are responsible for decoding the information contained in mRNA to produce proteins. By binding to the ribosome, aminoglycoside antibiotics disrupt protein production, which is often lethal for the bacterium.

As an final example, quinolone antibiotics impair an enzyme that unwinds the double helix of deoxyribonucleic acid (DNA). This unwinding must occur so that the genetic information can be used to make proteins and other bacterial components. These antibiotics kill bacteria at the genetic level.

■ Applications and Research

Every year, antibiotics continue to save millions of lives around the world. In less developed regions, where access to medical care can be limited, campaigns by the World Health Organization (WHO) and other agencies to distribute antibiotics have been invaluable in the response to epidemics of diseases such as cholera, plague, and yellow fever.

The discovery and manufacture of antibiotics continues. Screening of samples to uncover antibacterial properties has been automated; thousands of samples can be processed each day. Furthermore, the increased knowledge of the molecular details of the active sites of antibiotics and the ability to target specific regions have been exploited in the design of new antibiotics.

■ Impacts and Issues

In the decades after pencillin's discovery and use, many different antibiotics were discovered or synthesized and introduced for use. The control of bacterial infections became so routine that it appeared infectious diseases would become a problem of the past. However, that optimism has proven to be premature. Instead, some bacteria have developed resistance to a number of antibiotics. For example, bacterial resistance was first observed only about three years after the commercial introduction and widespread use of penicillin in the late 1940s. Penicillin-resistant staphylococcus bacteria were reported in 1944, and, by the 1950s, a penicillin-resistant strain of *Staphylococcus aureus* became a worldwide problem in hospitals. By the 1960s, most staphylococci were resistant to penicillin. Two decades ago it was rare to encounter methicillin-resistant *S. aureus* (MRSa). In

WORDS TO KNOW

ANTIBIOTIC: A drug, such as penicillin, used to fight infections caused by bacteria. Antibiotics act only on bacteria and are not effective against viruses.

ANTIBIOTIC RESISTANCE: The ability of bacteria to resist the actions of antibiotic drugs.

BACTERIOCIDAL: Bacteriocidal is a term that refers to the treatment of a bacterium such that the organism is killed. Bacteriostatic refers to a treatment that restricts the ability of the bacterium to grow. A bacteriocidal treatment is always lethal and is also referred to as sterilization.

BACTERIOSTATIC: Bacteriostatic refers to a treatment that restricts the ability of the bacterium to grow.

BROAD-SPECTRUM ANTIBIOTICS: Broad-spectrum antibiotics are drugs that kill a wide range of bacteria rather than just those from a specific family. For, example, Amoxicillin is a broad-spectrum antibiotic that is used against many common illnesses such as ear infections.

DISINFECTANT: Disinfection and the use of chemical disinfectants is one key strategy of infection control. Disinfectants reduce the number of living microorganisms, usually to a level that is considered to be safe for the particular environment. Typically, this entails the destruction of those microbes that are capable of causing disease.

NOSOCOMIAL: A nosocomial infection is an infection that is acquired in a hospital. More precisely, the Centers for Disease Control in Atlanta, Georgia, defines a nosocomial infection as a localized infection or one that is widely spread throughout the body that results from an adverse reaction to an infectious microorganism or toxin that was not present at the time of admission to the hospital.

2007, MRSa is a daily concern of a hospital's infection control challenge.

The effectiveness of an antibiotic to which bacteria have developed resistance can sometimes be restored by slightly modifying a chemical group of antibiotic. For example, the antibiotics ampicillin and amoxicillin are variants of penicillin. However, this strategy usually produces only a short-term benefit, since resistance to the altered antibiotic also develops.

One factor contributing to the growth of antibiotic resistance is the overuse or misuse of antibiotics. All the bacteria responsible for an infection may not be killed if an insufficient concentration of an antibiotic is used or if antibiotic therapy is stopped before the prescription has been used completely. The surviving bacteria may possess resistance to the antibiotic, which can sometimes be passed on to other bacteria. For example, tuberculosis has re-emerged as a significant health problem, especially for people whose immune systems are compromised, since the tuberculosis bacteria have developed resistance to the antibiotics used to treat them.

Acinetobacter baumannii is another bacterium that has developed resistance to many antibiotics. This bacterium is normally found in soil and water, and so is commonly encountered. While *Acinetobacter baumannii* infections were once confined to hospitals, where they accounted for about 80% of all nosocomial (hospital-acquired) infections, the bacterium now has become a growing problem for the military. Over 200 U.S. soldiers wounded in Iraq since 2003 have developed serious infections caused by multi-resistant *A. baumannii*, and military physicians have few treatment options for these infections.

New antibacterial drugs are expected to produce blockbuster sales for their manufacturers, as emerging resistant organisms push the development of new and efficient antibiotics into the forefront.

SEE ALSO *Antibiotic Resistance; Antimicrobial Soaps; MRSA.*

BIBLIOGRAPHY

Books

Bankston, John. *Joseph Lister and the Story of Antiseptics.* Hockessin, DE: Mitchell Lane Publishers, 2004.

Levy, Stuart B. *The Antibiotic Paradox: How the Misuse of Antibiotics Destroys Their Curative Powers.* New York: Harper Collins, 2002.

Thompson, Kimberly, and Debra Fulghum. *Overkill: Repairing the Damage Caused by Our Unhealthy Obsession with Germs, Antibiotics, and Antibacterial Products.* New York: Rodale Books, 2002.

Walsh, Christopher. *Antibiotics: Actions, Origins, Resistance.* Herndon, VA: ASM Press, 2003.

Brian Hoyle

Antibiotic Resistance

■ Introduction

Penicillin was the first antibiotic to be mass-produced for use in treating bacterial infections. Following its introduction during World War II (1939–1945), infections that had until then been difficult to treat became easy to cure. The next 20 years was a time of great optimism; scientists heralded that most, if not all, bacterial infections would be controlled by penicillin and additional antibiotics. In 1969, the U.S. Surgeon General William Stewart proclaimed, "It is time to close the book on infectious diseases. The war against pestilence is over."

This optimism proved to be premature. In fact, there had already been a hint of what was to come. Only three years after the introduction of penicillin, clinical infections caused by a penicillin-resistant form of the bacterium *Staphylococcus aureus* began to be reported. In the subsequent decades, antibiotic resistance has become a major concern in hospitals and in daily life. The problem does not have a single cause—bacteria have devised a number of ways to overcome antibiotics.

■ History and Scientific Foundations

By 1947, the antibiotic methicillin had been in widespread use for only two years. Nonetheless, resistance to this penicillin-related antibiotic by *S. aureus* was already known. This bacterium, since dubbed methicillin-resistant *S. aureus*, or MRSA, has become a huge problem, since it possesses resistance to a variety of other antibiotics commonly used to treat infections. As of 2007, about 50% of all infections caused by *S. aureus* in the United States are the result of MRSA.

Currently, there is only one antibiotic—vancomycin—that is effective against such multi-resistant bacteria. However, in 1997, a strain of *S. aureus* that also was resistant to vancomycin was reported in Japan. This resistant bacterium is now present in Europe and North America. While not yet as prevalent as MRSA, infection control experts warn that it is only a matter of time before the organism becomes more common.

Antibiotic resistance is present in other disease-causing bacteria as well. Acquisition of resistance has been a consequence of the use of antibiotics in hospitals. The selective pressure on a bacterium in a hospital is to develop antibiotic resistance, since the continued

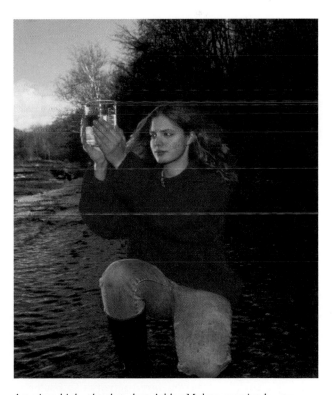

American high school student Ashley Mulroy examined water samples from the Ohio River and discovered the presence of antibiotics in the river and in the drinking water of her hometown. She observed that inefficient wastewater treatment, which results in antibiotic contamination, can lead to bacterial resistance. *Taro Yamasaki/Time Life Pictures/Getty Images.*

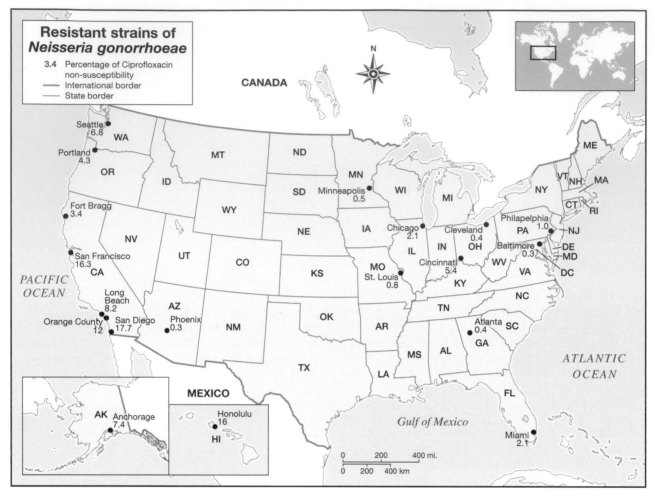

Resistant strains of
Neisseria gonorrhoeae

3.4 Percentage of Ciprofloxacin
non-susceptibility
—— International border
—— State border

Map showing Ciproflaxin resistance of strains of *Neisseria gonorrhoeae* in the United States, 2002. © *Copyright World Health Organization (WHO). Reproduced by permission.*

survival of the bacterium depends on its ability to thwart the antibiotic.

Bacteria can also become resistant to an antibiotic purely by chance. Changes in the bacterial deoxyribonucleic acid (DNA) can occur randomly. Portions of DNA may be inserted or removed, or there may be a substitution of some of the building blocks (nucleotides) of the DNA. If the change occurs in a portion of DNA that codes for a bacterial component, the result can be resistance to an antibiotic. For example, a change in the composition of the bacterial membrane may prevent an antibiotic from passing as easily to the inside of the cell, or the enhanced activity of a bacterial enzyme may degrade a particular antibiotic. This spontaneous antibiotic resistance is thought to be responsible for the appearance of drug resistance in the bacterium that causes tuberculosis, which has led to the resurgence of this lung infection.

A second way that antibiotic resistance can be acquired is by the transfer of some of the DNA from the chromosomes of one bacterium to another. This typically occurs when the two bacteria are connected to each other by a hollow tube (a sex pilus). DNA can pass down the tube from the donor bacterium to the recipient bacterium. The process can be interrupted by breaking the tube, and so the transfer of genetic material can often be incomplete.

The third means by which antibiotic resistance develops is the most worrisome. This also involves the transfer of DNA from one bacterium to another, but instead of the transfer of DNA from the chromosomes of the donor bacterium to the recipient bacterium, the DNA found in a circular piece of DNA—known as a plasmid—is transferred from donor to recipient. Transfer of the plasmid to a new bacterium can easily occur, and the inserted plasmid may not need to be part of the recipient's genome to produce whatever factor is responsible for antibiotic resistance.

Plasmid-mediated transfer can occur at a much higher frequency than the other types of DNA transfer, and, as a result, antibiotic resistance can spread quickly. Furthermore, the DNA transfer can be promoted by selection pressure. For example, the presence of antibiotics can encourage the transfer DNA coding for antibiotic resistance among populations of bacteria.

A plasmid may contain a number of genes that each code for resistance to a certain antibiotic, as well as the genetic information that enables all this information to be deciphered and the necessary resistance factors made. The plasmid only needs to get inside the recipient bacterium for that cell to become resistant to the antibiotics.

There are different mechanisms of antibiotic resistance. Change of the target site of an antibiotic can make the antibiotic less effective or completely ineffective. For example, some Gram-negative bacteria can become resistant to a class of antibiotics called beta-lactam antibiotics by a modification to proteins called penicillin-binding proteins. The modification keeps the beta-lactam antibiotics from disrupting the construction of peptidoglycan, a component that is vital to maintaining the structure of the bacterial membrane. Other mechanisms of antibiotic resistance include the increased ability of the bacterium to pump an antibiotic back out of the cell, and the production of enzymes by the bacteria that can destroy the incoming antibiotic.

Laboratory tests can determine whether the bacteria isolated from an infection are resistant to antibiotics; which antibiotics the microbe is resistant to; and, most importantly for treatment, which antibiotics can kill the microbe. Typically, this testing involves adding the bacteria to the surface of a solid nutrient. The bacteria are spread over the surface so that they will grow as a continuous layer (often called a lawn). At about the same time, discs of a paper-like material that have been soaked in various concentrations of antibiotics are positioned on the nutrient surface. When the bacteria eventually grow, there will be circular clear zones devoid of bacteria wherever the antibiotic has been effective in killing the bacterial cells. Measurement of the diameter of these so-called inhibition zones can be used to determine how sensitive a particular type of bacteria is to the particular antibiotic. An automated version of this test also exists, but the basic design of the test is similar.

■ Applications and Research

Antibiotic resistance now involves a race between the development and introduction of an antibiotic and the development of bacterial resistance to the drug. Antibiotic discovery or synthesis is a long and costly process. This has hampered antibiotic research, since a pharmaceutical company needs to have a reasonable expectation of recouping

WORDS TO KNOW

BACTERIOPHAGE: A virus that infects bacteria. When a bacteriophage that carries the diphtheria toxin gene infects diphtheria bacteria, the bacteria produce diphtheria toxin.

MRSA: Methicillin-resistant *Staphylococcus aureus* are bacteria resistant to most penicillan-type antibiotics, including methicillin.

PLASMID: A circular piece of DNA that exists outside of the bacterial chromosome and copies itself independently. Scientists often use bacterial plasmids in genetic engineering to carry genes into other organisms.

the hundreds of millions of dollars spent on drug development before the drug becomes clinically less useful.

For some antibiotics, effectiveness can be regenerated relatively easily by modifying the three-dimensional structure of the molecule. Even a slight alteration involving the replacement of one chemical group in the molecule by another can restore the potency of the drug. Unfortunately, this effectiveness tends to be short-term. Within several years, bacteria can adapt to the modified drug and once again become resistant.

Research continues to try and find new mechanisms of antibiotic resistance. By understanding how bacteria become resistant to antibiotics, researchers hope to discover or design drugs that will kill the bacteria without stimulating the development of resistance. One approach that is promising is the use of bacteriophages—viruses that specifically infect and make new copies inside of a certain type of bacteria. Different bacteriophages each infect a particular bacterium. Since bacteriophages have been around for millions of years without the development of resistance by the target bacteria, researchers have been experimenting with the use of bacteriophages to deliver a toxic payload of antibacterial compounds. As of 2007, the research seems promising.

■ Impacts and Issues

Antibiotic resistance is a problem that humans have created through the misuse and overuse of antibiotics. For example, it was once common practice to prescribe antibiotics for almost all illnesses, even those caused by viruses. Since viruses are not affected by antibiotics, this approach only served to exert a selection pressure favoring the development of resistance on the bacteria already present. In addition, antibiotics continue to be widely used in the poultry

IN CONTEXT: REAL-WORLD RISKS

Bacteria can adapt to the antibiotics used to kill them. This adaptation, which can involve structural changes or the production of enzymes that render the antibiotic useless, can make a particular bacterial species resistant to a particular antibiotic. Furthermore, a given bacterial species will usually display a spectrum of susceptibilities to antibiotics, with some antibiotics being very effective and others ineffective. For another bacterial species, the pattern of antibiotic sensitivity and resistance will be different. Thus, for diagnosis of an infection and for clinical decisions regarding the best treatment, tests of an organism's response to antibiotics are essential.

and cattle industries to enhance the weight gain of the birds or livestock. This practice involves giving antibiotics to healthy animals rather than using them to treat infections. It encourages the development of resistant bacteria, and this resistance can be passed to other bacterial populations.

Since 2000, the prevalence of community-associated MRSA (CA-MRSA) has been increasing. CA-MRSA infections are found in healthy people interacting normally in their community, not among those who have been hospitalized within the past year or had recent medical procedures, such as dialysis or surgery. This type of antibiotic resistance is especially challenging for health authorities, since it indicates that antibiotic resistance is capable of developing and spreading in the absence of antibiotic use. Recent outbreaks of community-associated MRSA occurred in Los Angeles county, California, and Chicago, Illinois, in 2004.

■ Primary Source Connection

In the following op-ed column published by the *New York Times* during the intense media coverage surrounding the 2001 anthrax attacks on the U.S. Postal Service, the Senate, and various media outlets, the authors Ellen K. Silbergeld and Polly Walker describe the dangers of the careless use of powerful antibiotics. At the time of publication, Ellen K. Silbergeld was professor of epidemiology at the University of Maryland School of Medicine. Polly Walker was associate director of the John Hopkins Center for a Livable Future.

What If Cipro Stopped Working?

Cipro, despite its current fame for preventing and treating anthrax, is in danger of becoming a casualty of what might be called the post-antibiotic age. Bayer, the maker of Cipro, also sells a chemically similar drug called Bay-

tril, which is used in large-scale poultry production worldwide. The widespread use of Baytril in chickens has already been shown to decrease Cipro's effectiveness in humans for some types of infections.

Bayer recommends that Baytril be used only to treat infected poultry and says it poses no threat to public health. But the use of antibiotics in agriculture is part of a serious public health problem in the United States. According to the Union of Concerned Scientists, as much as 70 percent of all antibiotics produced in the United States are fed to healthy livestock for "growth promotion" in other words, to increase their weight for market. Not only does this reduce their effectiveness in animals; it poses a real danger to humans.

The discovery and use of antibiotics to treat human disease and save lives is one of the greatest feats of modern medicine. Many of us are alive today because of antibiotics. Just 60 years ago, the discovery of antibiotics revolutionized medicine, tipping the balance in our favor against the sea of pathogens that surrounds us. Now, with the very real threat of biological terrorism, preserving the power of antibiotics is a matter of the highest urgency.

Bacteria have always adapted to our new drugs faster and more efficiently than we can adapt to their genetic changes. Through prudent use, we can preserve the effectiveness of our drugs for use in treating human disease while we search nature and chemistry for new defenses. Yet we are now squandering this precious resource by using powerful antibiotics carelessly for livestock and poultry— mostly for nontherapeutic reasons.

Agribusiness argues that nontherapeutic use of antibiotics is essential to the continued supply of cheap food. But many countries have demonstrated that food can be safely and efficiently produced without robbing the medicine chest. In the European Union, the nontherapeutic use of antibiotics in agriculture has been banned.

The use of antibiotics in food animal production increases the risks of contracting drug-resistant infections from eating animal products. Despite a national network for testing food, every year the Centers for Disease Control and Prevention reports incidents of food poisoning by drug-resistant bacteria. In addition, using antibiotics in agriculture can result in environmental pollution by both drugs and drug-resistant bacteria.

Last month, the New England Journal of Medicine reported that drug-resistant bacteria were present in meat purchased at supermarkets in the Washington, D.C., area. An accompanying editorial recommended that the use of nontherapeutic antibiotics in farm animals be prohibited.

We need better information and more government oversight in this arena. Opinions differ on the amount of antibiotics currently used in animal production. Creating a national tracking system to measure how much of each antibiotic is used and for what purposes—as proposed by the Food and Drug Administration—is a necessary first step. Mandatory reporting of antibiotic use was discussed in January at meetings sponsored by the F.D.A., but no actual legislation or regulations have been proposed.

For Bayer, the maker of Baytril, the need for action is clear. The use of Baytril falls into a gray area between growth promotion and treatment; it is common practice in the poultry industry to add Baytril to drinking water during the last weeks of a flock's life, even if no disease has been diagnosed. Last year, the F.D.A. asked Bayer and Abbott Laboratories, the two producers of the chicken drug, to withdraw their Cipro-like antibiotics from agricultural use voluntarily. Abbott agreed. Bayer did not.

Bayer has committed itself to supporting our national efforts to protect the public health by supplying Cipro at a reduced cost to the federal government. Voluntarily withdrawing Baytril from the market would show that the company is serious about its commitment to the public health.

Ellen K. Silbergeld
Polly Walker

SILBERGELD, ELLEN K., AND POLLY WALKER. "WHAT IF CIPRO STOPPED WORKING?" *NEW YORK TIMES* (NOVEMBER 3, 2001). AVAILABLE ONLINE AT <HTTP://QUERY.NYTIMES.COM/GST/ FULLPAGE.HTML?SEC=HEALTH&RES=9C0DEED91F30F93 0A35752C1A9679C8B63>.

SEE ALSO *Antibacterial Drugs; MRSA.*

BIBLIOGRAPHY

Books

Salyers, Abigail A., and Dixie D. Whitt. *Revenge of the Microbes: How Bacterial Resistance Is Undermining the Antibiotic Miracle.* Washington, DC: ASM Press, 2005.

Periodicals

Wickens, Hayley, and Paul Wade. "Understanding Antibiotic Resistance." *The Pharmaceutical Journal* 274 (2005): 501–504.

Zoler, Mitchel L. "Long-term, Acute Care Hospitals Breed Antibiotic Resistance." *Internal Medicine News* 37 (September 15, 2004): 51–52.

Brian Hoyle

Antimicrobial Soaps

■ Introduction

Antimicrobial soaps refer to solutions that are designed to lessen the number of living (viable) microorganisms on the surface of the skin. As they are usually rubbed on the skin during handwashing, the most common form of the antimicrobial product is a soap.

The main target of antimicrobial soaps are the bacteria that commonly live on (colonize) the surface of the skin. These include bacteria in the genera of *Staphylococcus* and *Streptococcus*. Normally, these bacteria are innocuous; they do not cause harm to the host. But, if they gain access to niches inside the body due to a cut or other injury, they can cause serious and even life-threatening diseases. An example is the contamination of implanted heart valves by *Staphylococcus aureus*, which can cause endocarditis. By handwashing with an antimicrobial soap for an adequate length of time (at least one minute) to lessen the number of living *S. aureus* on the skin prior to heart valve surgery, a surgeon can diminish the risk of infecting the patient.

Antimicrobial soaps are also a common part of the home. The ubiquitous bar of soap in the shower and by the bathroom sink is an example of an antimicrobial soap.

■ History and Scientific Foundations

The use of antibacterial soap began in the mid-nineteenth century. At that time, the Viennese physician Ignaz Semmelweiss (1818–1865) noted the markedly higher death rate among hospitalized patients who received care from medical students, versus patients cared for by midwives. Semmelweiss determined that it was a common practice for the students to come from dissection and teaching labs to the hospital ward without washing their hands. By instituting a handwashing pol-

icy, the previous high death rate was almost completely eliminated.

With time came the knowledge that bacteria and other disease causing microorganisms such as fungi could be transferred from person to person on the skin of the caregiver. The use of antimicrobial compounds in soaps gained credence in the several decades following World War II (1939–1945), with the expanded use of antibiotics to treat bacterial diseases. The initial overwhelming success of antibiotics made the incorporation of antimicrobials into other products a health priority.

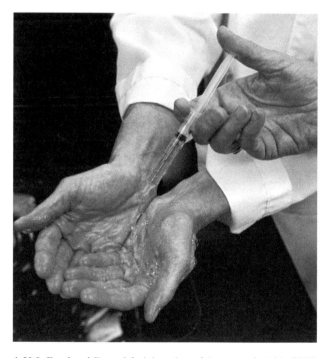

A U.S. Food and Drug Administration advisory panel said in 2005 that antibacterial soaps offer no more protection than regular soap and water in everyday use. In addition, the overuse of such soaps could potentially contribute to the development of bacteria resistant to antibiotics. *AP Images.*

The principle ingredient that has been most commonly used in antimicrobial soaps is triclosan. The compound contains a phenol ring structure to which are attached chlorine groups. The phenol ring is very difficult to break apart, which means that bacteria and fungi are less apt to be capable of degrading the triclosan molecule to a form that is inactive. As well, chlorine has a potent antibacterial and antifungal effect.

Triclosan has many sites of action in bacteria and fungi, which can vary depending on the applied concentration of the compound. For example, at the concentrations typically found in antibacterial soaps, triclosan binds to and inhibits the activity of a variety of proteins and other cell components both in the bacterial or fungal membranes and in the cytoplasm—the dense fluid that fills the interior of the microorganisms. The cytoplasmic targets are mainly enzymes—proteins that function to speed up chemical reactions, including those that are vital to cell survival. The multiple inactivations caused by triclosan are too much for the bacteria or fungi to overcome and they are rapidly killed.

Another antimicrobial compound used in soaps is triclocarban. This compound also has ring structures and chlorine groups, and its antimicrobial activity is similar to that of triclosan.

■ Applications and Research

Antibacterial soaps are a standard feature of hospitals and other health care facilities, where the need to control the spread of infections is essential. For example, the use of antibacterial soap or other type of skin wash is very important in controlling the spread of a type of bacteria designated methicillin resistant *Staphylococcus aureus* (MRSA) from ward to ward in hospitals. This is because MRSA is resistant to many antibiotics, and so can be difficult to treat once present in a hospital. A patient whose immune system is not functioning efficiently can become extremely ill or can die if infected with MRSA.

Other triclosan containing products have become more widely popular in everyday life. Examples of commercially available antimicrobial soaps include the facial wash marketed as Clearasil®, which is designed to lessen the development of acne, and Dial Complete® soap.

■ Impacts and Issues

While antimicrobial soaps have been very effective in controlling the spread of infectious diseases, their overuse or misuse may be promoting the development of bacteria that are resistant to triclosan. Studies with *Escherichia coli* have indicated that the genetic alterations that render the bacteria resistant to triclosan might also confer resistance to other antibacterial compounds including some antibiotics. Put another way, the use of

---

WORDS TO KNOW

COLONIZATION: Colonization is the process of occupation and increase in number of microorganisms at a specific site.

RESISTANT ORGANISM: Resistant organisms are bacteria, viruses, parasites, or other disease-causing agents that have stopped responding to drugs that once killed them.

TRICLOSAN: A chemical that kills bacteria. Most antibacterial soaps use this chemical.

IN CONTEXT: EFFECTIVE RULES AND REGULATIONS

Disinfection is a key strategy of infection control. Disinfection refers to the reduction in the number of living microorganisms to a level that is considered to be safe for the particular environment. Typically, this entails the destruction of those microbes that are capable of causing disease.

Disinfection is different from sterilization, which is the complete destruction of all microbial life on the surface or in the liquid. The steam-heat technique of autoclaving is an example of sterilization.

There are three levels of disinfection, with respect to power of the disinfection. High-level disinfection will kill all organisms, except for large concentrations of bacterial spores, using a chemical agent that has been approved as a so-called sterilant by the United States Food and Drug Administration. Intermediate level disinfection is that which kills mycobacteria, most viruses, and all types of bacteria. This type of disinfection uses a chemical agent that is approved as a tuberculocide by the United States Environmental Protection Agency (EPA). The last type of disinfection is called low-level disinfection. In this type, some viruses and bacteria are killed using a chemical compound designated by the EPA as a hospital disinfectant.

---

antimicrobial soaps may drive the bacteria to become more resistant and so a greater threat to health.

An important reason has been the expansion in the use of triclosan containing soaps in the home. Consumers have become more conscious of the possible health threat of microorganisms and the marketplace has responded by formulating products designed for everyday use. Unfortunately, if a microorganism is exposed to a sub-lethal concentration of triclosan, or not exposed to the compound long enough due to inadequate washing (the soap needs to be present on the skin for 30–45 seconds), the microbe

IN CONTEXT: PERSONAL RESPONSIBILITY AND PROTECTION

Improper handwashing can be dangerous. Particularly harsh soaps, or very frequent handwashing (for example, 20–30 times a day) can increase the acidity of the skin, which can counteract some of the protective fatty acid secretions. Also the physical act of washing will shed skin cells. If washing is excessive, the protective microflora will be removed, leaving the newly exposed skin susceptible to colonization by another, potentially harmful microorganism. Health care workers, who scrub their hands frequently, are prone to skin infections and damage.

IN CONTEXT: EFFECTIVE RULES AND REGULATIONS

In October 2005, a U.S. Food and Drug Administration panel advised that washing with popular antibacterial soaps and gels in the home was no more effective in preventing infections than washing with plain soap and water. The panel is currently considering recommendations for stricter rules in advertising and labeling of antibacterial products. The panel excluded alcohol-based antibacterial gels from the advisory, which were considered useful in preventing infections where adequate soap and water were not accessible.

may survive and become more resistant to the antimicrobial agent. If this resistance has been acquired because of a genetic alteration, the trait can be passed to future generations of microorganisms.

The link between triclosan resistance and resistance to other agents is contentious. While some studies published since 2003 have not found evidence of a link, other studies have. For example, triclosan has been demonstrated to be capable of blocking the manufacture of fatty acids, molecules vital to the construction of membranes. The altered membrane can make some bacteria resistant to antibiotics that formerly killed them.

The expanded and less controlled use of antimicrobial soaps is also a concern in light of a study published in 2006 that demonstrated that low doses of triclosan in the environment from domestic wastes cause hormonal alterations in the North American bullfrog. This indicates that there may be detrimental changes associated with the discharge of low levels of antimicrobial soaps into the environment.

SEE ALSO *Disinfection; Germ Theory of Disease; Handwashing; Resistant Organisms.*

BIBLIOGRAPHY

Books

Bankston, John. *Joseph Lister and the Story of Antiseptics.* Hockessin, DE: Mitchell Lane Publishers, 2004.

McDonnell, Gerald E. *Antisepsis, Disinfection, and Sterilization: Types, Action, and Resistance.* Washington, DC: ASM Press, 2007.

Tortora, Gerald J., Berdell R. Funke, and Christine L. Case. *Microbiology: An Introduction. 9th ed.* New York: Benjamin Cummings, 2006.

Web Sites

Centers for Disease Control and Prevention. "Antibacterial Household Products: Cause for Concern." <http://www.cdc.gov/ncidod/eid/vol7no3_supp/levy.htm> (accessed April 29. 2007).

Brian Hoyle

Antiviral Drugs

■ Introduction

Antiviral drugs are used to prevent or treat viral infections. They are antimicrobial compounds, as are antibiotics. However, antiviral compounds do not have the same mode of action as antibiotics. This is because most antibiotics rely on the ability of the bacteria to grow and divide. Bacteria grow and divide independently. In contrast, viruses must infect a host cell before they can exploit the host cell's genetic machinery to manufacture the components of new virus particles. Antibiotics are useless against viruses, both because viruses are localized inside of another cell or tissue, and because viruses are not alive in the absence of the host cell.

Antibiotics and antiviral drugs are similar in that specific drugs are designed for specific targets. For example, anti-retroviral drugs specifically inhibit infections caused by retroviruses, such as the human immunodeficiency virus (HIV). Other antiviral drugs specifically target other viruses, including herpes viruses and the various hepatitis viruses.

■ History and Scientific Foundations

The history of antiviral compounds dates back only to the 1960s. Prior to that time, a viral illness had to run its course. In the 1960s, antiviral drugs were developed to deal with herpes infections (which include cold sores, genital infection, chickenpox, mononucleosis, and Kaposi's sarcoma). At that time, the development of the drugs was more a trial-and-error process than a directed process. The process typically involved growing cultures of a particular type of cell and then infecting the cells with a particular virus. Successful infection is often apparent by a change in the appearance of the host cell. By adding compounds during the infection, researchers could monitor whether the visible signs of infection occurred or not. The absence of changes in the host cells was an indication that the particular compound was a potential antiviral agent.

This process was tedious and time-consuming. Beginning in the 1970s, advances in molecular biology made antiviral drug design more focused. The genetic sequences of disease-causing viruses began to be determined. In addition, it was learned that many viruses initiated infection by recognizing and binding to sites on the surface of host cells. As the three-dimensional

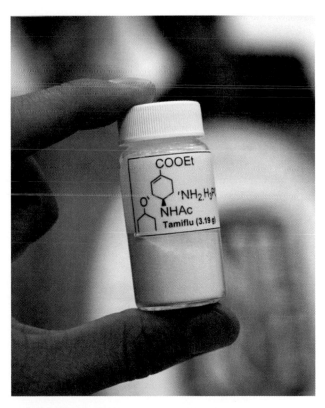

Several facilities worldwide are licensed to produce generic versions of the antiviral drug Tamiflu in preparation of a possible avian (bird) flu pandemic. © *Richard Chung/Reuters/Corbis.*

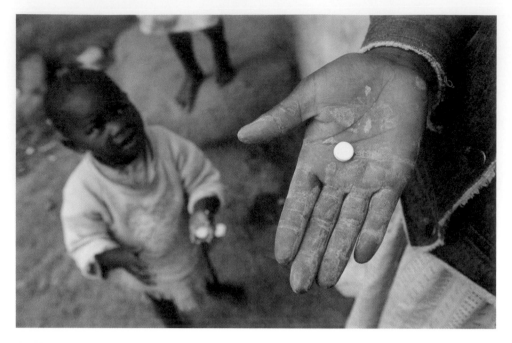

An HIV-positive mother takes a break from painting her house to take her ARV medication in South Africa. She is now able to use this generic fix-dose combination drug, Triomune, instead of three separate pills. This makes it easier for her to take all the needed medication. © *Gideon Mendel/Corbis.*

shapes of these host sites and the molecular details of the binding of the virus were clarified, it became possible to design compounds to block the binding.

The binding process can be blocked in two ways. In one approach, the target site on the host surface is occupied by an added molecule. Because the site is occupied, the virus is unable to bind to it. In the second approach, the viral recognition site is blocked by the addition of a molecule. The blocking molecule may be an antibody—a protein that is produced by the immune system—that has been produced in the laboratory. Then virus particles cannot gain access to the host cell; they are stranded outside the host cells and can be destroyed when they are recognized by the hosts' immune system, which causes antiviral immune molecules to be made and deployed.

This strategy of blocking viral infection very early in the infectious process is the basis of some viral vaccines. It can be very successful if the host or viral target sites do not change. However, in viral infections such as influenza, the viral site can change from year to year. A vaccine designed for the viral strain that dominates one year may be ineffective the next year, which is why new influenza vaccines need to be produced and administered prior to each flu season.

Some antiviral drugs operate slightly differently, by blocking the uptake of virus into the host cell. Other antiviral drugs prevent the infecting virus from using the host cell's genetic replication (duplication) mechanisms.

The numbers of infecting viruses are not reduced, but, because the infection process is blocked, new viruses are not made. Once again, the host's immune system can more easily deal with the stranded viruses.

Two antiviral drugs, idoxuridine and trifluridine, halt viral infection at the genetic level. These drugs act by replacing one of the units (a compound called thymidine) that forms the genetic material. The drugs are able to do this because their structure is similar to the structure of thymidine. The incorporation of either drug produces DNA that does not function. Other drugs mimic other compounds, and their incorporation produces the same result. However, the drugs can also be incorporated into the DNA of the host cells, which disrupts their function. This action can cause side effects, but if the infection is stopped it can be worthwhile in the longer term.

Other antiviral drugs, such as acyclovir, target an enzyme produced by the virus, usually early in the infection, that is vital for the replication of the genetic material. The drug binds to the enzyme, which prevents the enzyme from binding to its normal target. As a result, DNA formation stops. Acyclovir is used to treat infections due to herpes simplex viruses and Epstein-Barr virus.

Zidovudine (AZT) acts against HIV by blocking the activity of the reverse transcriptase enzyme. This enzyme makes it possible for the infecting virus to convert its RNA to DNA, and this DNA is subsequently used by the

60

INFECTIOUS DISEASES: IN CONTEXT

WORDS TO KNOW

ANTIBODY: Antibodies, or Y-shaped immunoglobulins, are proteins found in the blood that help to fight against foreign substances called antigens. Antigens, which are usually proteins or polysaccharides, stimulate the immune system to produce antibodies. The antibodies inactivate the antigen and help to remove it from the body. While antigens can be the source of infections from pathogenic bacteria and viruses, organic molecules detrimental to the body from internal or environmental sources also act as antigens. Genetic engineering and the use of various mutational mechanisms allow the construction of a vast array of antibodies (each with a unique genetic sequence).

ENZYME: Enzymes are molecules that act as critical catalysts in biological systems. Catalysts are substances that increase the rate of chemical reactions without being consumed in the reaction. Without enzymes, many reactions would require higher levels of energy and higher temperatures than exist in biological systems. Enzymes are proteins that possess specific binding sites for other molecules (substrates). A series of weak binding interactions allow enzymes to accelerate reaction rates. Enzyme kinetics is the study of enzymatic reactions and mechanisms. Enzyme inhibitor studies have allowed researchers to develop therapies for the treatment of diseases, including AIDS.

MESSENGER RIBONUCLEIC ACID (MRNA): A molecule of RNA that carries the genetic information for producing one or more proteins; mRNA is produced by copying one strand of DNA, but in eukaryotes is able to move from the nucleus to the cytoplasm (where protein synthesis takes place).

REPLICATION: A process of reproducing, duplicating, copying, or repeating something, such as the duplication of DNA or the recreation of characteristics of an infectious disease in a laboratory setting.

RESISTANCE: Immunity developed within a species (especially bacteria) via evolution to an antibiotic or other drug. For example, in bacteria, the acquisition of genetic mutations that render the bacteria invulnerable to the action of antibiotics.

STRAIN: A subclass or a specific genetic variation of an organism.

host cell's replication machinery to produce new viral constituents. The compound can become incorporated into the host cell DNA, which also blocks the replication of viral genetic material. AZT is beneficial in reducing the transmission of HIV from a pregnant woman to her developing fetus and to her newborn during labor or breastfeeding.

Still other antiviral drugs focus on translation—the process whereby the messenger ribonucleic acid (mRNA) (which is formed from instructions encoded in DNA) is used to manufacture compounds, such as protein. Some antiviral drugs block mRNA formation and disrupt the translation process. Antiviral therapy also involves molecular tools. The best example is oligonucleotides, which are sequences of the building blocks of genetic material that are deliberately made to be complimentary to a target sequence of viral genetic material. The term complimentary means that the two sequences are able to chemically associate with one another. When the oligonucleotide binds to a stretch of viral genetic material, it prevents that stretch from being used in viral replication. One oligonucleotide-based drug is available for the treatment of eye infections in patients with

acquired immunodeficiency syndrome (AIDS, also cited as acquired immune deficiency syndrome).

■ Applications and Research

The different mechanisms of action of different antiviral drugs have been useful in treating a variety of viral infections. For example, acyclovir, which was the first successful antiviral drug developed, is used to treat infections caused by herpes viruses, which include lesions on the genitals, in the mouth, and even in the brain, as well as treating chickenpox and shingles. The antiviral drug ganciclovir has been useful in the treatment of cytomegalovirus-mediated eye infections.

A well-known type of antiviral drug acts against retroviruses, in particular human HIV, the virus that causes AIDS. Most of the anti-retroviral drugs that have been developed have focused on combating HIV. The antiviral drug combination known as highly active antiretroviral therapy (HAART) is targeted at blocking the use of the HIV RNA to manufacture DNA (which is then used to make the viral components); blocking the integration of viral genetic material into the host genome; and blocking adhesion of the virus to host cells. This multi-pronged approach can delay the progression of AIDS.

Research is progressing on antiviral drugs to block enzymes that cut DNA or RNA or proteins. These enzymes are important in the viral manufacturing process, and so their disruption can stop viral replication. Researchers are also exploring ways to block the release of an assembled virus from the host cell. If release can be blocked, new host cells cannot be infected and the infection stops.

■ Impacts and Issues

Antiviral drugs are invaluable in the treatment of viral diseases. Millions of people infected with HIV or suffering from the symptoms of AIDS utilize them. The U.S. National Institutes of Health recommends HAART even if symptoms are absent. HAART is expensive, however. This has limited its use to those who can afford it, either because of personal finances or government assistance. In the regions that are most affected by AIDS, such as sub-Saharan Africa, HAART is far less available. Economics deprive those most in need of help. Organizations, including the International Center for Research on Health, are working to introduce HAART more widely in Africa, and to encourage its use.

Anti-retroviral drugs, such as those used in HAART, are urgently needed in sub-Saharan Africa, where more than 25 million people are infected with HIV. It has been argued that widespread availability and use of anti-retroviral drugs could make AIDS in Africa a treatable (although still chronic) disease, similar to the situation in Europe, Australia, and North America. However, such a large-scale humanitarian effort may be unrealistic, given that private industry would likely bear most of the economic burden.

Despite this gloomy picture, some hope can be drawn from a 2003 pilot project by Médecins Sans Frontières, which demonstrated that anti-retroviral programs could be implemented in regions as poor as rural Africa. Furthermore, a United Nations summit held in 2005 produced a pledge from the leaders of the economically advantaged Group of Eight countries to make access to anti-retroviral drugs universal by 2010. However, many challenges remain to realize this ambitious goal.

Another issue involving antiviral drugs is the risks posed by their use. One example is the reverse transcriptase inhibitor, AZT. While the use of AZT has reduced maternal transmission of HIV, research published in 2007, which utilized animal models of the infection and also the genetic examination of humans, indicates that this benefit may be accompanied by a risk of cancer later in the infant's life. Fetuses exposed to AZT were found to display markedly more mutations in their genetic material than those not exposed to the drug. Since many cancers are associated with mutations, the research has highlighted a previously unrecognized risk of AZT therapy.

A second example concerns the antiviral drug oseltamivir phosphate (sold as Tamiflu®). The drug, which is used to combat viral influenza and which is approved for Americans one year of age and older, has recognized side effects. The most common (nausea and vomiting) are relatively inconsequential, but Tamiflu has been anecdotally linked to instances of abnormal mental behavior in teenagers in Japan and 84 adverse events in Canada, including the deaths of 10 elderly people. Health Canada is monitoring its use and is prepared to take more stringent action if warranted, in light of the possibility that a flu epidemic could result in the use of Tamiflu® by millions of people worldwide.

In 2006, Tamiflu® resistance was reported in several people infected with the H5N1 strain of the influenza virus. H5N1 is the cause of a serious and sometimes lethal form of flu called avian influenza (bird flu). Resistance to drugs is always a concern, since over time and with the increased use of the particular drug, the resistant strain becomes predominant in a population, making the disease much harder, and usually more expensive, to treat. Since Tamiflu® is available at pharmacies, the possibility that the drug might be used improperly or inappropriately increases the likelihood that such resistance will develop. Monitoring by the U.S. Centers for Disease Control and Prevention (CDC) did not detect the resistant strain in the U.S. during 2006. However, surveillance is ongoing, since the global range of H5N1 is growing, and because the evolving ability of the virus to be more easily transmitted from person to person makes the possibility of a global epidemic increasingly likely.

SEE ALSO *Developing Nations and Drug Delivery; Pandemic Preparedness.*

BIBLIOGRAPHY

Books

Driscoll, John S. *Antiviral Drugs.* New York: Wiley, 2005.

Torrence, Paul F. *Antiviral Drug Discovery for Emerging Diseases and Bioterrorism Threats.* New York: Wiley-Interscience, 2005.

Periodicals

Monto, Arnold S. "Vaccines and Antiviral Drugs in Pandemic Preparedness." *Emerging Infectious Diseases* 12 (January 2006): 55–61.

Witt, Kristine L., et al. "Elevated Frequencies of Micronucleated Erythrocytes in Infants Exposed to Zidovudine in Utero and Postpartum to Prevent Mother-to-Child Transmission of HIV." *Environmental and Molecular Mutagenesis* 48 (April-May 2007): 322–329.

Brian Hoyle

Arthropod-borne Disease

■ Introduction

Arthropod-borne diseases are transmitted by arthropods, members of the invertebrate phylum Arthropoda, which includes insects, spiders, and crustaceans. Mosquitoes, fleas, ticks, lice, and flies are the arthropods that usually act as vectors for various pathogens (disease-causing microorganisms), including bacteria, viruses, helminths (parasitic worms), and protozoa. Transmission of these pathogens to humans by the arthropod vector can cause a variety of human diseases, including malaria, yellow fever, Chagas disease, and dengue fever. These and other arthropod-borne diseases can result in a wide range of effects, from mild flulike symptoms to death. Some survivors of arthropod borne diseases can suffer chronic, crippling aftereffects.

While arthropod-borne diseases are a major concern worldwide, developing countries are the most affected. These diseases tend to occur primarily in tropical countries—the endemic zones of the pathogens and the arthropods that harbor them. However, these diseases can also spread when people travel between infected and non-infected areas, or when infected arthropods are inadvertently transported. Natural disasters, wars, poverty, and overpopulation can facilitate outbreaks of disease, since they may create conditions that are ideal for transmission or may cause a breakdown in the health care and public health systems.

■ Disease History, Characteristics, and Transmission

Humans contract arthropod-borne diseases when a pathogen, such as a bacteria or virus, is transmitted from its reservoir (natural host) to a human via the arthropod vector. The most common arthropod vectors are flies, fleas, ticks, mosquitoes, and lice. Transmission from arthropod to human occurs either mechanically or biologically. In mechanical transmission, the arthropod deposits pathogens onto a surface from which a host either absorbs or ingests them. For example, a housefly may deposit bacteria onto food that is then eaten by a human. In biological transmission, the arthropod injects the pathogens directly into the body of the host; for example, when a mosquito bites a human.

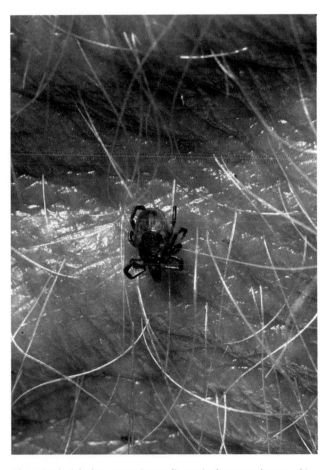

The nymph tick that causes Lyme disease is shown on human skin. Other arthropods that can transmit diseases to humans include certain species of mosquitoes, fleas, mites, lice, and flies. *Dr. Jeremy Burgess/Photo Researchers, Inc.*

The effects of arthropod-borne disease range from mild to severe. Arthropod-borne diseases, such as encephalitis and malaria, are characterized by symptoms such as headaches, fevers, weakness, and anemia. Some diseases can be fatal, and others, while not causing death, may have chronic effects that decrease quality of life.

Arthropod-borne diseases have shaped the course of history. From 1343–1351, several forms of plague caused by the bacterium *Yersinia pestis* were likely carried to humans by fleas on black rats. The event became known as the black plague or Black Death, which killed over two-thirds of the population of urban areas in Asia, one-third of the population of the Middle East, and between one-third and two-thirds of the population of Europe. Plague continued to ravage European cities sporadically, but never as it did during the Black Death. Isolated outbreaks of plague still occur, affecting under 5,000 people annually, but epidemic plague largely disappeared in Europe just before the turn of the nineteenth century—well before the advent of antibiotics. Scientists debate the reasons for its disappearance, but many point to increased sanitation and the possibility that *Yersinia pestis*-carrying fleas diminished as brown rat populations replaced black rats in Europe.

Until the mid-twentieth century, arthropod-borne diseases were an endemic health problem. American cities battled outbreaks of mosquito-borne yellow fever. Yellow fever, along with malaria, a disease involving a *Plasmodium* protozoan also transmitted by mosquitoes, stopped French construction of a canal through Panama during the 1880s when it claimed the lives of over 20,000 workers. The same diseases claimed an additional 5,000 lives when the United States completed the Panama Canal project two decades later.

Arthropod-borne diseases remain a threat, especially in less-developed countries. Malaria remains the most widespread arthropod-borne disease in the world, killing one to two million people and affecting between 250 and 500 million people per year (weather conditions can cause large changes in numbers of cases), almost exclusively in the developing world. Dengue fever, a viral disease transmitted by mosquitoes, increased in prevalence during the late 1990s and early 2000s. In 2005, it was endemic to over 100 countries, with about 50 millions cases of dengue fever occurring each year. Dengue hemorrhagic fever is a complication of dengue fever that is fatal in about 5% of cases.

■ Scope and Distribution

Arthropod-borne diseases occur worldwide, although they are more common in tropical areas such as are found in the Caribbean, Central and South America, Asia, the South Pacific, and Africa. Many regions in North America, Europe, and Australia are less affected by these diseases. Some arthropod-borne diseases are endemic to a particular country or locality, while others, such as malaria, are widely spread throughout the world.

Arthropod-borne diseases can be dispersed when infected individuals travel from a locality where they contracted the disease to an area where the disease is absent or less common. In addition, infected arthropods may be introduced to regions where the disease was previously absent, and, if conditions are favorable, the disease may gain a foothold in the new region. A variety of causes—from accidental transportation in food products to deliberate introduction of a species as a pest control agent—may be responsible for the transfer of an infected arthropod to an uninfected area.

■ Treatment and Prevention

The recommended treatment of an arthropod-borne disease depends upon the specific disease. Treatment often involves a course of antibiotics and, in some cases, a vaccine may be available for the specific disease. However, prevention measures are similar for all arthropod-borne diseases.

The most effective prevention method is to avoid being bitten by the arthropod vector in the first place. This can be achieved by wearing clothing that covers bare skin, using repellants to deter insects, avoiding outdoor activities at times when the arthropods are most active, and sleeping under mosquito netting. Travelers may want to avoid visiting tropical countries where certain arthropod-borne diseases are common, and anyone traveling to countries where these diseases are endemic certainly should take precautions to prevent being bitten. Vaccinations exist for some of these diseases to prevent development of the disease if transmission occurs. However, vaccinations are not available for all arthropod-borne diseases, and everyone does not have access to those vaccines that do exist.

For mechanically transmitted infections, prevention measures include excluding insects from areas where food is prepared and served, washing or thoroughly cooking any food that may have come into contact with an arthropod, and avoiding water bodies inhabited by arthropods. If these precautions are taken, ingestion or absorption of possible pathogens is unlikely.

■ Impacts and Issues

Arthropod-borne diseases spread rapidly when humans inhabit areas in high densities. This can occur during wars, where soldiers live in close quarters. It can also occur after natural disasters when homes are destroyed and people are forced to live close together in temporary shelters. It also occurs in poorer countries with large populations. An increase in the density of the human population leads to an increase in contact between humans and vectors, causing the rate of infection to rise.

Developing countries are most affected by arthropod-borne diseases. The World Health Organization estimates that up to 500 million cases of malaria occur each year, but fewer than 1,300 of these cases occur in the United States. An estimated one to two million people die every year due to malaria, and over 80% of the fatalities occur in Africa. This is primarily due to the poor living conditions—including lack of sanitation and the presence of stagnant water—that exist in many African regions. These conditions encourage the growth of arthropod populations. In addition, lack of access to high-quality health care in many areas limits prevention and treatment of disease, causing an increase in transmission, as well as, more serious outcomes when infection does occur.

Arthropod-borne diseases also have become a more significant risk in developed countries. For example, West Nile virus, a mosquito-borne disease, first emerged in the United States in 1999. This virus develops in birds and is transmitted to humans by mosquitoes. In 1999, 149 cases were reported in the United States. By 2003, over 9,000 cases were reported, including more than 250 fatalities. Methods to prevent the spread of West Nile virus focus on reducing the number of mosquitoes in an area and using personal protective measures (protective clothing, insect repellents, etc.) to prevent contact with mosquitoes.

One of the most common methods employed to combat arthropod-borne diseases is the use of insecticides to control the insect vectors. However, the sustainability of this method is questionable due to the emergence of insecticide-resistant arthropods. The widespread use of insecticides also can have unintended, negative environmental impacts. For example, the efficient insecticide DDT greatly reduced the number of malaria outbreaks in the 1950s and 1960s, but also

caused extensive die-off of bird populations and other negative effects on the natural environment. Today, the World Health Organization recommends the reuse of DDT, but proposes that this use be limited to targeted areas only where it can efficiently kill large populations of disease-bearing mosquitoes with minimal negative environmental effects.

The development of vaccines is a growing area of interest. The World Health Organization's Initiative for Vaccine Research (IVR) was established to guide the development of vaccines for various diseases, and this program supports research on various arthropod-borne diseases, including dengue fever, Japanese encephalitis, malaria, and West Nile virus. The Bill & Melinda Gates Foundation also established the Malaria Vaccine Initiative (MVI) in 1999, with the goal of developing a vaccine for malaria and making it available in developing countries, including Africa.

SEE ALSO *Animal Importation; Bacterial Disease; Chagas Disease; Cholera; Contact Precautions; Demographics and Infectious Disease; Dengue and Dengue Hemorrhagic Fever; Emerging Infectious Diseases; Host and Vector; Japanese Encephalitis; Lice Infestation (Pediculosis); Rickettsial Disease; Rift Valley Fever; Malaria; Microorganisms; Mosquito-borne Diseases; Sanitation; Travel and Infectious Disease; Tropical Infectious Diseases; Vaccines and Vaccine Development; War and Infectious Disease; West Nile; Yellow Fever.*

IN CONTEXT: SCIENTIFIC, POLITICAL, AND ETHICAL ISSUES

Based on data collected for a study on ectoparasitism and vector-borne diseases, Phillipe Brouqui, Didier Raoult, Andreas Stein, and other researchers at the *Maladies Infectieuses et Tropicales* argued that "[h]omeless people are particularly exposed to ectoparasites. The living conditions and the crowded shelters provide ideal conditions for the spread of lice, fleas, ticks, and mites." The researchers also argued that "exposure to arthropod-borne diseases has not been evaluated systematically."

A medical team visited shelters in Marseilles, France, for 4 consecutive years. Homeless volunteers were examined and received care during the study.

SOURCE: Brouqui, Phillipe, and Didier Raoult. "Arthropod-borne diseases in homeless." Ann N Y Acad Sci. (October 2006, 1078: 223-35) and Brouqui Phillipe, Andreas Stein, et al. "Ectoparasitism and vector-borne diseases in 930 homeless people from Marseilles." Medicine (Baltimore). (2005 Jan; 84(1): 61-8).

BIBLIOGRAPHY

Books

Centers for Disease Control and Prevention, et al. *Health Information for International Travel 2005–2006.* St. Louis, MO: Mosby, 2005.

Mandell, G.L., J.E. Bennett, and R. Dolin. *Principles and Practice of Infectious Diseases.* Vol. 2. Philadelphia, PA: Elsevier, 2005.

Periodicals

Hill, C.A., et al. "Arthropod-borne Diseases: Vector Control in the Genomics Era." *Nature Reviews Microbiology* 3 (March 2005): 262–268.

Web Sites

Bill & Melinda Gates Foundation. "Malaria Vaccine Initiative: Solving the Malaria Vaccine Puzzle." September 2005. <http://www.gatesfoundation. org/StoryGallery/GlobalHealth/SGGHMalaria MVI-011019.htm> (accessed January 31, 2007).

Centers for Disease Control and Prevention. "Dengue Fever." August 22, 2005. <http://www.cdc.gov/ ncidod/dvbid/dengue/> (accessed January 31, 2007).

Centers for Disease Control and Prevention. "Infectious Disease Information: Insect- and Arthropod-related Diseases." September 8, 2005. <http:// www.cdc.gov/ncidod/diseases/insects/special_ topics.htm> (accessed January 31, 2007).

Centers for Disease Control and Prevention. "West Nile Virus." January 25, 2007. <http://www.cdc.gov/ ncidod/dvbid/westnile/index.htm> (accessed January 31, 2007).

World Health Organization. "Dengue and Dengue Haemorrhagic Fever." April 2002. <http:// www.who.int/mediacentre/factsheets/fs117/en/> (accessed January 31, 2007).

Tony Hawas

Asilomar Conference

■ Introduction

The Asilomar Conference of 1975 was held to consider the possible biohazards of the then newly developed recombinant DNA technology. This technology involves selectively removing the genetic material (deoxyribonucleic acid or DNA) from one organism and inserting it into the DNA of a different organism. As a result of this recombination, the proteins encoded by the inserted genes are expressed in the host organism.

Following the development of recombinant DNA technology in the mid–1970s, researchers were soon able to successfully transfer DNA into target microorganisms, such as the bacterium *Escherichia coli*, thus enabling the target organism to produce the protein(s) encoded by the inserted DNA. Almost immediately, the researchers recognized the potential for the deliberate or accidental misuse of this technology to create an organism whose ability to cause disease was enhanced or even created anew.

The researchers took the extraordinary step of declaring a moratorium on recombinant DNA research until they could meet, discuss their concerns, and formulate guidelines to restore confidence in future research. The meeting took place in February 1975 in Asilomar, which is located on the northern coast of California near San Francisco.

■ History and Scientific Foundations

Recombinant DNA technology had its roots in the 1970 discovery by American microbiologist Hamilton Smith (1931–) of an enzyme dubbed a restriction enzyme. (In the decades that followed dozens of different restriction enzymes have been discovered.) Restriction enzymes function by recognizing a certain sequence (unique to each restriction enzyme) of nucleotides—the building blocks of DNA—and cutting the DNA at that site. The

cut is made in such a way that a portion of one of the two nucleotide strands that normally intertwine to form the DNA double helix is exposed. Activity of the restriction enzyme on another segment of DNA produces an exposed portion of the opposite strand. Because the exposed nucleotides on one exposed portion can bind to the corresponding nucleotide on the other exposed strand (the exposed nucleotide sequences are described

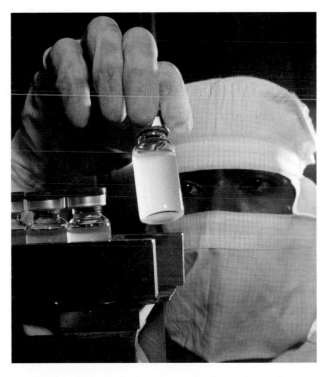

A technician checks the quality of a sample of recombinant hepatitis B vaccine. Traditional hepatitis vaccine contains the full virus, which could potentially become active and infect patients. A recombinant vaccine only contains a viral protein, and not the whole virus, so there is no risk of the virus becoming active. *Volker Steger/Photo Researchers, Inc.*

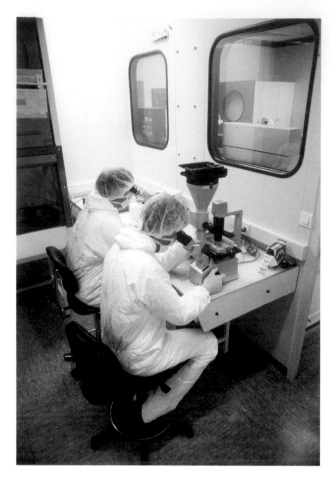

Laboratory technicians produce viral vectors for use in gene therapy. *Phanie/Photo Researchers, Inc.*

WORDS TO KNOW

DNA: Short for deoxyribonucleic acid, a double helix shaped molecule that is found in almost all living cells and that determines the characteristics of each organism.

RECOMBINANT DNA: DNA that is cut using specific enzymes so that a gene or DNA sequence can be inserted.

RESTRICTION ENZYME: A special type of protein that can recognize and cut DNA at certain sequences of bases to help scientists separate out a specific gene. Restriction enzymes recognize certain sequences of DNA and cleave the DNA at those sites. The enzymes are used to generate fragments of DNA that can be subsequently joined together to create new stretches of DNA.

as being complimentary to each other), segments of DNA from different sources could be made to meld together.

Following the discovery of restriction enzymes, progress in recombinant DNA technology occurred with astonishing swiftness. In 1972, Paul Berg (1926–) of Stanford University reported the manufacture of recombinant DNA consisting of an oncogene from a human cancer-causing monkey virus ligated (joined) into the genetic material of the bacterial virus lambda. The following year, Stanley Cohen (1935–) and Herbert Boyer (1936–) were successful in transferring foreign DNA into *E. coli*.

The rapid developments of recombinant DNA technology, combined with Bergs' demonstration that a potentially-harmful gene could be transferred into a new organism caused great concern. The specter of the malicious design of a deadly microorganism that was capable of person-to-person transmission, and the realization that the technology had outpaced knowledge of its potential pitfalls prompted the moratorium and the Asilomar conference.

■ Impacts and Issues

In February 1975, the leaders of the international molecular biology community—then just over 100 researchers, in contrast to the hundreds of thousands of molecular biology researchers in 2007—met at the Asilomar conference center in California. The purpose of the gathering was to establish at least a minimal set of guidelines for those engaged in recombinant DNA research. Then, anyone seeking to conduct recombinant DNA research would be required to follow these guidelines (a goal since achieved).

Conference delegates considered all the equipment and laboratory facilities that would be required to perform recombinant DNA research, and the type of research that might be done, to rate the risks of the research as minimal, low, moderate, or high. As the riskiness of the research increased (e.g., the organism being used was a known pathogen), the stringency of the precautions increased. For example, a low-risk research lab would not need any special ventilation, while high-risk research would require a facility designed to contain the organism in the event of a spill or other accident.

This task was very difficult, since guidelines were being formulated to some experiments that had yet to be done. Still, some realistic guidelines emerged. For example, the scientists decided that the bacteria used in the research should be incapable of surviving outside the controlled environment of the lab. This could be achieved by, as one example, genetically crippling the bacteria so that the cells could not make some vital nutrient. As a result, bacterial survival depended on the presence of the nutrient in the artificial food source on which they were grown. In this way, the chance of spread of the recombinant bacteria to the outside world would be extremely remote.

Other risk-related guidelines included a ban on food in a laboratory; wearing of protective gear, including a lab coat, gloves, and face mask; scrupulous clean up of work areas before and after an experiment to make sure surfaces and equipment was free of bacteria; and, at the highest risk level, the design of a laboratory that was self-contained and, as a result, completely separated from the outside world.

The guidelines banned certain types of experiments, such as the use of highly pathogenic organisms or genetic material known to encode a harmful product like a toxin. Then as now, it was recognized that scientists or organizations bent on the deliberate design of harmful organisms would circumvent the guidelines. However, the vast majority of the scientific community supported and have followed the guidelines developed at the Asilomar conference.

BIBLIOGRAPHY

Books

Clark, David P. *Molecular Biology Made Simple and Fun.* 3rd ed. St. Louis: Cache River Press, 2005.

Dale, Jeremy W., and Simon F. Park. *Molecular Genetics of Bacteria.* New York: John Wiley, 2004.

Periodicals

Berg, Paul., et al. "Summary Statement of the Asilomar Conference on Recombinant DNA Molecules." *Proceedings of the National Academy of Sciences of the United States of America* 72 (1975): 1981–1984.

Frederickson, Donald S. "The First Twenty-Five Years After Asilomar." *Perspectives in Biology and Medicine* 44 (2001): 170–182.

Brian Hoyle

RECOMBINANT FIRSTS

In 1972, Paul Berg of Stanford University was the first to create a recombinant DNA molecule. Berg isolated a gene from a human cancer-causing monkey virus, and then ligated (joined) the oncogene into the genome of the bacterial virus lambda. For this and subsequent recombinant DNA studies (which followed a voluntary one-year moratorium from his research while safety issues were addressed), he was awarded the 1980 Nobel Prize in chemistry.

In 1973, Stanley Cohen and Herbert Boyer created the first recombinant DNA organism, by adding recombinant plasmids to *E. coli.*

Since these firsts, advances in molecular biology techniques, in particular the development of polymerase chain reaction (PCR) techniques, make the construction of recombinant DNA swifter and easier.

IN CONTEXT: REAL-WORLD QUESTIONS

Potential applications of recombinant DNA technology include food crops engineered to produce edible vaccines. This strategy would make vaccination more readily available to children worldwide. Because of their use across many cultures and their ability to adapt to tropical and subtropical environments, bananas have been the object of considerable research effort. Transgenic bananas containing inactivated viruses that normally cause cholera, hepatitis B and diarrhea and transgenic potatoes carrying recombinant vaccines for cholera and intestinal disorders have been developed and evaluated, though their potential use remains controversial and the approach not yet fully accepted.

Aspergillosis

■ Introduction

Aspergillosis is a lung infection or allergic reaction that is caused by a type of fungus called *Aspergillus*. The fungus, which is found naturally on decaying organic material such as leaves, hay, and compost, can infect the lungs. Pulmonary aspergillosis can remain confined to the lungs or can spread to other parts of the body. The more widespread infection can be especially serious. It occurs most commonly in people whose immune systems are less capable of fighting off infections.

■ Disease History, Characteristics, and Transmission

Aspergillosis is most typically caused by *Aspergillus fumigatus* or *A. flavus*. Less commonly, the infection is caused by *A. terreus*, *A. nidulans*, and *A. niger*.

Inhalation of the spores of *Aspergillus* can lead to the growth of the fungus in the lungs. This growth can cause an allergic reaction called pulmonary aspergillosis. The infection, which can develop along with asthma, can diminish the ability of the lungs to function. Growth of the fungus also can produce a compact structure called a fungus ball. The ball tends to develop in an area of the lung that has previously been damaged by tuberculosis or some other infection that results in a localized build-up of fluid or infected material.

Pulmonary aspergillosis also can be more invasive, meaning the infection can move from the lungs to other parts of the body. This spread is promoted when the infection is less efficiently cleared due to a compromised immune system, as can occur during treatment for cancer and some other ailments, following organ transplantation to minimize rejection of the transplant, and in people with acquired immunodeficiency syndrome (AIDS, also cited as acquired immune deficiency syndrome).

The symptoms of aspergillosis include fever, a general feeling of tiredness, cough that can be combined with expelled blood or mucous, wheeziness when breathing, loss of weight, and periodic difficulty in breathing. Additional symptoms can be present in the more invasive type of aspergillosis. These include chills, headaches, chest pain, increased amount of expelled mucous, decreased amount of urine, bloody urine, bone pain, inflammation of nerve lining in the brain or spinal cord (meningitis), sinus infection, diminished vision, and heart trouble.

■ Scope and Distribution

Aspergillosis is global in scope because the fungus that causes the disease is a common environmental organism. The prevalence of aspergillosis is unclear, however, it tends

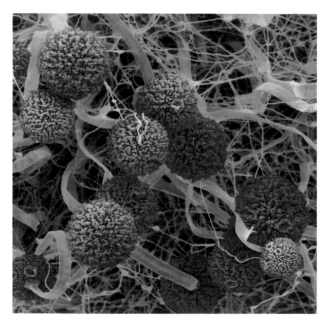

This magnified image shows *Aspergillus niger,* a mold that results in allergic reactions. It produces aflatoxins and can lead to the serious lung disease aspergillosis. *© Visuals Unlimited/Corbis.*

to be more prevalent in areas where the population includes more immunosuppressed people. For example, the city of San Francisco, which has a higher proportion of people with AIDS than some other metropolitan areas, may have a rate of aspergillosis of 1–2 people per 100,000 every year, according to data from the United States Centers for Disease Control and Prevention (CDC).

■ Treatment and Prevention

Aspergillosis is diagnosed by the detection of the lung infection. The infection can be imaged using x-ray or a technique called computed tomography (or CT). The fungus also can be obtained from a sample of expelled mucous or sputum and grown on various food sources. The food sources can be selected to help distinguish one type of fungus from another, and so can help identify the fungus as being from the genus *Aspergillus*. In addition, the sputum can be stained and examined using a light microscope to detect fungal cells. The staining method produces a less precise result; it reveals the presence of fungi, but is not refined enough to distinguish one genus of fungus from another. However, just knowing that the infection is caused by a fungus can be enough to initiate treatment.

Aspergillosis can also be diagnosed by detecting the presence of protein components of the fungus. The proteins function as antigens and stimulate the production of specific antibodies by the immune system. *Aspergillus* antigens can be detected by a skin-based reaction, or in a test tube or well of a plastic assay dish by the formation of a cloudy precipitate that is comprised of a complex (product) formed between a specific antigen and antibody.

Treatment for aspergillosis varies depending on the nature of the infection. When the infection involves a fungal ball, treatment can be withheld if the infection is not associated with bleeding into the lung. Then surgery is performed to remove the fungal mass. Aspergillosis that has spread more widely is treated for several weeks with an antifungal agent such as amphotericin B. Treatment is usually done intravenously to maintain a constant and effective level of drug in the body. *Aspergillus*-infected heart valves are usually removed, and extended treatment with an antifungal drug follows the surgery.

People whose illness is due to an allergic reaction to *Aspergillosis* do not benefit from the use of an antifungal drug. For them, treatment with prednisone, which dampens the immune system and so reduces the allergic reaction, is the typical approach.

Treatment of aspergillosis carries a risk. Extended use of amphotericin B can harm the kidneys. Use of the drug is a balance of the benefit obtained versus the risk imposed.

■ Impacts and Issues

The invasive form of aspergillosis can be life threatening. The seriousness of the infection is especially pronounced

in people with a malfunctioning immune system. This includes the millions of people around the world who are afflicted with acquired immunodeficiency syndrome (AIDS, also cited as acquired immune deficiency syndrome) and are vulnerable to opportunistic infections. Aspergillosis is yet another danger that confronts someone with AIDS. The death rate from the invasive form of aspergillosis is at least 50%.

Other issues that affect aspergillosis are the lack of a rapid test for the infection, and a lack of knowledge of risk factors that might be modified so as to reduce the risk of the infection. In the United States, research is underway in these areas specifically.

In addition to humans, aspergillosis can affect other species. For example, waterfowl populations can be decimated by aspergillosis outbreaks if the birds feed on decaying grain. Aspergillosis is a common and lethal infection in birds, such as parakeets and parrots.

SEE ALSO *Mycotic Disease; Nosocomial (Healthcare-Associated) Infections; Opportunistic Infection.*

BIBLIOGRAPHY

Books

Black, Jacquelyn. *Microbiology: Principles and Explorations.* New York: John Wiley & Sons, 2004.

DiClaudio, Dennis. *The Hypochondriac's Pocket Guide to Horrible Diseases You Probably Already Have.* New York: Bloomsbury, 2005.

Mader, Sylvia S. *Biology.* 8th ed. New York: McGraw-Hill, 2003.

Web Sites

Centers for Disease Control and Prevention. "Aspergillosis." <http://www.cdc.gov/ncidod/dbmd/diseaseinfo/aspergillosis_t.htm> (accessed March 25, 2007).

Brian Hoyle

Avian Influenza

▪ Introduction

Few phenomena in the field of infectious diseases have so captured world attention as avian (bird) influenza. From its onset in 2003, until this writing, only 310 cases were reported, resulting in 189 deaths—all limited to 12 countries. Indeed, during the same period, many times that number had died in those same countries of lightning bolts, jellyfish stings, and judicial beheadings. Not a single tourist has contracted the disease, and none of the thousands of health care workers involved in treatment and control has been infected. The few instances in which more than one family member developed avian influenza have been ascribed to common contact with infected birds, rather than human-to-human spread.

▪ Disease History, Characteristics, and Transmission

The term "avian influenza" is a misnomer, as virtually all strains (types) of the influenza virus pass through ducks or other birds before emerging into the human population. Influenza strains differ from one another according to the nature of two surface proteins:

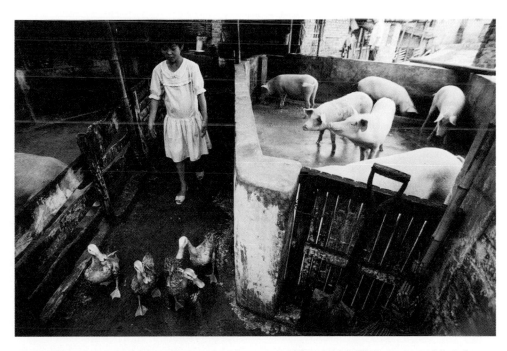

The close proximity of animals and humans in some regions of the world facilitates passage of the influenza virus among them. For example, here a girl in China is shown herding ducks through a pig pen. © *Karen Kasmauski/Corbis.*

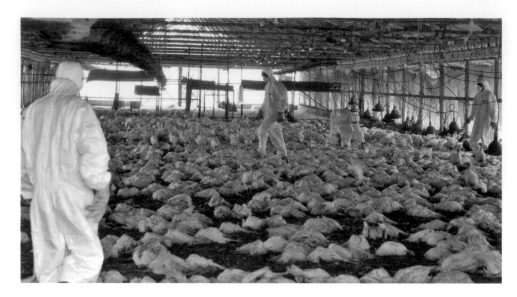

Workers wearing protective gear collect dead turkeys at a farm in Israel in March 2006 after poultry at several farms in the country were confirmed to have been infected with the H5N1 bird flu virus. Authorities believe Israel's migrating wild bird population poses a risk of spreading the disease, as the country is a major stopover for migrating birds to and from Eastern Europe, Central Asia, and Africa. © *Ammar Awad/Reuters/Corbis.*

hemagluttinin (H) and neuraminidase (N). There are 15 subtypes of the H antigen (a substance that induces an immune response).

The first recorded outbreak of influenza occurred in 1580, and an additional 31 pandemics (global epidemics) had been documented as of 2003. Twenty-one to 40 million deaths were estimated for the Spanish flu H1N1 pandemic of 1918–1919. The Asian flu (H2N2, 1957) and Hong Kong flu (H3N2, 1968) pandemics each resulted in one to four million deaths. Excess deaths attributable to influenza in the United States numbered 603,600 during the epidemics of 1918–1919, 1957–1958 and 1968–1969; and an additional 600,000 were estimated to have died in non-pandemic years during 1957 to 1990.

While most human infection is caused by types H1, H2 and H3, types H5 and H7 are known to be more virulent. In fact, before the current outbreak of H5N1 virus, small clusters of human infection by H7N7, H7N3, and even H5N1 had been reported on persons having close exposure to poultry in a variety of countries. Infections were generally mild, often limited to a mild cough and conjunctivitis (inflammation of the membranes of the eye). Nevertheless, prior outbreaks of H5N1 virus in Hong Kong during 1997–1998 resulted in six deaths. Antibody (a protein produced by the immune system in response to the presence of the specific H5N1 antigen) was demonstrated in 17.2 of poultry workers during the outbreak. Approximately 1.5 million chickens and other birds were slaughtered in attempts to control the virus, but the episode generated only passing interest.

H5N1 mutates rapidly and has a propensity to acquire genes from other animal species. Birds may excrete the virus from the mouth and cloaca (the excretory vent of a bird) for up to ten days. H5N1 virus was found to survive in bird feces for at least 35 days at low temperature (39.2°F, 4°C). At a much higher temperature (98.6°F, 37°C), H5N1 viruses have been shown to survive in fecal samples for 6 days.

■ Scope and Distribution

The current outbreak began in 2003, when one case of human H5N1 (fatal) was reported in China and 3 (fatal) in Vietnam. The following year, 17 cases (12 fatal) were reported in Thailand, and 29 (20 fatal) in Vietnam. Several asymptomatic (without symptoms) infections were subsequently reported in South Korea. In 2005, 20 cases (13 fatal) were reported in Indonesia, 5 (2 fatal) in Thailand, and 61 (19 fatal) in Vietnam. By the end of 2006, cases were being reported in Azerbaijan, Cambodia, China, Indonesia, Iraq, Turkey, and Africa (Djibouti and Egypt). As of 2007, the list of infected countries has expanded to include Laos and Nigeria.

In addition to human cases, numerous outbreaks limited to wild and domestic birds have been reported in Afghanistan, Albania, Austria, Azerbaijan, Bosnia and Herzegovina, Burkina Faso, Croatia, Cyprus, Czech Republic, Denmark, France, Georgia, Germany, Ghana, Greece, Hungary, India, Iran, Israel, Italy, Ivory Coast, Jordan, Kazakhstan, Kuwait, Malaysia, Mongolia, Myanmar, Netherlands, Niger, Nigeria, Pakistan, Poland, Philippines, Romania, Russian Federation, Saudi Arabia,

Scotland, Serbia, Slovakia, Slovenia, Spain, Sudan, Sweden, Switzerland, Ukraine, and the United Kingdom. In other words, the principal mode of spread among countries is in the intestines of migrating wild birds—and not in the potential human airplane passenger.

Perhaps more significantly, H5N1 infection has already appeared in a number of non-avian hosts, including pigs, tigers, leopards, dogs, civet cats and domestic cats, Cynomolgus macques, ferrets, New Zealand white rabbits, leopards, rats, mink, and stone marten. Indeed, infected blow flies (*Calliphora nigribarbis*) have been identified in the vicinity of poultry infected with H5N1 influenza virus in Japan.

A few words concerning the disease itself. Avian influenza is characterized by fever greater than 100.4°F (38°C), shortness of breath, and cough. The incubation period is two to four days. Some persons have reported sore throat, conjunctivitis, muscle pain, rash, and runny nose. Watery diarrhea or loose stools is noted in approximately 50% of the cases, a symptom that is uncommon in the more familiar forms of influenza. All patients reported to date have presented with significant lymphopenia (diminished concentration of lymphocytes, white blood cells, in the blood) and marked chest x-ray abnormalities consisting of diffuse, multifocal or patchy infiltrates (areas of inflammatory cells, foreign organisms, and cellular debris, often indicating pneumonia). Physical examination reveals the patient to be short of breath, with signs of lung inflammation. Myocardial (heart muscle) and hepatic (liver) dysfunction are also reported. Approximately 60% of patients have died, on an average of 10 days after the onset of symptoms.

■ Treatment and Prevention

Diagnosis depends on demonstration of the virus or serum antibody toward the virus in specialized laboratories. Because of intense media reporting (and misinformation) a given patient may be reported repeatedly; or a case of unrelated respiratory infection may be reported as "avian influenza." Thus, only reports issued by qualified centralized laboratories should be considered valid. As of 2007, only four anti-viral agents have been used for the treatment of influenza: Amantadine, Rimantadine, Oseltamivir, and Zanamivir. Although some success has been claimed in the use of Oseltamivir for the treatment of Avian Influenza H5N1, a large controlled clinical trial is not feasible. Vaccines against this strain are under development.

■ Impacts and Issues

So why has this text devoted precious space to a low incidence, non-contagious disease that primarily affects peripheral Asian communities? The answer might be

WORDS TO KNOW

ANTIBODY: Antibodies, or Y-shaped immunoglobulins, are proteins found in the blood that help to fight against foreign substances called antigens. Antigens, which are usually proteins or polysaccharides, stimulate the immune system to produce antibodies. The antibodies inactivate the antigen and help to remove it from the body. While antigens can be the source of infections from pathogenic bacteria and viruses, organic molecules detrimental to the body from internal or environmental sources also act as antigens. Genetic engineering and the use of various mutational mechanisms allow the construction of a vast array of antibodies (each with a unique genetic sequence).

ANTIGEN: Antigens, which are usually proteins or polysaccharides, stimulate the immune system to produce antibodies. The antibodies inactivate the antigen and help to remove it from the body. While antigens can be the source of infections from pathogenic bacteria and viruses, organic molecules detrimental to the body from internal or environmental sources also act as antigens. Genetic engineering and the use of various mutational mechanisms allow the construction of a vast array of antibodies (each with a unique genetic sequence).

CLOACA: The cavity into which the intestinal, genital, and urinary tracts open in vertebrates such as fish, reptiles, birds, and some primitive mammals.

HOST: Organism that serves as the habitat for a parasite, or possibly for a symbiont. A host may provide nutrition to the parasite or symbiont, or simply a place in which to live.

PANDEMIC: Pandemic, which means all the people, describes an epidemic that occurs in more than one country or population simultaneously.

STRAIN: A subclass or a specific genetic variation of an organism.

summed up in three words: potential for spread. We all suffer attacks of influenza, most of us repeatedly throughout our lives. Influenza is one of the most contagious of human diseases, and while rarely fatal, impacts on all of us in terms of numbers incapacitated and requiring medical care. The new avian influenza strain,

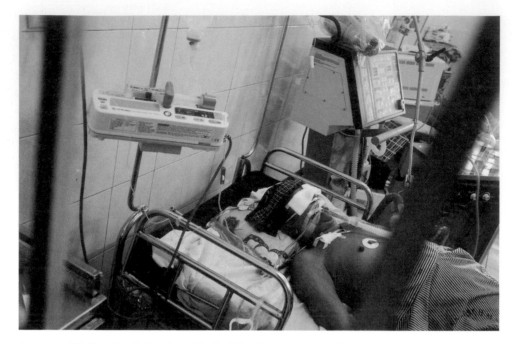

A person with the avian flu breathes with the help of a respirator in a Hanoi, Vietnam, hospital in November 2005. The mortality rate of those contracting H5N1 influenza during the first outbreak in Vietnam in early 2004 approached 100 percent. This occurred because few respirators were available; diagnostic testing was inadequate and slow; and a lack of personnel meant that family members often fed and cared for patients themselves. *© Dung Vo Trung/dung vo trung/politika/Corbis.*

while limited in time and place, is a very severe disease. The chance of dying of the better-known common strains is lower than one tenth of one percent; but the case-fatality rate for avian influenza is 61%. Thus, the fear of all those who deal with this outbreak is that the virus will one day revert to a contagious form, while retaining its high virulence ability to cause disease. At that point, we could be dealing with millions of cases . . . of a disease that carries a 61% mortality.

Another disturbing feature of the current outbreak is the age of infected persons. The common epidemic forms of influenza to date have had greatest impact among the elderly, with most deaths occurring in persons over age 65 with underlying heart or lung disease. Ninety percent of patients with the new H5N1 Avian influenza virus have been below age 40, with many deaths reported in children.

Primary source connection

The World Health Organization (WHO) publishes *Disease Outbreak News* reports to provide timely outbreak information and foster communication among various national and international public health organizations. As an example, the following report outlines WHO recommendations for combating the threat of pandemic Highly Pathogenic Avian Influenza H5N1.

Avian Influenza—Necessary precautions to prevent human infection of H5N1, need for virus sharing

WHO continues to be concerned by the simultaneous outbreaks of Highly Pathogenic Avian Influenza H5N1 in several Asian countries.

While these outbreaks thus far remain restricted to poultry populations, they nevertheless increase the chances of virus transmission and human infection of the disease, as well as the possible emergence of a new influenza virus strain capable of sparking a global pandemic.

In this context, WHO re-emphasizes the necessity of protecting individuals involved in the culling of H5N1-infected poultry. Workers who might be exposed to H5N1-infected poultry should have proper personal protective equipment (i.e. protective clothing, masks and goggles) since there is a high risk of exposure during the slaughtering process.

In addition to the use of personal protective equipment, WHO is recommending:

- To avoid the co-infection of avian and human influenza, which could allow for the emergence of a pandemic influenza virus, all persons involved in mass culling operations, transportation and burial/

incineration of carcasses should be vaccinated with the current WHO-recommended influenza vaccine.

- All persons exposed to infected poultry or to farms under suspicion should be under close monitoring by local health authorities. National authorities should also increase their surveillance of any reported clusters of influenza or influenza-like illness.

- Antiviral treatment should be available on an ongoing basis for treatment of a suspected human infection with a Highly Pathogenic Avian Influenza virus. If antivirals are available in sufficient quantities, prophylactic use should be considered.

Please see the full list of WHO's interim recommendations for the protection of persons involved in the mass slaughter of animals potentially infected with Highly Pathogenic Avian Influenza viruses.

WHO is also urging countries to work on standardized procedures for immediate sharing of all avian influenza virus strains responsible for outbreaks with WHO's international network of laboratories.

WHO is depending on the continued collaboration of the national health and agricultural services to establish routine procedures for immediate sharing of avian influenza virus samples. Without such virus samples, WHO will not be in a position to provide proper vaccine prototype strains and related guidance for vaccine producers.

World Health Organization

WORLD HEALTH ORGANIZATION, EPIDEMIC AND PANDEMIC ALERT AND RESPONSE (EPR). "AVIAN INFLUENZA—NECESSARY PRECAUTIONS TO PREVENT HUMAN INFECTION OF H5N1, NEED FOR VIRUS SHARING." *DISEASE OUTBREAK NEWS.* JULY 16, 2004.

SEE ALSO *Developing Nations and Drug Delivery; Emerging Infectious Diseases; H5N1; Influenza; Influenza, Tracking Seasonal Influences and Virus Mutation; Influenza Pandemic of 1918; Notifiable Diseases; Pandemic Preparedness; Vaccines and Vaccine Development.*

BIBLIOGRAPHY

Books

Bethe, Marilyn R. *Global Spread of the Avian Flu: Issues And Actions.* Hauppauge, NY: Nova Science, 2007.

U.S. Department of Health and Human Services *2006 Guide to Surviving Bird Flu: Common Sense Strategies and Preparedness Plans—Avian Flu and H5N1 Threat.* Progressive Management, 2006.

IN CONTEXT: REAL-WORLD RISKS

With regard to human transmission, as of May 2007, the Centers for Disease Control and Prevention (CDC) reports stated: "While there has been some human-to-human spread of H5N1, it has been limited, inefficient and unsustained. For example, in 2004 in Thailand, probable human-to-human spread in a family resulting from prolonged and very close contact between an ill child and her mother was reported. Most recently, In June 2006, World Health Organization (WHO) reported evidence of human-to-human spread in Indonesia. In this situation, 8 people in one family were infected. The first family member is thought to have become ill through contact with infected poultry. This person then infected six family members. One of those six people (a child) then infected another family member (his father). No further spread outside of the exposed family was documented or suspected. Nonetheless, because all influenza viruses have the ability to change, scientists are concerned that H5N1 virus one day could be able to infect humans and spread easily from one person to another. Because these viruses do not commonly infect humans, there is little or no immune protection against them in the human population. If H5N1 virus were to gain the capacity to spread easily from person to person, an influenza pandemic (worldwide outbreak of disease) could begin."

SOURCE: *Centers for Disease Control and Prevention*

Periodicals

Webster, R.G. and E.J. Walker. "The World is Teetering on the Edge of a Pandemic that Could Kill a Large Fraction of the Human Population." *American Scientist* 91 (2003): 122.

Web Sites

Centers for Disease Control and Prevention (CDC). "Avian Influenza (Bird Flu)." <http://www.cdc.gov/flu/avian/> (accessed May 10, 2007).

World Health Organization. "Avian Influenza." <http: http://www.who.int/csr/disease/avian_influenza/en/index.html> (accessed May 10, 2007).

Stephen A.Berger

B Virus (Cercopithecine herpesvirus 1) Infection

■ Introduction

B virus, also called Cercopithecine herpesvirus 1, is an infectious virus found in macaques (short-tailed monkeys), such as rhesus macaques, pig-tailed macaques, stump-tailed macaques, and cynomolgus monkeys. The virus—which is a member of the herpes group of viruses—possesses origins and causes disease similar to that of the herpes simplex virus in humans. When humans are infected with B virus from macaques, they can become ill with severe and sometimes permanent central nervous system (CNS) involvement or death from encephalomyelitis (inflammation of the brain).

The National Center for Infectious Diseases (NCID), of the U.S. Centers for Disease Control and Prevention (CDC), states that the mortality rate for undiagnosed/untreated B virus disease is historically almost 80%, mostly from complications of the disease. However, since antiviral therapy has become a treatment for B virus, the mortality rate has decreased.

B virus is also called herpes B virus, herpesvirus simiae, and monkey B virus. The last known fatality from B virus in the United States occurred in 1997 at the Yerkes National Primate Research Center, located at Emory University in Atlanta, Georgia. Biological material from a monkey infected the eye of a worker and, eventually, the infection killed the worker.

Because of this incident, the CDC formed a working group to devise recommendations for the evaluation, prevention, and treatment of B virus in humans. The group's report is called "Recommendations for Prevention of and Therapy for Exposure to B Virus (*Cercopithecine Herpesvirus 1*)." It was published in 2002 in the journal *Clinical Infectious Diseases*.

■ Disease History, Characteristics, and Transmission

The first medically documented case of human B virus infection occurred in 1932 when a researcher's hand was bitten by a rhesus macaque. The worker died two weeks later of encephalomyelitis.

Macaques are primates in the family Cercopithecidae (commonly called Old World monkeys), subfamily Cercopithecinae, and genus *Macaca*. The scientific name of the rhesus macaque is *Macaca mulatta*, the southern pig-tailed macaque is called *M. nemestrina*, the northern pig-tailed macaque is called *M. leonina*, the stump-tailed macaque (or bear macaque) is called *M. arctoides*, and the cynomolgus monkey (or crab-eating macaque) is called *M. fascicularis*.

Macaque monkeys infected with B virus usually become infected when oral or genital secretions from other monkeys contact their mucous membranes or skin. Infected monkeys usually have few or no symptoms. When symptoms are present, they usually consist of lesions on the face, genitals, lips, or mouth. Normally, the lesions heal themselves, however, they may re-appear repeatedly, especially during extended periods of stress or anxiety. This condition is called gingivostomatitis, which is a type of stomatitis, an inflammation of the mucous lining within the mouth (specifically on the tongue, lips, or gums). When the inflammation involves the gums (gingiva), it is called gingivostomatitis.

B virus infection in humans is rare. When it does occur, B virus usually comes from cells and tissues (such as in cultures) of monkeys, and less frequently from these animals' secretions (such as saliva), bites, or scratches. The incubation period is generally between two days and five weeks, although most symptoms appear in five days to three weeks. Symptoms usually limit themselves to the infected areas. They may include itching, numbness, skin lesions, and pain. However, some patients develop serious symptoms in the peripheral nervous system (PNS) or central nervous system (CNS). Some symptoms can initially include dizziness, headache, nausea, vomiting, and, later, seizures, respiratory failure, and coma.

Other patients have influenzalike (flulike) symptoms such as chills, fever, and muscle pain. Additional symptoms include itching, weakness, general pain, tingling, or numbness at the infection site. Often humans come down with acute encephalomyelitis (inflammation of the brain and spinal cord), which causes the death. Groups of people most at risk from B virus include laboratory workers, veterinarians, and other similar groups who have close contact with macaques or their cell cultures.

■ Scope and Distribution

B virus is found worldwide, but it is more likely to be found in areas inhabited by Asiatic monkeys of the genus *Macaca* or at locations where they are kept in captivity.

■ Treatment and Prevention

To prevent the transmission of the disease, protective equipment is recommended when working with macaque monkeys, especially virus-positive animals. Protective equipment includes eyewear (such as goggles or glasses with side shields), disposable head coverings, face shields (such as a welder's mask), gloves, disposable shoe covers, and disposable surgical scrubs or fluid-resistant cloth uniforms.

As recommended by the B Virus Working Group, which is headed by Jeffrey I. Cohen (National Institutes of Health, Bethesda, Maryland), bites, scratches, and any exposures to mucous membranes, including the eyes, must be cleansed immediately. Culture samples from the macaque and human should be sent for B virus diagnostic testing.

Specifically, the minutes after exposure are critical. The skin or mucosa affected by bites, scratches, or monkey fluids should be cleansed for a minimum of 15 minutes. If the eyes are contaminated, they should be irrigated with sterile saline solution or water for 15 minutes. Exposed skin should be washed with a chemical antiseptic (such as chlorhexidine or povidoneiodine) or detergent soap. After cleansing, wounds should be lightly massaged to increase the effectiveness of the cleaning agent. As soon as possible, antiviral medicine should be started in order to prevent severe disease or death from B virus.

■ Impacts and Issues

According to the CDC, workers who handle monkeys directly or handle cultures, bones, and other objects that originate from monkeys are potentially at risk for contracting B virus. Since this work is potentially hazardous, the CDC has written a set of guidelines for the care and maintenance of macaques titled "Guidelines for Prevention of Herpesvirus Simiae (B Virus) Infection in Monkey Handlers."

Although thousands of humans have handled macaques since B virus was first reported, only about 40 cases of human infection have been well-documented as of 2003. Even though only a few cases have been reported, CDC health officials feel that precautions

> ## WORDS TO KNOW
>
> **ENCEPHALOMYELITIS:** Simultaneous inflammation of the brain and spinal cord is encephalomyelitis.
>
> **HERPESVIRUS:** Herpesvirus is a family of viruses, many of which cause disease in humans. The *herpes simplex*-1 and *herpes simplex*-2 viruses cause infection in the mouth or on the genitals. Other common types of herpesvirus include chicken pox, Epstien-Barr virus, and cytomegalovirus. Herpesvirus is notable for its ability to remain latent, or inactive, in nerve cells near the area of infection, and to reactivate long after the initial infection. *Herpes simplex*-1 and -2, along with chickenpox, cause familiar skin sores. Epstein-Barr virus causes mononucleosis. Cytomegalovirus also causes a flu-like infection, but it can be dangerous to the elderly, infants, and those with weakened immune systems.
>
> **MACAQUE:** A macaque is any short-tailed monkey of the genus *Macaca*. Macaques, including rhesus monkeys, are often used as subjects in medical research because they are relatively affordable and resemble humans in many ways.

should be instituted to minimize health risks to monkey handlers since B virus is potentially deadly.

An effective vaccine for B virus, even after years of research, is still unavailable. Since the potential for human death from the B virus infection is high, and the handling and exposure to macaques is rising with increased use of the animals in laboratory settings, a better understanding of the infection is necessary. The mechanism by which the B virus lives within the macaque host is still unclear, and further research is needed to gain the knowledge necessary to combat this virus.

SEE ALSO *Antiviral Drugs; Personal Protective Equipment; Viral Disease; Zoonoses.*

BIBLIOGRAPHY

Books

Bannister, Barbara A. *Infection: Microbiology and Management.* Malden, MA: Blackwell Publishing, 2006.

Cohen, Jonathan, and William G. Powderly, eds. *Infectious Diseases.* New York: Mosby, 2004.

Ryan, Kenneth J., and C. George Ray, eds. *Sherris Medical Microbiology: An Introduction to Infectious Diseases.* New York: McGraw Hill, 2004.

Periodicals

Huff, Jennifer L., and Peter A. Barry. "B-Virus (*Cercopithecine herpesvirus* 1) Infection in Humans and Macaques: Potential for Zoonotic Disease." *Emerging Infectious Diseases* 9 (February 2003): 246–250. Also available online at: <http://oacu.od.nih.gov/UsefulResources/resources/emergindis2003.pdf>.

Web Sites

Centers for Disease Control and Prevention. "Recommendations for Prevention of and Therapy for Exposure to B Virus (*Cercopithecine Herpesvirus* 1)." November 15, 2002. <http://www.cdc.gov/ncidod/diseases/BVIRUS.pdf> (accessed April 16, 2007).

Georgia State University. "National B Virus Resource Center." <http://www2.gsu.edu/~wwwvir/> (accessed April 17, 2007).

Morbidity and Mortality Weekly Report. "Guidelines for Prevention of Herpesvirus Simiae (B Virus) Infection in Monkey Handlers." October 23, 1987. <http://www.cdc.gov/mmwr/preview/mmwrhtml/00015936.htm> (accessed April 18, 2007).

Babesiosis (Babesia Infection)

■ Introduction

Babesiosis (bab-EE-see-OH-sis), also known as *Babesia* infection, was first reported in humans in 1957 and first appeared in the United States in 1969. Since then, there have been at least 300 cases reported in the United States. As symptoms are either mild or do not arise in people with strong immune systems, some people are unaware they are infected. The majority of reported cases occur in people with weakened immune systems.

Infection occurs when humans are bitten by ticks infected with parasites of the genus *Babesia*. When symptoms arise from infection, they usually include fever, chills, muscle aches, and fatigue. In severe cases, liver and kidney damage can occur.

Babesiosis can be treated using a combination of antibiotics and anti-parasitic medications, and can be prevented by avoiding tick bites. This is done by covering up bare skin and wearing insect repellent.

■ Disease History, Characteristics, and Transmission

Babesiosis was first recognized in humans in 1957 after a Croatian cattle farmer contracted the disease. Prior to that case, babesiosis was thought to affect only animals. The biologist Victor Babes (1854–1926) first discovered the *Babesia* parasite in infected cattle. In 1893, Theobald Smith (1859–1934) and Frederick L. Kilbourne (1858–1936) determined that the parasite was transmitted via a tick vector, resulting in the disease babesiosis.

Babesiosis was first recorded in the United States in 1969 after an outbreak in Nantucket, Massachusetts. Since then, there have been further outbreaks throughout the U.S., mainly in the Northeast. Babesiosis outbreaks have also occurred in parts of Europe.

Babesiosis is caused by several species of parasites belonging to the genus *Babesia*. Although there are a number of species that cause the disease, the most com-

mon species that infect humans are *Babesia microti* and *B. divergens*. The parasite is transmitted from an infected animal to humans by ticks. The ticks feed off infected animals and ingest the parasite. When a tick bites a human, it transmits the parasite. The parasite then attacks

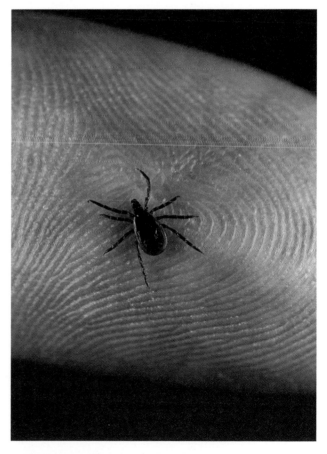

A female black-legged tick (*Ixodes scapularis*), formerly known as the deer tick (*Ixodes dammini*), is shown on a fingertip. These arthropods transmit diseases such as babesiosis and Lyme disease. *Scott Camazine/Photo Researchers, Inc.*

the host's red blood cells, which results in infection. The parasite remains in the bloodstream and can be transmitted to other humans by blood transfusions.

Symptoms of babesiosis include fever, chills, sweating, muscle aches, fatigue, an enlarged spleen, and hemolytic anemia. These symptoms may appear one to eight weeks after infection, and in some cases, an individual may not show symptoms for months or even years.

Scope and Distribution

Babesiosis occurs worldwide, although it is predominantly reported in the United States. The prevalence of this disease is unknown in malaria-endemic countries, since the *Babesia* parasite may be misidentified as *Plasmodium*, the parasite that causes malaria.

In the United States, the coastal areas of the Northeast, such as New York and Massachusetts, are the areas where babesiosis usually occurs. The parasite *B. microti* has been identified as the primary causal agent in these areas, although other species have been reported to cause infections in Washington, California, and Missouri. In Europe, the parasite *B. divergens* has been found to cause infection.

The majority of babesiosis cases involve people with weak immune systems, such as the elderly, very young children, people with immunodeficiencies, and people whose spleens have been removed. Severe complications such as low blood pressure, liver problems, anemia, and kidney failure may occur with this disease. Most people exhibit mild symptoms or show no symptoms at all. Symptoms often go unnoticed so that people are unaware they are infected.

Treatment and Prevention

Treatment of babesiosis usually requires removal of the parasites with anti-parasite medications in conjunction with antibiotic therapy. Two treatments are available. The first uses the drugs clindamycin and quinine, but these drugs sometimes are not well tolerated by patients. Another treatment uses the drugs atovaquone and azithromycin. Both treatments have been found to be equally effective. In some cases, no treatment is necessary for the infection to resolve.

No vaccine is available to protect humans from babesiosis. Avoiding contact with ticks is the most important way to keep from getting the disease. A variety of measures to avoid tick exposure can be used, including wearing protective clothing (such as long-sleeved shirts and long pants) and using insect repellents to discourage or kill ticks. If a tick has attached to a person's body, quick removal of the tick may prevent infection. Therefore, a thorough body check for ticks and the quick removal of any ticks discovered is a wise prevention strategy after any outdoor activity in a tick-infested area.

Impacts and Issues

Most known cases of babesiosis occur in the United States. However, it is likely that cases in malaria-endemic countries are not being identified due to similarities between the parasites causing each infection. Therefore, the distribution of this disease, and thus its impacts worldwide, may be understated.

In the United States, babesiosis is most common in the northeastern coastal states, including Massachusetts, Connecticut, Rhode Island, and New York. The disease is considered endemic in parts of these states. Babesiosis has also been reported in New Jersey, California, Georgia, Washington, and Minnesota. The increasing number of cases and increasing area of incidence indicates that babesiosis is an emerging disease.

The most common explanation for the increasing occurrence of babesiosis is an increase in the number of hosts for the parasite. The *Babesia* parasites reproduce in mice and other rodents, with the parasites being introduced into the mice while the tick feeds. While deer are not sites for parasite reproduction, they are a host for adult ticks. As a result, they have an indirect influence on the *Babesia* life cycle, since they ensure tick survival. Increased deer populations result in increased populations of ticks. This causes a higher likelihood that the parasite will be transmitted and a higher likelihood of human infection. In recent years, the size of deer populations in the United States has increased significantly, and this is thought to partially account for the increased incidence of babesiosis.

SEE ALSO *Arthropod-borne Disease; Emerging Infectious Diseases; Host and Vector; Immune Response to Infection; Immune System; Parasitic Diseases.*

BIBLIOGRAPHY

Books

Mandell, G.L., J.E. Bennett, and R. Dolin. *Principles and Practice of Infectious Diseases.* Vol. 2. Philadelphia, PA: Elsevier, 2005.

Periodicals

Herwaldt, B.L., et al. "Endemic Babesiosis in Another Eastern State: New Jersey." *Emerging Infectious Diseases* 9 (February 2003): 184–188.

Web Sites

Centers for Disease Control and Prevention. "Babesiosis." October 9, 2002. <http://www.dpd.cdc.gov/dpdx/HTML/Babesiosis.htm> (accessed February 1, 2007).

New York Department of Health. "Babesiosis." June 2004. <http://www.health.state.ny.us/diseases/communicable/babesiosis/fact_sheet.htm> (accessed February 1, 2007).

Stanford University. "History [of Babesiosis]." May 24, 2006. <http://www.stanford.edu/class/humbio103/ParaSites2006/Babesiosis/history.html> (accessed February 1, 2007).

Bacterial Disease

■ Introduction

Bacterial diseases refer to a large variety of diseases caused by bacteria or bacterial components that affect humans, domesticated animals, wildlife, fish, and birds. Most of these diseases are contagious—that is, they can be passed from one member of a species to another member, or, in a smaller number of instances, from one species to a different species. Depending on the organism, bacterial disease can be spread in different ways. Examples include contaminated food or water, air currents, infection of an environment that is not normally inhabited by the particular bacterium, and the possession or release of toxins by the bacteria.

■ Disease History, Characteristics, and Transmission

The history and characteristics of bacterial diseases are as varied as the diseases caused. *Bacillus anthracis*, the cause of anthrax, and *Yersinia pestis*, the cause of plague, have been present for millennia. Indeed, references to these diseases can be found in chapters of the Old Testament. Other bacterial infections have arisen only very recently. One example is the severe diarrheal and potentially kidney-destroying infection caused by the consumption of water or food that is contaminated by *Escherichia coli* strain O157:H7. The effects of O157:H7 are due to a cell-damaging toxin that can be released by the bacteria. Scientists who have studied this bacterium argue that this strain arose in the 1970s when *E. coli* residing in the intestinal tract (their normal environment) acquired genetic material that coded for the production of a destructive toxin from a related bacteria, *Shigella*.

Some bacterial diseases depend on the number of infecting bacteria present, and so are related to the growth of the bacteria. One example is the intestinal upset, diarrhea, and vomiting that results from the growth of *Campylobacter* following the ingestion of contaminated food or water. Poultry is a particularly important source of this infection, since the bacterium is a normal inhabitant of the intestinal tract of poultry. Release of intestinal contents during slaughter contaminates over 50% of the poultry sold each year in the United States, according to the U.S. Food and Drug Administration. The symptoms of *Campylobacter* can take a few days to develop, since the bacteria need time to reach sufficient numbers in the intestinal tract.

Other bacterial infections, particularly those involving toxins, require the presence of only a few bacteria, and growth of the bacteria is not necessary to produce the disease.

Bacterial diseases also vary in their methods of establishing infection. Some bacteria readily cause infections, since they are contagious—they can be easily passed from person-to-person, or can be easily spread to humans via a vector (another organism that transmits the bacteria from their normal host to a susceptible recipient). An example of a contagious bacterial disease is plague, which is caused by *Yersinia pestis*, and which is passed to people via the bite of an infected flea. Throughout history, plague has claimed millions of lives. In contrast, other bacteria cause infections opportunistically—that is, they are not normally infectious but can cause disease under certain circumstances. An example is *Pseudomonas aeruginosa*, a bacterium normally found in soil which is normally of little consequence to humans. However, in burn victims, the organism can infect the damaged skin. In addition, people who have cystic fibrosis and whose lungs can contain deposits of a thick mucus can be susceptible to recurring *P. aeruginosa* infections that can progressively compromise lung function.

Another means by which a few types of bacteria are able to cause infection is via their production of an environmentally hardy structure known as a spore. Similar to plant spores, bacterial spores are designed to help a bacterium survive tough environmental challenges, which can include temperatures that are too high or low for growth and lack of moisture. In a more hospitable

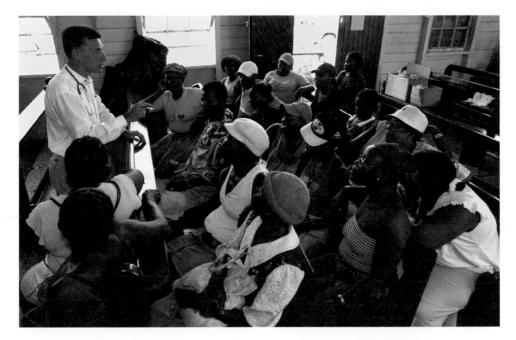

A medical doctor (above left), gives information about leptospirosis, a waterborne bacterial disease, to the residents of a village near Georgetown, Guyana, in 2005. After floods struck in January of that year, more than 20 people died from leptospirosis. *AP Images.*

environment, the spore can germinate and bacterial growth and division will resume. Bacteria in the genus *Bacillus* can form spores and, when they germinate, cause disease. A well known example is *B. anthracis*, which causes anthrax. Inhalation of only about 10 spores can be sufficient to cause pulmonary anthrax.

■ Scope and Distribution

Bacterial disease occurs virtually worldwide, with the exceptions of the far North and Antarctica and at very high altitudes. Even temperate waters can harbor disease-causing (pathogenic) bacteria, such as *Vibrio cholerae*, the cause of cholera.

■ Treatment and Prevention

Antibiotics are the standard treatment for bacterial infections caused by organisms sensitive to their actions. The type of antibiotic and the concentration required to kill the target bacteria depend on the organism. Frequently, bacteria develop resistance to a variety of antibiotics. Vaccines continue to be a valuable means of preventing bacterial diseases, such as diphtheria, meningococcal disease, and pertussis (whooping cough).

Bacterial diseases can be prevented in a variety of ways. Avoiding the source of the organism (for example, not drinking contaminated water), practicing good hygiene, such as regular handwashing with an antibacterial soap, and maintaining a balanced and healthy diet to keep the body's immune system efficient, are a few examples of good preventive measures.

■ Impacts and Issues

Bacterial diseases have been responsible for countless millions of deaths and continue to be a significant problem. Only a few decades ago, it was thought that many bacterial infections had been brought under control with the discovery or synthesis of a variety of antibiotics that were tremendously effective. However, this optimism has been short-lived. Antibiotic resistance is looming as one of the great medical challenges of the twenty-first century.

As of 2007, a number of vaccines that can be given orally are under development for several bacterial diseases. Vaccines against the intestinally damaging types of *Escherichia coli*, *Shigella*, and *Campylobacter* will hopefully lessen the occurrence of the diarrhea caused by these organisms. These and some other vaccines under development have the advantage of being stable at non-refrigeration temperatures, which would make them suitable for rural areas of underdeveloped and developing countries.

While progress is being made to lessen the occurrence of some bacterial diseases, the threat posed by the deliberate malicious use of disease-causing bacteria remains. Biological warfare has been practiced for centuries. In the twentieth century, a number of countries, including the United States, experimented with the use

WORDS TO KNOW

ANTIBIOTIC RESISTANCE: The ability of bacteria to resist the actions of antibiotic drugs.

RE-EMERGING DISEASE: Many diseases once thought to be controlled are reappearing to infect humans again. These are known as re-emerging diseases because they have not been common for a long period of time and are starting to appear again among large population groups.

SPORE: A dormant form assumed by some bacteria, such as anthrax, that enables the bacterium to survive high temperatures, dryness, and lack of nourishment for long periods of time. Under proper conditions, the spore may revert to the actively multiplying form of the bacteria.

of bacteria as a weapon. Now, this threat has moved from governments to organizations and individuals. The use of bacteria as a biological weapon has become part of the nightly news. As exemplified by the deliberate contamination of letters with *Bacillus anthracis* in Washington, D.C., in 2001, the danger posed by bioterrorism is real and difficult to prevent.

The specter of bioterrorism and the often frenzied reporting of bacterial disease outbreaks has spawned a growing apprehension in many people about diseases that are, in fact, not common. For example, the fear of the bacteria that cause necrotizing fasciitis, termed the

"flesh-eating bacteria" by the media, is out of proportion to the handful of cases that occur in North America each year.

What is a more realistic concern is the emergence or re-emergence of bacterial diseases that do pose a health threat. One example is the re-emergence of tuberculosis. The emerging strains are also more antibiotic resistant than their predecessors. In developing nations, multidrug resistant tuberculosis is considered an emergency by agencies such as the World Health Organization (WHO). WHO and other agencies, including the U.S. Centers for Disease Control and Prevention, have spearheaded surveillance and notification campaigns designed to detect and respond rapidly to such outbreaks.

SEE ALSO *Airborne Precautions; Antibiotic Resistance; Bioterrorism; Climate Change and Infectious Disease; Culture and Sensitivity; Emerging Infectious Diseases; Vaccines and Vaccine Development.*

BIBLIOGRAPHY

Books

Brunelle, Lynn, and Barbara Ravage. *Bacteria.* Milwaukee: Gareth Stevens, 2003.

Roemmele, Jacqueline A., and Donna Batdorff. *Surviving the Flesh-eating Bacteria: Understanding, Preventing, Treating, and Living with Necrotizing Fasciitis.* New York: Avery, 2003.

Web Sites

Centers for Disease Control and Prevention. "Division of Bacterial and Mycotic Diseases Home Page." May 12, 2006. <http://www.cdc.gov/ncidod/dbmd/index.htm> (accessed March 27, 2007).

Brian Hoyle

Balantidiasis

■ Introduction

Ingestion of the protozoan parasite *Balantidium coli* causes balantidiasis (ba-lan-ti-DYE-a-sis) infection. This parasite is transmitted from animal reservoirs to humans by oral contact with fecal matter. This transmission occurs when unwashed food or unclean water is ingested, or if hands are not washed after handling animals. While bal-antidiasis infection is rare, and most cases are asymptomatic, some cases result in diarrhea, dysentery, colitis, abdominal pain, weight loss, and fatalities. Treatment is effective and involves a short course of antibiotics, which eradicates the parasite.

Balantidiasis occurs worldwide, but is more common in areas in which humans live in close contact with livestock, and particularly in areas with poor sanitation or

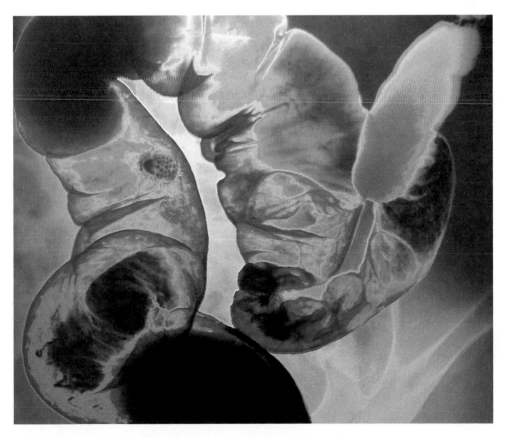

A colored barium X-ray shows the large intestine of a patient with balantidiasis. The disease is caused by the parasitic protozoan *Balantidium coli*, which is shown as a grey oval (center left). *Zephyr/Photo Researchers, Inc.*

other health problems. Infection is best prevented by treating water, washing food and hands, and reducing contact with livestock. Improving community sanitation standards, as well as educating communities on the importance of sanitation, can also help reduce infection.

Disease History, Characteristics, and Transmission

Balantidiasis is an intestinal infection caused by the parasite *Balantidium coli*. Humans are infected when they ingest *B. coli* cysts—immobile, protected forms of the parasite. Once in the body, these cysts break open and a mobile stage called a trophozoite is released. The trophozoite feeds on bacteria within the intestine, or enters the intestinal lining and secretes a tissue-destroying substance. As a result, sores (ulcers) and abscesses develop in the intestinal lining. New cysts are formed by the trophozoites and are excreted from the body in the feces. The cysts are well-protected and can remain outside the body under favorable conditions for many weeks.

B. coli are transmitted to humans from animal reservoirs such as livestock, rodents, and non-human primates. The most common reservoirs are pigs, which are often infected with *B. coli*, but tend to be asymptomatic. Transmission occurs when humans ingest food or water contaminated with the feces of infected animals, or when the mouth comes in contact with something contaminated with feces, such as unwashed hands.

Balantidiasis infection is uncommon in humans, and most cases are asymptomatic. However, asymptomatic humans are still capable of spreading the infection. When symptoms do appear, the most common symptoms are diarrhea, dysentery, abdominal cramps, and inflammation of the colon. In severe cases, perforation of the intestinal wall may occur, which can be fatal.

Scope and Distribution

Balantidiasis infection occurs worldwide, although it is more common in the tropics. It also is more common in regions where livestock, particularly pigs, is kept in conjunction with poor water systems and poor sanitation. Bolivia, the Philippines, and Papua New Guinea have all had outbreaks of balantidiasis, although the prevalence of the parasite *B. coli* is usually lower than 1%.

Treatment and Prevention

Medical treatment of balantidiasis is usually effective and is administered to both symptomatic and asymptomatic patients. Asymptomatic patients are treated in order to prevent them from spreading infection to others. Symptomatic patients are treated because untreated balantidiasis can become chronic and lead to dehydration, abdominal bleeding, and perforation of the intestinal wall, any of which—left untreated—can be fatal. Treatment usually involves oral administration of one of the following antibiotics: tetracycline, metronidazole, and iodoquinol. Tetracycline is the treatment of choice, but it is not recommended for pregnant women and children under the age of eight.

The most effective methods to prevent infection by *B. coli* involve improving sanitation. This includes boiling contaminated water prior to using it, washing hands after handling pigs or using the toilet, effectively washing and cooking food prior to eating, and preventing water sources from coming into contact with animal and human feces. As the most common mode of infection is from pigs to humans, reducing contact between pigs and humans will reduce infection. This can be achieved by preventing pigs from sharing human water sources, washing hands after handling pigs, and putting up barriers between pig and human living areas.

Impacts and Issues

Balantidiasis infection most commonly occurs in communities in which sanitation is poor. This situation often arises due to a lack of resources to provide adequate sanitation, as well as a lack of education about sanitary living. Infections by the parasite *B. coli* have also been found to cause more severe infection in people who are already debilitated. This may be due to malnourishment, coinciding parasitic infections, or a weakened immune system.

Efforts to improve sanitation and health in communities may lead to a reduction in the prevalence of infection. Installing hygienic measures such as potable water sources, toilets separate from living areas, and separate housing for livestock and humans will greatly reduce the likelihood of transmission of *B. coli* between animals and humans. In addition, educating people on the risks associated with poor hygiene may also help prevent transmission. Addressing other health issues within communities, such as coexisting parasitic infections and malnourishment, will help improve the overall health of the community and will aid in reducing the severity of any infections that do occur.

See Also *Dysentery; Handwashing; Parasitic Diseases; Sanitation.*

BIBLIOGRAPHY

Books

Mandell, G.L., J.E. Bennett, and R. Dolin. *Principles and Practice of Infectious Diseases.* Vol. 2. Philadelphia, PA: Elsevier, 2005.

Web Sites

Centers for Disease Control and Prevention. "Balantidiasis." May 6, 2004. <http://www.dpd.cdc.gov/dpdx/HTML/Balantidiasis.htm> (accessed February 2, 2007).

Stanford University. "The Parasite: *Balantidium coli.* The Disease: Balantidiasis." May 23, 2003. <http://www.stanford.edu/class/humbio103/ParaSites2003/Balantidium/Balantidium_coli_ParaSite.htm> (accessed February 2, 2007).

Baylisascaris Infection

■ Introduction

Baylisascaris (Bay-liss-AS-kuh-ris) is an intestinal infection caused by the *Baylisascaris procyonis* larvae of roundworms that infect raccoons, their primary host. According to the Centers for Disease Control and Prevention (CDC), the infection has also been diagnosed as secondarily infecting over ninety animal species, both domesticated and wild, including birds, mice, rabbits, and humans. Initially, raccoon roundworms grow within the intestine of raccoons. Millions of microscopic-sized eggs produced by the mature worms are passed with the raccoon's feces. The raccoon is not generally affected by being infested with the worms. However, infestation inside humans can cause serious illness or death.

Generally, two to four weeks after their fecal release into the environment, the eggs are considered to be infectious to animals and humans. The group of large raccoon roundworms is a very robust species, able to survive environments such as harsh cold and hot temperatures. With enough moisture, *Baylisascaris procyonis* can survive for years.

■ Disease History, Characteristics, and Transmission

According to the CDC, the first U.S. fatal human case was reported in 1984 in a ten-month-old infant living in rural Pennsylvania.

Common characteristics of adult *Baylisascaris* worms include a length from 5–8 inches (13–20 centimeters) and a width of about 0.5 inch (1.3 centimeter). Colored whitish-tan, they have a cylindrically shaped body that narrows at both ends.

Human transmission occurs when infective eggs are eaten within water, soil, or on objects contaminated with raccoon feces. Upon ingestion, eggs hatch into larvae within the intestines. They travel throughout the body, often affecting the muscles and organs, especially the brain.

Symptoms generally take from two to three weeks to appear, up to a maximum of two months. Common symptoms include skin irritations, nausea, tiredness, lack of muscle control, and inability to focus. More severe symptoms include brain and eye damage, liver enlargement, loss of muscle control, blindness, and coma. Ultimately, death can occur.

Symptom severity depends on the number of eggs ingested and where the larvae spread. Estimates show that around a few thousand eggs are needed to cause infection. A few eggs cause little or no symptoms, while large numbers can cause serious problems.

Raccoons are infected in two ways. In the direct cycle, raccoons, especially young ones, ingest the *Baylisascaris* eggs while feeding and grooming. In the indirect cycle, eggs are eaten by intermediate hosts such as armadillos, birds, chipmunks, dogs, mice, rabbits, and squirrels. Within the host, the eggs hatch, and the larvae travel into the intestines, liver, and lungs and, later, into the head, neck, or chest. Adult raccoons then eat the intermediate host, and the *Baylisascaris* larvae are released and sent to the intestine to mature.

There are usually no outward symptoms visible when raccoons are infected. Symptoms can be observed, however, when intermediate hosts are infected. When in their brains, larvae can cause behavioral changes, destroy the brain, or kill the host. Early symptoms include awkwardness in walking and climbing, sight problems, and a tilting head. Later symptoms includes loss of fear of humans; activities of rolling on the ground, laying on its side, and feet paddling; and finally, a comatose state and death.

■ Scope and Distribution

Raccoons are commonly found throughout the United States; however the occurrence of *Baylisascaris* infection is most prevalent in the Midwestern, Northeastern, Middle Atlantic, and West Coast states. Specifically, according to the CDC Division of Parasitic Diseases, the states with the most *Baylisascaris* infections are California, Illinois, Michigan, Minnesota, New York, Oregon, and Pennsylvania.

■ Treatment and Prevention

Baylisascaris can infect humans when contacting animal feces and when hands are not properly washed. Careful decontamination procedures after contact can aid in prevention. Droppings—dark, tubular, and with a strong odor—may contain infectious larvae even after months. Larvae can survive severe heat and cold environments and harsh chemicals.

To disinfect contaminated areas, feces should be immediately buried, burned, or isolated at a landfill. Wearing gloves, a facemask, and protective clothing can prevent further contamination. Known infected surfaces should be cleaned with high temperatures, such as with boiling water, or treated with strong disinfectants. Feeding and interacting with stray raccoons should also be avoided.

It is difficult to diagnose *Baylisascaris* infection. Medical professionals often first eliminate other infections with similar symptoms. There are no known treatments to lessen the illness.

Currently, no definitive commercial serologic (blood) test exists to diagnose the infection. Drugs and vaccines are not available to effectively kill larvae. Laser surgery has been successful in killing larvae within the eyes. However, damage already present is likely permanent.

■ Impacts and Issues

Baylisascaris infection is an emerging helminthic zoonosis (increasingly seen worm infection acquired from animals), and therefore, a growing public health concern. Due to time spent outdoors, it is becoming an increasing cause of severe human disease. In addition, due to increased encroachment of humans into raccoon habitat, raccoons have increasingly more contact with humans, which exacerbates the problem.

People most likely to become infected include children and persons who spend more time outdoors than other groups and are more likely to swallow infected substances. Hikers, taxidermists, veterinarians, trappers, wildlife handlers, and other similar groups who spend large amounts of time outdoors near raccoons and their habitats are also at increased risk.

According to the CDC, exposure and infection rates are in humans likely much larger than is medically reported. Rates of infected raccoons have been widely found in the United States to be up to 70% in adults and 90% in juveniles. Many veterinarians advise against keeping raccoons as pets, due to the widespread high rate of infection of the roundworm in raccoons. One adult female worm can produce hundreds of thousands of

eggs daily, and an infected raccoon can daily deposit as many as 45 million eggs.

Raccoons are among the most numerous wild animals in the U.S. Their close proximity to humans makes *Baylisascaris* infection a potentially major infectious disease. However, to date, the prevalence of infection in the U.S. population is not known and its identity as a growing public health problem is under-recognized.

Due to several factors, including the low infective dose, numerous availability of the host (raccoons), and lack of a definitive, effective treatment in human infection,

Baylisascaris procyonis is also considered a potential agent of bioterrorism.

SEE ALSO *Handwashing; Host and Vector; Public Health and Infectious Disease; Roundworm* (Ascariasis) *Infection.*

BIBLIOGRAPHY

Books

Samuel, William M., et al., editors. *Parasitic Diseases of Wild Mammals.* Ames, IA: Iowa State University Press, 2001.

Scheld, W. Michael, et al. *Emerging Infections.* Washington, D.C.: ASM, 2006.

Periodicals

Gompper, Matthew E. and Amber N. Wright. "Altered Prevalence of Raccoon Roundworm (*Baylisascaris procyonis*) Owing to Manipulated Contact Rates of Hosts." *Journal of Zoology.* (2005), 266: 215–219.

Sorvillo, Frank, et al. "*Baylisascaris procyonis*: An Emerging Helminthic Zoonosis." *Emerging Infectious Diseases.* (April 2002), 8, 4: 355–359.

Web Sites

Centers for Disease Control and Prevention. "Baylisascaris." <http://www.dpd.cdc.gov/dpdx/HTML/ Baylisascariasis.htm> (accessed March 4, 2007).

Centers for Disease Control and Prevention. "*Baylisascaris* Infection." September 23, 2004 <http://www.cdc.gov/ncidod/dpd/parasites/ baylisascaris/factsht_baylisascaris.htm> (accessed March 4, 2007).

Bilharzia (Schistosomiasis)

■ Introduction

Bilharzia (bill-HAR-zi-a), or schistosomiasis (SHIS-toe-SO-my-uh-sis), is an infection that usually results in organ damage and is caused by parasitic worms of the genus *Schistosoma*. This disease is mostly restricted to developing countries in which the parasites are endemic. However, infections have been recorded in developed countries, usually due to travel, immigration, or the entrance of refugees. Schistosomiasis can be acute, in which a common symptom is a fever appearing six to eight weeks following infection and disappearing within a few months; or chronic, in which organ damage occurs as a result of the immune system attacking parasite eggs retained in the body's organs. Chronic schistosomiasis is more common and usually does not appear until months or years after infection.

Treatment of schistosomiasis is effective and safe, involving a course of oral medications. Infection can be prevented by avoiding infected water bodies and by treating water before bathing or drinking. Attempts to treat infected populations and to control infection have had positive results within the past decade.

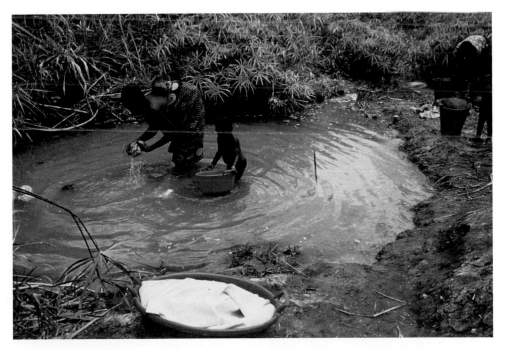

A woman and her children wash clothes at a pond containing snails in Tanzania. The snails carry fluke worms that cause schistosomiasis. The infective larvae are released by the snails into fresh water. *Andy Crump/TDR/WHO/Science Photo Library/Photo Researchers, Inc.*

WORDS TO KNOW

HOST: Organism that serves as the habitat for a parasite, or possibly for a symbiont. A host may provide nutrition to the parasite or symbiont, or simply a place in which to live.

SCHISTOSOMES: Blood flukes that infect an estimated 200 million people.

■ Disease History, Characteristics, and Transmission

Humans have suffered from schistosomiasis for thousands of years, with cases recorded in the period of the Egyptian pharaohs. However, the parasite causing this disease was not recognized until the nineteenth century. In 1851, Theodor Bilharz (1825–1862) first discovered a schistosome (a parasitic trematode worm) in infected people. Since then, a number of species of this parasite have been found to cause schistosomiasis, and their mode of infection and life cycle has been determined.

In humans, schistosomiasis is primarily caused by one of three types of *Schistosoma* parasites: *S. mansoni*, *S. haematobium*, and *S. japonicum*. There are also other, more localized species, such as *S. mekongi*, and *S. intercalatum*, which also cause human infections. While infection by these parasites usually results in some form of schistosomiasis, some species cause severe dermatitis, notably cercarial dermatitis.

There are both acute and chronic forms of this infection. Acute symptoms usually appear six to eight weeks after exposure to the parasite. The most common acute syndrome is called Katayama fever with symptoms including fever, loss of appetite, weight loss, abdominal pain, blood in the urine, weakness, headaches, joint and muscle pain, diarrhea, nausea, and cough. An initial symptom, usually occurring within days of exposure, is itchy skin. Acute symptoms usually disappear after a few weeks, although, some cases can be fatal. Chronic symptoms are more common than acute, and appear months to years after exposure. Chronic symptoms arise as a result of the body's immune system responding to the parasite's eggs. These eggs become lodged in various areas of the body depending on their species. Organ damage usually occurs as a result of the immune system responding to egg retention. The most commonly infected areas of the body are the urinary and intestinal systems, and damage to the bladder, intestines, spleen, and liver can occur. In rare cases, eggs may lodge in the spinal cord or brain, which can lead to seizures and paralysis.

Fresh water becomes contaminated with the eggs of *Schistosoma* parasite when a human who has the disease urinates or defecates in the water. The parasites hatch and are then ingested by freshwater snails, which are intermediate hosts during the parasite's life cycle. Following excretion from the snail, parasites can live in freshwater for 48 hours. During this time, they may come into contact with another human host and they can penetrate human skin within seconds. Once inside a host, the parasite develops into male and female worms that breed and lay eggs within blood vessels. While half of these eggs are excreted in urine or feces, the other half remain in the body and cause schistosomiasis symptoms. Excreted eggs hatch as soon as they enter fresh water, resulting in contamination of the water body. The cycle begins again if snails are present in the contaminated water.

■ Scope and Distribution

Schistosoma parasites are not found in the United States, but they are endemic to 74 developing countries. They are found in: Africa, the Caribbean, the Middle East, southern China, and Southeast Asia. Schistosomiasis is a major health risk, particularly within rural areas of Central China and Egypt. About 200 million people are estimated to be infected with *Schistosoma* parasites worldwide. While the majority of those suffering from this disease are found in countries where the parasite is endemic, some cases are found in other countries such as the United States and Great Britain as a result of travel, immigration, and entry of refugees into uninfected countries.

The majority of infected people tend to be rural agricultural workers who come into frequent contact with contaminated fresh water. In addition, a large number of children are infected. Across 54 countries, an estimated 66 million children are infected with the parasites. In one region alone, Lake Volta in Ghana, 90% of children in some villages are infected.

■ Treatment and Prevention

Treatment for schistosomiasis is effective and safe, usually involving a one to two day course of oral medications. Depending on the type of infection, one of three drugs is usually used. Praziquantal can be used for all forms of infection; oxamiquine is exclusively used for intestinal infections in Africa and South America; and metrifonate is used to treat urinary infections. Re-infection is possible after treatment, although the risk of serious organ damage is reduced as a result of treatment.

Because schistosomiasis is caused by a freshwater-borne parasite, the most effective prevention methods involve avoiding or treating contaminated water. Since the parasite penetrates the skin within seconds, avoiding contact with any potentially contaminated water bodies, such as lakes, rivers, and dams, will prevent infection. This includes avoiding swimming, bathing, and working in these water bodies. Fresh water that has been filtered, or heated to at least 150°F (65.5°C), is suitable for bathing. Water held in storage for 48 hours is also suitable for bathing as the parasite only lives without a host for this length of time. To ensure drinking water is free of parasites, filtering or boiling for at least one minute removes or kills the parasites.

Vigorous towel drying may also prevent parasite penetration, if the body has only been briefly submerged in contaminated water. However, this method is not recommended as a reliable means of prevention.

Long-term prevention of parasite infection involves controlling the occurrence of infection. Methods of control include educating people on parasite transmission; supplying clean water to regions where the parasite is endemic; diagnosing and treating infected people; controlling freshwater snails, the parasite's intermediate host; and increasing sanitation in infected regions.

■ Impacts and Issues

Schistosomiasis infection primarily occurs in developing countries. This is due to the fact that the parasites that cause schistosomiasis are endemic to developing countries, but the conditions of life in these regions also play an important role in the incidence and spread of the disease. Poverty; lack of awareness (both in terms of mode of infection and treatment methods); absent or inadequate of public health facilities; and unsanitary conditions all contribute to an increased risk of infection in developing countries. Furthermore, transmission of the disease to different areas is facilitated by the movement of populations and refugees. The World Health Organization (WHO) has stated that schistosomiasis is the second most important tropical disease, in terms of public health, following malaria. It is estimated that 200 million people worldwide are infected with the schistosomiasis parasite, and that 20,000 deaths are associated with the severe consequences of infection. In both rural Central China and Egypt, it poses a major health risk to populations.

Schistosomiasis can result in symptomatic infections, as well as fatalities. However, the majority of infected people show no symptoms, or only mild infections. In some cases, this disease has been found to cause reduced productivity in infected adults and decreased growth and school performance in infected children. Treatment in infected regions has resulted in an increase in the health of the population, suggesting that the treatment methods are effective.

The WHO has reported dramatic improvements in certain regions as a result of an increase in treatment administration, along with increased efforts to control infection. Objectives of these infection control programs have been met within two years of implementation in some regions. However, the WHO also

---

IN CONTEXT: SCHISTOSOME DISTRIBUTION

"Human contact with water is thus necessary for infection by schistosomes. Various animals, such as dogs, cats, rodents, pigs, horse and goats, serve as reservoirs for *S. japonicum*, and dogs for *S. mekongi*."

"*Schistosoma mansoni* is found in parts of South America and the Caribbean, Africa, and the Middle East; *S. haematobium* in Africa and the Middle East; and *S. japonicum* in the Far East. *Schistosoma mekongi* and *S. intercalatum* are found focally in Southeast Asia and central West Africa, respectively."

SOURCE: *The Centers for Disease Control & Prevention; National Center for Infectious Diseases. Division of Parasitic Diseases.*

---

emphasizes the need to maintain this control for the programs to be fully effective. Schistosomiasis is also one of the infections targeted as part of the WHO's Initiative for Vaccine Research. A variety of vaccine candidates have been tested, but, so far, none have been able to provide more than a partial reduction in the worm burdens of those vaccinated relative to non-immunized controls. Hopefully, better success can be achieved using mixture of recombinant antigens. Another approach to vaccination against schistosomiasis is to reduce egg secretion by targeting the fecundity of the female worm. Some success with this approach has been reported.

Another significant impact of schistosomiasis on human health is the likely link between urinary schistosomiasis infection and bladder cancer. In a number of infected regions, a significant correlation exists between the occurrence of bladder cancer in patients also showing urinary schistosomiasis. For example, the WHO reports that in some parts of Africa, schistosomiasis-linked bladder cancer has an occurrence 32 times greater than bladder cancer in the United States.

SEE ALSO *Cancer and Infectious Disease; Economic Development and Disease; Immigration and Infectious Disease; Immune Response to Infection; Parasitic Diseases; Swimmer's Ear and Swimmer's Itch (Cercarial Dermatitis); Travel and Infectious Disease; Water-borne Disease; World Health Organization (WHO).*

BIBLIOGRAPHY

Books

Arguin, P. M., P. E. Kozarsky, and A. W. Navin. *Health Information for International Travel 2005–2006.* Washington, DC: U.S. Department of Health and Human Services, 2005.

Web Sites

Centers for Disease Control and Prevention. "Schistosomiasis." August 27, 2004. <http://www.cdc.gov/ncidod/dpd/parasites/schistosomiasis/factsht_schistosomiasis.htm> (accessed January 30, 2007).

WebMD. "Schistosomiasis." March 31, 2005. <http://www.emedicine.com/emerg/topic857.htm> (accessed January 30, 2007).

World Health Organization. "Schistosomiasis." <http://www.who.int/vaccine_research/diseases/soa_parasitic/en/index5.html#vaccine> (accessed January 30, 2007).

Biological Weapons Convention

Introduction

The Biological Weapons Convention (also more properly, but less widely, known as the Biological and Toxin Weapons Convention) is an international agreement that prohibits the development and stockpiling of biological weapons. The language of the Biological Weapons Convention (BWC)—drafted in 1972—describes biological weapons as "repugnant to the conscience of mankind."

History and Scientific Foundations

The BWC broadly prohibits the development of pathogens—disease-causing microorganisms, such as viruses and bacteria—and biological toxins that do not have established prophylactic merit (i.e., no ability to serve a protective immunological role), beneficial industrial use, or use in medical treatment.

The BWC prohibits the offensive weaponization of biological agents (e.g., anthrax spores). The BWC also prohibits the transformation of biological agents with established legitimate and sanctioned purposes into agents of a nature and quality that could be used to effectively induce illness or death. In addition to offensive weaponization of microorganisms and/or toxins, prohibited research procedures include concentrating a strain of bacterium or virus, altering the size of aggregations of potentially harmful biologic agents (e.g., refining anthrax spore sizes to spore sizes small enough to be effectively and widely carried in air currents), producing strains capable of withstanding normally adverse environmental conditions (e.g., disbursement weapons blast), and/or the manipulation of a number of other factors that make biologic agents effective weapons.

The United States renounced the first-use of biological weapons and restricted future weapons research programs to issues concerning defensive responses (e.g., immunization, detection, etc.), by executive order in 1969.

Applications and Research

Although the BWC disarmament provisions stipulated that biological weapons stockpiles were to have been destroyed by 1975, most Western intelligence agencies openly question whether all stockpiles have been destroyed. For example, despite the fact that it was a signatory party to the 1972 Biological and Toxin Weapons Convention, the former Soviet Union maintained a well-funded and high-intensity biological weapons program throughout the 1970s and 1980s that worked to produce and stockpile biological weapons including anthrax and smallpox agents. United States intelligence agencies openly raise doubt as to whether successor Russian biological weapons programs have been completely dismantled.

Impacts and Issues

According to the United States Bureau of Arms Control, as of May 2007, there were 147 countries that were parties to the Biological Weapons Convention. An additional 16 countries were listed as signatory countries who had signed, but not yet ratified, the BWC.

Recent United States intelligence estimates compiled from various agencies provide indications that some countries are still actively involved in the development of biological weapons. The U.S. Office of Technology Assessment and the U.S. Department of State

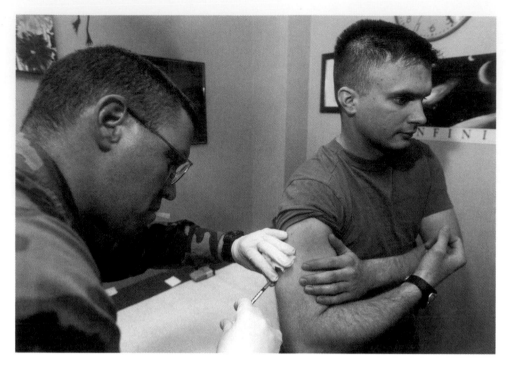

A U.S. Army soldier receives vaccinations to protect him against the potential biological threat of smallpox and anthrax. *AP Images.*

WORDS TO KNOW

BACTERIUM: Singular form of the term bacteria—single-celled microorganisms—bacterium refers to an individual microorganism.

EXECUTIVE ORDER: Presidential orders that implement or interpret a federal statute, administrative policy, or treaty.

SPORE: A dormant form assumed by some bacteria, such as anthrax, that enable the bacterium to survive high temperatures, dryness, and lack of nourishment for long periods of time. Under proper conditions, the spore may revert to the actively multiplying form of the bacteria.

STRAIN: A subclass or a specific genetic variation of an organism.

TOXIN: A poison that is produced by a living organism.

WEAPONIZATION: The use of any bacterium, virus, or other disease-causing organism as a weapon of war. Among other terms, it is also called germ warfare, biological weaponry, and biological warfare.

identify and report on states potentially developing biological weapons.

Although there have been several international meetings designed to strengthen the implementation and monitoring of BWC provisions, BWC verification procedures are currently the responsibility of an ad hoc commission of scientists. Broad international efforts to coordinate and strengthen enforcement of BWC provisions remains elusive.

SEE ALSO *Bioterrorism; War and Infectious Disease.*

BIBLIOGRAPHY

Books

Cole, Leonard A. *The Eleventh Plague: The Politics of Biological and Chemical Warfare.* New York: WH Freeman and Company, 1996.

Periodicals

DaSilva, E., "Biological Warfare, Terrorism, and the Biological Toxin Weapons Convention." *Electronic Journal of Biotechnology.* 3(1999):1–17.

Dire, D.J., and T.W. McGovern. "CBRNE - Biological Warfare Agents." *eMedicine Journal.* 4(2002): 1–39.

IN CONTEXT: TERRORISM AND BIOLOGICAL WARFARE

The USA PATRIOT Act (commonly called the Patriot Act) is an acronym for the Uniting and Strengthening America by Providing Appropriate Tools Required to Intercept and Obstruct Terrorism Act of 2001. The bill was signed into law by President George W. Bush on October 26, 2001. According to the act, research facilities that handled certain chemical and biological agents were required to institute new employee screening and security procedures.

The Patriot Act was introduced to improve counterterrorism efforts by providing law enforcement with new tools to detect and prevent terrorism. Section 817 of the USA Patriot Act is titled "Expansion of the Biological Weapons Statute" and expands on chapter 10 of title 18 in the United States Code, providing new laws designed to prevent terrorist acts involving biological weapons.

The specific changes made by the Patriot Act include making it unlawful to possess biological agents, toxins, or delivery systems unless there is a reasonably justified purpose and making it unlawful for a restricted person to possess biological agents, toxins, and delivery systems that are classified as select agents.

Laboratories that operate within the United States or that are funded by the U.S. must comply with the new regulations regarding prohibiting access to selected agents by restricted persons. Each organization is required to develop its own screening or application forms to obtain the required information on persons working (or seeking work) in their laboratories in order to certify their right to access to selected agents.

The Centers for Disease Control and Prevention (CDC) regulates "the possession, use, and transfer of select agents and toxins that have the potential to pose a severe threat to public health and safety. The CDC Select Agent Program oversees these activities and registers all laboratories and other entities in the United States of America that possess, use, or transfer a select agent or toxin."

The U.S. Departments of Health and Human Services (HHS) and Agriculture (USDA) published final rules for the possession, use, and transfer of select agents and toxins (42 C.F.R. Part 73, 7 C.F.R. Part 331, and 9 C.F.R. Part 121) in the Federal Register on March 18, 2005.

Web Sites

United States Department of State. "Parties and Signatories of the Biological Weapons Convention." <http://www.state.gov/t/ac/bw/fs/2002/8026.htm> (May 25, 2007).

Paul Davies

Bioterrorism

■ Introduction

After years of "back burner" low priority research, work on defensive measures against bioterrorism began in earnest in the United States soon after the anthrax attacks in 2001. Scientists are now developing strategies designed to protect the United States against a potentially limitless variety of biological weapons. The psychological impact of the anthrax attacks of late 2001 was enormous compared to the number of people actually killed and sickened during the episode. This is in keeping with the pattern of effective terror tactics in which expenditures of time, effort, and funds can be minimal, but impact on the target population is maximized.

■ History and Scientific Foundations

Since 2001, most defensive activity against bioterrorism threats has been focused on preventing or combating known "Class A" threats, including the organisms that cause anthrax, plague, smallpox, tularemia, and viral hemorrhagic fevers, as well as botulinum toxin. Activity to develop new drugs and vaccines is budgeted under Project Bioshield, which is directed by the Food and Drug Administration (FDA) and the Centers for Disease Control and Prevention (CDC).

Bioterrorism agents are essentially identical to biological warfare agents. Such agents may be classified operationally, as deadly or incapacitating agents, and as agents with or without the potential for secondary transmission (the ability to spread disease from one person affected by bioterrorism to another who was not exposed during the attack). Bioterrorism agents can also be classified according to their intended target, as when they are intended to sicken or kill people, animals, or vegetation such as crops; and according to type, including replicating pathogens (duplicating disease-causing organisms such as viruses, bacteria, or fungi), toxins, or biomodulators (immune system altering agents). Replicating pathogens and toxins are recognized as the greatest current threats.

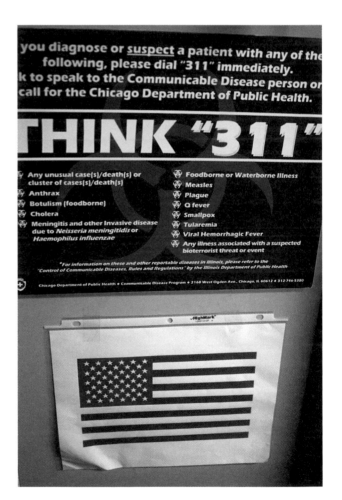

Signs, such as this, were hung in emergency rooms across the United States after the anthrax attacks of 2001. They encouraged physicians to watch for infectious diseases or signs of possible intentional biological contamination. *AP Images.*

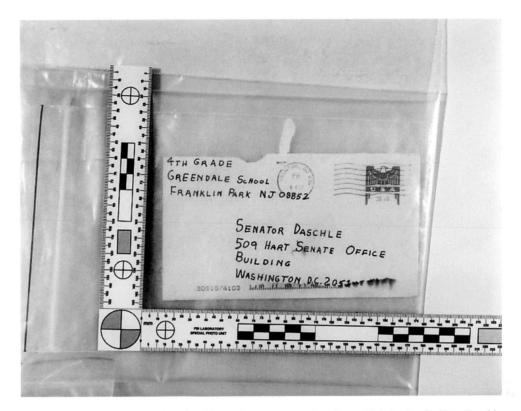

This envelope contained an anthrax-laced letter that was sent to then-Senate Majority Leader Tom Daschle in Washington, D.C., in October 2001. During the anthrax scare, two Washington, D.C., postal workers died from inhaled anthrax. Other anthrax-laden materials were sent to media centers in Florida and New York. Three others died from the disease as well. © *Reuters/Corbis.*

■ Applications and Research

Smallpox

Although many pathogens could be used to attack the U.S. population, only a few, including the smallpox virus, could cause illness or panic that could overwhelm existing medical and public health systems. The WHO authorizes two laboratories in the world to maintain stores of smallpox virus for research purposes, and authorities fear that additional smallpox virus may exist hidden away in laboratories other than the two WHO-designated repositories.

A new outbreak of smallpox could spread rapidly. The CDC strategy for controlling a new outbreak of smallpox incorporates principles that were used 30–40 years ago in eradicating the disease and have proven their effectiveness. They are based on knowledge that smallpox is mostly transmitted by close, face-to-face contact with infected individuals, while only a few cases could be transmitted by dry or aerosolized particles in close proximity to persons with the disease. New cases develop two weeks after exposure and take another two weeks to progress to pustules and scabs, giving a newly aware medical community some time to respond.

Smallpox vaccine is a live-virus vaccine composed of vaccinia virus that induces antibodies that also protect against smallpox. Smallpox vaccine production ceased in the early 1980s and current supplies of smallpox vaccine are limited. The CDC expects that new vaccines manufactured using cell cultures will be available within two to four years under the Bioshield program. Limited new supplies of the current vaccine are being manufactured under Bioshield.

After several years of considering mass vaccination as an alternative, CDC has settled on a ring vaccination strategy to combat a new smallpox outbreak. This includes isolation of confirmed and suspected smallpox cases with tracing, vaccination, and close surveillance of contacts to these cases as well as vaccination of the household contacts of the smallpox cases. Ring vaccination takes advantage of the relatively low infectivity of smallpox and focuses currently scarce vaccine resources where they will do the most good, minimizing adverse events, including rare deaths that could occur during indiscriminate mass vaccination.

Anthrax

Anthrax is an infectious disease caused by a spore-forming bacterium, the spores of which are very persistent and hard to break down in the environment, which makes anthrax a

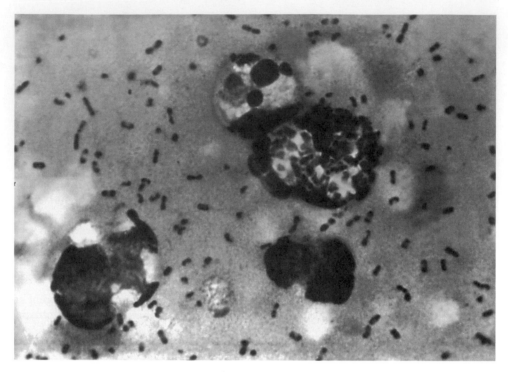

A bubonic plague smear, prepared from an adenopathic lymph node, or bubo, of a plague patient, shows the presence of the *Yersinia pestis* bacteria that causes the plague. The disease, considered a likely bioterrorist agent since it isn't difficult to make, is easily treatable with antibiotics if diagnosed early and properly. *Getty Images.*

persistent public health threat in spite of available treatment with familiar drugs.

There are three forms of anthrax infection: skin, gastrointestinal, and inhalational anthrax. Inhalational anthrax, with the highest death rates, occurs when spores are inhaled and infect the lungs. The treatments for all types of anthrax are the antibiotics ciprofloxacin, tetracycline drugs such as doxycycline, and some types of penicillin.

The anthrax vaccine is primarily given to people in the military and is only recommended for individuals considered to be at high risk of contracting the disease, such as scientists who handle anthrax bacteria. Current government efforts are focused on encouraging the development of new anthrax vaccines intended to prevent inhalational anthrax before and after exposure. The emergency response to anthrax consists of administration of antibiotics and spore cleanup by workers using personal protective equipment. Unvaccinated, exposed people and remediation workers begin taking preventative antibiotics at the time of their exposure and continue for at least 60 days.

Plague

Plague is caused by the bacterium *Yersinia pestis*. Bubonic plague is the most common type of naturally occurring plague, and is transmitted through the bite of an infected flea or exposure through a cut. Symptoms of bubonic plague include swollen, tender lymph nodes, headache, fever, and chills. If untreated, bubonic plague may result in death.

In pneumonic plague, the lungs are infected with the plague bacterium. People with pneumonic plague can transmit plague to other people, whereas bubonic plague cannot be spread from person to person. Antibiotics approved by the FDA to treat plague are streptomycin, doxycycline, and other tetracycline drugs. The public health response to pneumonic plague would be similar to that of anthrax, with the addition of quarantines that could impact sizable crowded geographic areas.

■ Impacts and Issues

The response to the 2001 anthrax attacks has been extensively analyzed as researchers attempt to model the optimal response to future attacks. The 2001 attacks were small-scale events, affecting a relatively few people in restricted geographic areas. In a recent study of a small-scale attack, Veterans Administration researchers conducted a cost-effectiveness analysis using a simulation model to determine the optimal response strategy for a small-scale anthrax attack against U.S. Postal Service distribution centers in a large metropolitan area. (A cost-effectiveness analysis compares the relative effectiveness of two or more alternatives in view of their costs and attempts to determine the best value for money.) The study compared three different strategies: (1) pre-attack vaccination of all U.S. distribution center postal workers, (2) post-attack antibiotic therapy followed by vaccination of exposed personnel, and (3) post-attack antibiotic therapy without vaccination of exposed personnel. The results showed that post-attack antibiotic therapy and vaccination of exposed postal workers is the most cost-effective response compared with post-attack antibiotic therapy alone. This was due to the greater prevention of death and disease when post-attack vaccination is combined with antibiotics. Pre-attack vaccination of all distribution center workers is less effective and more costly than the other two strategies. This is because vaccinating all postal employees would be very expensive, and the immunity conferred by the current vaccine is not perfect or always permanent, and the time between vaccination and an anthrax attack is indeterminate.

Some commentators have decried the resources and energy being poured into bioterrorism defense. According to this perspective, bioterrorism preparedness programs have wasted public health resources with little evidence of benefit. For example, several deaths and many serious illnesses have resulted from the smallpox vaccination program, but there is no clear evidence that any threat of smallpox exposure has existed since the eradication of the disease. Even the anthrax attacks were linked to secret U.S. military laboratories; without these laboratories the attacks probably would not have been possible. The huge effort to prepare the country against bioterrorist threats is seen by some critics as a great distraction from the need to allocate public health resources to address other health needs, and has been conducted at the expense of some vital programs.

Nevertheless, the anthrax attacks did demonstrate the havoc that malign individuals could wreak with sufficient determination, access to pathogens, and laboratory resources. As public protection will always be the primary responsibility of government, leaving the population totally unprepared for the eventuality of bioterrorism is simply not an option in the post-9/11 world. Accordingly, The Center for Law and the Public's Health at Georgetown and Johns Hopkins Universities drafted the Model State Emergency Health Powers Act (MSEHPA or Model Act) at the request of the CDC. The Model Act provides states with the powers needed to detect and contain either bioterrorism or a naturally occurring disease outbreak. To this extent, bioterrorism preparedness appears in sync with more conventional public health preparedness. Legislative bills based on the MSEHPA have been introduced in most states. This legislative effort has uncovered problems of state law obsolescence, inconsistency, and inadequacy. Most current state laws provide inadequate public protection whether a disease outbreak

WORDS TO KNOW

PATHOGEN: A disease-causing agent, such as a bacteria, virus, fungus, etc.

QUARANTINE: Quarantine is the practice of separating people who have been exposed to an infectious agent but have not yet developed symptoms from the general population. This can be done voluntarily or involuntarily by the authority of states and the federal Centers for Disease Control and Prevention.

RING VACCINATION: Ring vaccination is the vaccination of all susceptible people in an area surrounding a case of an infectious disease. Since vaccination makes people immune to the disease, the hope is that the disease will not spread from the known case to other people. Ring vaccination was used in eliminating the smallpox virus.

TOXIN: A poison that is produced by a living organism.

would be natural or intentional. They often date back to the early twentieth century and predate the immense changes in public health science over the past half century.

The Model Act is structured to support five basic public health functions to be facilitated by law: (1) preparedness, comprehensive planning for a public health emergency; (2) surveillance, measures to detect and track public health emergencies; (3) management of property, ensuring adequate availability of vaccines, pharmaceuticals, and hospitals, as well as providing power to abate hazards to the public's health; (4) protection of persons, powers to compel vaccination, testing, treatment, isolation, and quarantine when clearly necessary; and (5) communication, providing clear and authoritative information to the public. The act is also based on a legal framework to protect personal rights.

Use of Spectroscopy in Identifying Pathogens

Traditional detection of pathogens such as bacteria and viruses involves serologic (blood) testing in which potential pathogens in a tissue sample from an infected patient are cultured in the laboratory, and various stains and reagents are made to react with proteins of the pathogen's outer membrane. This is a slow and labor-intensive process. A new technique of rapidly identifying bacteria such as anthrax called desorption electrospray ionization recently developed at Purdue University could be used for homeland security. This technique enables the fast "fingerprinting" bacteria using a mass spectrometer. The analysis of bacteria and other microorganisms usually takes several hours. The spectrographic technique ionizes molecules outside of the spectrometer's vacuum chamber. Ionized molecules can then be manipulated, detected, and analyzed using electromagnetic fields. This technique is extremely sensitive, capable of detecting 1-billionth of a gram of a particular bacterium and identifying its subspecies, which is the level of accuracy required for detecting and monitoring infectious microorganisms. The technology can determine the subspecies and collect other information by observing the pattern of the pathogen's outer membrane proteins, and creates a sort of fingerprint as revealed by mass spectrometry. Such accuracy and timeliness makes the technology particularly apt for detecting bioterrorism agents, as word of an intentionally caused outbreak would need to be spread very soon after the appearance of suspected cases in order to prevent rapid transmission of the pathogen.

Involving the General Public in Preparedness

The public health emergency responses being fashioned by the CDC to a bioterrorist attack focus mainly on readying emergency and medical workers to cope with infection transmission, panic, and decontamination. While there has been some refinement in terms of how agencies and response personnel should coordinate their efforts, so far there have been few urgent instructions or preventive measures disseminated to the general public. On the other hand, promising new research on detection technologies, vaccines, and medicines to prevent or combat infections is now being funded under Project Bioshield.

Most bioterrorism policy discussion and response planning has been conducted among experts and has not involved much public participation. The capacity of the public to take an active role and even to lead in the response to bioterrorism is often discounted, or policymakers have assumed that local populations would get in the way of an effective response. This bias is based on fears of mass panic and social disorder. While no one really knows how the population will react to an extraordinary act of bioterrorism, experience with natural and technological disasters and disease outbreaks indicates that the public response would be generally effective and adaptive collective action. Therefore, the public should be viewed as a partner in the medical and public health response. Failure to involve the public in planning could hamper effective management of an epidemic and increase the likelihood of social breakdown. Ultimately, actions taken by nonprofessional individuals and groups could end up having the greatest impact on the outcome of a bioterrorism attack. Guidelines suggested for integrating the public into bioterrorism response planning include (1) treating the public as a capable ally in the

response to an epidemic; (2) enlisting civic organizations in practical public health activities; (3) anticipating needs for home-based patient care and infection control; (4) investment in public outreach and communication strategies; and (5) ensuring that planning reflects the values and priorities of affected populations.

■ Primary Source Connection

In an excerpt for the following journal article, the authors argue for a greater role for the biomedical research community in defense efforts against bioterrorism. Bradley T. Smith, PhD, is a Fellow, Thomas V. Inglesby, MD, is Deputy Director, and Tara O'toole, MD, MPH, is Director, all at the Johns Hopkins Center for Civilian Biodefense Strategies, Baltimore, Maryland.

Biodefense R&D: Anticipating Future Threats, Establishing a Strategic Environment

INTRODUCTION

The ultimate objective of the U.S. civilian biodefense strategy should be to eliminate the possibility of massively lethal bioterrorist attacks. A central pillar of this strategy must be an ambitious and aggressive scientific research, development, and production (R&D&P) program that delivers the diagnostic technologies, medicines, and vaccines needed to counter the range of bioweapons agents that might be used against the nation. A successful biodefense strategy must take account of the rapidly expanding spectrum of bioweapons agents and means of delivery made possible by 21st century advances in bioscientific knowledge and biotechnology. Meeting this challenge will require the engagement of America's extraordinary scientific talent and investments of financial and political capital on a scale far beyond that now committed or contemplated. The purpose of this article is to provide a brief analysis of the current biomedical R&D&P environment and to offer recommendations for the establishment of a national biodefense strategy that could significantly diminish the suffering and loss that would accompany bioterrorist attacks. In the longer term, a robust biodefense R&D&P effort, if coupled to substantial improvements in medical and public health systems, could conceivably render biological weapons ineffective as agents of mass lethality.

THE PROBLEM: 20TH AND 21ST CENTURY BIOWEAPONS

The advantage is now firmly with those who would seek to deploy offensive bioweapons; the state of biodefense is relatively weak. Following the terrorist attacks of

2001, the National Institute of Allergy and Infectious Diseases (NIAID) at the National Institutes of Health (NIH) received $1.7 billion to fund biodefense research projects. NIAID has since established a "roadmap" describing the scientific research needed to devise new "countermeasures" (i.e., diagnostic technologies, therapeutic drugs, and vaccines) for the pathogens thought to be the bioweapons agents of greatest concern. Much of the NIAID roadmap has, appropriately, focused on developing countermeasures for the six CDC Category A bioweapons threats (anthrax, smallpox, plague, botulism, tularemia, and the viral hemorrhagic fevers) for which there are striking gaps in available countermeasures..., and a selection of other bioweapons threats on the CDC's Category B and C lists (collectively termed "20th century bioweapons" in this article).

Growing numbers of people in the scientific community now recognize that looming just ahead is a far more daunting array of potential engineered bioweapon agents (collectively termed "21st century bioweapons" in this article). The life sciences are at the beginning of a revolutionary period. Scientific understanding of living systems and how to manipulate them is expanding exponentially, fueled by advances in computerization, the global dispersion of bioscientific expertise as well as biological databases, and substantial economic investment in biomedical and agricultural research and product development.

A prime example of these powerful advances was the identification in 2001 of the approximately 40,000 genes in the human genome. Scientists are rapidly learning how to translate this genomic "parts list" into a sophisticated understanding of how specific genes control human biological systems in the body. Such discoveries will bring great benefit to humankind, but they will also allow the development of a new constellation of powerful 21st century bioweapons.

There are already countless portents of the coming power of bioscience and how it will propel bioweapons developments. Scientists have shown that it is possible to create strains of the bacterium that causes anthrax to be resistant to the most powerful existing antibiotics. They have demonstrated the capacity to make viruses that can overcome vaccine-induced immunity. Viruses can be genetically modified to increase their ability to kill infected cells, or to become capable of attacking entirely new target species. Viruses and bacteria can be manipulated in ways that make them better able to survive environmental stress and to be disseminated over distances in the air as weapons. Technologies already exist that could be used to protect pathogens from detection or destruction by the human immune system. These are only a small sample of the developments ahead on the bioscience landscape.

The "dual use" aspect of bioscience does not pertain only to specific, isolated technological applications, as is the case in nuclear weapons work. Rather, it is biological knowledge itself that is the source of the power that can be applied toward beneficent or malevolent ends. The knowledge needed to engineer a more lethal viral or bacterial bioweapon is essentially the same as that needed to understand how that virus or bacteria causes disease and how to create an effective vaccine against it. The distinction between good biology and its "dark side" lies only in intent and application. With rare exception, it will be very difficult to sequester new bioscientific knowledge that might be applied to building biological weapons without simultaneously harming beneficial biomedical research and essential biodefense R&D&P.

Given the size, momentum, and global dissemination of the bioscientific enterprise and the great demand for the medical and agricultural products being created, the rapid global advance of bioscience is essentially unstoppable. A successful biodefense R&D&P strategy must accept that the growth and international diffusion of bio-scientific knowledge and technologies will continue at a phenomenal pace and must seek to leverage these powerful forces against the bioterrorist threat.

. . .

CONCLUSION

The full power of the nation's biomedical research, development, and production enterprise is not yet engaged in biodefense, and given the current environment, funding levels, priorities, and lack of clear vision for the biodefense R&D&P program, large numbers of the best biomedical scientists are unlikely to engage. Current biodefense initiatives, when compared to other U.S. government efforts to address top national security threats, suggest that the U.S. government either does not yet understand the grave nature and scope of the bioterrorist threat or is not prepared to commit fully to a robust biodefense research, development, and production effort. This must change if the nation is to counter the coming bioweapons threat and set the course to eliminate bioweapons as weapons of mass lethality.

Editor's note: Referenced citations omitted.

Bradley T. Smith, Thomas V. Inglesby, Tara O'toole

BRADLEY T. SMITH, THOMAS V. INGLESBY, AND TARA O'TOOLE. LDQUO;BIODEFENSE R&D: ANTICIPATING FUTURE THREATS, ESTABLISHING A STRATEGIC ENVIRONMENT.RDQUO; *BIOSECURITY & BIOTERRORISM.* 1(3):193–202, 2003.

SEE ALSO *War and Infectious Disease; Public Health and Infectious Disease.*

BIBLIOGRAPHY

Books

Fong, I.W., and Kenneth Alibek, eds. *Bioterrorism and Infectious Agents: A New Dilemma for the 21st Century.* New York: Springer, 2005.

Periodicals

Cohen H.W., R.M. Gould, V.W. Sidel. "The Pitfalls of Bioterrorism Preparedness: the Anthrax and Smallpox Experiences." *Am J Public Health*, (2004): 94:1667–1671.

Glass T.A., M. Schoch-Spana. "Bioterrorism and the People: How to Vaccinate a City against Panic." *Clinical Infectious Diseases* (2002) 34:217–23.

Gostin L.O., J.W. Sapsin, S.B. Teret, et al. "The Model State Emergency Health Powers Act: Planning for and Response to Bioterrorism and Naturally Occurring Infectious Diseases." *JAMA* (2002): 288:622–628.

Web Sites

Centers for Disease Control and Prevention (CDC). "Bioterrorism." <http://www.bt.cdc.gov/bioterrorism/> (accessed June 13, 2007).

Kenneth T. LaPensee

Blastomycosis

■ Introduction

Blastomycosis is a rare fungal infection caused by inhaling the fungal organism *Blastomyces dermatitidis* through the nose or mouth. The organism is usually found in habitats containing wood and soil. It lives commonly as a mold in warm, sandy soils located near water and within moist soil full of decomposing organic matter. The infection is restricted to humans, dogs, and other mammals in portions of North America. Human symptoms of the infection are similar to the influenzalike disease of the lungs called histoplasmosis (also called Darling's disease). Rarely, persons with blastomycosis develop chronic pulmonary infection or widespread disseminated infection.

When found in a host, *Blastomyces dermatitidis* lives as yeast. Because it lives as mold outside a host and as yeast inside, it is called a biphasic organism. Blastomycosis is commonly misdiagnosed as Valley fever (coccidioidomycosis), Lyme disease, or other viral infections.

■ Disease History, Characteristics, and Transmission

The first description of blastomycosis came in 1876 from French biologist Philippe Edouard Leon Van Tieghem (1839–1914). Later, in 1894, American dermatologist Thomas Gilchrist (1862–1927), from the University of Maryland School of Medicine, described it more thoroughly. At that time, Gilchrist isolated and proved the cause of the human infection. Because of this description, it is often called Gilchrist's disease or Gilchrist's mycosis. It is also sometimes called Chicago disease and North American blastomycosis.

Transmission of the fungus is by inhalation of airborne spores after contaminated soil has been disturbed. Persons, such as forestry workers, campers, hunters, and farmers, located near wooded sites are at increased risk.

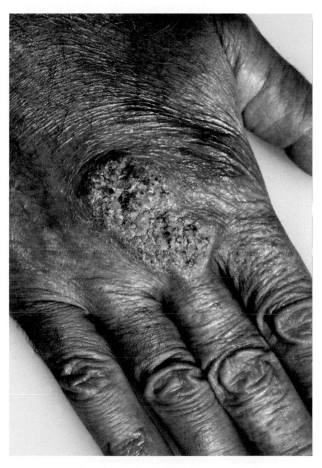

Skin lesions are typical of blastomycosis, a fungal disease that affects the skin and lungs. This infection is characterized by multiple inflammatory lesions of the internal organs, mucous membranes, or skin. *Scott Camazine/Photo Researchers, Inc.*

People who have compromised immune systems also are at high risk.

According to the Centers of Disease Control and Prevention Division of Bacterial and Mycotic Diseases,

WORDS TO KNOW

HOST: Organism that serves as the habitat for a parasite, or possibly for a symbiont. A host may provide nutrition to the parasite or symbiont, or simply a place in which to live.

MYCOTIC DISEASE: Mycotic disease is a disease caused by fungal infection.

SPORE: A dormant form assumed by some bacteria, such as anthrax, that enable the bacterium to survive high temperatures, dryness, and lack of nourishment for long periods of time. Under proper conditions, the spore may revert to the actively multiplying form of the bacteria.

symptoms occur in about 50% of all cases. Common symptoms, which sometimes parallel symptoms of influenza (flu), include a nonproductive cough, fever, chills, headache, and pain or stiffness in muscles or joints. When it resembles bacterial pneumonia, symptoms include high fever, chills, a productive cough with brown or bloody-looking sputum, and chest pain of the lungs. When it looks like tuberculosis or lung cancer, symptoms include a low-grade fever, productive cough, night sweats, and weight loss. Other symptoms can include shortness of breath, sweating, tiredness, overall discomfort and ill-feeling, rash, skin and bone lesions, and problems with the bladder, kidney, prostate, and testes.

Once the infection is inside the lungs, it grows rapidly, becoming noticeable in the blood, brain, bone, lymphatic system, skin, and genital and urinary systems. The incubation period is generally 30 to 100 days. No symptoms occur in about half the infections. The death rate from the infection is about 5%.

■ Scope and Distribution

Blastomycosis is concentrated in parts of North America, especially in the central southern, midwestern, and southeastern parts of the United States and the northwestern part of Ontario in Canada. Infection is more frequent in the basin areas around the Ohio River and Mississippi River and in the areas surrounding the Great Lakes. It occurs in about one to two people out of 100,000 in these North American regions.

Some cases are reported in Central America, South America, and Africa. Although anyone can contract the infection, it more commonly affects people with com-

promised immune systems. Males are more likely to become infected than are females.

■ Treatment and Prevention

Once identified, the diagnosis can be confirmed with cellular and tissue tests such as the KOH test. The KOH test is a procedure performed with a microscope that uses potassium hydroxide (KOH) to dissolve skin tissue and reveal fungal cells. Other diagnostic tests employed may include chest x-rays to show nodule growth or pneumonia; skin, organ or tissue biopsies; and blood and sputum cultures. When other tests fail, a urine antigen test usually identifies the disease.

Blastomycosis in the lungs does not always require drug treatment to eliminate it. However, when the infection spreads outside the lungs or has become severe within the lungs, amphotericin B (such as Abelcet® and Fungisome®), itraconazole (such as Sporanox®), or other antifungal medicines may be prescribed orally or intravenously. Amphotericin B is usually reserved for severe cases. While it is more effective than other antifungals, it also is more toxic. Periodic follow-up by a physician is recommended to detect any recurrences. Cure rates are high, however, treatment often takes many weeks or months.

People with minor irritations of the skin and lungs usually recover without suffering permanent problems. Major complications—such as large abscesses, relapses, or recurrences of the disease and negative side effects of drugs—can lead to complications. If patients do not recover, they may develop chronic lung infection or widespread infection of the bones, skin, and genitourinary tract. On occasion, the fungus affects the meninges, the protective covering of the brain and spinal column. If left untreated, severe cases can progress rapidly and eventually cause death.

■ Impacts and Issues

Blastomycosis has not been accurately and reliably reported by the medical community in the past. This is largely due to the fact that national reporting is not required in Canada and the United States and that its occurrence has been restricted to North America. However, the disease is becoming better defined as more research is performed. Unfortunately it is still not completely understood. Lack of information about the disease is primarily due to the difficulty in isolating the causative organism from its natural environment.

Most medical practitioners consider blastomycosis to be an important mycotic disease (fungal disease or infection). According to the *Canadian Medical Association Journal* (CMAJ), its prevalence (or endemicity) may be more extensive than previously thought. The CMAJ suggests that physicians include it in the potential diagnoses of unexplained granulomatous pulmonary (relating to the lungs) disease and cutaneous (relating to the skin) disease.

Currently, a number of uncertainties still surround the origins, characteristics, causes, and other important medical facts (that is, the epidemiology) of blastomycosis. A greater understanding of the epidemiology of this disease will allow it to be more effectively combated in the future.

SEE ALSO *Coccidioidomycosis; Histoplasmosis; Mycotic Disease.*

BIBLIOGRAPHY

Books

Al-Doory, Yousef, and Arthur F. DiSalvo, eds. *Blastomycosis.* New York: Plenum, 1992.

Korting, H. C., ed. *Mycoses: Diagnosis, Therapy and Prophylaxis of Fungal Diseases.* Berlin, Germany: Blackwell Science, 2005.

Sobel, Jack D. *Contemporary Diagnosis and Management of Fungal Infections.* Newtown, PA: Handbooks in Health Care, 2003.

Periodicals

Lester, Robert S., et al. "Novel Cases of Blastomycosis Acquired in Toronto, Ontario." *Canadian Medical Association Journal* 163 (November 14, 2000): 1309–1312.

Ross, John J., and Douglas N. Keeling. "Cutaneous Blastomycosis in New Brunswick: Case Report." *Canadian Medical Association Journal* 163 (November 14, 2000): 1303–1305.

Web Sites

Canadian Medical Association. "Blastomycosis." November 4, 2000. <http://www.cmaj.ca/cgi/content/full/163/10/1231> (accessed March 11, 2007).

Centers of Disease Control and Prevention. "Blastomycosis." October 6, 2005. <http://www.cdc.gov/ncidod/dbmd/diseaseinfo/blastomycosis_t.htm> (accessed March 11, 2007).

Blood Supply and Infectious Disease

■ Introduction

In the 1980s, thousands of patients with hemophilia around the world contracted HIV/AIDS through contaminated blood. Many have since died. This tragedy led to new measures to ensure the safety of the blood supply to protect those needing transfusions or blood products. The use of unpaid, voluntary, regular donors is encouraged, and all donated blood units are tested for the presence of transfusion-transmissible infections (TTIs), like HIV and hepatitis, a viral infection of the liver. These changes have meant a dramatic decrease in the risk of contracting a TTI. For the vast majority of people in the United States and Europe, the medical benefits of blood transfusion or blood products now outweigh the risk from infection. However, this is not the case in many developing countries, where lack of resources and infrastructure mean that donors and donated blood may not be screened as carefully.

■ History and Scientific Foundations

The major TTIs spread by bloodborne pathogens are HIV, hepatitis B (HBV), and hepatitis C (HCV); in some regions, malaria, syphilis, and Chagas disease might also be transmitted through blood. HIV was first identified in the early 1980s, and a test that could be used for screening blood was discovered in 1985. Before this time, anyone who received blood from an HIV positive donor would have been at risk of getting infected themselves. People with hemophilia, a blood clotting disorder, were especially at risk of HIV, because they depend upon receiving Factor VIII (a protein which helps their blood clot normally) made from pooled blood donations. Over 1,200 people in the United Kingdom developed HIV through contaminated Factor VIII before standardized testing; many have since died of AIDS. According to a 1993 report by the Centers for Disease Control (CDC), more than half the hemophiliacs living in the United States in the early 1980s were similarly infected. A similar situation developed in the general population with HCV, a chronic liver infection that can lead to liver cancer, through exposure before 1990, when little was known of the virus and no test was available. Up to 200,000 Americans may have been infected with HCV through blood transfusion before testing began.

■ Applications and Research

To minimize the risk of TTIs, the World Health Organization (WHO) has developed a two-fold approach to blood safety. First, blood services are encouraged to use only voluntary unpaid donors who have a low risk of carrying a TTI, and use them regularly. Therefore, potential donors answer various health-related questions before blood is taken from them. After this, each unit of donated blood is tested for the most common of the TTIs. In the United States, the Food and Drug Administration (FDA), which controls blood safety, mandates tests for HIV, HBV, HCV, human T-lymphotrophic virus (which can cause leukemia and diseases of the brain and nervous system), and syphilis. In the United Kingdom, the Department of Health requires donated blood to be tested for HIV, HBV, and HCV.

These measures for improving the safety of the blood supply do work. The American Red Cross says that the risk of contracting HIV from blood is now one in 1.5 million units. This risk is 2,000 times lower than it was 1982–1984, when donors and donations could not be screened because there was no test available. Donated blood is generally screened for TTIs using tests that detect either the infectious agent (viruses, in the case of HIV, HBV, or HCV) or antibodies to the infectious agent. Generally, the test results are in the form of a color response, which is read as positive or negative by computer, and the whole procedure is fast enough not to disrupt the supply of blood to those who need it.

■ Impacts and Issues

HIV took the world by surprise, and there is always the possibility of a new infection that might threaten the blood supply. At present, there is concern over variant Creutzfeld-Jakob disease (vCJD), a rare, fatal brain disease that was first identified in the United Kingdom in 1995. Three cases, out of a total of 158 cases (as of December 2006), have come from contaminated blood. There is currently no test for the prion protein, which is the infective agent in vCJD, so donations cannot be screened. The American Red Cross is dealing with the threat that vCJD could pose to the U.S. blood supply by disqualifying potential donors who have spent periods of time in the U.K. and some other European countries, in case they are infected.

Meanwhile, the safety of blood continues to be a global issue. Many developing countries have not yet adopted the WHO rules. Family or paid donors, known to carry a higher risk of TTIs, account for more than 50% of blood donated in developing countries. The populations in these countries are also at risk from the use of untested blood in transfusions. WHO has a number of projects underway aimed at building and supporting the blood supply around the world, so that everyone has access to safe transfusions and blood products.

SEE ALSO *Bloodborne Pathogens; Hepatitis B; Hepatitis C; HIV.*

BIBLIOGRAPHY

Web Sites

American Red Cross. "Blood Donation Eligibility Guidelines." March 21, 2005. <http://www.redcross.org/services/biomed/0,1082,0_557_,00.html> (accessed January 16, 2007).

World Health Organization. "Blood Transfusion Safety." <http://www.who.int/bloodsafety/en/> (accessed January 16, 2007).

Susan Aldridge

WORDS TO KNOW

BLOODBORNE PATHOGENS: Disease-causing agents carried or transported in the blood. Bloodborne infections are those in which the infectious agent is transmitted from one person to another via contaminated blood.

CREUTZFELDT-JAKOB DISEASE (CJD): Creutzfeldt-Jakob disease (CJD) is a transmissible, rapidly progressing, fatal neurodegenerative disorder related to bovine spongiform encephalopathy (BSE), commonly called mad cow disease.

TRANSFUSION-TRANSMISSIBLE INFECTIONS: Any infection that can be transmitted to a person by a blood transfusion (addition of stored whole blood or blood fractions to a person's own blood) is a transfusion-transmissible infection. Some diseases that can be transmitted in this way are AIDS, hepatitis B, hepatitis C, syphilis, malaria, and Chagas disease.

IN CONTEXT: PERSONAL AND SOCIAL RESPONSBILITY

Blood donation is the process in which a person (called a blood donor) voluntarily gives (or donates) blood that will be securely stored at a designated place (often times called a blood bank) for some future use, often times for a blood transfusion. People sometimes donate blood for themselves, particularly when they know that they are scheduled for surgery at a near future point in time.

Transfusion is the medical process of transferring whole blood or blood components from one person (donor) to another (recipient) in order to restore lost blood, to improve clotting time, and to improve the ability of the blood to deliver oxygen to the body's tissues. Whole blood is used exactly as it was received from the donor. Blood components are parts of whole blood, such as red blood cells (RBCs), plasma, platelets, clotting factors, immunoglobulins, and white blood cells. Use of blood components is a more efficient way to use the blood supply, because blood that has been processed (fractionated) into components can be used to treat more than one person. On average, one pint of blood components is used for three patients. Transfusions have saved countless numbers of people around the world. Each year in the United States, about 4.5 million people are in need of blood transfusions.

Bloodborne Pathogens

■ Introduction

Bloodborne pathogens are microscopic disease-causing organisms that are present in the blood of humans with certain infections that can cause disease in other humans who come in contact with the infected blood. The three major bloodborne pathogens are: hepatitis B virus (HBV), hepatitis C virus (HCV), and the human immunodeficiency virus (HIV), although other diseases can be transmitted via the bloodborne route of infection. Exposure to blood containing any of these pathogens carries a risk of transmission of the infection.

Healthcare workers, including doctors, dentists, and nurses, can become exposed through needlestick injuries, which occur if they are accidentally pricked with a needle that has been used on an infected person. Drug users who share needles can also become infected with bloodborne pathogens, and this is a major route of transmitting HCV. In the past, people receiving blood transfusions and blood products were also at risk of infection by bloodborne pathogens. Reducing the risk from bloodborne pathogens depends upon people following the strict precautions laid down by the Occupational Safety & Health Administration

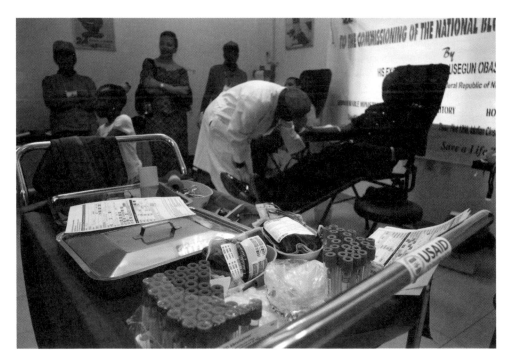

With help from the United States, Nigeria set up the National Blood Transfusion Service, which became the first planned transfusion center in the country. Created to help the nation move away from relying on blood sellers and other questionable sources for blood exchange, it is designed to prevent the spread of blood-borne diseases such as AIDS and Hepatitis B. *AP Images.*

(OSHA) in the United States and equivalent organizations in other countries.

History and Scientific Foundations

When HIV was identified in the early 1980s, it soon became clear that transmission through infected blood was a real possibility. Indeed, thousands of people with the blood clotting disorder hemophilia became infected with HIV because of their dependence on blood products. Now that blood and donors are screened in many countries—and there are efforts on the part of the World Health Organization (WHO) to make this a global practice—this route of exposure to HIV and the two other major bloodborne pathogens HBV and HCV has become less significant.

However, there is still a risk of transmission of bloodborne pathogens to those who become exposed to infected blood, either through their occupation or through their lifestyle. For healthcare workers, a major risk of exposure comes from needlestick injury (NSI), which occurs if a healthcare worker is pricked with a needle that has been used to in an injection or to take blood from an infected person. A NSI can occur either during the procedure itself, or during disposal of the needle. A similar risk exists from cuts occurring from sharp instruments, like scalpels, that have been contaminated with infected blood. Instruments that can cause this kind of injury are generally known as sharps. Splashes of infected blood to the eye, nose, mouth or skin also carry a risk. According to the National Institute for Occupational Safety and Health (NIOSH), there are between 600,000–800,000 NSIs each year in the United States, with nurses being most at risk. And around one third of all NSIs take place during sharps disposal.

HBV is the most easily transmitted of the bloodborne pathogens. However, there is now a vaccine against HBV that is made available to those at risk. Without vaccination, there is a one-in-three chance of contracting HBV through a needlestick injury. For HCV, there is around a 2% risk of infection through NSI. The general risk of contracting HCV through exposure via a blood splash is not known, but there has been one case of infection through a splash in the eye and one from a splash into broken skin. Around 1% of healthcare workers have HCV infection, compared to around 3% of the general United States population. But it is not known how many of the healthcare worker HCV infections arose through occupational exposure.

For HIV, the risk of becoming infected through a needlestick injury is about one in three hundred, although the risk is higher when a person with advanced AIDS is the source of the infected blood. Deep injections, and instruments that are obviously contaminated with blood also carry a higher risk of infection. The risk

WORDS TO KNOW

BLOODBORNE ROUTE: Via the blood. For example: Bloodborne pathogens are pathogens (disease-causing agents) carried or transported in the blood. Bloodborne infections are those in which the infectious agent is transmitted from one person to another via contaminated blood. Infections of the blood can occur as a result of the spread of an ongoing infection caused by bacteria such as *Yersinia pestis, Haemophilus influenzae*, and *Staphylococcus aureus*.

NEEDLESTICK INJURY: Any accidental breakage or puncture of the skin by an unsterilized medical needle (syringe) is a needlestick injury. Healthcare providers are at particular risk for needlestick injuries (which may transmit disease) because of the large number of needles they handle.

PATHOGEN: A disease-causing agent, such as a bacteria, virus, fungus, etc.

POSTEXPOSURE PROPHYLAXIS: Postexposure prophylaxis is treatment with drugs immediately after exposure to an infectious microorganism. The aim of this approach is to prevent an infection from becoming established.

STANDARD PRECAUTIONS: Standard precautions are the safety measures taken to prevent the transmission of disease-causing bacteria. These include proper hand washing; wearing gloves, goggles, and other protective clothing; proper handling of needles; and sterilization of equipment.

following HIV-infected blood splashes is around one in a thousand. There have been no documented cases of HIV transmission due to an exposure involving contact of infected blood with intact skin.

Applications and Research

Commonsense precautions, such as protecting the hands, eyes, and mouth when dealing with blood from patients potentially infected with HBV, HCV, and HIV, can go a long way to reducing the risk of transmission of these bloodborne pathogens. It is also important to use properly trained staff (phlebotomists) to take blood samples. Simply reducing the number of times needles are used on patients, for injections, placing catheters, and taking blood samples, also reduces the risk of transmitting bloodborne pathogens, by cutting down on the number of occasions on which accidents can take place.

Science and technology have also contributed towards reducing the risk of transmission of bloodborne pathogens. For instance, the Centers for Disease Control and Prevention (CDC) say that the annual number of HBV infections has decreased more than 90% since the introduction of the vaccine in 1982. In 1983, there were more than 10,000 such infections in the United States every year and by 2001, this was down to fewer than 400. Unfortunately, there are no such vaccines against HCV or HIV, although research is ongoing. Postexposure prophylaxis (PEP) can be used to protect someone who may have been exposed to HIV through infected blood. This involves giving the antiretroviral drugs used to treat HIV/AIDS patients as soon as possible after exposure. Some studies have suggested this may reduce the risk of HIV transmission, although it is not universally recommended because the drugs have side effects and the risk of infection remains small.

■ Impacts and Issues

OSHA reports that 5.6 million workers in the United States are at risk of exposure to bloodborne pathogens. In 1991, OSHA issued the Bloodborne Pathogens Standard Prevention Act, which was updated in 2001. This law encompasses the "universal precautions" philosophy of CDC, now called standard precautions, and affects many aspects of the way healthcare, and other workers, carry out their day-to-day tasks. Basically, all persons receiving care are considered potentially contaminated with bloodborne pathogens unless proven otherwise, and therefore, using protective measures to avoid contact with blood is now standard procedure for healthcare workers.

Prevention of exposure involves physical protection of the worker with gloves, masks, and eye shields during surgery or other procedures where there is a potential for contact with blood. Safe devices such as retractable or sheathed needles must be used when taking blood, and any NSIs must be reported and followed up. Protection

from infection depends upon all those who may be at risk taking this code seriously and following it before, during, and after handling blood from potential sources of bloodborne pathogen risk.

The advent of safer devices, such as needle-less injectors, has also been an important advance. CDC reports a 62–88% reduction in NSIs from the introduction of better devices. For injecting drug users at risk of bloodborne infections, especially HCV, education in harm reduction and needle exchange schemes may also reduce the incidence of new infections. However, it is difficult to document this, as there is often a lengthy time lag between exposure and evidence of infection.

SEE ALSO *Blood Supply and Infectious Disease; Hepatitis B; Hepatitis C; HIV; Infection Control and Asepsis; Standard Precautions.*

BIBLIOGRAPHY

Books

American Academy of Orthopedic Surgeons. *Bloodborne Pathogens.* 5th ed. New York: Jones and Bartlett, 2007.

Web Sites

Centers for Disease Control and Prevention (CDC). "Exposure to Blood: What Healthcare Personnel Need to Know." July 2003 <http://www.cdc.gov/ncidod/dhqp/pdf/bbp/Exp_to_Blood.pdf> (accessed Feb 8, 2007).

Centers for Disease Control and Prevention (CDC). "Infection Control Guidelines." <http://www.cdc.gov/ncidod/dhqp/guidelines.html> (accessed February 8, 2007).

U.S. Department of Labor Occupational Safety & Health Administration. "BloodbornePathogens and Needlestick Prevention OSHA Standards." <http://www.osha.gov/SLTC/bloodbornepathogens.standards.html> (accessed February 8, 2007).

Susan Aldridge

Botulism

■ Introduction

Botulism is a disease that is caused by a bacterial toxin. The toxin is one of seven (A-G) made and released by the bacterium *Clostridium botulinum*. Botulism toxin types A, B, E, and F cause botulism in humans. Another bacterium called *Clostridium baratii* can also produce a disease-causing toxin, but this bacterium is rarely encountered, and is responsible for far fewer cases of botulism than is *C. botulinum*.

Botulism toxins are powerful neurotoxins; they affect nerves and can produce paralysis. One microgram of toxin—a millionth of a gram—can kill a person. Paralysis from botulism affects the functioning of organs and tissues, and when botulism is fatal, it is usually due to failure of the respiratory muscles.

■ Disease History, Characteristics, and Transmission

Botulism was first described in 1735 in an illness outbreak that was traced to the consumption of contaminated German sausage. Indeed, the word botulism was derived from the Latin word *botulus*, meaning sausage.

C. botulinum are commonly found in soil. They can be present on vegetables and other food grown in soil, and can be eaten if the food is not completely washed free of bacteria. Fortunately, under these conditions where oxygen is present, the bacteria do not produce the toxin and so are harmless when eaten. Botulism is not a contagious disease—it cannot be spread from person to person. Rarely, botulism occurs as the result of a wound infected with *C. botulinum*.

The toxin is produced when the bacterium grows in the absence of oxygen. Growth of the bacteria in, for example, the low-oxygen and slightly acidic environment (the bacteria cannot grow above pH 5) of some canned foods is associated with the production of gas. Canned foods can bulge due to the build-up of the gas. Discard-

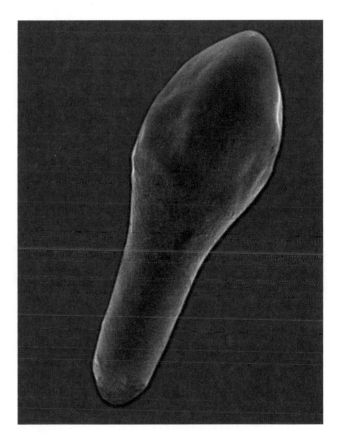

The spore stage of *Clostridium botulinum,* a gram-positive, endospore-forming, rod bacteria that causes botulism (food poisoning) and wound infections, is shown. *© Visuals Unlimited/ Corbis.*

ing a bulging unopened can is always a wise precaution. With foodborne botulism, growth of the bacteria in the food may occur, but is not mandatory for developing botulism, as the presence of the toxin alone is sufficient to cause illness. Because the toxin causes the illness, foodborne botulism is often described as a food intoxication.

Rarely, botulism can also be caused by the infection of *C. botulinum* in an open wound. Growth of the bacteria deep in the tissues leads to the production of the toxin, which then spreads via the bloodstream.

Symptoms of botulism are produced when the toxin enters the bloodstream. The toxin blocks the production of a neurotransmitter called acetylcholine, a chemical that bridges the physical gap between nerve cells and so aids in the transmission of impulses from nerve to nerve. As nerves are affected and paralysis occurs, a person experiences difficulty seeing, talking, and swallowing, and can become nauseous.

C. botulinum is one of a few types of bacteria that can produce a structure known as a spore. A spore is a form of the bacterium that is non-growing but which can persist in that form for a long time and in conditions of excess heat, dryness, and other harsh environments that would kill the normally growing cell. The spore form allows the organism to survive inhospitable conditions and then, when conditions improve, such as in canned food or inside the body, the bacteria can resume growth, division, and toxin production.

■ Scope and Distribution

Botulism is a fairly rare illness. In the United States, for example, only about 100 cases have been reported each year since the 1990s. Most cases are due to the improper canning of foods at home.

The different forms of the botulism toxin display some differences in their geography. In the United States, type A botulism, which is the most severe, occurs most often in western regions, particularly in the Rocky Mountains. Type B toxin, whose symptoms tend to be less severe, is more common in the eastern United States. Type E toxin is found more in the bacteria that live in fresh water sediments. The reasons for their different distributions is not clear.

■ Treatment and Prevention

Diagnosis of botulism is complicated by the fact that the disease is infrequently seen. A physician may have little experience in dealing with the illness. As well, in its early stages, botulism has symptoms that are similar to other ailments such as Guillain-Barré syndrome and stroke. Both of these considerations sometimes lead to a delayed diagnosis of botulism.

Diagnosis involves the detection of toxin in the infected person's blood, which can be accomplished using specific immune components, or antibodies. An antibody to the specific botulism toxin will react with the toxin, producing a visible clump of material. As well, sometimes living bacteria can be recovered from the feces.

Treatment for botulism often involves the administration of an antibody-containing antitoxin that blocks the binding of the toxin to the nerve cells. With time, paralysis fades. However, recovery can take many weeks. If botulism is suspected soon after exposure to the bacteria, the stomach contents can be emptied to remove potentially contaminated undigested food. When lung muscles have been affected, a patient may need mechanical assistance in breathing.

■ Impacts and Issues

A century ago, botulism was frequently a death sentence—one of every two people who became ill with it died. In 2007, of the approximately 100 people predicted to become ill with botulism in the United States, eight will die. In contrast to some other diseases that take a toll on the underdeveloped of the world, botulism is more prevalent in developed regions, particularly where food is processed, canned, and sold.

Botulism does have significance in its potential as a bioterrorist threat. This potent killing power of the *Clostridium* neurotoxins has been recognized for decades. During World War II (1939–1945), several nations including the United States and Canada experimented with the development of botulism toxin-based weapons. Sprays that contained the spore form of *C. botulinum* were developed and tested. The idea was that inhalation of the spores would lead to resumed growth of the bacteria and production of the lethal neurotoxin. The sprays were never used in battle.

Botulinum toxin A is exploited cosmetically as a means of lessening wrinkles. Injection of Botox® relaxes muscles, which can produce a more youthful appearance. The American Society of Aesthetic and Plastic Surgery (ASAPS) estimates that the worldwide market for Botox® is around 900 million dollars annually, and over two million Botox® procedures are performed per year. Botulinum toxin A has also shown promise in lessening dystonia (muscle spasms) that occurs in cerebral palsy, and in treating crossed eyes (strabismus).

In 1976, a form of botulism was recognized in infants in the United States that stemmed from babies ingesting *C. botulinum* spores, which colonized their intestinal tract (an infant's intestinal tract is less acidic than that of an adult) and eventually produced botulinum toxin. Evidence indicated that honey was linked with both the reservoir of the bacteria and the resulting disease. Since that time, honey-linked infant botulism has been reported in other countries, prompting recommendations from the American Academy of Pediatrics for all infants less than 12 months of age not to receive foods containing honey.

As botulism is a rare occurrence, The Centers for Disease Control and Prevention (CDC) maintains a central supply of antitoxin against botulism. State health departments consult with the CDC for release of the antitoxin when a case has been reported to them. Fast action is essential, as the antitoxin reduces the severity of the symptoms only if given early.

When a food source of botulism is discovered, the Food and Drug Administration (FDA) issues a class-1 recall of the product. Class-1 recalls are reserved for dangerous or defective products that could cause serious health problems or death, and involve communication between the FDA, manufacturer or supplier, and the public to remove the product from the market, or remove the food source from the food supply. For instance, in February 2007, the FDA issued a warning against consumption of Earth's Best Organic 2 Apple Peach Barley Breakfast baby food because of the risk of contamination with *Clostridium botulinum*. The manufacturer initiated a recall of the food, and working in conjunction with the FDA, removed the potentially contaminated baby food jars from store shelves, began an awareness campaign, and tracked and corrected the source of the contamination. As of March 2007, a potential outbreak of infant botulism was prevented, and no cases of infant botulism were reported from ingesting Earth's Best Organic baby food.

IN CONTEXT: BOTULINUM TOXIN AS A BIOLOGICAL WEAPON

According to the CDC, aerosolized botulinum toxin is a possible mechanism for a bioterrorism attack. As yet inhalational botulism cannot, however, be clinically differentiated from the naturally occurring forms. What factors might assist or complicate the definitive initial determination of such an attack?

Key clinical or epidemiological factors assisting the determination of an intentional attack:

- Inhalational botulism does not occur naturally.
- Botulism is not transmissible from person-to-person.
- Indications of intentional release of a biologic agent aerosolized botulinum toxin might include an unusual geographic clustering of illness (e.g., persons who attended the same public event or gathering).
- Symptoms begin within six hours to two weeks after exposure (often within 12 to 36 hours).

SOURCE: *Centers for Disease Control and Prevention (CDC)*

SEE ALSO *Bacterial Disease; Food-borne Disease and Food Safety.*

BIBLIOGRAPHY

Books

Prescott, Lansing M., John P. Harley, Donald A. Klein. *Microbiology.* New York: McGraw-Hill, 2004.

Tortora, Gerard J., Berell R. Funke, Christine L. Case. *Microbiology: An Introduction.* New York: Benjamin Cummings, 2006.

Websites

U.S. Food and Drug Administration. "*Clostridium botulinum.*" <http://www.cfsan.fda.gov/~mow/chap2.html> (accessed March 1, 2007).

Brian Hoyle

Bovine Spongiform Encephalopathy ("Mad Cow" Disease)

■ Introduction

Bovine spongiform encephalopathy (BSE) is a progressive infection of the brain and nervous system found in cattle. It is often known as "mad cow" disease, because of the way affected animals stagger. There is much evidence that BSE can be transmitted from cattle to humans via the consumption of infected beef, resulting in an invariably fatal brain disorder called variant Creutzfeldt-Jakob disease (vCJD). An epidemic of BSE in the United Kingdom (U.K.) in the 1980s and 1990s has been linked to several cases of the human form of vCJD, mainly among younger people. The impact of BSE on Britain's farmers and beef industry was severe, as countries rushed to boycott imports of meat that might have come from infected cows. Although the BSE epidemic has largely died away, occasional cases still appear around the world. Meanwhile, many scientific questions on how BSE is transmitted remain unanswered.

■ Disease History, Characteristics, and Transmission

BSE is a relatively new disease of cattle which was first identified in the United Kingdom in 1986. It proved to be one of a group of diseases called the transmissible spongiform encephalopathies (TSEs). On post-mortem examination with a light microscope, the brain tissue of an animal with a TSE shows a characteristic spongy appearance because the pathology of the disease creates holes within the brain tissue—hence the term "spongiform."

TSEs affect other animals, including humans. For instance scrapie, a TSE found in sheep, has been known since the eighteenth century and is found at a low level in many parts of the world. The name comes from the tendency of animals with the disease to scrape their fleece against trees and bushes. TSEs have also been found in mink (transmissible mink encephalopathy)

and in mule, deer, and elk (chronic wasting disease). CJD is the most significant TSE in humans; it is very rare, usually occurring at a rate of around one per million of the population. The cases that arose from exposure to

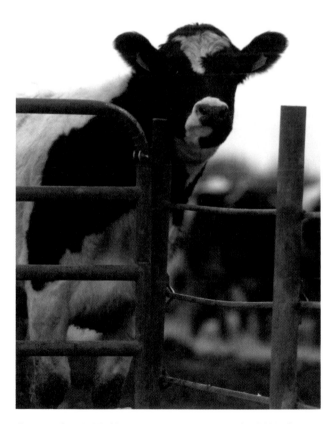

Cows at a farm in Washington state were quarantined in 2003 after one of them was found to have bovine spongiform encephalopathy (BSE), better known as "mad cow" disease. Meat from the infected cow was processed and sold to consumers before the positive test results were received, prompting a recall of the meat. © Kevin P. Casey/Corbis.

BSE in the United Kingdom from the mid–1990s represent a new form of CJD.

BSE occurs in adult animals of both sexes. The incubation period—the time lag from exposure to the appearance of symptoms—of TSEs is usually measured in years. Therefore the disease is rarely seen in very young animals, even though they may be infected. Animals with BSE exhibit abnormalities of movement and posture and changes in mental state which an experienced vet or farmer would be able to detect. The disease lasts for several weeks and is invariably both progressive and fatal.

TSEs can be transmitted from one animal to another. However, there is a species barrier, which means that transmission within species is more likely than transmission between species. For instance, there are no known instances of scrapie being transmitted to humans.

It is widely (but not universally) accepted that BSE arose in cattle from exposure to feed derived from sheep infected with scrapie. Adding protein from the carcasses of ruminants (sheep and cows) to animal feed is a long-established practice. The U.K. BSE Inquiry, which was set up to look at the underlying causes of the BSE epidemic, concluded that changes in the way the feed was processed probably allowed infectious material to survive and infect the cattle consuming it. From the time the BSE epidemic first took hold there were fears that the disease might be transmitted to humans through exposure to meat and meat products (such as hamburgers) from infected animals. These fears were realized with the announcement of the first case of variant CJD in 1996.

However, it has been hard to prove for certain that exposure to BSE causes variant CJD. This is because the infective agent in TSEs is an unusual entity known as a prion. Research on infected tissue has shown that prions are not destroyed by either heat (which would destroy bacteria) or ultra-violet light (which would destroy viruses). Prions are an abnormal form of a protein that is found normally in the brain. When it infects the brain, the prion corrupts the normal prion protein molecules. These newly formed abnormal prion protein molecules go on to corrupt further normal prion molecules, beginning a cascade effect. The accumulation of more and more abnormal prion molecules triggers the brain damage that produces the symptoms of TSEs.

■ Scope and Distribution

By September 1, 2006, approximately 183,139 cases of BSE had been confirmed in the United Kingdom, according to the Department for Environment, Food and Rural Affairs. The epidemic peaked in 1992, with 36,680 confirmed cases in that year. In 2006, there were only 15 cases.

Although BSE has reached epidemic levels only in the United Kingdom, it has affected other countries too. The World Organization for Animal Health collects data on BSE. While there have been no cases, to date, in

WORDS TO KNOW

ENCEPHALOPATHY: Any abnormality in the structure or function of the brain.

PRIONS: Prions are proteins that are infectious. Indeed, the name prion is derived from "proteinaceous infectious particles." The discovery of prions and confirmation of their infectious nature overturned a central dogma that infections were caused by intact organisms, particularly microorganisms such as bacteria, fungi, parasites, or viruses. Since prions lack genetic material, the prevailing attitude was that a protein could not cause disease.

TRANSMISSION: Microorganisms that cause disease in humans and other species are known as pathogens. The transmission of pathogens to a human or other host can occur in a number of ways, depending upon the microorganism.

ZOONOSES: Zoonoses are diseases of microbiological origin that can be transmitted from animals to people. The causes of the diseases can be bacteria, viruses, parasites, and fungi.

Australia, New Zealand, Africa and much of Asia, there have been several in European countries such as France, Germany, Ireland, and Portugal. As of August 23, 2006, there had been twelve confirmed cases of BSE in North America, nine in Canada, and three in the United States.

■ Treatment and Prevention

There is no treatment for BSE, but much has been done to prevent its spread—both to other cattle in a herd and to humans. The government of the United Kingdom has introduced a number of measures to keep BSE under control. In July 1988, it imposed a ban on feeding cattle with potentially infected material. This measure kept animals that were not already infected from becoming infected and has been adopted in many countries, including those who are currently BSE-free. This measure alone made a major contribution to halting the growth of the U.K. BSE epidemic. However, because BSE has a long incubation time, there was a lag between introducing this ban and a fall in the number of cases. This is why the number of cases continued to rise from 1988, despite the ban. In 1997, the U.K. also began a selective cull—slaughtering those animals that were at risk of contracting BSE. This further reduces the risk of the spread of infection.

IN CONTEXT: EFFECTIVE RULES AND REGULATIONS

Variant CJD (vCJD) is the human form of bovine spongiform encephalopathy (BSE) disease that emerged in Britain in the mid–1990s. The vCJD outbreak in Britain echoed the emergence in the 1950s of a strange and invariably fatal condition called kuru (meaning "trembling with fear") among the Fore people of New Guinea. After years of living among the group, American doctor Carlton Gajdusek (1923–)—who went on to win the Nobel Prize for Medicine or Physiology in 1976—came to the conclusion that the disease was transmitted in the ritualistic eating of the brains of the deceased, a Fore funeral custom. He suspected that one of these brains, at least, must have belonged to someone with sporadic or familial CJD. There were some striking parallels between the emergence of vCJD and its links with the earlier epidemic bovine spongiform encephalopathy (BSE or mad cow disease), one of the transmissible spongiform encephalopathies (TSEs) found in cattle. The latter prompted a public enquiry to investigate the cause of the outbreak.

The picture that emerged from the inquiry was, briefly, that vCJD is, indeed, the human form of BSE (mad cow disease). The Inquiry concluded that infected material—either from sheep infected with scrapie (a sheep TSE) or from BSE-infected cattle—was incorporated into cattle feed. Further, it was found that changes in the processing of carcasses used for animal feed were the likely cause of this contamination. Fortunately, the epidemic, though tragic for the victims and their families, was limited by steps such as the wholesale slaughtering of infected cattle and a ban on imports of British beef.

The inquiry led to a variety of developments. For example, in an attempt to restore public confidence, a Food Standards Agency was set up in the United Kingdom to advise on food safety issues. Regulatory authorities are moving towards eliminating animal products from the manufacture of medicines and other items destined for human consumption. The BSE inquiry also led to changes in the supply of blood and blood products, in an attempt to screen out donors that are, unknowingly, carrying vCJD.

The spread of BSE to humans has been limited by restricting imports of meat and meat products that might be infected. In 1996, cattle over 30 months old were no longer allowed to enter the food chain—instead, they were incinerated after slaughter. This ban has now been lifted and replaced by BSE testing—only meat that tests negative can enter the food supply.

■ Impacts and Issues

The BSE epidemic hit British farmers and the United Kingdom meat industry hard. In 1996, the government of the U.K. admitted a link between BSE and variant CJD, and shortly afterward, France and many other European countries announced a ban on imports of British beef and related products. South Africa, Singapore, and South Korea soon joined in. The Meat and Livestock Commission stated that the bans had caused half of the U.K.'s slaughterhouse workers to lose their jobs. The import bans were gradually lifted over the next few years, as the BSE epidemic began to die down. But it has taken many years for British beef sales to begin to recover, both at home and abroad.

In 1998, a public inquiry into BSE and variant CJD began. This concluded with lessons to be learned to stop such a catastrophe from happening again. People in Britain and elsewhere are now more aware of safety issues around food. They wish to know where their food comes from and what is in it. In 2000, the government of the United Kingdom set up the Food Standards Agency, a department that looks after public health and consumer interests with respect to food. This was a response to public distrust generated by the way the government was seen to have handled the BSE crisis. Formerly, food and agriculture had been the responsibility of the same department, which many felt marginalized the interests of the consumer.

BSE has substantial economic impact. During the 1990s BSE outbreak in the United Kingdom, hundreds of animals were destroyed. Quarantined farms and slaughterhouses lost business. New regulations governing cattle feed and BSE testing programs proved expensive to implement. However, in most nations where BSE is detected, the most significant economic impact is the loss of revenue from the export of beef products. Beginning in 2001, several nations restricted the import of American beef products, concerned that the United States beef industry lacked sufficient testing and identification methods for BSE. In 2003, when the U.S. Department of Agriculture announced that BSE had been discovered in one cow in Washington state, approximately 60 nations temporarily banned the import of U.S. beef. The infected cow was later traced to a herd in Canada, but the discovery of BSE in the North American herd resulted in approximately $4.7 billion in beef industry losses that year.

SEE ALSO *Creutzfeldt-Jakob Disease-nv; Prion Disease; Zoonoses.*

BIBLIOGRAPHY

Web Sites

BSE Inquiry. "The BSE Inquiry: The Report." <http://www.bseinquiry.gov.uk/report/index.htm> (accessed January 26, 2007).

Centers for Disease Control and Prevention (CDC). "BSE (Bovine Spongiform Encephalopathy, or Mad Cow Disease)." January 4, 2007 <http://www.cdc.gov/ncidod/dvrd/bse> (accessed January 26, 2007).

Department for Environment, Food and Rural Affairs. "BSE: Frequently Asked Questions." October 3, 2006 <http://www.defra.gov.uk/animalh/bse/faq.html> (accessed January 26, 2007).

Food Standards Agency. "BSE." <http://www.food.gov.uk/bse> (accessed January 26, 2007).

Meat and Livestock Commission. "Beef Information." October, 2005 <http://www.meatmatters.com/sections/britishmeat/beef_information.php> (accessed January 26, 2007).

U.S. Food and Drug Administration (FDA). "Commonly Asked Questions about BSE in Products Regulated by FDA's Center for Food Safety and Applied Nutrition (CFSAN)." September 14, 2005 <http://www.cfsan.fda.gov/~comm/bsefaq.html> (accessed January 26, 2007).

Susan Aldridge

Brucellosis

■ Introduction

Brucellosis (broo-sell-OH-sis) is a disease that is caused by a variety of bacteria in the genus *Brucella*. Swine, cattle, and sheep can be directly infected by brucellosis. Humans can develop brucellosis indirectly by contact with infected animals (brucellosis is a zoonotic infection) or by consuming milk or dairy products that are contaminated with the bacteria.

Vaccination of animals born and raised in the United States against brucellosis is required, which helps protect both the nation's livestock and humans most at risk of being secondarily infected. However, monitoring of imported livestock is necessary to prevent introducing brucellosis into a population of animals, as vaccination programs are not in effect in every country.

■ Disease History, Characteristics, and Transmission

Brucellosis was named after David Bruce, a researcher who isolated the organism in 1887 from five sick British soldiers stationed on the island of Malta. The designation of brucellosis as Malta fever recognizes this origin as

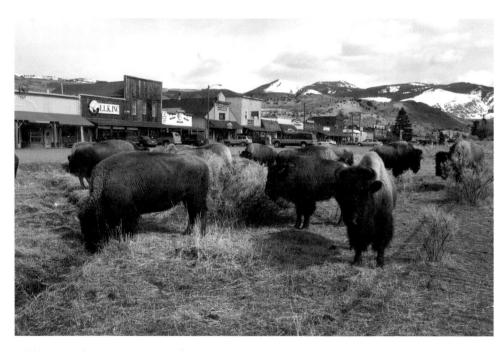

Wild bison are shown grazing in a small Montana town near the border of Yellowstone National Park. Bison are captured as they try to leave the park, and those testing positive for brucellosis are sent to slaughter. Humans who come into contact with infected animals can contract brucellosis. © *William Campbell/Sygma/Corbis.*

well as the 1905 description of human brucellosis cases in Malta from *Brucella*-contaminated unpasteurized milk. The disease is also known as undulant fever, as the fever tends to increase and decrease with time. Brucellosis dates back much further than these formal descriptions. Descriptions from the time of Hippocrates (Greek physician and philosopher born around 460 BC) are now thought to refer to brucellosis.

A number of different species of the bacterium are responsible for the disease in various livestock. *Brucella melitensis* infects goats and sheep, *B. suis* infects pigs and in caribou, *B. abortus* causes the disease in cattle, bison, and elk, *B. ovis* also infects sheep, and *B. canis* causes the disease in dogs.

Brucella are shaped somewhat like a football. In contrast to many disease-causing bacteria that have an outer coating called a capsule, *Brucella* lack a capsule. A capsule can help shield a bacterium from host defenses such as antibodies. Lacking a capsule, *Brucella* would be exposed to the body's defenses if not for its infection strategy. Instead, the bacteria cause infection by entering host cells. Within host cells, the bacteria are shielded and are able to grow and multiply.

The species of *Brucella* that are capable of causing brucellosis in humans are *B. melitensis*, *B. abortis*, and *B. suis*. The infection that develops in dogs is not transmitted to humans. Humans acquire the infection indirectly, usually by handling infected animals or even a carcass; if a person has a cut or abrasion in the skin, especially on the hands, the bacteria easily gain access to the bloodstream. However, entry is possible even in the absence of a wound, as the bacteria are able to invade skin cells and reach the bloodstream. Another route of infection is via contaminated moist soil and hay. In these environments, the bacteria can remain alive and capable of infection for months. As well, people are infected by drinking unpasteurized milk, or eating cheese or ice cream that has been made from unpasteurized milk. Finally, the organism can be inhaled and the bacteria spread to the bloodstream following invasion of lung cells.

Person-to-person spread via breastfeeding and during sex can occur, but is rare. It is possible that the transplantation of contaminated tissue could cause brucellosis.

When the bacteria enter the bloodstream, they migrate to lymph nodes. Normally, lymph nodes such as those located in the neck and the armpit function to destroy invading bacteria and viruses. However, *Brucella* circumvents this and invades the lymph node cells. From there, the bacteria can spread to the spleen, bone marrow, and liver. Tissue irritation and organ damage occurs. In severe cases, the lining of the heart can be infected.

The time from exposure to the appearance of symptoms is usually around three weeks. Symptoms include general feelings of weakness and tiredness, muscle pain, chills, and fever. The fever and chills can subside and recur during the illness. Brucellosis is lethal in about 10% of cases, usually because of heart infection.

WORDS TO KNOW

CULL: A cull is the selection, often for destruction, of a part of an animal population. Often done just to reduce numbers, a widespread cull was carried out during the epidemic of bovine spongiform encephalopathy (BSE or mad cow disease) in the United Kingdom during the 1980s

NOTIFIABLE DISEASES: Diseases that the law requires must be reported to health officials when diagnosed, including active tuberculosis and several sexually transmitted diseases; also called reportable diseases.

ZOONOSES: Zoonoses are diseases of microbiological origin that can be transmitted from animals to people. The causes of the diseases can be bacteria, viruses, parasites, and fungi.

■ Scope and Distribution

The prevalence of human brucellosis is related to the prevalence of the infection in domestic and wild animal populations. In countries such as the U.S. and Canada, where stringent monitoring and infection control measures are in place and where vaccination programs have been operating for years, brucellosis in both livestock and humans is rare. Culling (slaughtering) of infected animals in some North American wild elk and bison populations has been carried out to ensure that the infection does not spread from the wild populations to livestock.

Infection is most common in those who come into frequent contact with domestic and wild animals; veterinarians, cattlemen, and workers in slaughterhouses. In the U.S., there are about 100 of human brucellosis cases per year, representing one out of every three million Americans.

Elsewhere in the world, brucellosis is more frequent in countries where agriculture involves more people in closer contact with unvaccinated livestock, and where infection control precautions are not as stringent. Areas considered to be high risk according to the U.S. Centers for Disease Control and Prevention (CDC) are China, India, Peru, Mexico, Eastern Europe, the Mediterranean, the Caribbean, and the Middle East.

Age and race do not influence the occurrence of brucellosis. In developing countries where mostly women tend livestock, the disease is initially more prevalent in women. In developing countries where mostly men tend livestock, the situation is reversed.

IN CONTEXT: PERSONAL RESPONSIBILITY AND PROTECTION

The Coordinating Center for Infectious Diseases/Division of Bacterial and Mycotic Diseases states that "direct person-to-person spread of brucellosis is extremely rare. Mothers who are breast-feeding may transmit the infection to their infants. Sexual transmission has also been reported. For both sexual and breast-feeding transmission, if the infant or person at risk is treated for brucellosis, their risk of becoming infected will probably be eliminated within 3 days. Although uncommon, transmission may also occur via contaminated tissue transplantation."

To prevent infection the CCID and CDC recommend that travelers "do not consume unpasteurized milk, cheese, or ice cream while traveling. If you are not sure that the dairy product is pasteurized, don't eat it. Hunters and animal herdsman should use rubber gloves when handling viscera of animals."

As of 2007 there is no vaccine available for humans.

SOURCE: *Coordinating Center for Infectious Diseases/Division of Bacterial and Mycotic Diseases, Centers for Disease Control and Prevention (CDC)*

IN CONTEXT: TRENDS AND STATISTICS

In October 2005, The Coordinating Center for Infectious Diseases/Division of Bacterial and Mycotic Diseases stated that "for previous 10 years, approximately 100 cases of Brucellosis per year have been reported."

California, Florida, Texas, and Virginia account for most cases.

"In 2001, the National Brucellosis Eradication Program reported only 3 newly affected cattle herds, compared to 14 herds identified in 2000."

SOURCE: *Centers for Disease Control and Prevention (CDC)*

■ Treatment and Prevention

Brucellosis is suspected based on the symptoms and a history of contact with animals. Confirmation of the infection relies on the recovery of the bacteria from blood samples, bone marrow, or liver tissue. The confirmation step can take months, since *Brucella* grows slowly during laboratory culture. This also poses a hazard for lab personnel, who may be exposed to the bacteria during the incubation period. A quicker means of detecting the bacteria is by the presence of antibodies produced against the infecting bacteria. Antibody pro-

duction by the host may not be efficient, since the infection takes place inside host cells. But commercially available antibodies can be used to test blood for the presence of the corresponding bacterial component.

Human brucellosis that is caused by *B. abortus* is usually mild and may not require treatment. In contrast, the disease caused by *B. melitensis* and *B. suis* can produce severe, prolonged symptoms if not treated.

Treatment typically involves antibiotics; for adults, different antibiotics are given orally and by injection for several weeks. The intramuscular injections are necessary to allow the antibiotic to penetrate into the host cells to the site of infection.

Prevention is possible because of vaccines. Typically, vaccination of animals is the norm. Control of the disease in animals controls the disease in humans. In fact, two vaccine formulations used for animals contain live but weakened bacteria, and are capable of causing brucellosis if accidentally given to a person.

Multiple episodes of brucellosis among laboratory workers have been reported in the past, mostly from inhaling the bacteria in the confined space of a laboratory. In order to prevent exposure in the laboratory, scientists now study the bacteria using biosafety level three precautions, including gowns, gloves, and performing tests under a biosafety cabinet.

■ Impacts and Issues

In North America, brucellosis is prevalent in wild elk and bison herds. Trap and slaughter campaigns of affected animals have been accomplished in Montana and in Wood Buffalo National Park, which straddles the Canadian provinces of Alberta and British Columbia. Ironically, the national park was created in the 1920s to protect the declining bison population. The culls, which have been controversial, are aimed at keeping cattle and swine herds free of brucellosis.

While brucellosis in commercial livestock is unusual in North America, the continent is at risk if infected animals or food products are imported. Preventive measures include the vaccination of all animals that are raised for food. An individual can minimize their risk of brucellosis by not eating animal products from suspect countries and not eating unpasteurized diary products.

Brucellosis is also recognized as a potential biological threat because it can be spread through the air. There is a historical basis for this categorization. Following World War II (1939–1945), the United States military developed a weapon that would disperse *B. abortus* and *B. suis* upon detonation. The weapon, which was the first biological weapon developed by the U.S., was intended in part to cripple an enemy's livestock-based agriculture. The weapons program was ended by President Richard Nixon in 1967. Today, scientists are working to develop a rapid diagnostic test for brucellosis in the event of a suspected biological attack, and brucellosis remains among the list of nationally notifiable diseases.

SEE ALSO *Animal Importation; Bacterial Disease; Bioterrorism; Public Health and Infectious Disease; Zoonoses.*

BIBLIOGRAPHY

Books

Drexler, Madeline. *Secret Agents: The Menace of Emerging Infections.* New York: Penguin, 2003.

Hart, Tony. *Microterrors: The Complete Guide to Bacterial, Viral and Fungal Infections that Threaten Our Health.* Tonawanda: Firefly Books, 2004.

Periodicals

Kozukeev, Turatbek, B., S. Ajeilat, M. Favorov. "Risk factors for Brucellosis - Leylek and Kadamjay districts, Batken Oblast, Kyrgyzstan, January - November, 2003." *Morbidity and Mortality Weekly.* 55(SUP01): 31–34 (2006).

Brian Hoyle

Burkholderia

■ Introduction

Burkholderia refers to a genus of bacteria. The genus is important from the standpoint of infectious disease because several species cause illness in humans and animals. *Burkholderia cepacia* can cause a lung infection in people who have cystic fibrosis. *B. pseudomallei* causes melioidosis, an infection of the blood that can result in pain and tissue destruction at different sites in the body. *B. mallei* causes an illness known as glanders, a respiratory illness that occurs primarily in horses, mules, and donkeys and can be transmitted to humans. Glanders infection is often lethal in people.

Infections such as melioidosis are reaching epidemic levels in various regions of the world, and the respiratory infection caused by *B. cepacia* is a main health threat in those with cystic fibrosis. Adding to the concern about *Burkholderia*, several species are worrisome because of their documented use as biological warfare agents.

■ Disease History, Characteristics, and Transmission

B. cepacia was discovered in the 1940s by Cornell University researcher Walter Burkholder during an investigation into a disease outbreak in New York State. By the 1980s, the organism was recognized as being able to colonize and form an infection in the lungs of people with cystic fibrosis. Then, the infection was regarded as being minor, compared to that caused by *Pseudomonas aeruginosa*. Indeed, at first the organism was not recognized as a unique genus, and was called *Pseudomonas cepacia*. However, only a decade later, the uniqueness and seriousness of *B. cepacia* in cystic fibrosis had been recognized.

The lung infection caused by *B. cepacia* can become chronic. Over years, even decades, the infection will alternately become severe, leading to difficulty in breathing, and less severe, when it is managed more effectively by antibiotics and other forms of therapy. The lung infection is not contagious.

Glanders is another lung infection that, in contrast, can be spread from person to person by coughing. If not treated, the infection can be lethal within days. A less invasive form of the infection can require months from which to fully recover.

Glanders is not a significant health concern currently in North America and Europe, as imported livestock is monitored for the disease. However, it is still prevalent in

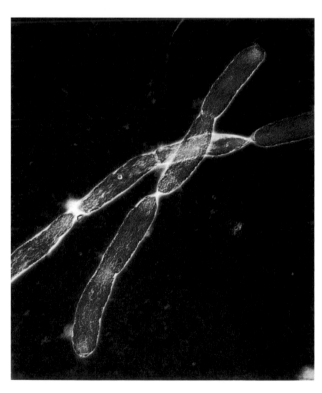

Burkholderia mallei, the bacterium that causes glanders, is shown. An infectious disease, glanders primarily affects horses, donkeys, and mules. *Eye of Science/Photo Researchers, Inc.*

Africa, Asia, the Middle East, Central America, and South America.

Melioidosis is a third *Burkholderia*-mediated disease that is caused by *B. pseudomallei*. It is also a disease of the respiratory tract; indeed, it displays symptoms that are similar to glanders. However, melioidosis and glanders differ in how they are acquired.

Melioidosis is prevalent in tropical climates. For example, the disease is endemic—it is frequently present year-round—in the Southeast Asian countries of Cambodia, Thailand, Vietnam, Laos, Malaysia, and Myanmar, and is also prevalent in the northern portion of Australia. As well, the disease is present but less prevalent in the South Pacific, India, Africa, and the Middle East.

Elsewhere in the world, melioidosis does occur, but only sporadically. Cases have been reported from Mexico, Equador, Panama, Haiti, Brazil, Peru, and in the U.S. states of Hawaii and Georgia. In the U.S., only a few cases are reported each year, according to the Centers for Disease Control and Prevention, and these typically involve people who have been traveling in areas where melioidosis is prevalent.

Many animals are susceptible to melioidosis including horses, sheep, cattle, goats, dogs, and cats. The disease can be transferred from the infected animals to humans, hence it is a zoonosis. As well, the disease can be spread from person to person. The disease can also be acquired by drinking contaminated water or coming into contact with contaminated water in a crop field.

Melioidosis can occur just in the respiratory tract or, if the blood becomes infected, can become more widespread in the body. The symptoms of fever, muscle or bone ache, headache, and weight loss may appear in only a few days, or may take years to become evident.

■ Scope and Distribution

Burkholderia are common environmental organisms and so are common in many areas of the world.

Some types of *Burkholderia* infections are at epidemic proportions in tropical regions and are less common, but nevertheless present, elsewhere in the world. The distribution of *B. cepacia* is global. It is a health threat in persons with cystic fibrosis worldwide.

■ Treatment and Prevention

Melioidosis is diagnosed by isolating the organism from the blood, urine, sputum, or from sores on the skin. The illness is treated using antibiotics. As of 2007, no vaccine exists to protect people from melioidosis. Prevention consists of minimizing contact with potential sources of the organism.

Similarly, *B. cepacia* lung infections and glanders are treated using appropriate antibiotics and, in the case of

---

WORDS TO KNOW

ANTIBIOTIC RESISTANCE: The ability of bacteria to resist the actions of antibiotic drugs.

BIOLOGICAL WARFARE: Biological warfare, as defined by The United Nations, is the use of any living organism (e.g. bacterium, virus) or an infective component (e.g., toxin), to cause disease or death in humans, animals, or plants. In contrast to bioterrorism, biological warfare is defined as the "state-sanctioned" use of biological weapons on an opposing military force or civilian population.

COLONIZE: Colonize refers to the process where a microorganism is able to persist and grow at a given location.

ZOONOSES: Zoonoses are diseases of microbiological origin that can be transmitted from animals to people. The causes of the diseases can be bacteria, viruses, parasites, and fungi.

IN CONTEXT: BIOLOGICAL WEAPON THREATS

B. mallei and *B. pseudomallei* are considered potential biological weapons. Horses and other animals used in the transport of troops and military gear were deliberately infected with glanders during World War I (1915–1918), and it was used by the Japanese to infect prisoners during World War II (1939–1945).

---

cystic fibrosis, other treatments designed to lessen the clogging of the lungs with the overproduced mucous.

■ Impacts and Issues

Melioidosis is an important disease in some tropical regions of the world. The more persistent form of the illness can be debilitating, disrupting family life and making it impossible for a person to work.

B. cepacia is an important disease-causing organism for millions of people who have cystic fibrosis. The lung infection can persist for decades, and the long-term attempts by the host's immune system to destroy the infection can progressively damage the lungs to such an extent that survival is threatened.

B. cepacia lung infections also can similarly and progressively lessen lung function. Additionally, the attempts to eradicate the infection using antibiotics can be less than effective, which can result in the development of bacteria that are resistant to the antibiotics being used. This can make subsequent treatment more difficult and, as more potent antibiotics may be necessary, increasingly expensive.

B. mallei and *B. pseudomallei* are considered potential biological weapons. Both organisms can be resistant to a variety of antibiotics, which can make it more difficult to treat the infections they cause. Also, because they can infect both livestock and humans, they have been exploited during wartime.

Some species of *Burkholderia* are beneficial. In particular, *B. cepacia* and *B. fungorum* are able to degrade certain pesticides that otherwise tend to persist in the environment and cause ecological damage. This environmental benefit comes with the risk that those exposed to, for example, sprays containing the organisms, could be at risk to develop illness. However, under controlled conditions of use, *Burkholderia* can be useful in reducing pesticide contamination.

SEE ALSO *Bacterial Disease; Bioterrorism; Glanders (Melioidosis); Opportunistic Infection.*

BIBLIOGRAPHY

Books

Black, Jacquelyn. *Microbiology: Principles and Explorations.* New York: John Wiley & Sons, 2004.

DiClaudio, Dennis. *The Hypochondriac's Pocket Guide to Horrible Diseases You Probably Already Have.* New York: Bloomsbury, 2005.

Websites

Centers for Disease Control and Prevention. "What You Should Know about *Burkholderia cepacia* infection." <http://www.cdc.gov/ncidod/dbmd/diseaseinfo/blastomycosis_t.htm> (accessed March 25, 2007).

Brian Hoyle

Buruli (Bairnsdale) Ulcer

■ Introduction

Buruli ulcer, also called Bairnsdale ulcer, is a chronic, infectious disease caused by the bacterium *Mycobacterium ulceranus*. This bacterium is a member of the family Mycobacteriaceae, the same family that includes the bacteria responsible for tuberculosis and leprosy.

Infection from the disease leads to deformation and destruction of blood vessels, nerves, soft skin tissues, and, occasionally, bones. Large ulcers often form on the body, usually on the legs or arms. The name Buruli is often associated with the infection because of its widespread incidence during the 1960s in Buruli County (now Nakasongola District) of Uganda.

■ Disease History, Characteristics, and Transmission

Buruli ulcer disease was first discovered in Africa. It was described by Scottish explorer James Augustus Grant (1827–1892) in the book *A Walk Across Africa* that he published after his equatorial African journeys. During an expedition, Grant described his infected leg as being stiff and swollen and, later, discharging bodily fluids. His account is considered the first factual description of the disease.

In the late 1890s, British physician Sir Albert Cook described skin ulcers found on Uganda natives and, in the late 1940s, Australian professor Peter MacCallum described the disease in the Bairnsdale district of southwestern Australia. These two scientists are credited with first discovering that *M. ulceranus* caused the disease.

The *M. ulceranus* bacterium is commonly found in still or slowly moving water sources (such as swamps, ponds, and lakes), during flooding, and in small aquatic animals (such as insects). Humans are infected by contact with insects or with contaminated materials from water sources. Scientists have not yet determined the mode of transmission. According to the World Health Organization (WHO), infections occur in all ages and genders, however, most infections occur in children under 15 years of age, probably because they spend more time swimming in bodies of water.

Infection usually begins as a nodule within subcutaneous fat (the pre-ulcerative stage). Eventually, fat cells die due to exposure to countless numbers of mycobacteria (any rod-shaped bacteria of genus *Mycobacterium*). The infection can also occur as a skin ulceration—a pimple, or nodule, on the skin (dermis). In both cases, the infection is usually painless and without fever.

Later, larger lesions develop on the skin (the ulcerative stage). The infection may heal on its own, but more commonly the disease slowly progresses with more ulcers and resultant scarring. As much as 15% of the body can be covered eventually with ulcers. As this happens, destructive and dangerous toxins called mycolactone attack the immune system and destroy skin, tissues, and bones. According to the WHO, scarring of the skin can create permanent disabilities—most commonly, restricted movement of limbs.

This disease primarily affects the limbs, but also can occur on other exposed areas. The WHO states that about 90% of lesions occur on the limbs and almost 60% occur on the lower limbs. Buruli ulcers do not occur on the hands or feet of adults. In children, the disease can occur anywhere. A painful form of the disease produces severe swelling of limbs and fever. The infection, in this case, can occur anytime—after simple wounds to more serious physical traumas. Patients not treated early often suffer long-term disabilities, such as impaired joint movement and disfiguring cosmetic problems.

■ Scope and Distribution

Historically, Buruli ulcer has occurred in over 30 countries, primarily those with subtropical and tropical climates. These countries are in central and western Africa (such as Benin, Cameroon, Congo, Ghana, the Ivory Coast, Liberia, Nigeria, Uganda, and Zaire), Central

WORDS TO KNOW

BACTERIOLOGICAL STAIN: A bacterial subclass of a particular tribe and genus.

HISTOPATHOLOGY: Histopathology is the study of diseased tissues. A synonym for histopathology is pathologic histology.

LESION: The tissue disruption or the loss of function caused by a particular disease process.

MYCOBACTERIA: *Mycobacteria* is a genus of bacteria that contains the bacteria that causes leprosy and tuberculosis. The bacteria have unusual cell walls that are harder to dissolve than the cell walls of other bacteria.

PCR (POLYMERASE CHAIN REACTION): The polymerase chain reaction, or PCR, refers to a widely used technique in molecular biology involving the amplification of specific sequences of genomic DNA.

TOXIN: A poison that is produced by a living organism.

IN CONTEXT: DISEASE IN DEVELOPING NATIONS

Due to its increased frequency in western Africa and other poorer parts of the world, the WHO, in 1998, highlighted the plight of Buruli ulcer patients with its Global Buruli Ulcer Initiative (GBUI). In 2004, the World Health Assembly resolved to improve the research, detection, and control of Buruli ulcer.

SOURCE: *World Health Organization*

and South America, the western Pacific (including Australia and New Guinea), and Southeast Asia. In recent years, the disease is becoming more frequent in under-developed countries, specifically, in the countries of western Africa. In fact, in such areas *M. ulceranus* is the third leading cause of mycobacterial infection in healthy people.

■ Treatment and Prevention

Diagnosis of Buruli ulcer is usually made from the ulcer that appears in an infected area. Tests performed to confirm a diagnosis of Buruli ulcer include polymerase chain reaction (PCR, a technique that copies a specific DNA [deoxyribonucleic acid] sequence), Ziehl-Neelsen stain (a bacteriological stain that identifies mycobacteria), culture of *M. ulceranus* (ulcer or tissue biopsies), and histopathology (tissue biopsies).

The treatment of Buruli ulcer usually involves the surgical removal of the lesion. This treatment is normally successful when performed early in the infection. Treatment that occurs in later stages of the infection may require long-term care with extensive skin grafting. The WHO recommends that rifampicin and streptomycin, two antibiotic drugs, be used together for eight weeks to reduce the need for surgery. According to WHO statistics, such treatment leads to complete healing of the lesion in nearly 50% of the cases. Currently, experimental drugs are being tested. These include diarylquinoline, epiprim and dapsone, rifampicin, and sitafloxacin. Besides antibiotic therapy, surgery to remove necrotic tissue, repair skin defects, and correct deformities is often performed.

A bacille Calmette-Guérin (BCG) vaccination, according to the WHO, provides short-term, but limited, protection. Medical scientists are investigating more advanced forms of vaccinations. For the time being, once Buruli ulcer disease has reached an advanced stage, medical professionals can only help to reduce suffering and disabilities.

■ Impacts and Issues

Buruli ulcer disease is one of the most ignored tropical diseases. Unfortunately, it is also one of the most treatable tropical diseases. The family of bacteria that cause Buruli ulcer also cause other serious diseases in mammals, including leprosy and tuberculosis. However, these diseases have garnered much more attention that Buruli ulcer disease. Although Buruli ulcer disease is found around the world, there is limited knowledge about the infection. Such ignorance of the disease is most likely due to the fact that it primarily affects the poorest of rural areas, coupled with insufficient knowledge among health workers and the general public about the disease and inaccurate diagnoses. As a result, only limited reporting of the disease occurs.

In February 2007, a team of researchers lead by Australian scientist Tim Stinear published the entire genome sequence of *M. ulceranus*. Such important information should help to stimulate new research into diagnostic tests, drug treatments, and vaccines. In fact, scientists are currently developing a diagnostic test that can be used locally so that treatment can be done quickly and inexpensively.

SEE ALSO *Bacterial Disease; Emerging Infectious Diseases; Tropical Infectious Diseases; World Health Organization (WHO).*

BIBLIOGRAPHY

Books

Cohen, Jonathan, and William G. Powderly, eds. *Infectious Diseases.* New York: Mosby, 2004.

Lee, Bok Y., ed. *The Wound Management Manual.* New York: McGraw Hill, 2005.

Periodicals

Amofah, George, et al. "Buruli Ulcer in Ghana: Results of a National Case Search." *Emerging Infectious Diseases* 8 (February 2002): 167–170. Also available online at: <http://www.cdc.gov/ncidod/eid/vol8no2/pdf/01-0119.pdf>.

Web Sites

Armed Forces Institute of Pathology. "Buruli Ulcer." February 4, 2004. <http://www.afip.org/Departments/infectious/bu/> (accessed April 24, 2007).

World Health Organization. "Global Buruli Ulcer Initiative (GBUI)." <http://www.who.int/buruli/en/> (accessed April 24, 2007).

Campylobacter Infection

■ Introduction

The infection that is caused by the group of bacteria in the genus *Campylobacter* is called campylobacteriosis. The infection, which occurs in the intestinal tract of humans, causes abdominal pain and diarrhea. *Campylobacter jejuni* is responsible for more bacterial diarrhea in the United States than any other bacteria, and estimates are that upwards of 14% of all diarrhea worldwide is due to campylobacteriosis.

Campylobacter infections typically result from eating contaminated food or drinking contaminated water. The bacteria need time to grow to numbers that produce the symptoms of the infection; this is usually two to five days after the contaminated food or water has been ingested.

■ Disease History, Characteristics, and Transmission

It has been known for decades that *Campylobacter* bacteria are pathogenic, that is, they are capable of causing illness. For example, the capability of the bacteria to cause disease in animals has been known since the first decade of the twentieth century. But, the identity of *Campylobacter* as human pathogens has only been known since the 1980s.

According to the United States Centers for Disease Control and Prevention (CDC), more than 10,000 *Campylobacter* infections are reported each year. Considering that the symptoms of nausea, fever, abdominal cramps, vomiting, and diarrhea are often not reported or are not even diagnosed, the actual number of cases is not doubt much higher. Indeed, CDC's own estimate is that the number of infections in the U.S. number in the millions each year.

The symptoms of *Campylobacter* infections are not usually life-threatening in the developed world, where the level of health and sanitary conditions are better than

in underdeveloped and developing countries. Most people who become infected recover in about a week or less without the need of medical aid. Still, even in countries such as the United States, severe *Campylobacter* infections occur, producing bloody diarrhea (as intestinal cells are

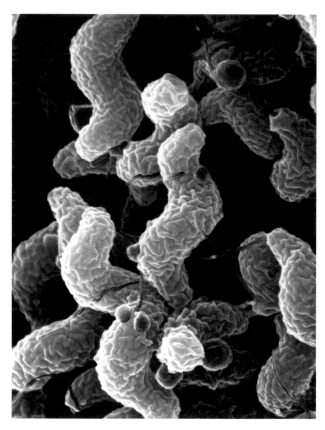

Campylobacter bacteria are the number one cause of food-related gastrointestinal illness in the United States. To learn more about this pathogen, ARS scientists are sequencing multiple *Campylobacter* genomes. This scanning electron microscope image shows the characteristic spiral, or corkscrew, shape of *C. jejuni* cells and related structures. *Science Source.*

damaged). Some people can have abdominal cramps for several months after an infection. The fluid loss from the diarrhea can dehydrate a person if enough fluids are not taken in; in severe cases that require hospitalization, the fluid may need to be supplied intravenously. Very rarely, a high fever that accompanies an infection will trigger a seizure. Also, in an estimated one case in every 1,000, *Campylobacter* infection contributes to a neurological disorder called Guillain-Barré syndrome, where a person's own immune system attacks the nerves, producing paralysis.

■ Scope and Distribution

Campylobacter infections are an example of a zoonosis—an illness or disease that is transmitted to humans by animals or animal products. This is because *Campylobacter* is a natural resident in the intestinal tracts of creatures including swine, cattle, dogs, shellfish, and poultry. The animals harbor the bacteria without any ill effect. The bacteria also naturally inhabit the soil.

■ Treatment and Prevention

Campylobacter is readily susceptible to fairly conventional antibiotics. Treatment is not routinely done, as symptoms usually ease within a few days.

Preventing infection from the ingestion of contaminated food or water is a greater challenge. Poultry are an important source of the infection. Over 50% of raw chicken is contaminated with *Campylobacter*. During slaughter, the intestinal contents (including *Campylobacter*) can contaminate the carcass. If the chicken is undercooked, the bacteria can survive and can cause an infection after being ingested. Fortunately, the bacteria do not tolerate temperatures that are even slightly above room temperature (approximately 68°F [20°C]). Proper cooking of food kills the bacteria. Washing a cutting board after exposure to poultry, refrigeration of raw meat and poultry, and the thawing of meat in the refrigerator or microwave are efficient ways to prevent the transfer of *Campylobacter* to other foods.

■ Impacts and Issues

Research into *Campylobacter* infections consists primarily of genetic studies that are aimed at detecting genes of particular importance in the infection process. It is hoped that this knowledge will led to strategies to block the infection or to rapidly detect the presence of the bacteria on food products. One example of the latter approach is the incorporation of a detection system into food packaging. The presence of living bacteria is evident as a color change in an indicator strip in the packaging.

WORDS TO KNOW

MYCOTIC: Mycotic means having to do with or caused by a fungus. Any medical condition caused by a fungus is a mycotic condition, also called a mycosis.

PATHOGENS: Agents or microorganisms causing or capable of causing disease.

ZOONOSES: Zoonoses are diseases of microbiological origin that can be transmitted from animals to people. The causes of the diseases can be bacteria, viruses, parasites, and fungi.

IN CONTEXT: PERSONAL RESPONSIBILITY AND PREVENTION

The Division of Bacterial and Mycotic Diseases, Centers for Disease Control and Prevention (CDC) recommends the following tips for preventing Campylobacteriosis:

Cook all poultry products thoroughly. Make sure that the meat is cooked throughout (no longer pink), any juices run clear, and the inside is cooked to 170°F (77°C) for breast meat, and 180°F (82°C) for thigh meat.

If you are served undercooked poultry in a restaurant, send it back for further cooking.

Wash hands with soap before handling raw foods of animal origin. Wash hands with soap after handling raw foods of animal origin and before touching anything else.

Prevent cross-contamination in the kitchen:

- Use separate cutting boards for foods of animal origin and other foods. Carefully clean all cutting boards, countertops, and utensils with soap and hot water after preparing raw food of animal origin.
- Avoid consuming unpasteurized milk and untreated surface water.
- Make sure that persons with diarrhea, especially children, wash their hands carefully and frequently with soap to reduce the risk of spreading the infection.
- Wash hands with soap after having contact with pet feces.

SOURCE: *Centers for Disease Control and Prevention (CDC)*

The United States Department of Agriculture carries out research on how to prevent *Campylobacter* infection from poultry. Organizations, including the CDC, maintain surveillance programs that help determine how often *Campylobacter* disease occurs, and factors that favor development of the infection.

In 1982, Centers for Disease Control and Prevention (CDC) began a national *Campylobacter* surveillance program in 1982. The program was revised in 1996 to further identify risk factors. In 2005 the Food and Drug Administration (FDA) revised its Model Food Code with hopes that the guide could reduce the risk of exposure to contaminated chicken. Exposure is not only risky and costly to those infected, but can potentially ruin or severely impact business and earnings for a commercial food establishment (and impact the people employed, etc.).

As with other pathogenic bacteria, researchers work to discover or manufacture antibiotics that are more adept at killing the bacteria without promoting the development of resistance to the antibiotic by the target bacteria.

SEE ALSO *Food-borne Disease and Food Safety.*

BIBLIOGRAPHY

Books

Ketley, Julian. *Campylobacter*. New York: Taylor & Francis, 2005.

Periodicals

Durham, Sharon. "Finding Solutions to *Campylobacter* in Poultry Production." *Agricultural Research*. 54 (2006): 10–11.

Price, Lance B., Elizabeth Johnson, Rocia Vailes, Ellen Silbergeld. "Fluoroquinolone-resistant *Campylobacter* Isolates from Conventional and Antibiotic-free Chicken Products." *Environmental Health Perspectives*. 113 (2005): 557–561.

Web Sites

Food and Drug Administration. "Model Food Code: 2005 Recommendations of the United States Public Health Service Food and Drug Administration." <http://www.cfsan.fda.gov/~dms/fc05-toc.html> (accessed April 2007).

Brian Hoyle

Cancer and Infectious Disease

■ Introduction

Cancer is not normally considered an infectious disease. Yet there is an important link between some infectious agents and certain cancers. Research has shown that chronic infection with certain viruses, and at least one bacterium, can increase the risk of these cancers. For example, human papillomavirus (HPV) is the leading cause of cervical cancer, while chronic hepatitis B virus or hepatitis C virus infection may develop into liver cancer. These viruses are now listed as carcinogens (cancer-causing substances) by the U.S.—and other—governments. Viruses have a number of ways of causing changes in cells that

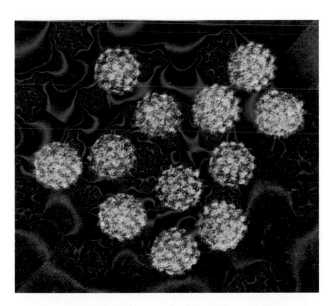

A colored transmission electron micrograph (TEM) shows human papilloma viruses (HPV), the cause of warts. Warts commonly grow on the hands and soles of the feet, on the mucous membranes, and on the genitals. Papilloma viruses belong to the papovavirus group, most of whose members are capable of inducing non-malignant tumors. HPV has been implicated in certain skin and cervical cancers. *Dr Linda Stannard, Uct/Photo Researchers, Inc.*

can cause them to divide uncontrollably, leading to the formation of a tumor. The recognition that infection can play a role in cancer is leading to new approaches to prevention and treatment. For instance, vaccination against HPV is now being introduced for girls and young women, because there is now good evidence that it protects them against cervical cancer in later life.

■ History and Scientific Foundations

It has long been known that certain viruses can cause cancer in animals. Danish researchers Wilhelm Ellermann and Oluf Bang discovered a virus that spreads leukemia among chickens in 1908. Then, in 1911, Peyton Rous (1879–1970) of the Rockefeller Institute in New York identified a virus responsible for sarcoma (a cancer of a connective tissue, like bone or cartilage) in chickens. By the 1930s, it was recognized that viruses played a role in several animal cancers. However, the significance of Rous's work for human cancer was not appreciated for many years; he was finally awarded a Nobel Prize in physiology or medicine in 1966.

The first discovery of a human cancer virus came from research carried out in Uganda in the 1950s by the Irish surgeon Denis Burkitt (1911–1993). He discovered a type of cancer of the jaw that affected young children. The disease became known as Burkitt's lymphoma, and it is still the most common tumor among African children. Tumor samples were analyzed by Anthony Epstein back in London, who discovered the presence of a new type of herpes virus, named Epstein-Barr virus (EBV). Originally, it looked as if EBV was carried by mosquitoes, because Burkitt's lymphoma was found in areas where malaria is endemic. EBV infection is very common, affecting around 90% of the world's population, most of whom do not get Burkitt's lymphoma. It is not transmission by mosquitoes, but it is exposure to malaria in combination with EBV infection

WORDS TO KNOW

CARCINOGEN: A carcinogen is any biological, chemical, or physical substance or agent that can cause cancer. There are over one hundred different types of cancer, which can be distinguished by the type of cell or organ that is affected, the treatment plan employed, and the cause of the cancer. Most of the carcinogens that are commonly discussed come from chemical sources artificially produced by humans. Some of the better-known carcinogens are the pesticide DDT (dichlorodiphenyltrichloroethane), asbestos, and the carcinogens produced when tobacco is smoked.

RETROVIRUS: Retroviruses are viruses in which the genetic material consists of ribonucleic acid (RNA) instead of the usual deoxyribonucleic acid (DNA). Retroviruses produce an enzyme known as reverse transcriptase that can transform RNA into DNA, which can then be permanently integrated into the DNA of the infected host cells.

the early 1980s that first alerted the medical community to the existence of HIV. Before the emergence of HIV, KS was rare in the West, although it was known in central Africa and the Middle East. HHV-8 is isolated from most KS tumors. Meanwhile, the human T-lymphotrophic virus (HTLV-1) is associated with a blood cancer called adult T-cell leukemia (ATL). Like HIV, HTLV-1 is a retrovirus—a type of virus whose genetic material is made of RNA rather than DNA. Both HIV and HTLV-1 are related to retroviruses known to cause leukemia in animals.

Finally, infection with the bacterium *Helicobacter pylori* increases the risk of stomach cancer. *H. pylori* is unusual because it can survive the acid conditions of the stomach. Infection causes inflammation of the stomach lining, increasing the risk of both stomach ulcers and stomach cancer. About one-third of the U.S. population has evidence of *H. pylori* infection. Although around one-half of all cases of stomach cancer are linked to the infection, most of those who do carry the infection will not develop cancer.

■ Applications and Research

Viruses and bacteria can raise the risk of cancer in various ways. They can cause chronic inflammation of the tissue they infect. Or, like HIV, they may suppress immunity and allow cancer-causing viruses to take hold. Immune suppression after an organ transplant is an important cause of HBV-associated lymphoma, for example. Some viruses can invade cells directly and alter their genetic machinery, disrupting normal control over cell division. But infection is only ever one link in a chain of events leading to tumor formation. Other factors, such as smoking, diet, or genetic disposition, may be equally important. The chain may be broken using a vaccine, which prevents infection, or by an antibiotic, which eliminates it. The introduction of a vaccine against HBV in Taiwan 25 years ago led to reduced rates of liver cancer in the country. There is, however, no vaccine against HCV—although research is ongoing. More recently, vaccines against HPV have been developed. In some clinical trials, this has provided girls and young women with 100% protection from infection. One of these, Gardasil, is now approved in some countries for use in females aged nine to 26, to protect them from cervical cancer. Eliminating *H. pylori* with antibiotics can prevent new stomach cancers from developing in patients who have had superficial stomach cancers removed.

The viruses described above, and *H. pylori*, have a well established link to cancer. The possibility that the role of infection in cancer may be even wider is being investigated. For example, there is evidence that infection with *Chlamydia trachoma* could increase the risk of cervical cancer, and a related species, *Chlamydia psittaci*, could be linked to a rare cancer of the eyes known as mucosa-associated lymphoid tissue lymphoma. A monkey

that allows cancer to develop. This fits what scientists now understand about cancer—that it develops in stages, over a long period of time, under the influence of a combination of different risk factors, both genetic and environmental. EBV has also been linked to other cancers, including nasopharyngeal cancer, which affects the area at the back of the nose, and it also is found in around half of Hodgkin's lymphoma cases.

The human papillomaviruses (HPVs) are a large group of viruses that can cause warts on the skin, mouth, and genitals. HPV infection is very common among people who are sexually active, and certain strains can cause cervical cancer. Most women who have cervical cancer show signs of infection with one of these strains. The risk of contracting HPV infection increases with the number of sexual partners a woman has.

Hepatitis B virus (HBV) and Hepatitis C virus (HCV) may cause chronic viral hepatitis, an infection of the liver that is linked to an increased risk of hepatocellular (liver) cancer. In the United States, about one-third of cases of liver cancer are related to HBV and HCV.

The human immunodeficiency virus (HIV) does not, in itself, increase the risk of cancer. However, HIV infection does increase the risk of infection by the human herpes virus 8 (HHV-8), which can lead to a skin cancer called Kaposi's sarcoma (KS). Indeed, it was the appearance of KS among homosexual men in the United States in virus called SV40 has been linked to mesothelioma, a cancer of the lining of the chest wall, in which asbestos exposure is another risk factor. Researchers in England have even suggested that common infections contracted either in the womb or during childhood may lead to clusters of childhood cancers that have previously been attributed to other environmental factors, such as overhead power lines.

■ Impacts and Issues

Most viruses and bacteria are not known to be a risk factor for cancer, and cancer is not, in itself, contagious. Moreover, the majority of people infected with agents known to be carcinogenic will not actually contract cancer; the presence of one or more other risk factors is necessary for cancer to develop.

Worldwide, infection is linked to 15 to 20% of all cancers. Other important contributing factors include smoking, diet, sunlight exposure, and genetics. In developed countries, the cancers that can be linked to infection tend to be much less common than they are in developing countries. For example, cervical cancer is becoming rare in the West because of the availability of the Pap smear, a test that checks for changes in the cells of a woman's cervix and the basis of national screening programs. Cure rates of cases caught at an early stage are very high. But cervical cancer is still the second most common cancer among women worldwide. Vaccination or screening, if it could be afforded, could help cut the global toll from the disease. Nasopharyngeal cancer is more common in Africa and Southeast Asia. In China, a high consumption of salt combines with EBV to increase the risk of this disease. HBV and HCV infection, and hepatocellular cancer, are all more common in developing countries, while ATL is found mainly in southern Japan, the Caribbean, Central Africa, and Latin America. Meanwhile, stomach cancer is the fourth most common cancer worldwide.

In 2007, Texas became the first state to consider mandatory vaccination against HPV for girls entering the sixth grade. The vaccine, Gardasil®, was approved for use in girls and women ages nine to 26 in 2006; it protects against the four types of HPV that are responsible for causing 70% of cervical cancers. After concerns regarding parental rights, vaccine availability, and the high cost of the vaccine arose, plans to mandate vaccination against HPV were put on hold. Costing over $350 for the three-injection series, Gardasil® is one of the most expensive vaccines ever produced. This expense makes distributing the vaccine to young women in developing countries impractical at the present time without corporate, government, or philanthropic action. The Bill and Melinda Gates Foundation and Merck, the manufacturer of the vaccine, plan a cooperative effort to distribute and administer Gardasil® to women in developing countries throughout the world.

IN CONTEXT: MONITORING DISEASE

Congress established the National Program of Cancer Registries (NPCR) with the Cancer Registries Amendment Act in 1992. The Centers for Disease Control and Prevention (CDC) administers the program and collects data related to the occurrence, type, extent, location, and treatment of cancers.

Cancer registries based in individual U.S. states within the United States also collect and analyze data related to cancers.

IN CONTEXT: DISEASE BURDEN OF CANCER

According to the National Institutes of Health *Fact Book Fiscal Year 2004*: "Cancer costs (the United States) an estimated $210 billion overall in 2005, including nearly $136 billion for lost productivity and more than $70 billion for direct medical costs."

SEE ALSO *Epstein-Barr Virus; HPV (Human Papillomavirus) Infection;* Helicobacter pylori; *Hepatitis B; Hepatitis C.*

BIBLIOGRAPHY

Books

Wilson, Walter R., and Merle A. Sande. *Current Diagnosis & Treatment in Infectious Diseases.* New York: McGraw Hill, 2001.

Periodicals

Boseley, S. "Can You Catch Cancer?" *The Guardian* (January 24, 2006).

Crawford, D. H. "An Introduction to Viruses and Cancer." *Microbiology Today* 56 (2005): 110–112.

Web Sites

American Cancer Society. "Infectious Agents and Cancer." October 17, 2006. <http://www.cancer.org/docroot/PED/content/PED_1_3X_Infectious_Agents_and_Cancer.asp? sitearea=PED> (accessed February 19, 2007).

National Institutes of Health. "List of Cancer-Causing Agents Grows." January 31, 2005. <http://www.nih.gov/news/pr/jan2005/niehs-31.htm> (accessed February 19, 2007).

Susan Aldridge

Candidiasis

■ Introduction

Candida is a group, or genus, of closely related species of yeast that occur naturally in the skin and gastrointestinal tract. They are the major fungal component of human flora—that is, the community of microbes that lives within the human body. If the flora remain in a healthy balance with their human host, then they do not cause disease. But various factors, such as antibiotic use or a weakened immune system, may upset this balance and lead to infection by species within the flora. Infection caused by *Candida* is known as candidiasis (can-di-DYE-a-sis), and is the most common fungal infection, or mycotic disease, that arises from the human flora. Candidiasis ranges from mild to severe and even life-threatening, depending upon its location. The most common forms of candidiasis affect the mouth, esophagus, vagina, and the bloodstream. Candidiasis does respond to antifungal drugs, although these must be carefully prescribed as some *Candida* species have developed resistance to specific drugs.

■ Disease History, Characteristics, and Transmission

There are over 150 different species of *Candida*. Most of these do not cause disease. Of those that do, *Candida albicans* is the most common cause of human mycoses,

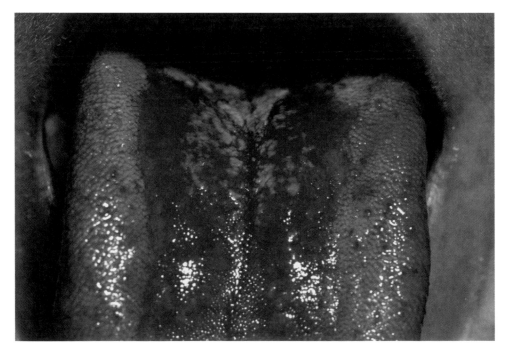

Close-up of the tongue of a woman with thrush (candidiasis) shows the back of her tongue covered in white patches of *Candida albicans*, a yeast-like fungus. *Dr P. Marazzi/Photo Researchers, Inc.*

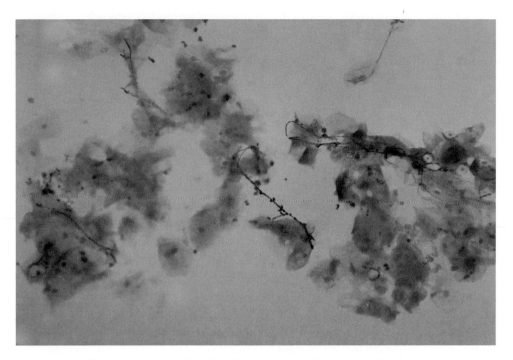

A micrograph of a vaginal smear of *Candida albicans* is shown. This fungus, which is common in most people, can cause an infection called candidiasis (also known as a yeast infection), when an imbalance occurs. © *CDC/PHIL/Corbis.*

including blood infections. However, infections from so-called non-*albicans Candida* (NAC) species, such as *C. glabrata* and *C. krusei*, are becoming more common. *C. albicans* is distinguished from NAC species under the microscope by the appearance of tiny cylindrical projections, called germ tubes, that appear within two to four hours of incubating a sample under investigation.

When the immune system is healthy and the skin and mucous membranes of the gastrointestinal and vaginal tract are intact, the existence of *Candida* will not cause any health problems. When these conditions do not hold, then *Candida* may become pathogenic, causing infection and leading to various types of illness.

One of the most important factors causing candidiasis is weakened immunity, which occurs in HIV/AIDS, after cancer chemotherapy (which depletes the white cells that fight infection), and after bone marrow or organ transplantation. Patients having transplants must take medication to stop rejection of the new organ for the rest of their lives. Unfortunately, this also impairs their immune systems and puts them at increased risk of infection, including candidiasis. Other causes of candidiasis include antibiotic use, which can alter the balance of the intestinal flora; the contraceptive pill; pregnancy; old age; malnutrition; and diabetes. In hospitals, the use of intravenous and urinary catheters, which are tubes inserted into the body to deliver fluids and medication and drain the bladder, respectively, often lead to candidiasis. Although *Candida* can be transmitted via the hands of caregivers and healthcare workers, most cases of candidiasis are endogenous—that is, the patient is infected *Candida* already present within the body.

■ Scope and Distribution

The most common sites of candidiasis are the mouth, the esophagus, the skin, the vagina, and the bloodstream. Oral and esophageal candidiasis are often also known as thrush (or oropharyngeal candidiasis [OPC]). Oral thrush is common among people with weakened immunity, especially those with HIV/AIDS. It causes white patches on the tongue and inside the mouth and may be associated with soreness and a burning sensation. Esophageal thrush is also found in HIV/AIDS; it may not cause any symptoms, but some people have difficulty in swallowing, pain, nausea, and vomiting.

Vulvovaginal candidiasis is also very common, affecting three quarters of all women at some stage in their lives. It causes genital itching and burning, with or without a "cottage cheese"-like discharge. Candidiasis can occur when the normal acidity of the vagina changes or with hormonal changes, both of which can encourage the overgrowth of *Candida*. Risk factors include pregnancy, diabetes, use of broad-spectrum antibiotics, and steroid medications. Men can get a form of the disease—genital candidiasis, which causes an itchy rash on the penis. However, transmission of thrush through sexual intercourse is rare; most infections are endogenous.

INTERTRIGO: Intertrigo, sometimes called eczema intertrigo, is a skin rash, often occurring in obese persons on parts of the body symmetrically opposite each other. It is caused by irritation of skin trapped under hanging folds of flesh such as pendulous breasts.

PATHOGENIC: Something causing or capable of causing disease.

FLORA: In microbiology, flora refers to the collective microorganisms that normally inhabit an organism or system. Human intestines, for example, contain bacteria that aid digestion and are considered normal flora.

MYCOTIC DISEASE: Mycotic disease is a disease caused by fungal infection.

NOSOCOMIAL: A nosocomial infection is an infection that is acquired in a hospital. More precisely, the Centers for Disease Control in Atlanta, Georgia, defines a nosocomial infection as a localized infection or one that is widely spread throughout the body that results from an adverse reaction to an infectious microorganism or toxin that was not present at the time of admission to the hospital.

PATHOGENIC: Something causing or capable of causing disease.

IN CONTEXT: REAL-WORLD RISKS

The Division of Bacterial and Mycotic Diseases, Centers for Disease Control and Prevention (CDC) warns that "Over-the-counter treatments for yeast infections/Vulvovaginal Candidiasis (VVC) are becoming more available. As a result, more women are diagnosing themselves with VVC and using one of a family of drugs called 'azoles' for therapy. However, misdiagnosis is common, and studies have shown that as many as two-thirds of all OTC drugs sold to treat VVC were used by women without the disease. Using these drugs when they are not needed may lead to a resistant infection. Resistant infections are very difficult to treat with the currently available medications for VVC."

SOURCE: *Coordinating Center for Infectious Diseases / Division of Bacterial and Mycotic Diseases, Centers for Disease Control and Prevention.*

Candidiasis of the skin is sometimes called intertrigo and produces a rash in warm, moist areas such as the armpit, groin, and under the breast. Diaper rash is often a form of candidiasis that affects babies in the area where the diaper comes into contact with the skin. Sometimes, especially in people with HIV/AIDS, candidiasis may also affect the nails. Oral, esophageal, vaginal, and skin candidiasis can all clear up with antifungal treatment, with no lasting effects on health, although they may recur. They may cause some discomfort, even pain, but are relatively mild infections in their own right (although the patient may be suffering from serious disease, such as HIV/AIDS or diabetes, that has allows candidiasis to develop).

Invasive candidiasis, however, can be very serious, even life-threatening. It occurs when *Candida* invades the bloodstream, and it is dangerous because it may then spread throughout the body, reaching the liver, kidneys, spleen, and other organs. Patients with cancer, depletion of white cells from cancer treatment, or major burns are at risk, as are those who have had organ transplants, abdominal surgery, or broad-spectrum antibiotics. Patients with catheters are also at risk of invasive candidiasis. The death rate from invasive candidiasis can be as high as 50%. Therefore, if *Candida* is found in a blood culture from a patient, especially if they have fever, then it can be assumed that candidiasis may be spreading through the whole body and prompt treatment is essential.

■ Treatment and Prevention

Candida species cannot be avoided or eliminated, as they occur naturally in the human body. Therefore, prevention depends on dealing with the risk factors that make people vulnerable to candidiasis. For instance, the introduction of the latest treatment for HIV/AIDS (HAART, highly active antiretroviral therapy), has reduced the incidence of esophageal candidiasis in this group. There are also antifungal drugs that can be applied either topically, as a cream or powder, or orally, as a tablet. Vaginal thrush can be treated with antifungal suppositories inserted into the vagina. The main antifungal drugs used in the treatment for candidiasis are amphotericin B, fluconazole, and nystatin, and there are several new drugs at the research stage. Meanwhile, patients with invasive candidiasis must have catheters removed or replaced, as these can be a major source of further infection.

The Division of Bacterial and Mycotic Diseases, Centers for Disease Control and Prevention (CDC), recommends that "because genital candidiasis / Vulvovaginal Candidiasis (VVC) and urinary tract infections share similar symptoms, such as a burning sensation when urinating, it is important to see a doctor and obtain laboratory testing to determine the cause of the symptoms and to treat effectively. Symptoms, which may be very uncomfortable, may persist. There is a chance that the infection may be passed between sex partners."

■ Impacts and Issues

Infections acquired in hospitals, also known as nosocomial infections from the Greek word for hospital (*nosocomium*), are an increasing public health problem. Those affected are often already very sick and are unable to fight an infection the way a healthy person would, because their immune system is weak. Added to this, many organisms that cause nosocomial infections are becoming resistant to antibiotics, so treatment may be ineffective. *Candida*, which is normally either harmless or the cause of only mild infection, is the fourth leading cause of nosocomial bloodstream infection, according to the Centers for Disease Control and Prevention (CDC). Such infections occur at a rate of five to ten per 10,000 hospital admissions and carry a mortality rate of 40–50%. Even if a patient survives, hospital stays are prolonged and this involves significant extra health care costs, which may run to thousands of dollars. Once found mainly in cancer and bone marrow transplant units, nosocomial infections, including *Candida*, now appear in all parts of the hospital and are on the increase. An aging population, more frequent use of invasive therapies involving catheters, and overuse of antibiotics are among the contributing factors.

SEE ALSO *Mycotic Disease; Nosocomial (Healthcare-Associated) Infections.*

IN CONTEXT: REAL-WORLD RISKS

The Division of Bacterial and Mycotic Diseases, Centers for Disease Control and Prevention (CDC) warns that overuse of antifungal medications to treat candidiasis of the mouth and throat (also known as a "thrush" or oropharyngeal candidiasis (OPC), "can increase the chance that they (antifungal medications) will eventually not work (the fungus develops resistance to medications). Therefore, it is important to be sure of the diagnosis from before treating with over-the-counter or other antifungal medications."

SOURCE: *Division of Bacterial and Mycotic Diseases, Centers for Disease Control and Prevention*

BIBLIOGRAPHY

Books

Gates, Robert. *Infectious Disease Secrets,* 2nd ed. Philadelphia: Hanley & Belfus, 2003.

Wilson, Walter, and Merle A. Sande. *Current Diagnosis & Treatment in Infectious Diseases.* New York: McGraw Hill, 2001.

Web Sites

Centers for Disease Control and Prevention (CDC). "Division of Bacterial and Mycotic Diseases: Candidiasis." Oct 6, 2005. <http://www.cdc.gov/ncidod/dbmd/diseaseinfo/default.htm> (accessed Jan 27, 2007).

Susan Aldridge

Cat Scratch Disease

■ Introduction

Cat scratch disease is an infection caused by the bacterium *Bartonella henselae*. It is most often transmitted to humans by the bite or scratch of a cat.

■ Disease History, Characteristics, and Transmission

Cat scratch disease was first described in 1889. Recognition that the cat is important in the spread of the disease came in 1931, but the bacterium responsible for cat scratch disease was not identified until 1985. This bacterium was initially identified as *Rochalimaea henselae* (the bacterium that causes a disease called trench fever); it was later reclassified as *Bartonella henselae*. It took such a long time to identify *B. henselae* as the cause of cat scratch disease because the bacterium is difficult to grow in artificial lab media, due to its specific nutrient requirements. In addition, the bacterium grows slowly in the laboratory even in the presence of the appropriate food sources.

The first sign of cat scratch disease is a mild infection at the site of the bite or scratch. Often, this injury does not receive much attention, since it is minor, but if the injured area is not cleaned, the bacteria can enter the bloodstream. Characteristics of the resulting infection include soreness at the wound site (which may take days to develop), expansion of the wound site and the production of pus, swelling of the lymph nodes near the wound (generally those in the underarm and neck) to an inch or more in size, loss of appetite, headache, moderate fever, bone and joint pain, rash, sore throat, and a feeling of weakness that persists.

A domestic cat can carry the bacteria in its saliva, but not display any symptoms of infection (a condition called colonization), making it impossible for those who handle the cat to know that it can infect them. For many people, there is no need to worry, since the body's immune system can successfully fight off the infection. However, if a person is immunocompromised—the immune system is not functioning efficiently—cat scratch disease can develop. In addition, some immunocompromised individuals can develop more severe symptoms

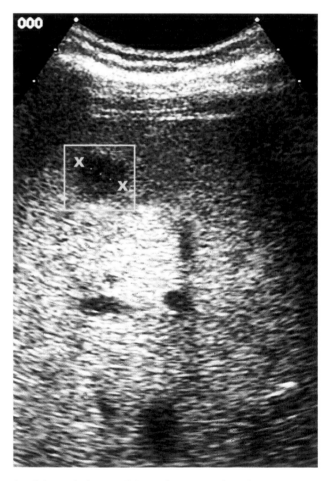

An abdominal ultrasound shows damage to a liver due to cat scratch disease. *James Cavallini/Photo Researchers, Inc.*

when they contract cat scratch disease, including infections of the spleen, liver, lungs, and eyes. A compromised immune system is sometimes a natural result of the aging process or can arise as the result of a disease that affects the immune system, such as infection with human immunodeficiency virus (HIV). The immune system also may be suppressed deliberately in patients who have received an organ transplant to avoid rejection of the transplanted organ.

Cat scratch disease cannot be passed from person to person, and usually does not require medical treatment. Once a person has had this infection, he or she is immune to the bacterium for life.

■ Scope and Distribution

About 40% of domestic cats will carry *B. henselae* at some time in their lives. The bacteria tend to be associated with younger cats, especially those who have fleas in their fur.

In the United States, more than 20,000 cases of cat scratch disease are diagnosed every year. Most cases involve people under the age of 21, with many of these being children who have been scratched or bitten by their family cat during play with the pet.

■ Treatment and Prevention

Cat scratch disease is typically diagnosed by the detection of swollen lymph nodes when the individual has been bitten or scratched by a cat. The infection tends to be resolved without treatment. However, immunocompromised patients may require treatment with antibiotics. If necessary, the swollen lymph nodes can be drained by inserting a needle into the node and withdrawing the fluid.

The risk of cat scratch disease is minimized by properly handling cats. Anyone who is scratched or bitten by a cat should wash the wound with soap and water to disinfect the area. Also, since cats can harbor the bacteria in their saliva, they should not be allowed to lick a person's face or a cut. Treating cats to reduce flea infestations is also a wise preventative strategy.

■ Impacts and Issues

With a population of more than 60 million domestic cats in the United States, there is ample opportunity for the spread of cat scratch disease. For most people, the consequences of the diseases are not serious and the disease does not require medical treatment. However, for about 10% of those who contract the disease, the result can be more serious, with consequences such as an altered mental state, loss of vision, and even pneumonia.

WORDS TO KNOW

COLONIZED: Colonized is the past tense of colonize, and refers to a surface that has been occupied by microorganisms.

IMMUNOCOMPROMISED: A reduction of the ability of the immune system to recognize and respond to the presence of foreign material.

ZOONOSES: Zoonoses are diseases of microbiological origin that can be transmitted from animals to people. The causes of the diseases can be bacteria, viruses, parasites, and fungi.

IN CONTEXT: PERSONAL RESPONSIBILITY AND PREVENTION

The National Center for Infectious Disease, Healthy Pets Healthy People published guidelines to reduce risk of cat scratch disease recommends:

- Avoid "rough play" with cats, especially kittens. This includes any activity that may lead to cat scratches and bites.
- Wash cat bites and scratches immediately and thoroughly with running water and soap.
- Do not allow cats to lick open wounds that you may have.
- Control fleas.
- If you develop an infection (with pus and pronounced swelling) where you were scratched or bitten by a cat or develop symptoms, including fever, headache, swollen lymph nodes, and fatigue, contact your physician.

SOURCE: *National Center for Infectious Disease and the Centers for Disease Control and Prevention (CDC)*

Cat scratch disease is seasonal. More than 90% of the cases occur in the autumn and early winter. This may be due to the fact that many kittens are born during the summer, and this population of new kittens has been infested with bacterium-carrying fleas by autumn. In addition, in more northern climates, the cooler months of the year usually bring people into closer contact with their house cats. In both cases, treating the pet for fleas and handwashing after petting kittens will reduce the chances of contracting the disease.

In addition to its close association with cat bites and scratches, cat scratch disease has been linked to the bites of dogs and even monkeys. This link between the disease and monkeys can put zoo staff and some veterinarians at risk for the disease in western countries, and larger populations at risk in developing countries where monkeys and humans come into contact.

SEE ALSO *Bacterial Disease; Vector-borne Disease; Zoonoses.*

BIBLIOGRAPHY

Books

Torrey, E. Fuller, and R.H. Yolken. *Beasts Of The Earth: Animals, Humans, And Disease.* Rutgers, NJ: Rutgers University Press, 2005.

Van Der Merwe, Jacob I.T. *Survival of the Cleanest: A Common Sense Guide to Preventing Infectious Disease.* Victoria, BC: Spicers Publishing, 2005.

Periodicals

Finn, Robert. "Fever of Unknown Origin? Consider Cat Scratch Disease." *Family Practice News* 35 (September 1, 2005): 67.

Web Sites

Centers for Disease Control and Prevention. "Cat Scratch Disease." <http://www.cdc.gov/healthypets/diseases/catscratch.htm> (accessed March 16, 2007).

Brian Hoyle

CDC (Centers for Disease Control and Prevention)

◼ Introduction

The Centers for Disease Control and Prevention (CDC) is part of the federal government's U.S. Department of Health and Human Services. Its headquarters are in Atlanta, Georgia. By maintaining viable relationships with state health departments and other related organizations, the CDC researches all aspects of diseases, along with developing and applying disease prevention and control, environmental health, and health education activities for all citizens of the United States. CDC also participates in international infectious disease research and response.

CDC has about 15,000 employees and 6,000 contractors in various positions, including biologists, behavioral and social scientists, physicians, veterinarians, microbiologists, statisticians, chemists, economists, engineers, epidemiologists, statisticians, and various other scientists and support personnel. CDC's headquarters coordinates its operations across the United States and Puerto Rico, including regional offices in Alaska, Colorado, Ohio, Maryland, North Carolina, Pennsylvania, Washington State, Washington D.C., and West Virginia. Other CDC employees are located in about 45 countries around the world.

◼ History and Scientific Foundations

The CDC was established on July 1, 1946, in Atlanta, Georgia, under its original name: the Communicable Disease Center (CDC). At that time, it had fewer than 400 employees. Its founder was U.S. public health official Joseph Walter Mountin (1891–1952).

The organization was established out of the U.S. military agency called the Office of Malaria Control in War Areas, which was active during World War II (1939–1945). By taking over the military office, the

CDC gained access to over six hundred military bases and related establishments in order to combat mosquitoes carrying malaria, which was still prevalent in the

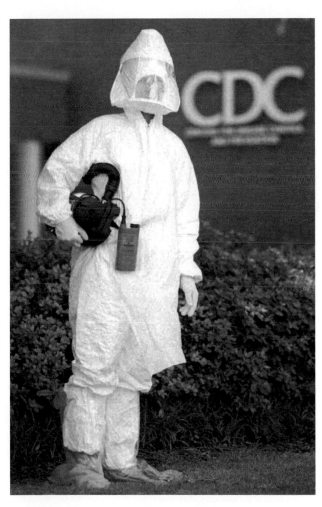

A nurse with the Centers for Disease Control and Prevention (CDC) in Atlanta wears a protective suit and respirator like those that researchers use when investigating cases of Ebola virus infection. *AP Images.*

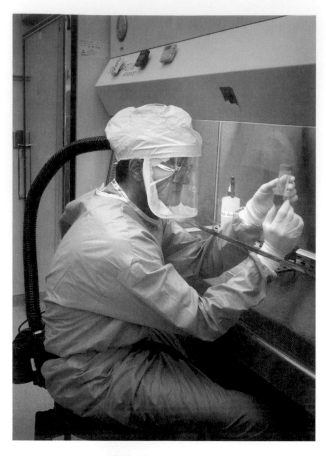

A scientist exams a sample of cultured influenza viruses in a sealed laboratory. This influenza virus strain caused the Spanish flu pandemic in 1918, which infected one-fifth of the world's population and killed between 20 and 50 million people. In 2005 CDC scientists reconstructed the virus hoping to identify the traits that made it so deadly. This allows scientists to develop new vaccines and treatments for future pandemic influenza viruses. *CDC/Photo Researchers, Inc.*

southern states. Besides malaria, the fledgling organization also worked with typhus and other infectious diseases.

The agency hired engineers, entomologists (scientists that study insects), and physicians to research and develop ways to combat infectious health problems. These professionals of the Communicable Disease Center, a part of the U.S. Public Health Service, fought mosquito-carrying malaria with the use of the insecticide DDT that is now restricted in the United States and many other countries of the world. In those years, the organization sprayed millions of homes for malaria.

By 1947, Mountin was promoting his organization as an effective organization to pursue additional public health issues such as birth defects, chronic diseases, communicable diseases, health statistics, injuries, occupational health, and toxic chemicals. The organization expanded its operations when fifteen acres of Emory University land in Atlanta, Georgia, was donated by Robert Woodruff,

chairman of the board of the Coca-Cola Company. The campus included two Biosafety Level 4 laboratories and other scientific facilities. Branches were established in Morgantown, West Virginia; Cincinnati, Ohio; Fort Collins, Colorado; and locations overseas.

Over the next sixty years, the organization expanded its expertise in the control and prevention of diseases. In 1970, its name was changed to the Center for Disease Control in order to include all of its work with communicable diseases such as AIDS (acquired immunodeficiency syndrome); chronic diseases such as cancer and heart disease; emerging diseases; birth defects such as those caused by lead poisoning; occupational illnesses and disabilities; injury control; workplace hazards; blood supply; environmental health threats; and bioterrorism.

In 1980, with expansion of the organizational structure, its name was changed to the Centers for Disease Control. Twelve years later, in 1992, its current name was adopted: the Centers for Disease Control and Prevention. The U.S. Congress requested that the organization maintain the initials CDC when its new, longer name was adopted.

■ Applications and Research

The hierarchy of the CDC begins with the Office of the Director and the National Institute for Occupational Safety and health. The Office of the Director manages and coordinates the activities of the CDC by providing overall direction to its scientific and medical programs and by providing leadership and assessment of administrative management activities. The National Institute for Occupational Safety and Health, which joined the CDC in 1973, ensures safety and health for all people in the workplace.

Six coordinating centers concentrate on specific areas of concern. Three of its coordinating centers are the: (1) Coordinating Center for Environmental Health and Injury Prevention (National Center for Environmental Health and National Center for Injury Prevention and Control); (2) Coordinating Center for Health Information Service (National Center for Health Marketing, National Center for Health Statistics, and National Center for Public Health Informatics); and (3) Coordinating Center for Health Promotion (National Center on Birth Defects and Developmental Disabilities, National Center for Chronic Disease Prevention and Health Promotion, and Office of Genomics and Disease Prevention).

Further, its other three coordinating centers are the: (4) Coordinating Center for Infectious Diseases (National Center for HIV/AIDS, Viral Hepatitis, STD, and TB Prevention, National Center for Immunization and Respiratory Diseases, National Center for Zoonotic, Vector-Borne, and Enteric Diseases, National Center for Preparedness, Detection, and Control of Infectious Diseases); (5) Coordinating Office for Global Health; and

(6) Coordinating Office for Terrorism Preparedness and Emergency Response.

CDC began a reorganization of its Coordinating Center for Infectious Diseases (CCID) on March 13, 2007. Various research centers were reorganized—or created anew—to better combat emerging and endemic global health threats.

CDC's reorganization also acknowledges the impact of globalization on infectious disease. Travel, migration, and trade have increased incidence of some infectious diseases. Disease outbreaks frequently cross state and national borders, requiring increased communication and coordinated response among various public health agencies and governments. Increased education of health care providers is necessary to help recognize, report, and respond to infectious diseases in regions where various diseases are rare or had been eliminated. The Coordinating Center for Infectious Diseases works with other CDC branches (such as the Coordinating Office for Global Health) and international health agencies such as the World Health Organization (WHO) to research infectious diseases worldwide.

Under the umbrella of the Coordinating Center for Infectious Diseases, the National Center for Preparedness, Detection, and Control of Infectious Diseases works with researchers, public health organizations, and government agencies to track, study, and respond to infectious disease. Part of its mission is to develop United States policy on infectious disease including travel advisories and restrictions, quarantine and isolation laws, and epidemic preparedness requirements.

The National Center for Zoonotic, Vector-Borne, and Entric Diseases (NCZVED) will assist international efforts to prevent and treat diseases caused by animal and insect vectors as well as food and waterborne diseases. The center will play a key role in international efforts to combat neglected tropical diseases such as malaria and emerging threats in the United States such as rodent-borne hantavirus.

In response to the increasing global incidence of HIV/AIDS and reemerging tuberculosis (TB), CDC's National Center for HIV/AIDS, Viral, Hepatitis, STD and TB Prevention (NCHHSTP) will focus on research, prevention, and intervention initatives to combat TB and sexually transmitted diseases (STDs), including HIV/AIDS. Research at the new center will assist treatment and education programs, as well as aid vaccine development.

The Coordinating Office for Terrorism Preparedness and Emergency Response works with federal, state, and local officials in the United States to develop emergency preparedness and response plans. While CDC efforts focus on response to bioterrorism events, it also advises officials on possible health concerns following a conventional terrorist event of natural disaster.

CDC also publishes several journals intended to relay information throughout the international public

WORDS TO KNOW

EPIDEMIOLOGY: Epidemiology is the study of various factors that influence the occurrence, distribution, prevention, and control of disease, injury, and other health-related events in a defined human population. By the application of various analytical techniques including mathematical analysis of the data, the probable cause of an infectious outbreak can be pinpointed.

NEGLECTED TROPICAL DISEASES: Many tropical diseases are considered to be neglected because despite their prevalence in less-developed areas, new vaccines and treatments are not being developed for them. Malaria was once considered to be a neglected tropical disease, but recently a great deal of research and money have been devoted to its treatment and cure.

VECTOR: Any agent, living or otherwise, that carries and transmits parasites and diseases. Also, an organism or chemical used to transport a gene into a new host cell.

VECTOR-BORNE DISEASE: A vector-borne disease is one in which the pathogenic microorganism is transmitted from an infected individual to another individual by an arthropod or other agent, sometimes with other animals serving as intermediary hosts. The transmission depends upon the attributes and requirements of at least three different living organisms: the pathologic agent, either a virus, protozoa, bacteria, or helminth (worm); the vector, which are commonly arthropods such as ticks or mosquitoes; and the human host.

health community. *Emerging Infectious Diseases* is published by CDC's Coordinating Center for Infectious Diseases and compiles articles and announcements on infectious diseases worldwide. *Morbidity and Mortality Weekly Report*, commonly known as the *MMWR*, collects and publishes reports from state public health agencies. Both publications foster communication and share up-to-date information among various health organizations.

The CDC has the main Biosafety Level 4 laboratories in the United States in its Special Pathogens Branch. A Biosafety Level 4 laboratory is one of a select few laboratories whose scientists and technicians are allowed to work with dangerous and unusual agents that have the highest potential for individual health risks and life-threatening diseases.

The Centers for Disease Control and Prevention is also the only repository of smallpox in the United States. Smallpox is a highly contagious disease that is acquired only by humans. It is caused by two virus variants: *Variola major* and *Variola minor*.

The CDC also provides health information to various sectors of the U.S. economy. Working with state and local organizations, the organization collects and analyzes data to detect disease outbreaks and health threats, researches effective measures for disease and injury control and prevention, and identifies risk factors and causes of diseases and injuries. Along with actively protecting health and safety, the CDC provides information to individuals making personal health decisions and organizations making professional decisions affecting larger populations of people.

In general, CDC conducts research both in the field and in the laboratory. Several CDC centers maintain field response teams to aid in the identification and surveillance of infectious diseases. International health agencies may request CDC assistance in identifying or studying disease outbreaks.

CDC participates in several international efforts to identify, research, and respond to infectious disease. For example, CDC's international outreach includes participation in the Integrated Disease Surveillance and Response (IDSR) program. IDSR seeks to strengthen local public health surveillance of and response to infectious disease outbreaks. The program goals also include increasing communication between various health agencies, sharing accurate and timely information about outbreaks, and collecting samples and utilizing laboratory research to assist further disease surveillance.

■ Impacts and Issues

The CDC has made dramatic impacts into the health of U.S. citizens throughout its existence. Two important CDC accomplishments have been identifying the causes of toxic shock syndrome (TSS, a rare disease in which *Staphylococcus aureus* bacteria infect human skin, oral cavities, and vagina) and Legionnaires' disease (a serious type of pneumonia caused by the bacterium *Legionella pneumophila* that was first recognized in July 1976 at an American Legion convention in Philadelphia, Pennsylvania).

Today, the CDC is working to find solutions for many global health threats, from malaria to HIV/AIDS. CDC is committed to education and outreach efforts promoting food and water safety, sanitation, nutrition, wellness, and personal hygiene as means of fighting infectious disease.

CDC's broad international experience and close relations with other public health agencies also aids the fight against infectious diseases within the United States. In 1993, a mysterious illness appeared in the Four Corners region of the southwestern United States (the area at the borders of the states of Arizona, Colorado, New Mexico, and Utah). The CDC quickly identified the illness as a new form of hantavirus. Government laboratories once associated with the Department of Defense collected information on hantaviruses, especially Korean hemorrhagic fever with renal syndrome (HFRS), after outbreaks among troops during the Korean War (1950–1953). CDC researchers were able to compare the emerging outbreak in the Four Corners area with previous studies on hantaviruses in Asia, thus quickly diagnosing hantavirus pulmonary syndrome (HPS), a new health threat never-before recognized in the Western Hemisphere. HPS remains an emerging health threat. The hantavirus is routinely found in rodent populations, the vector (transmitter) of the disease, in the U.S. southwest, occasionally sickening humans. CDC continues to research HPS and disseminate information on identification and prevention to local health officials.

CDC is currently participating in WHO's Global Alliance for Vaccines and Immunization (GAVI) initiatives to identify the sources of disease in underdeveloped and developing nations, as well as increase development of and access to vaccines and therapeutic medications. CDC's commitment to GAVI includes assisting the disease identification, control, elimination, and eradication efforts through field and laboratory research. CDC is also participating in GAVI research programs on microbial resistance, antibiotic usage, and pandemic influenza preparedness planning.

SEE ALSO *Bacterial Disease; Emerging Infectious Diseases; Travel and infectious disease; African Sleeping Sickness (Trypanosomiasis).*

BIBLIOGRAPHY

Books

Dowell, Scott F. *Protecting the Nation's Health in an Era of Globalization: CDC's Global Infectious Disease Strategy.* Atlanta, GA: Department of Health and Human Services, Centers for Disease Control, 2002.

Web Sites

U.S. Centers for Disease Control and Prevention (CDC). "Home Website of the CDC." May 4, 2007 <http://www.cdc.gov/> (accessed May 4, 2007).

William Arthur Atkins

Chagas Disease

■ Introduction

Chagas (SHA-gus) disease is caused by infection with the parasite *Trypanosoma cruzi*, which is transmitted from an animal reservoir to a human or other animal host by insects. Chagas disease occurs mostly in Latin America and is endemic (occurs naturally in a region) to rural areas in Mexico, Central America, and South America. However, through migration and other mass movements of people, the disease has been spread all over the world. Since parasites can be transmitted via the bloodstream, another mode of infection is via exposure to infected blood. This is the main mode of infection in non-endemic countries.

Drug treatment for Chagas disease is usually only effective during acute stages of the disease and is aimed at removing the parasite. However, during the chronic stages treatment targets the effects of the disease, such as damaged organs. Chagas disease is best prevented through avoidance of insects that may be infected with *T. cruzi*, or through preventing infection from contaminated blood.

■ Disease History, Characteristics, and Transmission

Chagas disease was first identified in 1909 by the Brazilian physician Carlos Chagas. This disease, also known as

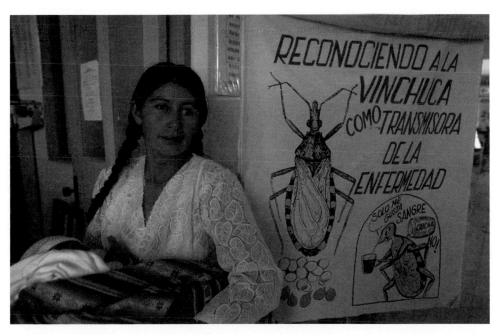

A mother and child visit a clinic during an outbreak of Chagas disease in Bolivia in 1997. The poster in the background illustrates how the disease is contracted from the bite of a parasite-infected triatomine insect, also called the kissing bug, found mainly in Central America, South America, and Mexico. *© Balaguer Alejandro/Corbis Sygma.*

American trypanosomiasis, is caused by the parasite *Trypanosoma cruzi*, which is transmitted to animals and humans by an insect vector (*Triatoma infestans*).

Human infection usually occurs in one of two ways—parasites in the feces of insects enter the body by ingestion or through the skin, or parasites are passed from an infected bloodstream into an uninfected bloodstream. In endemic areas, contact with an insect vector is the source of most infections. When blood-sucking insects feed on infected animals, they become infected with the parasites. These insects then bite another animal or human and leave behind feces. These feces are usually rubbed into the open bite wound or into mucous membranes, such as are found in the eyes or mouth, when the animal or human scratches the area. The parasite enters the bloodstream of the host and infects tissue cells.

Transmission can also occur when blood from an infected person is introduced into an uninfected person. Such infections can occur during blood transfusions, between mothers and babies, during organ transplants, and from blood exposure in laboratories.

Chagas disease is characterized by acute and chronic stages, both of which can be symptom-free. Though the acute phase tends to be symptom-free, some people experience fever, fatigue, body aches, headaches, rashes, diarrhea, vomiting, and loss of appetite during this phase. Swelling can also occur in areas where the parasite entered the body. The most common swelling is known as Romana's sign—a swelling of the eyelid on the side of the face closest to the site of the parasite's entry. Symptoms usually fade, although infection persists if untreated.

The chronic phase usually occurs many years after infection, although some people never develop this chronic phase of the disease at all. The most common chronic problems are cardiac, including an enlarged heart, heart failure, altered heart rate, or cardiac arrest; and intestinal effects, such as an enlarged esophagus or colon, which causes problems eating or passing stool.

■ Scope and Distribution

Since Chagas disease can be transmitted by infected blood as well as by insect vectors, it can exist outside endemic areas. However, vector-borne infections of Chagas disease generally occur only in endemic areas from the southern United States to southern Argentina. Rural areas in Mexico, Central America, and South America are the principle locations of vector-borne infections.

The human populations at highest risk for developing Chagas disease are low-income people living in rural areas. Housing is often of poor quality and provides ideal habitats for insects carrying the disease. Rural areas in Central and South America, where houses are often built of mud, adobe, or thatch, have a high incidence of infection. It is estimated that as many as 11 million people in Mexico, Central America, and South America are infected with Chagas disease.

As populations have begun to make large-scale migrations, Chagas disease has spread from rural areas into previously uninfected areas. This has increased its global distribution and given rise to other modes of infection, resulting in a need to adopt new infection control strategies. Countries into which the disease is introduced must take steps to identify infected persons in order to prevent the spread of the disease. Any activities that involve potential mixing of blood, such as transfusions, require stringent monitoring.

■ Treatment and Prevention

Chagas disease can be effectively treated with medication during the acute stages of infection. The drugs most commonly used to treat Chagas disease are benznidazole and nifurtimox. These are antiparasitic drugs aimed at killing the parasite. However, they are toxic and must be taken under medical supervision, since they may cause adverse side effects. Chemotherapy can also be used in an attempt to remove the parasite, although this treatment is not 100 percent effective.

Treatment during the chronic stages of Chagas disease focuses on controlling the effects of the disease, such as cardiac and intestinal complications. This may include insertion of a pacemaker, to control the heart's rhythm and to prevent chronic heart failure; or surgery on enlarged organs, such as the esophagus or colon. Organ transplants are also sometimes performed to replace damaged organs.

As there is no vaccine or drug available to prevent infection, prevention efforts focus on preventing parasite transmission. In terms of vector-borne infection, avoiding rural areas in which the disease is likely to exist, or treating houses, clothes, and bodies with insect repellants may prevent contact with a vector. Feces-contaminated food can also carry the parasite. Therefore, careful handling and preparation of food, plus an awareness of whether insects have been near the food, may prevent infection.

Bloodborne transmission of Chagas disease can also occur. Therefore, medical procedures, such as blood transfusions and organ transplants, require strict screening to prevent transmission of the parasite. In addition, mothers infected with Chagas disease can potentially pass the parasite to their babies while breastfeeding, if the skin around the nipple is broken. Avoiding breastfeeding when the nipples have broken skin can prevent infection.

■ Impacts and Issues

Large-scale population movements have led to an increased risk of Chagas disease in areas outside Latin America where the disease is not endemic. In nonendemic areas, the disease is largely spread by infected blood, making strict screening of the blood supply imperative. However, some countries do not perform routine tests for Chagas disease in their blood banks, and, thus, the risk of infection is high in those countries. The World Health Organization ranks the infection rate for Chagas disease from Latin American blood banks higher than HIV, hepatitis B, and hepatitis C.

T. cruzi, the parasite that causes Chagas disease, has also been discovered in wild animals in some American states. This discovery suggests that wild reservoirs of this parasite may exist in the United States, raising the possibility of an outbreak of vector borne infections, if insects feeding on these wild animals come in contact with humans.

Transmission between a vector and human is less likely to occur in densely vegetated habits, such as rainforests, or in city areas. However, regions in which the habitat is thinned out and the abundance of fauna is reduced while the human population increases are hotspots for an outbreak of Chagas disease. In these areas, a decrease in the abundance of animals drives the vector insects to seek a new food source, and the growing human population provides a ready target. Deforestation of the Amazon and other areas of tropical rainforest in Central and South America may create just such hotspots, and more people may be infected with Chagas disease as a result.

SEE ALSO *Arthropod-borne Disease; Blood Supply and Infectious Disease; Bloodborne Pathogens; Economic Development and Disease; Host and Vector; Immigration and Infectious Disease; Parasitic Diseases; Vector-borne Disease; Zoonoses.*

BIBLIOGRAPHY

Books

Arguin, P.M., P.E. Kozarsky, and A.W. Navin. *Health Information for International Travel 2005–2006.* Washington, DC: U.S. Department of Health and Human Services, 2005.

Periodicals

Aufderheide, A.C., et al. "A 9,000-year Record of Chagas' Disease." *Proceedings of the National Academy of Sciences of the United States of America* 101 (2004): 2034–2039.

Web Sites

Centers for Disease Control and Prevention (CDC). "Chagas Disease (American Trypanosomiasis)." December 13, 2006. <http://www.cdc.gov/ncidod/dpd/parasites/chagasdisease/factsht_chagas_disease.htm> (accessed January 31, 2007).

Directors of Health Promotion and Education. "Chagas Disease." <http://www.dhpe.org/infect/Chagas.html> (accessed January 31, 2007).

Pan American Health Organization. "Chagas Disease (American Trypanosomiasis)." <http://www.paho.org/english/ad/dpc/cd/chagas.htm> (accessed January 31, 2007).

Chickenpox (Varicella)

■ Introduction

Chickenpox is a viral disease primarily of children, although it can infect any non-immune person. Infection is caused by the varicella-zoster virus (VZV), which is stored in human hosts and is transmitted via direct contact, as well as by inhalation of contaminated airborne particles. Infection with this virus results in the formation of an itchy rash that is sometimes accompanied by a fever. Treatment usually centers on the symptoms of the infections—the rash and fever—rather than on the virus itself. However, antiviral medication may be adminis-

tered in severe cases. Complications such as bacterial infections, brain infections, viral pneumonia, and even death occur rarely. Following recovery from chickenpox, the virus remains in the body and can be reactivated, causing a new disease called shingles.

Chickenpox is a worldwide disease and most people will develop it by adulthood. Immunity develops after the infection. However, there is a vaccine available that is 80–90% effective. If a vaccinated person develops chickenpox, the vaccination appears to lessen the severity of infection.

Children develop chickenpox most frequently, although adults tend to have more severe infections. High-risk

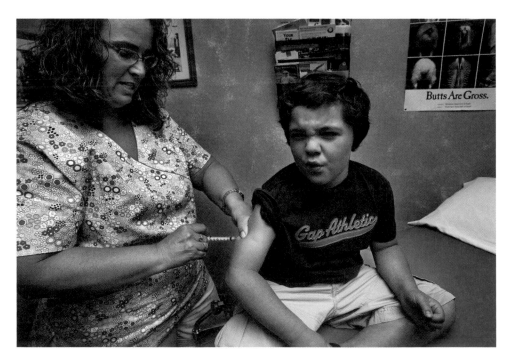

A medical assistant is shown vaccinating a child for chickenpox in Washington state in 2006. The vaccination is required in Washington and most other states for children entering kindergarten and sixth grade, as well as children over 19 months of age who are in preschool or licensed child care. *AP Images.*

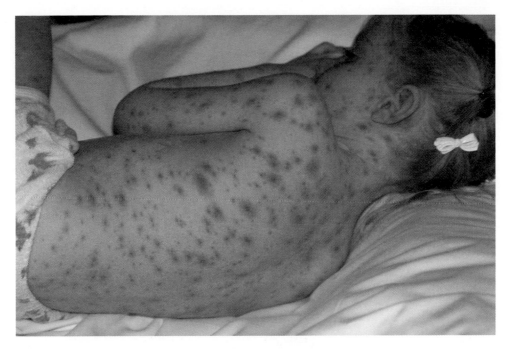

A girl displays the signs of chickenpox.   © *Lester V. Bergman/Corbis.*

groups include those with compromised immune systems, newborns, and pregnant women. Individuals in these groups are also unable to use the vaccine due to the risk of developing the disease from the vaccine.

■ Disease History, Characteristics, and Transmission

Chickenpox has existed for centuries. Originally, doctors were aware of the disease without knowing its cause. Similarities between chickenpox and smallpox, a deadly disease that no longer occurs in humans, made it hard for practitioners to differentiate between the two. The first description of chickenpox on record was made by the Italian scientist Giovanni Filippo during the 1500s. Subsequently, English physician Richard Morton identified the disease in the 1600s, as did the English physician William Heberden in the 1700s. Heberden first demonstrated that chickenpox and smallpox are different diseases.

Chickenpox is a viral disease that arises when humans become infected with the varicella-zoster virus (VZV), which is a type of human herpes virus. Humans are a reservoir for VZV and the virus is very contagious among humans. Transmission occurs when airborne particles from infected people are inhaled, or when direct contact occurs between infected and non-infected people. Therefore, coughing and sneezing spreads the virus, as does touching the open lesions of infected persons. There is a 70–80% chance that a person who has no history of chickenpox will get the disease following exposure to an infected person.

VZV has an incubation period of about 14–16 days after which the first symptoms appear. Chickenpox is characterized by the formation of itchy blisters that break out most commonly on the scalp, face, and torso. These blisters form vesicles that contain an infectious fluid, and within a day of developing, the blisters break and crust over. Blisters tend to continually form over a period of five to 10 days and the outbreak is over when all sores have formed a crust. Scratching the blisters may cause scarring. Accompanying symptoms include mild fever and weakness.

A person is contagious approximately one to two days prior to the rash developing, and he or she remains contagious until all the blisters have crusted over. Since the incubation period is two to three weeks, a person may be unaware they have contracted the disease until weeks after contact with an infected person.

While most cases of chickenpox are not considered serious, and recovery is likely, the disease potentially can be fatal in both children and adults. Complications can arise, such as bacterial infections under the skin, within bones and tissue, in the lungs, and in the blood. The virus can also cause complications directly, such as encephalitis and viral pneumonia. Prior to the development of a vaccine, approximately 100 people died from chickenpox in the United States every year.

Following recovery from chickenpox, the varicella virus remains in the body and settles among nerve fibers. The virus tends to remain dormant, but it can be

WORDS TO KNOW

IMMUNOCOMPROMISED: A reduction of the ability of the immune system to recognize and respond to the presence of foreign material.

POSTHERPETIC NEURALGIA: Neuralgia is pain arising in a nerve that is not the result of any injury. Postherpetic neuralgia is neuralgia experienced after infection with a herpesvirus, namely *Herpes simplex* or *Herpes zoster*.

VACCINE: A substance that is introduced to stimulate antibody production and thus provide immunity to a particular disease.

VARICELLA ZOSTER IMMUNE GLOBULIN (VZIG): Varicella zoster immune globulin is a preparation that can give people temporary protection against chickenpox after exposure to the varicella virus. It is used for children and adults who are at risk of complications of the disease or who are susceptible to infection because they have weakened immunity.

VESICLE: A membrane-bound sphere that contains a variety of substances in cells.

reactivated and result in a different infection known as shingles or zoster. This infection generally occurs in older people and is characterized by a painful rash, fever, headache, body aches, and general feelings of illness. While recovery is likely from shingles, many patients suffer ongoing complications, in particular, post-herpetic neuralgia. Post-herpetic neuralgia is nerve pain that arises most likely as a result of the virus becoming active within the nerve fibers and damaging them. This pain can vary from mild to severe and may be present for only three months, or for life. In general, people do not suffer a second case of chickenpox, but there have been some exceptions.

■ Scope and Distribution

Chickenpox is a worldwide virus. Its prevalence within society is so high that by adulthood almost all people will have contracted the disease. While children contract the highest number of cases, anyone who comes in contact with an infected person, and has not previously had the disease, is at risk of becoming infected with the virus. In the United States, approximately 4 million cases of chickenpox are reported annually, and despite vaccinations, fatalities still occur.

When children of school age contract the virus, they are required to stay home from school until they are no longer contagious. However, due to the high infectiousness of this disease, outbreaks are hard to prevent, and despite policies that keep infected children at home, outbreaks are likely to occur.

Adults also contract the virus, although the number of adult cases is much lower than the number of cases among children. Despite this, prior to the release of a vaccine in the United States, half of all fatalities were adults. This statistic highlights the fact that adults tend to develop more severe cases of chickenpox.

There are also groups of high risk people within society. These include immunocompromised people, pregnant women, newborn babies, and healthcare workers. Immunocompromised people include cancer and AIDS patients, as well as transplant recipients. Their immune systems are less able to fight off infection, making them more likely to contract the virus. Chickenpox infection during pregnancy may result in complications with the fetal development. These complications may include growth retardation, such as underdevelopment of limbs and lack of growth in some parts of the brain. In addition, a chickenpox infection during pregnancy may lead to miscarriage, premature labor, or infection of the fetus with the virus. Newborn babies have an increased fatality rate if they contract the disease and do not receive treatment. Healthcare workers and people taking care of sick family members are also at risk of contracting the virus.

The development of a second bout of chickenpox is rare and does not seem to be predetermined by any condition. However, the occurrence of shingles tends to be more likely in people 50 years old or older and in immunocompromised people. Shingles is not as common as chickenpox, but still has an annual rate of 1 million cases annually in the United States. Of these, approximately 20% will develop post-herpetic neuralgia. However, shingles does not spread from person to person, but arises in people who already have the varicella-zoster virus in their bodies. And, although shingles can cause chickenpox in non-infected people, it is not as contagious as chickenpox and usually requires contact with the blister fluid in order for transmission to occur. As of May 2006, a vaccine against shingles was approved and is recommended by the CDC for all adults over the age of 60.

■ Treatment and Prevention

Most cases of chickenpox do not require treatment for recovery to occur. In general, treatment is provided for the symptoms, namely the fever and rash. Fever is treated with non-aspirin medications, such as acetaminophen, since aspirin is linked with the development of Reye's syndrome. The rash is generally treated with calamine lotion, cool compresses, or oatmeal baths to alleviate the itching.

However, in some cases, more specific treatment is employed. Antiviral medication may be given to adults or to children at risk of developing a serious illness. In addition, bacterial infections may arise when blisters are scratched and opened, and anti-bacterial medication may be necessary. Bacterial infections can be prevented by avoiding scratching the blisters, and keeping them clean.

After infection with the chickenpox virus, most patients have a lifelong immunity to the disease. This reduces their chances of contracting the virus again, but it does not keep them from developing shingles. Newborn babies receive immunity from immune mothers, but this immunity lasts only for the first few months of their lives.

A vaccine is available to prevent chickenpox. The vaccine was developed in Japan and the United States and was first released in the United States in 1995. Vaccination is recommended for children between the ages of 12 and 18 months, since this ensures the best protection, but the vaccine can also be given to people older than 18 months. In children under 13 years old, one dose of the vaccine is necessary, whereas those 13 years old and older require two doses administered four to eight weeks apart. Some people do develop chickenpox after being vaccinated, but they tend to have very mild cases of the disease. Vaccination is recommended for almost everyone who has not had chickenpox with the exceptions noted below.

Some individuals should not be vaccinated against chickenpox, including newborns, children with leukemia or lymphoma, people with immune problems, people taking drugs that suppress the immune system, and pregnant women, because of the risk that they may develop the disease as a result of the vaccination. However, if a person in one of these categories is exposed to the virus, they can receive a temporary protective vaccine known as varicella zoster immune globulin (VZIG). VZIG acts to prevent the development of the disease or to modify the disease after exposure. The protection conferred by VZIG is only short term and the treatment is expensive. As a result, it is only administered to people at high risk of developing severe chickenpox when they are exposed to the virus.

During an outbreak of chickenpox, disease transmission can be minimized by separating those with the disease from others and by limiting the duration of any contact that must occur between infected and non-infected individuals. Since chickenpox is highly contagious, anyone who is not immune to the disease should avoid inhaling contaminated air and touching open lesions on infected people. Protection from shingles patients is less difficult due to the fact that transmission occurs via contact with rash fluid only. If these rashes are well covered, risk of transmission is greatly reduced.

IN CONTEXT: REAL-WORLD QUESTIONS

Questions sometimes arise as to whether varicella vaccine should be administered to a healthy child who has intimate personal contact with an immunocompromised individual (e.g., a sibling with leukemia, or an immunocompromised individual in their household). With regard to this issue, the Centers for Disease Control and Prevention, National Immunization Program states that the, "ACIP (Advisory Committee on Immunization Practices) and the American Association of Pediatrics (AAP) recommend that healthy household contacts of immunocompromised persons be vaccinated. This is the most effective way to protect the immunocompromised person from varicella. However, because of the small risk of household transmission of vaccine virus, vaccinees who develop a vaccine-related rash should avoid contact with immunocompromised persons while the rash is present. If a susceptible immunocompromised person is inadvertently exposed to a person with a vaccine-related rash, varicella zoster immune globulin (VZIG) need not be given because disease associated with this type of transmission would be expected to be mild. It is preferable to expose the immunocompromised person to the much lower risk of severe disease due to vaccine virus than to wild virus in household contacts."

SOURCE: *Centers for Disease Control and Prevention, National Immunization Program*

■ Impacts and Issues

Despite the availability of an effective vaccine, many people are still not vaccinated against chickenpox for a number of reasons. The benefits associated with vaccination must be weighed against such factors as the cost, importance, and likely impact the vaccination will have. In developing countries, there are many diseases with high rates of morbidity and mortality that can be prevented by vaccination. Vaccination against chickenpox may not be as high a priority as vaccinations against other diseases, especially when funding is limited and the health care delivery system is overburdened.

In countries where the vaccine is affordable, generally available, and of significant benefit to the public health, many still avoid getting vaccinated. People may remain unvaccinated voluntarily because of misconceptions surrounding the seriousness of this disease. Many people are under the impression that chickenpox is a relatively mild virus that all people will encounter and recover from during their lives. However, complications and deaths occur from chickenpox infections, even in healthy individuals. Prior to the vaccine being made available in the United States, 100 people died annually from this disease. These people were not all high-risk patients, but rather, most were healthy individuals. Since vaccination was introduced, the Centers for Disease Control and Prevention

(CDC) was still reporting deaths during 1999 and 2000 among healthy, unvaccinated people.

Vaccination appears to be a more cost-effective option for many populations, since the costs of preventing cases of chickenpox often outweigh the costs of combating an outbreak and treating those who contract the disease.

■ Primary Source Connection

In this newspaper article appeared in the *Washington Times* during the 2003 school year. The author, Denise Barnes, describes the actions that were taken after hundreds of students in Washington, D.C., failed to provide proof of their immunization status to school officials. Vaccination for chickenpox is required by the school district when students cannot verify that they have had the disease.

Time's Up on School Shots; 434 Students Sent to Court

D.C. public school officials yesterday referred 434 students to truancy court after they failed to provide updated immunization records after 30 days of school. Officials reminded their parents that they could face fines and jail time.

"We're going to court," said Ralph Neal, assistant schools superintendent. "It's been a whole month."

Mr. Neal said the D.C. Compulsory School Attendance Amendment Act of 1990 states that principals must refer students to truancy court if they fail to provide proof of immunizations by Oct. 1. He also said Superintendent Clifford B. Janey told principals yesterday to begin the legal process.

"Parents, if convicted, could be fined $100 or [spend] up to 10 days in jail," Mr. Neal said.

The biggest problems remain in middle, junior and high schools, which have 379 of the students. Among them, 285 are in senior high schools and 94 are in junior highs or middle schools.

The remaining 55 students are in elementary schools and special education centers. The District has 60,799 students in about 200 schools, including specialty schools and programs.

Officials estimated in mid-August that about 5,000 students were still without the mandatory shots and said they would know more when school started Sept. 1. They reported in mid-September that the number had been reduced to 1,190 students.

The school system in August 2003 had about 11,000 students without shots, which means the number of noncompliant students was reduced by more than 50 percent this summer, said Dr. Karyn Berry of the city's Department of Health.

The students who did not receive their shots or provide up-to-date proof were allowed inside schools but were kept in designated areas such as auditoriums or classrooms.

The required shots are DPT (for diphtheria, pertussis and tetanus), OPV (oral polio vaccine), MMR (measles, mumps and rubella), HIB (haemophilus influenza type B), HepB (hepatitis B), and varicella immunizations, if students have not had chicken pox.

"We've worked collaboratively with parents, and we are pleased that more than 60,000 parents have worked along with us," Mr. Neal said. "But we have [about] 400 students [without shots.] And the law states they must be immunized. Students not attending school are truant. Being a truant means that you are in violation of the law. We need to hold everyone accountable, and we need the cooperation of parents."

The District has improved the situation, in part, by offering free shots at clinics.

Vera Jackson, a spokeswoman for the city's Department of Health, said six clinics remain open, and no appointment is necessary.

"We're still working very hard to make sure everybody gets immunized," she said.

Denise Barnes

BARNES, DENISE, "TIME'S UP ON SCHOOL SHOTS; 434 STUDENTS SENT TO COURT." *THE WASHINGTON TIMES* (OCTOBER 2, 2003).

SEE ALSO *AIDS (Acquired Immunodeficiency Syndrome); Cancer and Infectious Disease; Childhood Infectious Diseases, Immunization Impacts; HIV; Meningitis, Viral; Shingles (Herpes Zoster) Infection; Smallpox; Vaccines and Vaccine Development; Viral Disease.*

BIBLIOGRAPHY

Books

Mandell, G. L., J. E. Bennett, and R. Dolin. *Principles and Practice of Infectious Diseases.* 6th ed. Philadelphia, PA: Elsevier, 2004.

Web Sites

Centers for Disease Control. "Varicella Disease (Chickenpox)." May 26, 2005. <http://www.cdc.gov/nip/diseases/varicella/default.htm> (accessed March 8, 2007).

Centers for Disease Control. "Varicella Vaccine (Chickenpox)." April 25, 2005. <http://www.cdc.gov/nip/vaccine/varicella/faqs-gen-vaccine.htm> (accessed March 8, 2007).

U.S. Department of Health and Human Services. "FDA Licenses Chickenpox Vaccine." March 17, 2005. <http://www.fda.gov/bbs/topics/NEWS/NEW00509.html> (accessed March 8, 2007).

World Health Organization. "Immunization, Vaccines, and Biologicals: Varicella Vaccine." May 2003. <http://www.who.int/vaccines/en/varicella.shtml#vaccines> (accessed March 8, 2007).

Chikungunya

■ Introduction

Chikungunya (chick-un-GUNE-ya) is an arthropod-borne virus transmitted to humans via a mosquito bite. Transmission of the disease is known to occur in regions within India, Africa, Southeast Asia, the Philippines, and the Caribbean. However, since 2000, infections have occurred worldwide as travelers have contracted chikungunya from infected mosquitoes while traveling through endemic regions (areas where the disease exists normally), and then imported the disease when they traveled home.

Infection usually results in a range of symptoms including fever, aches, joint pains, nausea, vomiting, and chills. However, a full recovery is common following treatment involving rest, fluids, and drugs for fever or joint pains. There have been a large number of outbreaks between the years of 2004 and 2007, particularly in

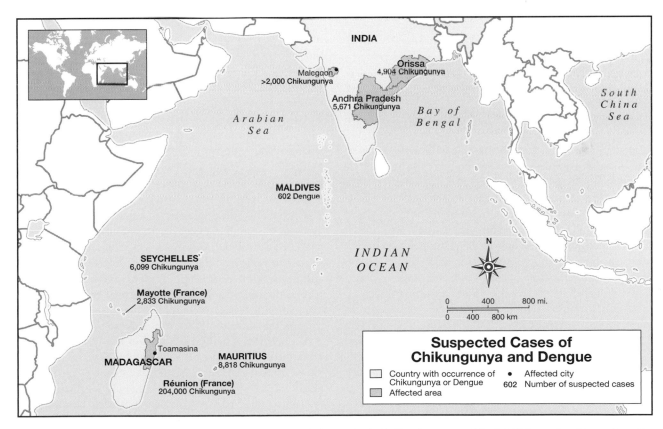

Map showing the number of suspected cases of chikungunya and dengue in the Indian Ocean area, March 2006. *© Copyright World Health Organization (WHO). Reproduced by permission.*

157

India and groups of islands in the Indian Ocean. Because of these outbreaks, the World Health Organization considers chikungunya an important re-emergent disease (a disease capable of causing large outbreaks after a period of relatively few occurrences).

There is no vaccine available to protect against infection with the chikungunya virus, therefore, the best prevention method is avoidance of mosquitoes. This is achieved by using insect repellants, wearing long-sleeved clothing, using mosquito nets, and removing stagnant water bodies where mosquitoes breed.

Disease History, Characteristics, and Transmission

Chikungunya virus infection was first described during the 1950s by scientists Marion Robinson and W.H.R. Lumsden. The first known outbreak occurred during 1952 in Africa, and the first outbreak in India was in 1963 in Calcutta.

Infection is transmitted to humans via a bite from mosquitoes in the genus *Aedes*. These mosquitoes are also responsible for the transmission of dengue and yellow fever. Mosquitoes pick up the infection when they feed on infected people or non-human primates. This virus is from the family Togoviridae and the genus *Alphavirus*. Infection is not thought to be transmitted directly from person to person.

Chikungunya manifests itself in humans one to 12 days (usually about a week) after being bitten by an infected mosquito. Most cases result in a range of symptoms, although there have been some asymptomatic cases. The most common symptoms are: fever, headache, joint pain, swelling of joints, arthritis of the joints, chills, nausea, and vomiting. A rash may also occur, and in rare cases, bleeding and hemorrhaging result. Acute fever usually lasts from a few days to two weeks, and some people with chikungunya experience prolonged fatigue. The symptoms of chikungunya are similar to dengue fever, and as a result, the disease is sometimes misdiagnosed. Life-long immunity is thought to occur following chikungunya infection.

Scope and Distribution

Chikungunya first appeared in Africa in 1952 and was first discovered in India ten years later. The virus is distributed around Africa and Asia. Outbreaks have been reported in India, Central and South Africa, Africa, Southeast Asia, the Philippines, and the Caribbean.

In 2005, there was a reemergence of chikungunya in India with 180,000 cases reported between 2005 and 2007. In early 2005, an outbreak occurred in the Comoro Islands. Since this outbreak, other islands in the Indian Ocean have reported infections. On the island of Réunion, chikungunya infection was first identified in March 2005, with 150,000 cases identified before February 2006. Among the other islands in the Indian Ocean, 300,000 suspected cases were reported before May 2006. The chikungunya outbreak in this region constitutes the largest known outbreak since scientists began tracking the disease.

Transmission of chikungunya has not yet been found to occur in Europe or other non-endemic areas. However, there are an increasing number of travelers being infected while in regions with chikungunya outbreaks and then returning to non-infected regions. Between 2005 and 2006, the Centers for Disease Control and Prevention (CDC) diagnosed 12 travelers from the United States infected with chikungunya after traveling to known infected areas.

Treatment and Prevention

Treatment of chikungunya is aimed at relieving symptoms. No vaccine or specific antiviral treatment is available. The most common treatments for symptoms include rest, fluids, and anti-inflammatory/analgesic drugs such as ibuprofen, naproxen, acetaminophen, or paracetamol. These treatments help relieve fever, aches, joint pains, and arthritis. In most cases, people recover fully from chikungunya, often in a few days. However, in rare cases, joint pain can persist, or prolonged fatigue may be experienced. Death is unlikely, although there are a few reported deaths related to bleeding from this infection. Some deaths appear to be the result of using aspirin to treat symptoms, which may be linked with bleeding in persons with chikungunya.

As this infection is transmitted via mosquitoes, the best prevention method is to avoid the bite of infected mosquitoes. This can be achieved by eliminating mosquito breeding grounds, such as stagnant water bodies; using insect repellants on the body and clothing; using mosquito nets; and wearing long-sleeved clothing. In addition, to prevent infection from being spread to more mosquitoes, the above prevention methods should be used by infected people as well.

■ Impacts and Issues

Although chikungunya transmission is confined to endemic countries, infection can occur worldwide as travelers to infected regions become infected and return to their home countries. This has a potential impact on the distribution of this disease. The distribution of one chikungunya disease vector, the mosquito *Aedes aegypti*, is almost worldwide. Therefore, the risk for large geographic expansion of endemic areas of the disease is possible. Mosquitoes from non-infected regions could become infected by feeding on infected travelers, or could be imported within shipping containers, thus potentially spreading chikungunya to previously uninfected regions.

Distinguishing between chikungunya and dengue fever is sometimes difficult, as they have similar symptoms and are transmitted via the same vector. Therefore, the occurrence of chikungunya may be misrepresented due to misdiagnosis. The CDC suggests that the possibility that cases of chikungunya have been misdiagnosed as dengue fever could potentially mean that the number of chikungunya cases is higher than previously assumed.

French authorities received media criticism for a perceived slow response to the Réunion Island (an overseas department of France) outbreak in 2005. By February 2006, the French government took measures to eliminate mosquito breeding grounds on the island, and formed a task force to study re-emerging infectious diseases, especially chikungunya. Researchers in France are currently working to test a preliminary vaccine developed for chikungunya in the 1980s by United States Army scientists.

SEE ALSO *Arthropod-borne Disease; Dengue and Dengue Hemorrhagic Fever; Mosquito-borne Diseases; Travel and Infectious Disease; Vector-borne Disease; Yellow Fever.*

BIBLIOGRAPHY

Periodicals

Hochedez P., S. Jaureguiberry, M. Debruyne, P. Bossi, P. Hausfater, G. Brucker, F. Bricaire, and E. Caumes. "Chikungunya Infection in Travelers." *Emerging Infectious Diseases.* vol. 12, no. 10 (2006): 1565–1567.

Web Sites

Centers for Disease Control and Prevention (CDC). "Chikungunya Fever." Jan. 16, 2006 <http://www.cdc.gov/ncidod/dvbid/Chikungunya/index.htm> (accessed February 8, 2007).

Centers for Disease Control and Prevention (CDC). "Chikungunya Fever Diagnosed Among International Travelers—United States, 2005–2006." Sep. 29, 2006 <http://www.cdc.gov/mmwr/preview/mmwrhtml/mm5538a2.htm> (accessed February 8, 2007).

Public Health Agency of Canada. "Material Safety Data Sheet—Infectious Substances." Apr. 23, 2001 <http://www.phac-aspc.gc.ca/msds-ftss/msds172e.html> (accessed February 8, 2007).

Childhood Infectious Diseases, Immunization Impacts

■ Introduction

Less than 100 years ago in the United States, a quarter of children died before their fifth birthday. Most of those died before reaching one year old. Today, the diseases that caused these deaths are rare in developed countries, and many American doctors have never treated a child with measles, polio, or diphtheria. The practice of immunizing children can claim a great deal of the credit for the miraculous reduction in childhood suffering and death during the last century.

■ History and Policy Response

The primary cause of infant and child deaths throughout recorded history has been infectious disease. For centuries, attempts to control infections included bloodletting, purging, use of leeches, or swallowing various concoctions of herbs and poisons. The epidemics of smallpox, measles, diphtheria, and pneumonia ignored these remedies and continued killing children.

In 1798, Edward Jenner (1749–1823) proved the effectiveness of vaccination as a strategy in preventing smallpox, and in 1956, the World Health Organization (WHO) in conjunction with national governments began a immunization program to eradicate smallpox from the world. The campaign was successful. In 1977, health officials in Somalia reported the last natural case of smallpox, and the WHO declared victory over smallpox in 1979.

The success of the smallpox campaign proved that effective immunization strategies could eradicate disease. Elimination of polio from North America in 1991 provided further proof that immunization is a powerful weapon for combating infectious diseases. While construction and production of vaccines can be quite complex, the idea behind how vaccines provide protection from disease is quite simple.

For centuries, medical practitioners knew that contracting a mild form of certain diseases protected against more severe forms of the same or similar diseases. The discovery that microorganisms caused infectious diseases provided a scientific foundation for this immunity phenomenon. When exposed to these microorganisms, the immune system will create specific neutralizing agents called antibodies. If the immune system produces

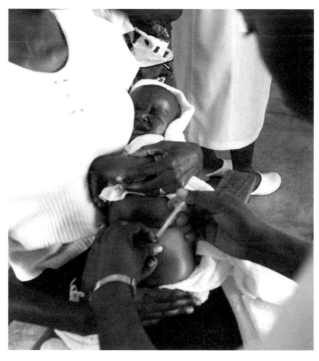

A two-month-old baby receives a vaccine against diphtheria, tetanus, whooping cough, and hepatitis B in Mozambique during an international drive to immunize thousands of the world's impoverished children. The initiative, largely funded by Microsoft co-founder Bill Gate's foundation, aims to prevent the spread of the deadly but preventable diseases that kill 3 million people annually. *AP Images.*

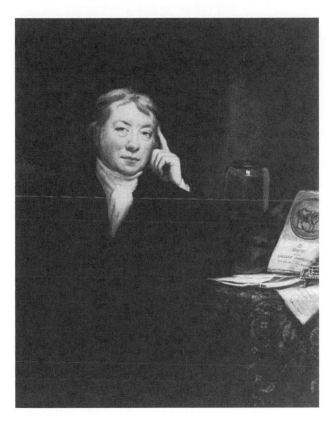

Edward Jenner (1749–1823) discovered a vaccine for smallpox in the late 1790s. *The Library of Congress.*

antibodies fast enough, the body survives. Some micro organisms spread too rapidly however, and the body is overwhelmed before the immune system can react. At times the immune system does eventually stop the spread of the microorganism, but the body is so weakened that it never fully recovers. In some children, a second disease develops soon after the first, and the weakened body succumbs. Immunization primes the immune system to react quickly.

Active immunization is the process of inducing immunity without causing disease. A vaccine is a substance that when administered, induces the immune system to produce protective antibodies. Vaccines may be purified toxins, specific bacterial or viral proteins, genetically engineered pieces of the organism, or even whole-killed bacteria. The vaccine mimics the disease-causing microorganism but does not cause disease. The vaccine fools the immune system to produce antibodies with little or no discomfort to the person. The immunity acquired may be life-long or may need repeated vaccine boosters to maintain protection.

Using the techniques developed early in the nineteenth century, vaccines for diphtheria, pertussis, tuberculosis, and tetanus entered the medical arsenal in the

1920s. When Jonas Salk (1914–1995) perfected injectable polio vaccine in 1955, parents waited in long lines to have their children vaccinated against polio. In the 1960s, an oral polio vaccine became available followed quickly by vaccines against measles, mumps, and rubella.

Despite the relative crude nature of the early vaccines, they provided effective control of many diseases and further refinement in vaccine design reduced side effects and reactions to the vaccines. Nations around the globe began widespread immunization programs in the latter part of the twentieth century. In 1962, the United States established a vaccination program coordinated by the federal government, and this program remains in existence, providing support to finance and administer a complete series of childhood vaccines. The Expanded Program on Immunization begun in 1974 by the WHO provides similar support worldwide for childhood vaccination.

While only smallpox has been eradicated, the impact of many diseases is a shadow of prior centuries. Immunization programs have virtually eliminated tetanus, diphtheria, measles, mumps, rubella, and *Haemophilus influenzae* type b meningitis from the United States. Experts at WHO estimate that the use of vaccines prevented more than two million childhood deaths in 2003.

These successes derive from the practices of giving vaccines to many children early in life. In many countries, school immunization laws facilitate active immunization of children against a core group of diseases prior to school entry. While the specific vaccinations vary from country to country, this core group recommended by WHO includes measles, polio, tetanus, pertussis, hepatitis B, and tuberculosis. Additionally, children receive vaccination against *Haemophilus influenzae* type b meningitis, rubella, and yellow fever in many countries.

■ Impacts and Issues

Success in defeating infectious diseases depends on obtaining and sustaining high rates of immunization in children. No vaccine is 100% effective. Even if every child received vaccinations against all diseases, some children would remain susceptible. A phenomenon called "herd immunity" helps to protect those children who remain susceptible after vaccination. Herd immunity helps to halt the spread of disease by surrounding those susceptible children with many children who are immune. Immune children shield the susceptible children. Diseases do not spread effectively if most children are protected and only a few are not.

Immunization of children is extremely cost effective. Children are easy to find and gather in groups. Actual contact time with the medical provider is minimal. Immunization requires no change in lifestyle. The current

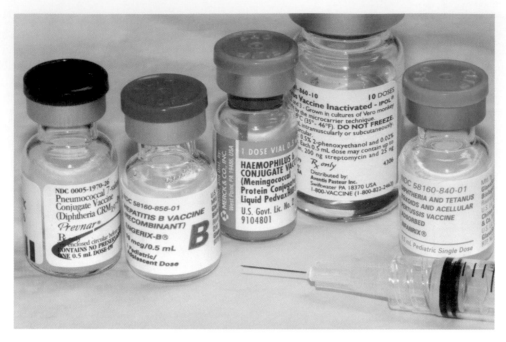

The immunizations typically given to a two-month-old child in the United States include those for diphtheria, hepatitis B, meningitis, and tetanus.   *David Davis/Photo Researchers, Inc.*

widely used vaccines produce few side effects or reactions. In the United States, every dollar invested saves between $2 and $27 in medical costs to treat infectious diseases.

Immunization programs do save lives, yet major efforts remain. An estimated 1.4 million children died worldwide in 2002 from vaccine-preventable diseases. Measles accounted for a third of the deaths and *Haemophilus influenzae* another third, while pertussis and neonatal tetanus killed most of the remainder. Many more children die from diseases potentially preventable by vaccines. For example, rotavirus causes the most common type of diarrheal disease worldwide. A new vaccine has recently become available to prevent rotavirus diarrhea that, if used worldwide, would prevent about 500,000 childhood deaths in developing nations annually. Use of a vaccine to prevent childhood pneumonia would save the lives of about two million children annually. Researchers work diligently to produce vaccines for the diseases such as malaria and HIV that are ravaging both adults and children. New forms of old diseases continue to emerge, and continued surveillance and research is a high priority.

Some problems have developed while trying to continue the remarkable success of immunization programs obtained in the twentieth century. Many citizens of developed countries consider themselves safe because so few get sick from epidemic diseases such as polio or diphtheria, and vaccination rates have been dropping in developed countries as a result. Until a disease disappears from the world, no country can consider itself safe. No disease is more than an airplane trip away from anyone. If the percentage of immune individuals declines, the risk of epidemic disease skyrockets.

Compared to a century ago, the practice of immunization has reduced the burden of infectious disease worldwide. Children have benefited the most, with millions more children surviving to adulthood. The challenges for the twenty-first century include maintaining the progress, expanding the scope, and moving toward eventual eradication of infectious diseases. Complacency only benefits the disease-causing organisms in this war.

■ Primary Source Connection

In the following article in *Atlantic Monthly* magazine, Arthur Allen relates the story of a community in Colorado that has experienced outbreaks of pertussis (whooping cough) and other preventable diseases after parents chose not to vaccinate their children according to state recommendations.

As most of a population becomes vaccinated, a herd-immunity effect provides some protection to those who are unvaccinated. As Allen relates, this herd immunity is not enough to prevent outbreaks of infectious disease. Arthur Allen, a Washington-based journalist, is also the author of *Vaccine: The Controversial Story of Medicine's Greatest Lifesaver.*

This schedule indicates the recommended ages for routine administration of currently licensed childhood vaccines, as of December 1, 2006, for children aged 0-6 years.

Vaccines ▼ Age ▶	Birth	1 month	2 months	4 months	6 months	12 months	15 months	18 months	19-23 months	2-3 years	4-6 years
Hepatitis B	HepB	HepB		see footnote 1		HepB				HepB Series	
Rotavirus			Rota	Rota	Rota						
Diptheria, Tetanus, Pertussis			DTaP	DTaP	DTaP		DTaP				DTaP
Haemophilus influenzae type b			Hib	Hib	Hib[4]	Hib		Hib			
Pneumococcal			PCV	PCV	PCV	PCV				PCV PPV	
Inactivated Poliovirus			IPV	IPV		IPV					IPV
Influenza						Influenza (Yearly)					
Measles, Mumps, Rubella						MMR					MMR
Varicella						Varicella					Varicella
Hepatitis A						HepA 2 (doses)				HepA Series	
Meningococcal										MPSV4	

Range of recommended ages

Catch-up immunization

Certain high-risk groups

1. Hepatitis B vaccine (HepB). (Minimum age: birth)
At birth:
• Administer monovalent HepB to all newborns before hospital discharge.
• If mother is hepatitis surface antigen (HBsAg)-positive, administer HepB and 0.5 mL of hepatitis B immune globulin (HBIG) within 12 hours of birth.
• If mother's HBsAg status is unknown, administer HepB within 12 hours of birth. Determine the HBsAg status as soon as possible and if HBsAg-positive, administer HBIG (no later than age 1 week).
• If mother is HBsAg-negative, the birth dose can only be delayed with physician's order and mother's negative HBsAg laboratory report documented in the infant's medical record.

After the birth dose:
• The HepB series should be completed with either monovalent HepB or a combination vaccine containing HepB. The second dose should be administered at age 1–2 months. The final dose should be administered at age ≥24 weeks. Infants born to HBsAg-positive mothers should be tested for HBsAg and antibody to HBsAg after completion of ≥3 doses of a licensed HepB series, at age 9–18 months (generally at the next well-child visit).
4-month dose:
• It is permissible to administer 4 doses of HepB when combination vaccines are administered after the birth dose. If monovalent HepB is used for doses after the birth dose, a dose at age 4 months is not needed.

Centers for Disease Control and Prevention (CDC) chart listing the recommended immunization schedule for children from birth to age six in the United States in 2007. *Centers for Disease Control and Prevention. Recommended immunization schedules for persons aged 0-18 years—United States, 2007. MMWR 2006;55(51&52):Q1-Q4./CDC.*

Bucking the Herd: Parents Who Refuse Vaccinations for Their Children May Be Putting Entire Communities at Risk

Boulder, Colorado, a university town of 96,000, lies in a sequestered valley on the western edge of the Great Plains. Both geographically and culturally it is a place apart. Ralph Nader won more than 10 percent of Boulder's vote in the most recent presidential election. Natural-food groceries outnumber Safeways; chiropractors' offices line the main drag; and the city council recently declared that dog owners would henceforth be referred to as "dog guardians." A popular bumper sticker reads, WELCOME TO BOULDER, 20 SQUARE MILES SURROUNDED BY REALITY. Boulder is, in short, an experiment-oriented city.

A particularly interesting experiment, from a public-health perspective, has taken shape at the Shining Moun-

tain Waldorf School, a campus of one-story wooden buildings set amid cottonwood and willow trees hard by the foothills of the Rockies. By their parents' choosing, nearly half of the 292 students at Shining Mountain have received only a few, and in some cases none, of the twenty-one childhood vaccinations mandated by Colorado state law in accordance with federal guidelines. The shunning of one of the vaccines, against diphtheria, tetanus, and pertussis, has resulted in a revival of whooping cough, the illness that occurs when colonies of the bacteria *Bordetella pertussis* attach to the lining of the upper respiratory passages, releasing toxins that cause inflammation and a spasmodic cough. The high-pitched whoop is a symptom heard mainly in younger children; it's the sound of a desperate attempt to breathe.

Shining Mountain exemplifies a growing movement in American life: the challenge to childhood vaccination. According to a survey published in the November 2000

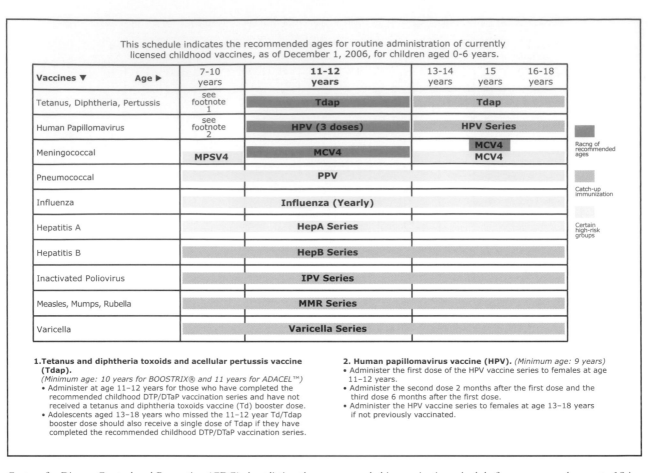

This schedule indicates the recommended ages for routine administration of currently licensed childhood vaccines, as of December 1, 2006, for children aged 0-6 years.

Vaccines ▼ Age ▶	7-10 years	11-12 years	13-14 years	15 years	16-18 years
Tetanus, Diphtheria, Pertussis	see footnote 1	Tdap	Tdap		
Human Papillomavirus	see footnote 2	HPV (3 doses)	HPV Series		
Meningococcal	MPSV4	MCV4		MCV4 / MCV4	
Pneumococcal		PPV			
Influenza		Influenza (Yearly)			
Hepatitis A		HepA Series			
Hepatitis B		HepB Series			
Inactivated Poliovirus		IPV Series			
Measles, Mumps, Rubella		MMR Series			
Varicella		Varicella Series			

Racng of recommended ages

Catch-up immunization

Certain high-risk groups

1. Tetanus and diphtheria toxoids and acellular pertussis vaccine (Tdap).
(Minimum age: 10 years for BOOSTRIX® and 11 years for ADACEL™)
• Administer at age 11–12 years for those who have completed the recommended childhood DTP/DTaP vaccination series and have not received a tetanus and diphtheria toxoids vaccine (Td) booster dose.
• Adolescents aged 13–18 years who missed the 11–12 year Td/Tdap booster dose should also receive a single dose of Tdap if they have completed the recommended childhood DTP/DTaP vaccination series.

2. Human papillomavirus vaccine (HPV). *(Minimum age: 9 years)*
• Administer the first dose of the HPV vaccine series to females at age 11–12 years.
• Administer the second dose 2 months after the first dose and the third dose 6 months after the first dose.
• Administer the HPV vaccine series to females at age 13–18 years if not previously vaccinated.

Centers for Disease Control and Prevention (CDC) chart listing the recommended immunization schedule for persons aged seven to 18 in the United States in 2007. *Centers for Disease Control and Prevention. Recommended immunization schedules for persons aged 0-18 years—United States, 2007. MMWR 2006;55(51&52):Q1-Q4.*

issue of *Pediatrics*, one fourth of all parents are skeptical of some or all of the standard vaccines. Some states grant exemptions to the law so that parents can refuse vaccinations for their children. In Colorado, parents who don't want their children vaccinated have only to sign a card stating as much. In Oregon, the rate of religious exemptions—which are granted to all parents who choose not to have their children immunized for philosophical reasons—tripled, from 0.9 percent in the 1996-1997 school year to 2.7 percent in 2001.

Those skeptical of vaccines have various reasons. Some argue that vaccines are responsible for otherwise unexplained increases in conditions such as autism, asthma, and multiple sclerosis. Others, including the conservative activist Phyllis Schlafly, see government attempts to track and enforce immunization as an intrusion on privacy. Still others—parents whose recollections of their own bouts of chickenpox or measles are bathed in nostalgia—argue that the elimination of traditional childhood illnesses is an attack on childhood itself. The

parents at Shining Mountain are influenced by the philosophy of Rudolf Steiner, a turn-of-the-century Austrian philosopher who founded the Waldorf movement. Steiner (who was not a medical doctor) argued that children's spirits benefited from being tempered in the fires of a good inflammation.

The critics have concluded that the dangers of vaccination outweigh the risks of vaccine-preventable disease. Like all medical interventions, vaccination entails some risk, although the extent and gravity of potential side effects are matters of debate. For example, febrile seizures occur in roughly one in 10,000 children—perhaps 1,000 a year in the United States—who receive the current whooping-cough vaccine. Such seizures rarely, if ever, lead to permanent brain damage, however, and in any case febrile seizures are triggered just as easily by a run-of-the-mill infection as by a vaccine. Suspicions that mercury preservatives used in vaccines inflicted neurological damage on children are worrisome but unproved. (Mercury has largely been phased out of vaccines over the past three years.)

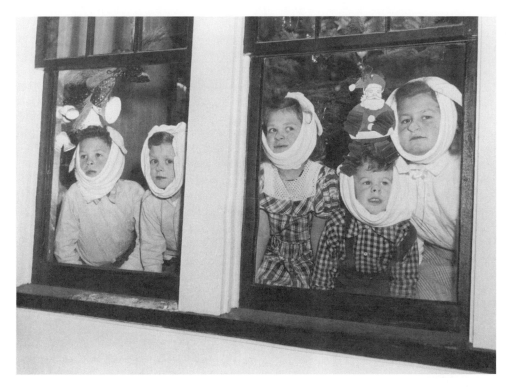

Children with mumps watch from the windows of their home as other youngsters play outside in the snow in New York, 1948. With routine vaccinations, measles, mumps, and other diseases formerly associated with childhood dramatically decreased in the twentieth century. © *Bettmann/Corbis.*

To some extent vaccination is a victim of its own success. Owing to vaccination campaigns, smallpox no longer exists in humans, and polio has been driven from the Western Hemisphere. Measles, diphtheria, and invasive *Hemophilus* bacterial disease (such as meningitis) are rare in the United States, and even whooping cough is unusual enough that few parents consider it a threat. All these diseases, with the exception of smallpox, still infest various corners of the world, but in most of the United States even those who have not been vaccinated against them, or in whom the vaccine is not effective, are protected, because most of the people we meet have been vaccinated. Epidemiologists call this phenomenon "herd immunity": the more vaccinated sheep there are, the safer an unvaccinated one is. When vaccination rates drop, disease returns.

Precisely at what point herd immunity fails is difficult to calculate, but there is ample evidence that it does. Since the collapse of the Soviet public-health system diphtheria has returned to Russia with a vengeance, killing thousands. Sweden suspended vaccination against whooping cough from 1979 to 1996 while testing a new vaccine. In a study of the moratorium period that was published in 1993, Swedish physicians found that 60 percent of the country's children got whooping cough before they were ten. However, close medical monitor-

ing kept the death rate from whooping cough at about one per year during that period.

Boulder, which has the lowest schoolwide vaccination rate in Colorado, has one of the highest per capita rates of whooping cough in the United States. The problem started in 1993, when fifty-two people in Boulder County contracted the disease. Since then the county has seen an average of eighty-one cases a year. Although unvaccinated children are six times as likely as vaccinated children to get whooping cough during an outbreak, about half the cases in Colorado have involved vaccinated children; the whooping-cough vaccine sometimes fails to produce effective immunity, and even successful pertussis immunity generally wanes by age ten. "At first we called it an outbreak; then we started calling it a sustained outbreak; now we just say it's endemic," Ann Marie Bailey, the county nurse epidemiologist when I visited Boulder last year, told me.

To many in Boulder, endemic pertussis is no cause for alarm. Shining Mountain's director, Robert Schiappacasse, says that his daughter, who had been immunized, got whooping cough but suffered no lasting effects. He became a little concerned, he told me, when the baby of one of the school's secretaries "coughed himself into a hernia" after visiting the school during an outbreak. Still, "parents here," Schiappacasse said, apparently including himself in the category, "are more

WORDS TO KNOW

ANTIBODY: Antibodies, or Y-shaped immunoglobulins, are proteins found in the blood that help to fight against foreign substances called antigens. Antigens, which are usually proteins or polysaccharides, stimulate the immune system to produce antibodies. The antibodies inactivate the antigen and help to remove it from the body. While antigens can be the source of infections from pathogenic bacteria and viruses, organic molecules detrimental to the body from internal or environmental sources also act as antigens. Genetic engineering and the use of various mutational mechanisms allow the construction of a vast array of antibodies (each with a unique genetic sequence).

ERADICATE: To get rid of; the permanent reduction to zero of global incidence of a particular infection.

HERD IMMUNITY: Herd immunity is a resistance to disease that occurs in a population when a proportion of them have been immunized against it. The theory is that it is less likely that an infectious disease will spread in a group where some individuals are less likely to contract it.

likely to be worried about fumes from a new carpet than they are about any infectious disease."

I also spoke with Johnnie Egars, a Shining Mountain parent whose three children, all unvaccinated, got whooping cough in 1994. Her youngest child was particularly sick. Egars's description of the experience was harrowing. "It was a loud cough that went down to her toes, and the whoop was a sharp intake of breath," she recalled. "She coughed and coughed until she threw up; then she slept an hour or two. Then she'd wake up and start over again." The daughter, who was two at the time, was undergoing treatment for cancer; she was hospitalized for three days in the infectious-diseases ward of Children's Hospital in Denver. Nonetheless, Egars is comfortable with her decision not to vaccinate her children. A niece was hospitalized with febrile seizures following a pertussis vaccination, and in her view, "immunization just weakens the immune system." She adds, "We have a history of cancer in my family, so we try to do everything we can to strengthen the immune system."

From its reservoir in the undervaccinated population of Boulder, pertussis has branched out: neighboring Jefferson and Denver Counties had more cases in 2000 than Boulder did. Some of the people who live near Boulder are angry. "There is a constant presence of whooping cough here, and it's because of Boulder Valley," says Kathy Keffeler, the chief school nurse for Longmont, a growing city just north of Boulder.

Pertussis is on the rise not just in Colorado but across the country: there were 7,600 cases last year, as compared with 4,600 in 1994. It can be fatal, especially in countries—like ours—with spotty health-care coverage. In 2000, it killed seventeen people in the United States, including two Colorado babies, both of whom were taken to the hospital too late. "It was very sad," Tina Albertson, a pediatric resident who cared for one of the infants, told me. "She was a six-week-old girl with a sister and a brother, four and six. The family had chosen not to immunize, and the week she was born, her siblings both had whooping cough. When they're real little, the babies don't whoop—they just stop breathing. This little girl was septic by the time they got her here."

Like most in Boulder, Ann Marie Bailey, the nurse epidemiologist, is tolerant of the alternative health-care scene; she cedes nonvaccinating parents the right to decide what's best for their children. But she gently points out that they're fooling themselves if they think no one else is affected by their decisions. "We've been able to show very definitely that whooping cough spreads from these pockets in small communities. If they lived in a vacuum at Shining Mountain—if they never went out to go swimming or to church or the YMCA or the Boy Scouts—it would be a different ball game," she told me.

Jia Gottlieb, a family practitioner who offers acupuncture and breathing exercises along with traditional medicine, said, "When I get parents who don't vaccinate, I tell them, 'When your boy gets a vaccination he takes on a risk for the public good, just like the firemen [at the World Trade Center] who went back into the buildings.'" But Gottlieb's words usually fall on deaf ears. "These are probably people who donate a lot of money to good causes," he said, "but their view is 'I'm going to let everyone else's child take a risk but not my own.' That's not avant-garde. That's not enlightened. It's pretty primitive. And ironically, in a town like Boulder the selfish strategy is probably not in the best interests of your child either."

Arthur Allen

ALLEN, ARTHUR. "BUCKING THE HERD: PARENTS WHO REFUSE VACCINATIONS FOR THEIR CHILDREN MAY BE PUTTING ENTIRE COMMUNITIES AT RISK." *ATLANTIC MONTHLY* 290, 2 (SEPTEMBER 2002).

SEE ALSO *Developing Nations and Drug Delivery; Immune Response to Infection; Polio Eradication Campaign.*

BIBLIOGRAPHY

Books

Oshinsky, David. *Polio: An American Story.* New York: Oxford University Press, 2006.

Periodicals

Cohen, Stuart A. "On the Precipice: Private-Sector Vaccine Delivery." *Pediatric News* 40 (April 1, 2006).

Web Sites

Centers for Disease Control and Prevention. "National Immunization Program." <http://www.cdc.gov/nip> (accessed June 1, 2007).

Lloyd Scott Clements

Chlamydia Infection

■ Introduction

Chlamydia trachomatis is the most common cause of sexually transmitted disease (STD) around the world. Any sexually active individual is at risk of chlamydia, as this infection is often known. Because the majority of cases produce no symptoms, people often do not realize they are infected and go on to infect others. Chlamydia can have serious consequences for a woman's reproductive health and often leads to infertility. Certain strains of *C. trachomatis* cause an eye disease called trachoma, which is responsible for about six million cases of infectious blindness in the developing world. In addition, *C. psittaci* is a *Chlamydia* species carried by birds that occasionally infects humans, resulting in an unusual form of pneumonia. The other important *Chlamydia* species is *C. pneumoniae*, which infects approximately one half of the world's population and sometimes causes upper and lower respiratory tract infections. All of these infections can be treated successfully with antibiotics, but many people go undiagnosed or do not have access to treatment.

■ Disease History, Characteristics, and Transmission

The three main *Chlamydia* species are among the world's most prevalent microbial pathogens (disease-causing organisms) and are a significant cause of ill health. When *C. trachomatis* infects the genital tract it often produces no symptoms at all, but women may report a burning sensation on urination and a vaginal discharge. Men may experience a discharge from the penis, as well as itching and a burning sensation. Chlamydia infection, if left untreated, can cause extensive damage to the female reproductive system, leading to pelvic inflammatory disease and infertility. It can also lead to ectopic pregnancy, a potentially fatal condition where a fertilized egg begins to develop within one of the fallopian tubes instead of in the womb. Women with chlamydia are also up to five times more likely to become infected with HIV if exposed to it.

Trachoma is a chronic inflammation of the conjunctiva, which are the membranes covering the inside surfaces of the eyelids, the white of the eye, and the cornea. The infection leads to blindness through scarring of these tissues. *C. psittaci* causes a pneumonia of gradual

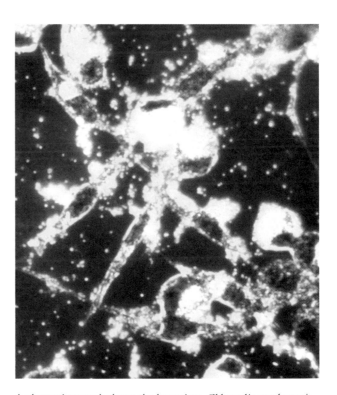

A photomicrograph shows the bacterium *Chlamydia trachomatis*. The bacterium causes a variety of ocular and urogenital diseases, including trachoma, one of the most common infectious causes of blindness worldwide. Chlamydia is the most frequently reported bacterial sexually transmitted disease in the United States. © *Mediscan/Corbis.*

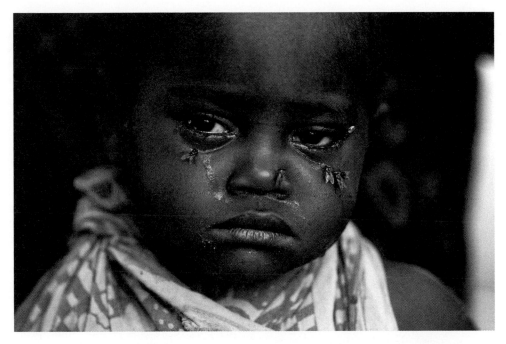

In 2006 the World Health Organization estimated that some 80 million people worldwide have trachoma, which leads to blindness. It is most common in poor, remote, and dry regions of the world, in places such as Africa, Asia, and the Middle East, among others. Children infected with the disease spread the ailment as they play. Flies are also carriers from one child to another. *Joe McNally/Getty Images.*

onset over one to two weeks, with severe headache and a cough that may result in spitting up blood. *C. pneumoniae* can cause a range of infections including sinusitis, pharyngitis (throat infection), bronchitis, and pneumonia. It is responsible for up to 12% of cases of community-acquired pneumonia.

C. trachomatis is transmitted from person to person through genital, oral, and anal sexual intercourse, and can affect anyone who is sexually active. Young women are especially at risk, because the infection is more likely to take hold where the cervix is not fully matured. *C. trachomatis* can also be transmitted from mother-to-child during childbirth. Newborns exposed to *C. trachomatis* from their mother's cervix may develop conjunctivitis or pneumonia. The strains of *C. trachomatis* that cause trachoma are transmitted from hand-to-hand and also by handling fomites, objects that have been used by an infected person. Common fomites include sheets, crockery, clothing, books, and papers. Trachoma is more common in conditions of poor hygiene and overcrowding; it is often found in arid countries where access to water is limited. Reinfection between family members is common. Finally, *C. pneumoniae* is spread from hand-to-hand and by coughs and sneezes.

■ Scope and Distribution

Chlamydia is the most frequently reported bacterial sexually transmitted disease in the United States, according to the Centers for Disease Control and Prevention (CDC), with nearly one million cases reported in 2004. The true number is probably much greater than this—maybe three to five million cases per year—because so many people are unaware that they are infected. World Health Organization (WHO) data gathered from screening programs show that chlamydia is a significant public health problem the world over. In Australia, for

WORDS TO KNOW

FOMITE: A fomite is an object or a surface to which an infectious microorganism such as bacteria or viruses can adhere and be transmitted. Transmission is often by touch.

SEXUALLY TRANSMITTED DISEASE (STD): Sexually transmitted diseases (STDs) vary in their susceptibility to treatment, their signs and symptoms, and the consequences if they are left untreated. Some are caused by bacteria. These usually can be treated and cured. Others are caused by viruses and can typically be treated but not cured. More than 15 million new cases of STD are diagnosed annually in the United States.

matis that can cause trachoma. Despite ongoing efforts at control, there are still more than 500 million people at high risk of infection, over 140 million infected, and six million trachoma-blinded individuals in Africa, the Middle East, Central and Southeast Asia, and certain countries in Latin America, according to WHO data.

■ Treatment and Prevention

Treatment of chlamydia infections is straightforward, using antibiotics, such as tetracylines, macrolides, or fluoroquinolones. Resistance of the bacterium to these drugs is uncommon. However, diagnosis of the sexually acquired infection requires laboratory equipment that is not often available in less developed countries. Diagnosis involves a urine test and sometimes a swab of fluids from the cervix or penis. The sexual partners of those infected should also be tested and treated, if necessary, to prevent reinfection. Moreover, persons with chlamydia should abstain from sexual intercourse until treatment is completed. Condoms provide some protection against transmission of the bacterium.

Screening, that is, testing people who do not have symptoms, is an important part of monitoring the prevalence of chlamydia. Many countries have adopted screening programs. The CDC recommends annual screening for all sexually active women aged 25 or younger. Older women with risk factors, such as a new sex partner or multiple sex partners, are often advised to have an annual screening as well, as should all pregnant women.

According to the WHO, a vaccine against *C. trachomatis*, administered prior to adolescence and which would be effective through the childbearing years, would be the best way to halt the toll of the infection globally. There are two such vaccines currently in development.

■ Impacts and Issues

The greatest impact of sexually transmitted *C. trachomatis* is the silent nature of the infection. Three-quarters of those infected are unaware of the fact because they have no symptoms. This means they can infect others and continue to do so until the disease is diagnosed. For women, the damage that untreated chlamydia inflicts on the reproductive system is also silent. Over one-third of women with untreated chlamydia develop pelvic inflammatory disease and can lose fertility, often without even being aware of the reason why. Screening is important so that infection can be dealt with before permanent damage to the uterus, fallopian tubes, and the surrounding tissues develops.

The control of chlamydia and other sexually-transmitted diseases, like HIV, involves education aimed at reducing risky sexual behaviors. Both sexual abstinence

instance, it is the most common sexually transmitted disease, while in Europe, rates among pregnant women range from 2.7% in Italy, to 6.2% in the United Kingdom, 6.7% in Denmark, and 8% in Iceland. In African countries, rates of chlamydia infection among pregnant women range 6–13%. Globally, the WHO estimates there are around 92 million new cases of chlamydia infection each year, about 50 million of which are among women.

In some parts of the developing world, 90% of the population is infected with one of the strains of *C. tracho-*

and having sexual intercourse only with a partner who is not infected are effective ways of avoiding infection with *C. trachomatis*. Having sex with multiple partners increases the risk. International health officials attempt to offer advice and present facts about sexual behaviors and their link to sexually transmitted diseases such as chlamydia in a non-judgmental manner, taking into account cultural differences in differing populations.

The impact of trachoma in less developed countries has important social and economic implications. Loss of vision from trachoma often starts in middle life, although the infection may be present much earlier. It is also two to three times more common among women, probably due to the fact that women generally spend a greater time in close contact with small children, who are the main reservoir of infection. Middle-aged women often make an important contribution to the family income and, therefore, disability in this group has a severe economic impact. That is one of the reasons why the WHO launched a global health alliance in 1997 with the goal of eliminating trachoma as a blinding disease by 2020.

SEE ALSO Chlamydia pneumoniae; *Psittacosis; Sexually Transmitted Diseases; Trachoma.*

BIBLIOGRAPHY

Books

Wilson, Walter, and Merle A. Sande. *Current Diagnosis & Treatment in Infectious Diseases.* New York: McGraw Hill, 2001.

Web Sites

Centers for Disease Control and Prevention (CDC). "Chlamydia—CDC Fact Sheet." April 2006. <http://www.cdc.gov/std/chlamydia/STDFact-Chlamydia.htm> (accessed January 28, 2007).

World Health Organization Department of HIV/AIDS. "Global Prevalence of Selected Curable Sexually Transmitted Infections: Chlamydia." <http://www.who.int/docstore/hiv/GRSTI/003.htm> (accessed January 29, 2007).

World Health Organization Initiative for Vaccine Research (IVR). "Sexually Transmitted Diseases." <http://www.who.int/vaccine_research/diseases/soa_std/en/index.html> (accessed January 28, 2007).

World Health Organization Prevention of Blindness and Visual Impairment. "Trachoma." <http://www.who.int/blindness/causes/priority/en/index2.html> (accessed February 14, 2007).

Susan Aldridge

Chlamydia pneumoniae

■ Introduction

Around half of the world's population is infected with *C. pneumoniae*, although it does not cause any obvious health problems in the majority. *C. pneumoniae* can, however, cause upper and lower respiratory tract infections, ranging from mild to severe and life-threatening. As the name suggests, pneumonia is the most common infection associated with *C. pneumoniae*. It can be difficult to diagnose, and there is, as yet, no standard diagnostic method for identifying its presence. Fortunately, however, it does respond to standard antibiotic treatment. In recent years, research has also suggested that *C. pneumoniae* infection may have a long-term impact on health, possibly playing a role in the development of heart disease.

■ Disease History, Characteristics, and Transmission

C. pneumoniae infection may affect both the upper and the lower respiratory tract. Bronchitis and pneumonia are the most common forms of *C. pneumoniae* infection. Sinusitis, pharyngitis (infection of the throat), and laryngitis (infection of the larynx or voice box) are less likely. Pneumonia may develop gradually with fever, hoarseness, and cough, although sometimes fever may be absent. *C. pneumoniae* may also make asthma symptoms worse. Transmission of *C. pneumoniae* is by hand-to-hand contact or by exposure to the aerosols created by coughing and sneezing.

■ Scope and Distribution

C. pneumoniae infection is common, and school-age children seem to be most susceptible. The Centers for Disease Control and Prevention (CDC) reports that about 50% of adults are affected by the time they are

20 years old. Reinfection throughout life is also common. Older adults are most at risk for complications from *C. pneumoniae* infection, which may account for

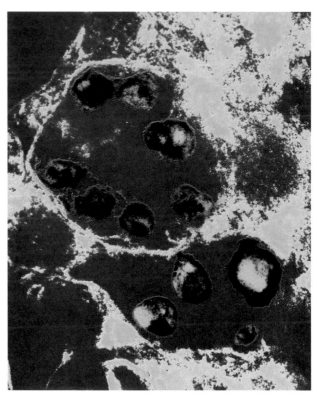

A colored transmission electron micrograph (TEM) of a coronary artery of the heart shows pear-shaped structures (brown) believed to be *Chlamydia pneumoniae* bacteria. The bacteria are in vacuole spaces of a foam or fat-filled cell (yellow). Foam cells are found in atheroma plaque that coats arteries in the disease of atherosclerosis. *C. pneumoniae* may increase plaque formation and scarring of the diseased arteries as the immune system fights the bacteria. By contributing to atherosclerosis, *C. pneumonia* may be a cause of heart attack and stroke. If so, antibiotic drugs may be used to prevent heart attacks. *C.C. Kuo, University of Washingon, Seattle/Photo Researchers, Inc.*

6–12% of all community-acquired pneumonia (CAP)—that is, as the name suggests, pneumonia acquired in the community (including retirement homes) rather than in hospital. Unlike influenza, *C. pneumoniae* is not seasonal in nature and does not "peak"in the winter months. Because *C. pneumoniae* is not easy to diagnose with certainty, there are neither precise figures for its incidence nor any definitive information about trends—that is, whether or not it is becoming more common. *C.pneumoniae* is not currently a notifiable infection.

■ Treatment and Prevention

Treatment of *C. pneumoniae* includes antibiotics in the tetracycline, macrolide, or fluoroquinolone classes. Like all infections spread by hand-to-hand contact or aerosol exposure, the best approach to prevention is frequent and thorough handwashing.

■ Impacts and Issues

C. pneumoniae is a significant contributor to CAP, which is a major public health problem. In the United States, pneumonia is the leading cause of death due to infectious disease and the sixth leading cause of death overall. Nearly half of all deaths from infection are caused by pneumonia and other respiratory infections, and most of these occur in people over the age of 65. There are 2–5 million cases of CAP in the United States each year, leading to around half a million hospitalizations, with associated healthcare costs. If a person with pneumonia is admitted to the hospital, the death rate from the disease goes up from one percent to 14%. For those admitted to intensive care, the mortality rate from pneumonia can be as high as 40%.

Research has suggested that *C. pneumoniae* may have other consequences for health. Atherosclerotic plaques are fatty deposits that are found lining the inner walls of the coronary and carotid arteries, the vessels serving the heart and brain, of those with heart disease. *C. pneumoniae* infection has been located within these plaques, possibly because the bacterium can infect many of the cells that make up the deposits. Research indicates that *C. pneumoniae* may aid in creating the inflammation and immune reaction within blood vessel walls that contribute to heart attacks and strokes. There is no definitive evidence, as yet, that a *C. pneumoniae* infection actually causes heart disease, merely that it is associated with it. There have been several clinical trials aimed at testing whether antibiotics can prevent heart disease by wiping out *C. pneumoniae* infection. So far it appears that antibiotic therapy does not reduce overall mortality from heart disease or the overall rate of heart attack or stroke. The potential role of *C. pneumoniae* in heart disease continues to be explored, while significantly and for

the first time, evidence points to an infectious agent as a risk factor for the number one killer in the U.S.

Other research has suggested that *C. pneumoniae* could also play a role in Alzheimer's disease, asthma, and arthritis.

SEE ALSO Chlamydia *Infection; Pneumonia; Psittacosis.*

BIBLIOGRAPHY

Books

Gates, Robert H. *Infectious Disease Secrets,* 2nd ed. Philadelphia: Hanley and Beltus, 2003.

Wilson, Walter R., and Merle A. Sande. *Current Diagnosis & Treatment in Infectious Diseases.* New York: McGraw Hill, 2001.

CHLAMYDIA PNEUMONIAE AND *CHLAMYDOPHILA PNEUMONIAE*

The bacterium *Chlamydia pneumoniae* is one of the *Chlamydia* genus, a group that also includes *C. trachomatis* and *C. psittaci.* Together, these species are among the most common microbial pathogens (disease-causing organisms) in the world, although *C. pneumoniae* was only identified as such in 1983. A name change to *Chlamydophila pneumoniae* has been proposed for the bacterium to highlight its distinctiveness from other *Chlamydia* species associated with sexually transmitted disease (e.g. chlamydia infection).

Periodicals

Andraws, R., J.S. Berger, and D.L. Brown. "Effects of Antibiotic Therapy on Outcomes of Patients with Coronary Artery Disease: A Meta-analysis of Randomized Controlled Trials." *Journal of the American Medical Association*. no. 293 (2005): 2641–2647.

Web Sites

Centers for Disease Control and Prevention (CDC). "Chlamydia pneumoniae." Oct 6, 2005. <http://www.cdc.gov/ncidod/dbmd/diseaseinfo/chlamydiapneumonia_t.htm> (accessed Jan 30, 2007).

Cholera

■ Introduction

Cholera, sometimes called Asiatic cholera or epidemic cholera, is a disease with roots in antiquity that remains a global threat. Many parts of the world have been hit by major epidemics over the course of human history. Cholera is an acute intestinal infection caused by the bacterium *Vibrio cholerae*. It can cause very rapid dehydration of the body, which can be fatal. Cholera is transmitted by contaminated food and water. It is endemic—that is, present all the time—in countries where there is inadequate access to clean water. Treatment of cholera is simple and relies on restoring the fluids lost by the body. However, even this simple treatment may not be available in very poor countries. The best approach to preventing cholera lies in better sanitation—improving public health through adequate sewage disposal and cleaning up the water supply. In many less developed countries, this is a difficult challenge to meet, since it requires political stability and increased investment in the national infrastructure.

■ Disease History, Characteristics, and Transmission

V. cholerae belongs to the *Vibrio* genus of Gram-negative bacteria. The term Gram-negative refers to the way in which a bacterium absorbs visualizing stains under a microscope for identification purposes. *Vibrio* species exist as straight or curved rods in watery environments. These bacteria use a whiplike projection called a flagellum to propel themselves. (The flagellum is an extension to the bacterial cell body.) *Vibrio* species prefer marine environments and grow best in the presence of salt. They are one of the most common organisms in the surface waters of the world.

There are 139 serotypes of *V. cholerae*—they are basically all the same species, but are distinguished by the number and type of antigen (protein) molecules on their cell surfaces. Most cholera infections are caused by the *V. cholerae* 01 serotype, but others have been found in specific outbreaks or epidemics. For instance, the *El Tor* serotype was first isolated in the quarantine station of the same name in Sinai in 1906, and was linked to an outbreak among pilgrims returning from Mecca. It seems to survive for longer than the 01 serotype, which is killed by 15 minutes of heating. In 1992, the 0139 serotype was first identified in Madras and was responsible for outbreaks in Bangladesh and Thailand during the following year.

Most people infected with *V. cholerae* do not actually become ill, although the bacterium is present in their feces for seven to 14 days, which means they may contaminate food or water. However, *V. cholerae* 01 and a few other serotypes produce a potent toxin that affects the mucosal lining of the small intestine, causing severe diarrhea, with very rapid onset. The incubation period of *V. cholerae* ranges from just a few hours to five days. In most cases, the illness is difficult to distinguish from other diarrheal diseases. But, in severe cholera, the diarrhea is copious—the patient may lose more than a quart (liter) of fluid every hour. Microscopic examination of stool samples reveals the presence of *V. cholerae* as "shooting stars"—as the bacteria use their flagella to dart through the sample. Pathologists may call a sample "rice-water stool" due to its appearance—clear, but flecked with mucus and cells. The diarrhea may be accompanied by vomiting, but pain and fever are minimal and certainly out of proportion to the severity of the diarrhea.

Severe cholera can lead to dehydration, through a combination of diarrhea and vomiting. The patient may enter a state of shock due to massive fluid loss and electrolyte imbalance, suffering seizures, kidney failure, heart rhythm abnormalities, and unconsciousness. Death from dehydration and shock may occur within hours. As a result, cholera is always considered a medical emergency and, indeed, it is one of the most rapidly fatal illnesses ever known. Left untreated, severe cholera has

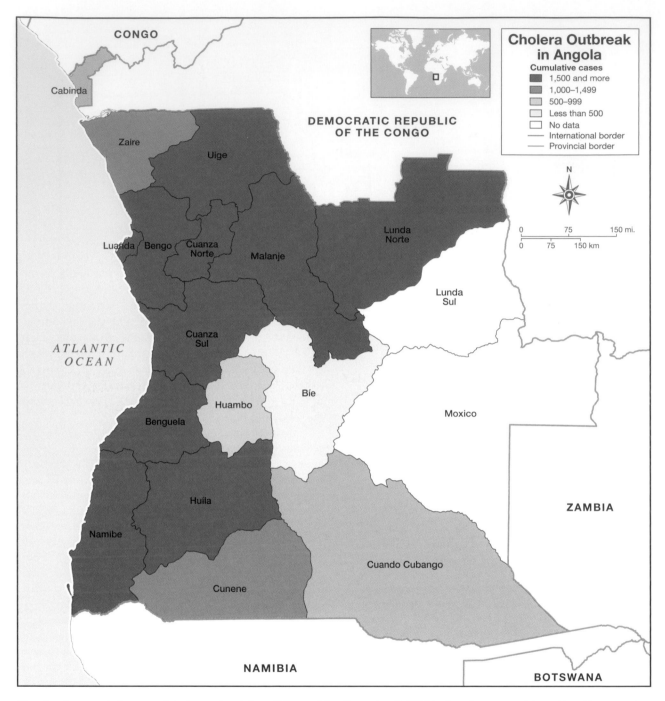

Map showing cumulative cases of cholera outbreak from February 13 to December 7, 2006 in Angola. *© Copyright World Health Organization (WHO). Reproduced by permission.*

a death rate of 30–50%, but when treated promptly, mortality falls to less than 1%.

Transmission of *V. cholerae* is through the fecal-oral route, which, in practical terms, means the consumption of, or contact with, contaminated food and water. *V. cholerae* is hard to avoid in places where sanitation is poor and access to clean water for drinking or washing is limited or non-existent. Imported foodstuffs are only a

rare cause of cholera, and the risk can be kept at bay through high standards of food handling hygiene.

■ Scope and Distribution

Cholera affects many countries around the world. According to the latest data from the World Health

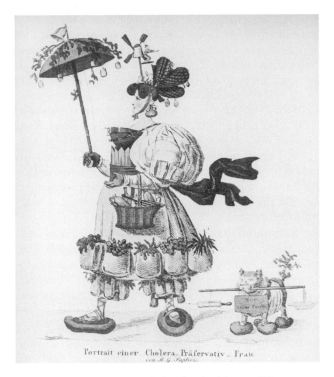

This costume was recommended to frantic citizens of Vienna during a 19-century cholera epidemic. The woman has a cholera band around her body, and her skirt is weighted down by bags of aromatic herbs. Her shoes are of double width and size to prevent infections from the street. The small windmill on her hat was to chase away evil winds. Her cat is dressed in similar attire. © *Bettmann/Corbis.*

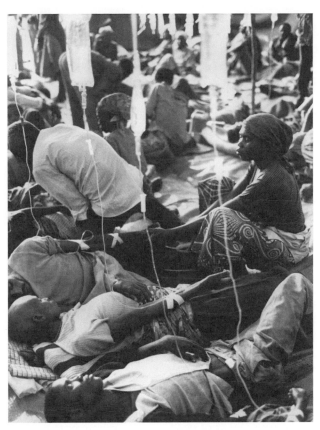

Rwandan refugees with cholera are given saline drips at a Médecins sans Frontières (Doctors without Borders) emergency hospital in a refugee camp in Zaire (now the Democratic Republic of the Congo) in 1994. © *Howard Davies/Corbis.*

Organization (WHO), there were 131,943 cases reported in 2005, including 2,272 deaths, from 52 countries. This represents a 30% increase over 2004, although the number of countries reporting cholera was down from 56. The 2005 increase can be largely accounted for by a series of outbreaks in 14 countries in West Africa, including Senegal, Guinea-Bissau, Ghana, Guinea, and Mauritania. The latter, and Gambia, had previously been free from cholera for over a decade, so this is a downturn for them. Indeed, Africa accounted for about 95% of all cholera cases, although the number of cases from Asia also increased by 18%. The Indian subcontinent accounted for nearly half of all the Asian cases. There were 12 cases in the United States—four of them related to Hurricane Katrina—and ten in Europe. Globally, WHO admits that the toll from cholera is much higher, because surveillance and reporting systems are far from perfect. Some countries only report laboratory-confirmed cases, and there is often confusion over what is and is not cholera.

Cholera is rare in areas where basic hygiene standards can be assured. However, there has been a source of cholera present in the Gulf of Mexico since at least 1973. This has led to sporadic cholera cases in Texas, Louisiana, Georgia, and Florida, linked to eating crabs, shrimp, or oysters that were not properly cooked or stored.

■ Treatment and Prevention

The most important treatment for cholera is fluid and electrolyte (salt) replacement to treat the losses caused by diarrhea and vomiting. Oral rehydration fluid, containing glucose and salt dissolved in water, is the most convenient form of this treatment. Eighty percent of all cases of cholera can be treated in this way, and the treatment needs to be continued until the diarrhea stops. Intravenous administration of rehydration fluid sometimes may be necessary. In countries where oral rehydration fluid is not available, water in which rice has been boiled provides a good alternative. Where antibiotic treatment is needed, tetracycline is the drug of choice and has been shown to shorten the duration of the disease. Ampicillin is a suitable alternative for children and pregnant women.

Clean water and effective sanitation are the most effective preventive measures against cholera. Chlorination of water, boiling of water in households, and the

WORDS TO KNOW

ELECTROLYTES: Compounds that ionize in a solution; electrolytes dissolved in the blood play an important role in maintaining the proper functioning of the body.

FECAL-ORAL ROUTE: The transmission of minute particles of fecal material from one organism (human or animal) to the mouth of another organism.

construction and maintenance of latrines are basic measures that can help achieve these goals. High standards of personal hygiene and food preparation can also reduce the spread of the disease. Accurate and ongoing surveillance of outbreaks and epidemics can help reduce the toll from cholera.

There are now three oral vaccines against cholera, and research has shown them to be safe, effective, and capable of mounting an immune response against the disease. They are suitable for travelers, but WHO is also carrying out trials of mass vaccinations among vulnerable populations. Trials of one vaccine that have been carried out in Bangladesh and Peru show that it gives protection for at least six months among all age groups. A second cholera vaccine is being produced and tested in Vietnam, and there are plans to use this vaccine in India. The results on the third vaccine, not currently being produced, have been less convincing, although it has been shown to be safe.

■ Impacts and Issues

Cholera is one of the great killers of all time. The characteristic symptoms of the disease were described by the Greek physician Hippocrates (c.460–c.357 BC), and the disease is also mentioned by early Indian and Chinese writers. Epidemic cholera was first described in 1563 by Garcia del Huerto, a Portuguese physician working in Goa, India. The natural "home" of cholera appears to be the Ganges plain and delta in northern India and Bangladesh. From here, it spread along trade routes, although for many centuries the disease was generally confined to India. Beginning in the nineteenth century, cholera began to spread around the world as trade expanded. Between 1817 and 1923, there were six pandemics. It was the second pandemic, beginning in 1824, that brought cholera to England (1831), North America (1832), and the Caribbean and Latin America (1833).

The seventh pandemic of cholera, caused by the *El Tor* serotype, began in 1961 and affected the Far East,

although most of Europe was spared. During the 1980s, outbreaks of cholera were common in refugee camps and city slums in famine and war-stricken countries such as Ethiopia and Sudan. The disease, carried by the *El Tor* serotype, returned to the Western Hemisphere in the early 1990s, beginning in Peru—where it had been absent for over 100 years—and spreading outwards through Latin America. In 1992, a large epidemic in Bangladesh was attributed to the newly identified 0139 serotype.

The rapid onset and high mortality of cholera brought great fear to populations during the nineteenth century, as it affected many areas for the first time. Many people thought the cause of cholera—and other diseases—was "miasma" or "bad air." Therefore, the standard treatment was to burn huge bonfires to cleanse the air. However, some blamed cholera on low morals and drunkenness. The belief that "cleanliness is next to Godliness" at least led to the beginnings of an interest in public health in England and America. Social reformers began to campaign for piped water, drains, and proper sewage disposal. Although these changes took many years to bring about, they eventually made a significant contribution towards cutting the death toll from cholera and many other infectious diseases.

It was the English physician John Snow (1813–1858) who suggested that contaminated water, rather than bad air, caused the transmission of cholera. He carried out a serious scientific investigation during the 1848 epidemic in London. His classic work on the subject is titled "On the Mode of Communication of Cholera." In August 1854, there was a fresh outbreak of cholera in and around Broad Street, near Snow's own home. He suggested removing the handle from the Broad Street pump, since this was the probable source of the outbreak. This was done and thereafter there were no more major cholera outbreaks in London.

Snow also accepted the germ theory of disease, put forward by the Louis Pasteur (1822–1895) and Robert Koch (1843–1910). In 1882, Koch discovered the bacillus that causes tuberculosis—also a major killer—and the following year, working in Egypt, he identified *V. cholerae* as the cause of cholera.

Thanks to Snow, Koch, and other researchers, cholera is a well-understood disease in scientific and clinical terms. The causative agents have been discovered, an effective cure is known, and there are vaccines against the disease. Its continuing existence is not due to a lack of scientific understanding or effective treatment and prevention options but to the economic and political factors in many countries that affect their level of development. Today, WHO says that most developing countries face the threat of a cholera outbreak or epidemic. According to WHO and its Global Task Force on Cholera Control, improvements in sanitation and access to clean water represent the only sustainable approach to cholera prevention and control. These factors are more important than drugs to treat the disease or vaccines to protect against it. In areas of the world afflicted by poverty or war (or both), the high standards of public health that are taken for granted in the West are too often hard to achieve and sustain.

The response to cholera is too often reactive—that is, dealing with an outbreak or epidemic once it has occurred. Fighting the threat of cholera requires a multi-disciplinary approach involving a country's agriculture, water, health, and education sectors. Investment in infrastructure, including construction of water and sewage treatment plants, is key to improving public health. Long-term planning is needed so that attention is given not just to responding to cholera when it happens—although that is important—but also to prevention and surveillance. There is a need for far more openness and transparency on surveillance and reporting. Some countries fear that reporting a cholera outbreak will lead to travel and trade restrictions that will hurt their economy.

Because the above goals may be difficult to achieve in many countries, especially in urban slums and in crisis situations, the use of oral cholera vaccines as a complementary management tool is becoming more popular. For example, in 2002–2003 a mass vaccination campaign—the first in an endemic setting—was carried out in Beira, Mozambique, where there are yearly outbreaks. Vaccinated people were shown to have a high level of protection from cholera. Other mass vaccinations have been carried out in emergency settings—in Darfur in Sudan in 2004, for example. These campaigns are challenging, since they are costly and hard to implement, but WHO regards the experience gained as encouraging.

Cholera often is a seasonal disease, occurring each year during the rainy season. For example, in Bangladesh, where it is endemic, cholera comes after the monsoons. This is related to an increase in the growth of algae during the rainy season in the watery environment inhabited by *V. cholerae*. The algae and the bacteria form a symbotic (mutually beneficial) relationship, which allows the bacteria to survive indefinitely in contaminated water. Cholera is also associated with floods and cyclones and often spreads in times of war, especially in refugee camps, because upheaval and overcrowding cause the breakdown of basic facilities, such as water supply. For example, about 45,000 people died of cholera in refugee camps during the war in Rwanda in 1994.

The Global Task Force on Cholera Control has been considering how to improve the use of vaccination as a control tool. It is looking for ways to identify the populations most at risk and protocols for proper use of vaccines in complex emergency settings. Many countries are making significant efforts to control the spread of cholera. For example, there was an outbreak of 1,133 cases in Iran in 2005, including 11 deaths, but this outbreak was rapidly brought under control because the

BOIL IT, COOK IT, PEEL IT, OR FORGET IT

The Division of Bacterial and Mycotic Diseases at the Centers for Disease Control and Prevention (CDC) states that "when simple precautions are observed, contracting the disease (cholera) is unlikely" and offers the following recommendations for travelers to lower their risk of cholera.

All travelers to areas where cholera has occurred should observe the following recommendations:

- Drink only water that you have boiled or treated with chlorine or iodine. Other safe beverages include tea and coffee made with boiled water and carbonated, bottled beverages with no ice.
- Eat only foods that have been thoroughly cooked and are still hot, or fruit that you have peeled yourself.
- Avoid undercooked or raw fish or shellfish, including ceviche.
- Make sure all vegetables are cooked. Avoid salads.
- Avoid foods and beverages from street vendors.
- Do not bring perishable seafood back to the United States.

A simple rule of thumb is "Boil it, cook it, peel it, or forget it."

SOURCE: *Centers for Disease Control and Prevention (CDC)*

government was able to mount an effective emergency response. However, there are also increasing numbers of vulnerable people living in unsanitary conditions. For instance, in Afghanistan there was a recent outbreak of more than 150,000 cases of an acute watery diarrhea that WHO considers to be cholera. In the future, global warming may lead to more frequent droughts, which have also been linked to cholera outbreaks.

■ Primary Source Connection

Sometimes the fear of disease can be as captivating as the reality. Although rare in industrialized nations for more than a century, cholera still raises a powerful and feared specter, especially following disasters that devastate local sanitation resources. The essay below reflects on the fear of widespread cholera following Hurricane Katrina's landfall in along the Mississippi Gulf Coast and the devastation of New Orleans by flooding after levee breaks. The author, Steven Shapin, is Franklin L. Ford Professor of the History of Science at Harvard University. Shapin previously served as Professor of Sociology at the University of California, San Diego, and at Edinburgh University. He is a frequent contributor to the *The New Yorker* magazine.

IN CONTEXT: ACCESS TO IMPROVED SANITATION

The list below reflects selected data from the World Health Organization (WHO) that demonstrates the wide disparity in results reported by WHO as of February 2007 for the relative percentage of the population of a country reported to have access to improved sanitation.

- Afghanistan 8% of the population (year reported: 2002)
- Chad 8% (2002)
- Congo 9% (2002)
- Eritrea 9% (2002)
- Niger 12% (2002)
- India 30% (2002)
- Nigeria 38% (2002)
- Uganda 41% (2002)
- Viet Nam 41% (2002)
- Rwanda 41% (2002)
- China 44% (2002)
- Romania 51% (2002)
- Guatemala 61% (2002)
- Mexico 77% (2002)
- Iraq 80% (2002)
- Iran (Islamic Republic of) 84% (2002)
- Russian Federation 87% (2002)
- Tonga 97% (2002)
- Cuba 98% (2002)
- Ukraine 99% (2002)
- Canada 100% (2002)
- United States of America 100% (2002)
- United Arab Emirates 100% (2002)

SOURCE: *World Health Organization (WHO)*

Sick City

After Katrina, cholera. On August 31, 2005—two days after the hurricane made landfall—the Bush Administration's Health and Human Services Secretary warned, "We are gravely concerned about the potential for cholera, typhoid, and dehydrating diseases that could come as a result of the stagnant water and other conditions." Around the world, newspapers and other media evoked the spectre of cholera in the United States, the world's hygienic superpower. A newspaper in Columbus, Ohio, reported that New Orleans was a cesspool of "enough cholera germs to wipe out Los Angeles." And a paper in Tennessee, where some New Orleans refugees had arrived, whipped up fear among the locals with the headline "KATRINA EVACUEE DIAGNOSED WITH CHOLERA."

There was to be no outbreak of cholera in New Orleans, nor among the residents who fled. Despite raw sewage and decomposing bodies floating in the toxic brew that drowned the city, cholera was never likely to happen: there was little evidence that the specific bacteria that cause cholera were present. But the point had been made: Katrina had reduced a great American city to Third World conditions. Twenty-first-century America had had a cholera scare.

Cholera is a horrific illness. The onset of the disease is typically quick and spectacular; you can be healthy one moment and dead within hours. The disease, left untreated, has a fatality rate that can reach fifty per cent. The first sign that you have it is a sudden and explosive watery diarrhea, classically described as "rice-water stool," resembling the water in which rice has been rinsed and sometimes having a fishy smell. White specks floating in the stool are bits of lining from the small intestine. As a result of water loss—vomiting often accompanies diarrhea, and as much as a litre of water may be lost per hour—your eyes become sunken; your body is racked with agonizing cramps; the skin becomes leathery; lips and face turn blue; blood pressure drops; heartbeat becomes irregular; the amount of oxygen reaching your cells diminishes. Once you enter hypovolemic shock, death can follow within minutes. A mid-nineteenth-century English newspaper report described cholera victims who were "one minute warm, palpitating, human organisms—the next a sort of galvanized corpse, with icy breath, stopped pulse, and blood congealed—blue, shrivelled up, convulsed." Through it all, and until the very last stages, is the added horror of full consciousness. You are aware of what's happening: "the mind within remains untouched and clear,—shining strangely through the glazed eyes … a spirit, looking out in terror from a corpse."

You may know precisely what is going to happen to you because cholera is an epidemic disease, and unless you are fortunate enough to be the first victim you have probably seen many others die of it, possibly members of your own family, since the disease often affects households en bloc. Once cholera begins, it can spread with terrifying speed. Residents of cities in its path used to track cholera's approach in the daily papers, panic growing as nearby cities were struck. Those who have the means to flee do, and the refugees cause panic in the places to which they've fled. Writing from Paris during the 1831–32 epidemic, the poet Heinrich Heine said that it "was as if the end of the world had come." The people fell on the victims "like beasts, like maniacs."

Cholera is now remarkably easy to treat: the key is to quickly provide victims with large amounts of fluids and electrolytes. That simple regime can reduce the fatality rate to less than one per cent. In 2004, there were only five cases of cholera reported to the Centers for Disease Control, four of which were acquired outside the U.S., and none of which proved fatal. Epidemic cholera is now almost exclusively a Third World illness—often appearing in the wake of civil wars and natural disasters—and it is a major killer only in places lacking the infrastructure for effective emergency treatment. Within the last several years, there has been cholera in Angola, Sudan (including Darfur), the Democratic Republic of the Congo, and an arc of West African countries from Senegal to Niger. In the early nineteen-nineties, there were more than a million cases in Latin America, mass deaths from cholera among the refugees from Rwandan genocide in 1994, and regular outbreaks in India and Bangladesh, especially after floods. The World Health Organization calls cholera "one of the key indicators of social development." Its presence is a sure sign that people are not living with civilized amenities.

Of course, this is a state that continues to elude much of the world—including all those underdeveloped countries which are currently experiencing what epidemiologists call the Seventh Pandemic. The problem is no longer an incorrect understanding of the cause: around the world, people have known for more than a century what you have to do to prevent cholera. Rather, cholera persists because of infrastructural inadequacies that arise from such social and political circumstances as the Third World's foreign-debt burdens, inequitable world-trade regimes, local failures of urban planning, corruption, crime, and incompetence. Victorian London illustrates how much could be done with bad science; the continuing existence of cholera in the Third World shows that even good science is impotent without the resources, the institutions, and the will to act.

Steven Shapin

SHAPIN, STEVEN. "SICK CITY." *THE NEW YORKER* (NOV 6, 2006).

See Also *Public Health and Infectious Disease; Sanitation; War and Infectious Disease; Water-borne Disease.*

BIBLIOGRAPHY

Books

Gates, Robert H. *Infectious Disease Secrets.* 2nd ed. Philadelphia: Hanley and Beltus, 2003.

Lock, Stephen, John M. Last, and George Dunea. *The Oxford Illustrated Companion to Medicine.* Oxford: Oxford University Press, 2001.

Porter Roy, ed. *Cambridge Illustrated History of Medicine.* Cambridge: Cambridge University Press, 1996.

Wilson, Walter R., and Merle A. Sande. *Current Diagnosis & Treatment in Infectious Diseases.* New York: McGraw Hill, 2001.

Periodicals

"Cholera 2005." *World Health Organization Weekly Epidemiological Record* 81 (August 4, 2006): 297–308. This article can be found online at <http://www.who.int/wer/2006/wer8131/en/index.html>.

Web Sites

Centers for Disease Control and Prevention. "Cholera." October 6, 2005. <http://www.cdc.gov/ncidod/dbmd/diseaseinfo/cholera_g.htm> (accessed February 13, 2007).

University of California, Los Angeles. School of Public Health. Department of Epidemiology. "John Snow." <http://www.ph.ucla.edu/epi/snow.html> (accessed February 13, 2007).

World Health Organization. "Cholera." <http://www.who.int/topics/cholera/en/> (accessed February 13, 2007).

Susan Aldridge

Climate Change and Infectious Disease

■ Introduction

Climate change is any change in the weather pattern over a given area that lasts longer than a single season. It may be local or worldwide; it may mean higher or lower average temperatures, higher or lower average rainfall, more or less frequent storms, or other shifts. Climate change can take place on a time scale of a few years, like the El Niño climate oscillation, which recurs every three to eight years, or long-term and non-reversing, like the global climate change now being caused by human fuel-burning and unsustainable agricultural practices. Climate change can interact in complex ways with infectious disease. It may encourage or discourage the growth of mosquitoes or other animals that spread disease, change the seasonal availability of hosts for pathogens (disease-causing organisms) that can infect human beings, stimulate the evolution of new pathogens, or change temperatures or precipitation rates to make it more difficult to raise food or obtain clean drinking water. Scientists forecast that the global prevalence of some infectious diseases will increase in years to come.

■ History and Scientific Foundations

The connection between climate and disease has long been suspected. Over two thousand years ago, Greek physician Hippocrates (c. 460-370 BC) taught that weather was related to epidemics of infectious disease. In trying to understand such epidemics, doctors should, he said, have "due regard to the seasons of the year, and the diseases which they produce, and to the states of the wind peculiar to each country and the qualities of its waters." In the seventeenth century, English naturalist Robert Plot (1640-1696) wrote that if humans could make weather observations over widely separated parts of the world at one time, they might "in time thereby learn to be forewarned certainly of divers emergencies

(such as heats, colds, deaths, plagues, and other epidemical distempers)."

Better understanding of the complicated relationships between climate, weather, and human health has been possible since the development of the germ theory of disease in the nineteenth century and of the science of ecology (the study of the relationships among communities of living things) in the twentieth century. Extreme weather events such as drought, flood, and heat waves have obvious, direct effects on human health; for example, the 2003 heat wave in Europe caused approximately 44,000 deaths. Such events can also cause death indirectly by triggering outbreaks of infectious diseases such

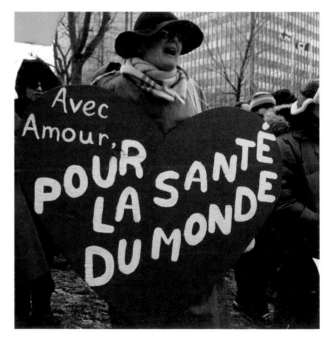

A protester carries a sign reading "With Love, For the Health of the World" during a demonstration against global warming in December 2005 in Montreal, Canada. *AP Images.*

as cholera. Long-term climate shifts can be accompanied by increased numbers of extreme weather events, but can also change the infectious disease picture in less obvious ways. Today, scientists are increasingly concerned with these subtle, long-term relationships between global climate change and infectious disease.

Global climate change is the shifting of climate and weather patterns over the whole world. Such changes are definitely happening—recently scientists have measured faster melting of glaciers and ice caps, rising sea levels, warmer winters, and hotter summers. Specific locations still experience occasional cold, but the cold is usually not as intense or does not last as long. The years 1995 to 2006 contained 11 of the 12 warmest years since 1850, when record-keeping began; from 1960 to 2003, sea levels rose at an average rate of .07 in (1.8 mm) per year. Rainfall has increased in some parts of the world and decreased in others.

Global climate change can occur naturally and has done so many times in the history of Earth. However, the phrase "global climate change" is most often used to refer to changes caused by human beings. Humans change climate by releasing gases into the atmosphere from agriculture and burning fossil fuels. These gases, especially carbon dioxide (CO_2), methane (CH_4), and nitrous oxide (NO), absorb infrared radiation (heat) radiated by the Earth's surface, preventing the Earth from losing heat to space. In effect, the atmosphere acts like a blanket wrapped around the Earth, and increased greenhouse gas concentrations make it a warmer blanket. The atmospheric concentration of carbon dioxide, the most significant greenhouse gas, has increased by about 35% since the beginning of the Industrial Revolution in the mid-1700s. As of 2007, the majority—estimated at 95%—of scientists who study climate agreed not only that global climate change is occurring, but that it is mostly caused by human activity.

Some of climate change's predicted effects include hotter and more frequent heat waves, more frequent and violent weather events such as hurricanes, warmer weather, and increased or decreased precipitation (rain and snow), depending on location. These changes affect the environmental pathways by which organisms contaminate food and drinking water supplies. They also affect human activities and settlement patterns (how people live and where they live). These changes, in turn, can affect the prevalence of diseases borne by water, insects, and rodents. Diseases such as acquired immunodeficiency syndrome (AIDS, also cited as acquired immune deficiency syndrome), which involve organisms that are usually transmitted directly from person to person, are usually less likely to be affected by climate change. Disease organisms that spend a significant part of their life-cycle outside the human body, such as the malaria parasite, are most likely to be affected by climate change.

WORDS TO KNOW

EPIDEMIC: *Epidemic,* from the Greek meaning "prevalent among the people," is most commonly used to describe an outbreak of an illness or disease in which the number of individual cases significantly exceeds the usual or expected number of cases in any given population.

PATHOGEN: A disease-causing agent, such as a bacteria, virus, fungus, etc.

PREVALENCE: The actual number of cases of disease (or injury) that exist in a population.

RE-EMERGING DISEASE: Many diseases once thought to be controlled are reappearing to infect humans again. These are known as re-emerging diseases because they have not been common for a long period of time and are starting to appear again among large population groups.

VECTOR: Any agent, living or otherwise, that carries and transmits parasites and diseases. Also, an organism or chemical used to transport a gene into a new host cell.

■ Research

That global warming might someday be caused by human-released greenhouse gases was first proposed in 1890 by Swedish scientist Svante Arrhenius (1859-1927). The idea was revived by American physicist Stephen Schneider (1945-), among others, in the mid-1970s. By the 1990s, climate scientists were in broad agreement that global warming is real and primarily human-caused. This view has been supported by on-the-ground weather and temperature observations and by satellite measurements of Earth's heat output. Many computer models of Earth's weather have been used to research global climate change; for example, the 2007 report of the International Panel on Climate Change concluded, partly on the basis of 14 different computer climate models, that there is "very high confidence" that human activity is causing Earth to warm.

As the reality of global climate change became clearer in the 1990s, scientists saw that it might have implications for infectious disease. Malaria, which kills between one and three million people per year, was studied intensively. Both the malaria parasite and the mosquitoes that transmit it to humans are affected by temperature; mosquito populations are also affected by rainfall. (Mosquitoes require stagnant water in which to breed.) A computer-based study reported in 1999 that climate change would likely have two primary effects on malaria. First, increasing warmth in temperate zones such as North America, Europe, and central Asia would allow mosquitoes to transmit the disease in previously unaffected areas. Second, decreased rainfall in some areas, such as the Amazon basin in South America, might shorten the infection season in those areas (a positive effect). A similar study published in 2004 confirmed the core findings of the 1999 study. It predicted that by the year 2080, about 80 million additional people would be at risk of malaria because of climate change.

■ Impacts and Issues

Uncertainties

It is difficult to predict accurately the impact of climate change on human health for two basic reasons. First, predicting climate change itself is uncertain, especially over specific parts of the continents: where will more rain fall, where less? How many heat waves, droughts, or floods will there be, and when and where? Such forecasts can only be made using computer models, and these predictions always carry some level of uncertainty when the system being modeled is as complex as the weather of Earth. Predictions of average, global effects (or continent-wide effects) are less uncertain but are also less useful in predicting the effects of climate change on infectious diseases.

Second, infectious disease patterns depend not only on climate but on human population size, population density, poverty, government prevention policies, and medical advances. For example, spending money to provide village water pumps in some African villages would tend to decrease disease from water-borne organisms and might offset some or all the negative effects (that is, those effects relating to water-borne disease) of decreased rainfall. Or, the development of a cheap, effective vaccine for malaria would alter predictions of malaria's future prevalence.

Certain large-scale issues, however, are not in doubt. For example, extreme weather events such as severe hurricanes are predicted by climate models to become more common, and such events can cause outbreaks of infectious disease. In 1998, for example, Hurricane Mitch dropped 6 ft (1.8 m) of rain over much of Central America. Besides the 11,000 people killed directly by flooding, there were 30,000 cases of malaria and 1,000 cases of dengue fever in Honduras in the aftermath of the rains. In 2005, torrential rain in the area of Mumbai (formerly Bombay), India, triggered epidemics of malaria, dengue fever, cholera and other forms of diarrhea, and leptospirosis (a bacterial disease spread by the urine of infected animals, particularly rats).

Some of the infectious-disease effects of climate change are likely to involve drinking water. As of 2007, lack of clean drinking water (water free of significant quantities of microbes, toxins, and parasites) was already one of the worst health problems in the world. At that time, over one billion people had no access to clean drinking and washing water, while some 2.6 billion lacked adequate sanitation. Water-borne infectious diseases kill approximately 3.2 million people per year; about two million of those deaths are children. Diarrhea, which is generally caused by food- and water-borne pathogens such as cholera and *Escherichia coli*, already kills 2.2 million people per year, the majority under five years old. The World Health Organization (WHO) predicts that the number of cases of diarrhea in third-world countries will have increased by 2–5% by 2020 as a result of climate change.

Some infectious diseases are already apparently increasing in prevalence or range because of climate change, and more quickly than has been predicted. Physician Paul Epstein of Harvard University has said, "things we projected to occur in 2080 are happening in 2006." In 2005, a group of scientists including Epstein reported that because of warming climate, organisms that act as vectors (that is, as carriers of disease to humans), including mice, ticks, and mosquitoes, were already spreading to larger areas around the world.

Malaria, West Nile Virus, Lyme Disease

Forty percent of the world's population is vulnerable to infection by malaria, and malaria is already a worsening problem due to movements of population into malarial areas, destruction of forests, evolution of resistance to pesticides by mosquitoes and to antimalarial drugs by malaria parasites, and the breakdown of public-health facilities in some poor countries. Global warming is also contributing to the increasing prevalence of malaria and is likely to become a more important factor over the next few decades. Warmer temperatures can cause mosquitoes to mature more rapidly, breed over a longer season, bite more often, and speed up the growth of malaria parasites in the insect's digestive system. In Africa and Latin America, malaria is already spreading to higher elevations in mountainous regions as the climate at those altitudes warms. In 2005, the Harvard group projected that the percentage of the area of Zimbabwe that is climatically suitable for malaria would grow from less than one fourth today to about 90% by 2100. As a consequence, the percentage of the Zimbabwean population at risk for malaria would grow from about 45% to nearly 100%. Major climate-driven spread of malarial areas is also expected in other African countries, including Ethiopia and South Africa, and in highland regions of Latin America and Asia. On the other hand, it has been shown by projects such as the Lubombo Spatial Development Initiative in South Africa, Mozambique, and Swaziland that house-to-house insecticide spraying, systematic surveillance to detect malaria outbreaks, and improved medical care can greatly reduce malaria infection and death rates.

As noted above, AIDS is sometimes cited as typical of those diseases unlikely to be affected by climate change. However, in 2007 researchers reported that infection with malaria tends to increase the amount of HIV (human immunodeficiency) virus in a person with AIDS and to make HIV more easily transmitted to a sexual partner. Not only does malaria help AIDS spread, but AIDS helps malaria spread: AIDS weakens the immune system, making it more likely that a person will catch malaria. As malaria (probably) becomes more widespread because of climate change, the AIDS pandemic may thus be amplified along with it.

West Nile virus claims fewer lives than many other infectious diseases but has received intense publicity in North America due to its sudden re-emergence in 1999 and rapid spread since that time. The virus probably evolved about 1,000 years ago and was first identified in 1937. Outbreaks of West Nile have occurred since 1990 in Eastern Europe, Africa, and North America. Infection with the virus is most often asymptomatic (that is, without signs), but in a minority of cases it causes a debilitating or fatal infection of the central nervous system. In 2003 and 2004, West Nile cases in North America were concentrated in Colorado, Texas, Arizona, and California—regions that had undergone spring droughts. The southwestern and central parts of the United States are predicted by climate forecast models to experience more drought in the years to come because of global climate change, which increases the likelihood that West Nile will be a chronic and growing problem in these and similar states.

Lyme disease is a bacterial disease transmitted to humans by the bites of ticks (a type of blood-sucking insect). Lyme disease is found in North America, Europe, China, and Japan. Although rarely fatal, it can be severely debilitating. Ticks require wild populations of deer and mice in order to thrive and to pass Lyme disease to human beings: colder temperatures limit tick survival away from the mammal host (over 90% of the tick's life cycle), so warmer climates will allow larger tick populations and tend to spread Lyme disease to areas formerly protected by cold winters. In the United States, regrowth of forests in formerly agricultural areas has been the primary culprit so far in the increase of tick populations and the spread of Lyme disease, but scientists predict that climate change will play an increasing role in spreading Lyme disease. In the northeast and central United States and southeastern Canada, a 213% increase in tick habitat area by 2080 is predicted.

Mitigation

There is ongoing controversy over how to respond to climate change. Since change is already occurring, adaptation—

changes in human practices that respond to the effects of changing climate, including new infectious disease challenges—is also already occurring. Many countries have agreed, at least in principle, to mitigate (lessen) climate change by stabilizing the amount of greenhouse gases in the atmosphere. This would require burning less fossil fuel or using new technologies to isolate the carbon dioxide released during such burning (e.g., injecting CO_2 from burning coal deep into the ground, where it cannot affect the climate). Other nations, including China, among the largest producers of greenhouse gases, have opposed mandating new industrial practices or energy efficiency in the home or on the road, because many of these changes would be costly. Nevertheless, in 2006, the WHO estimated that each year at least 150,000 deaths are already attributable to climate change.

SEE ALSO *Dengue and Dengue Hemorrhagic Fever; Lyme Disease; Malaria; Re-emerging Infectious Diseases.*

BIBLIOGRAPHY

Books

Climate Change and Human Health: Risks and Responses, edited by A.J. McMichael, et al. Geneva, Switzerland: World Health Organization, 2003.

Committee on Climate, Ecosystems, Infectious Diseases, and Human Health, Board on Atmospheric Sciences and Climate, National Research Council (U.S.A.). *Under the Weather: Climate, Ecosystems, and Infectious Disease.* Washington, DC: National Academy Press, 2001.

Periodicals

Haines, A., et al. "Climate Change and Human Health: Impacts, Vulnerability, and Mitigation." *The Lancet* 367 (2006): 2101-2110.

Martens, Pim, and Susanne C. Moser. "Health Impacts of Climate Change." *Science* 292 (2001): 1065–1066.

McMichael, A.J., Rosale E. Woodruff, and Simon Hales. "Climate Change and Human Health: Present and Future Risks." *The Lancet* 367 (2006): 859-861.

Struck, Doug. "Climate Change Drives Disease to New Territory: Viruses Moving North to Areas Unprepared for Them, Experts Say." *Washington Post* (May 5, 2006).

van Lieshout, M., et al. "Climate Change and Malaria: Analysis of the SRES Climate and Socio-Economic Scenarios." *Global Environmental Change* 14 (2004): 87–99.

Web Sites

Harvard Medical School Center for Health and the Global Environment. "Climate Change Futures: Health, Ecological and Economic Dimensions." 2005

<http://chge.med.harvard.edu> (accessed May 26, 2007).

International Panel on Climate Change (United Nations). "Climate Change 2007: Impacts, Adaptation and Vulnerability." 2007 <http://www.ipcc.ch/SPM13apr07.pdf> (accessed May 26, 2007).

International Panel on Climate Change (United Nations). "Climate Change 2007: The Physical Science Basis." 2007 <http://ipcc-wg1.ucar.edu/wg1/docs/WG1AR4_SPM_PlenaryApproved.pdf> (accessed May 26, 2007).

World Health Organization (United Nations). "Health Adaptation to Climate Change." 2005 <http://www.who.int/globalchange/climate/gefproject/en/index.html> (accessed May 26, 2007).

Larry Gilman

Clostridium difficile Infection

■ Introduction

Clostridium difficile is an anaerobic, spore-forming bacterium that is part of the normal human flora, that is, the normal community of microbes that lives within the human body. It accounts for around three percent of the bacteria in an adult gut, and 66% in the infant gut. *C. difficile* does not usually cause problems in children or healthy adults. However, certain strains of *C. difficile* can produce toxins that are a major cause of both antibiotic-associated diarrhea (AAD) and nosocomial diarrhea, a hospital-acquired infection. Sick people, especially if they are on long-term antibiotic treatment, are vulnerable to *C. difficile* infections, which may cause severe colitis, that is, inflammation of the colon. In the elderly, or those with weakened immunity, *C. difficile* infection may prove fatal. There have been various outbreaks of *C. difficile* infection in hospitals and nursing homes, which have been investigated by health authorities. Often, poor hygiene on the part of healthcare workers—lack of regular handwashing, for instance—has been the underlying cause of the outbreak.

■ Disease History, Characteristics, and Transmission

Prolonged use of antibiotics can alter the balance of the intestinal flora and it is under these circumstances that *C. difficile* infection may take hold, causing AAD. Symptoms include watery diarrhea, fever, loss of appetite, nausea, and abdominal pain and tenderness. Symptoms can start during antibiotic treatment or after it has ended. Nearly all antibiotics can cause AAD, and the condition is also associated with the use of certain anticancer drugs such as fluorouracil and methotrexate. Sometimes AAD leads to a complication called pseudomembranous colitis, where inflamed, patchy deposits form on the inner lining of the colon.

C. difficile bacteria are found in feces, and people can spread infection if they touch items or surfaces that are contaminated and then touch their mouth or eyes.

C. difficile also forms spores that can survive for long periods on surfaces and clothes, so re-infection is common.

■ Scope and Distribution

The elderly are particularly susceptible to *C. difficile* infection, with over 80% of cases being found in those aged over 65. Outbreaks are especially common in nursing

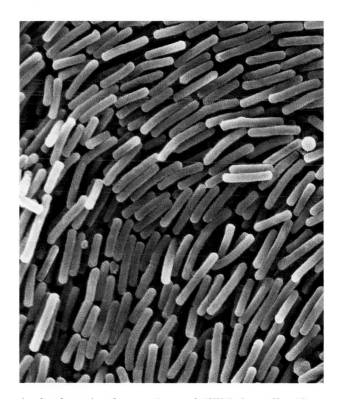

A colored scanning electron micrograph (SEM) shows *Clostridium difficile* bacteria. These rod-shaped bacteria cause antibiotic-associated diarrhea and pseudomembranous colitis, one of the most common hospital-acquired infections. *Biomedical Imaging Unit, Southampton General Hospital/Photo Researchers, Inc.*

WORDS TO KNOW

ANAEROBIC BACTERIA: Bacteria that grow without oxygen, also called anaerobes. Anaerobic bacteria can infect deep wounds, deep tissues, and internal organs where there is little oxygen. These infections are characterized by abscess formation, foul-smelling pus, and tissue destruction.

NORMAL FLORA: The bacteria that normally inhabit some part of the body, such as the mouth or intestines, are normal flora. Normal flora are essential to health.

NOSOCOMIAL: A nosocomial infection is an infection that is acquired in a hospital. More precisely, the Centers for Disease Control in Atlanta, Georgia, defines a nosocomial infection as a localized infection or one that is widely spread throughout the body that results from an adverse reaction to an infectious microorganism or toxin that was not present at the time of admission to the hospital.

TOXIN: A poison that is produced by a living organism.

homes and among hospitalized patients. Long term, or inappropriate, use of antibiotics is another strong risk factor for infection.

Although the incidence of *C. difficile* worldwide is unknown, many health authorities now collect data on outbreaks of *C. difficile* infection. For example, the United Kingdom Health Protection Agency reported an outbreak at a hospital in Nottinghamshire in November 2006 that led to the temporary closure of wards and the deaths of nine elderly people. Another hospital in the same area experienced a simultaneous outbreak, which contributed to the deaths of three patients. Emergency funds were made available by England's Health Secretary to track, study, and combat the outbreak of *C. difficile*.

■ Treatment and Prevention

In AAD, the aim of treatment is to restore the balance of the intestinal flora. This usually involves discontinuing or changing the antibiotic that has triggered the condition. If this is not successful, then further antibiotic treatment is used to get the infection under control. Vancomycin and metronidazole are the two antibiotics most commonly prescribed for *C. difficile*. Sometimes vancomycin is avoided because there is a risk of encouraging the growth of vancomycin-resistant enterococci, a species of gut bacteria that may lead to an infection that is no longer responsive to antibiotic treatment. Diarrhea often leads to dehydration, so it is also important to restore fluids and salts. Non-antibiotic treatment may sometimes be used to restore the intestinal flora. These may include *Lactobacillus* (as found in bioactive yogurts) and the yeast, *Saccharomyces boulardii*.

Anyone infected with *C. difficile* can spread the infection to others, whether or not they have become ill themselves. Transmission can be prevented by washing hands with soap and water, especially after using the bathroom and before eating. Surfaces in bathrooms, kitchens, and other areas should be kept clean with detergent and disinfectant on a regular basis.

■ Impacts and Issues

C. difficile infection highlights the potential dangers of long-term broad-spectrum antibiotic treatment. Although these drugs can play a valuable role in bringing infectious diseases under control, they can also upset the natural balance of the normal intestinal flora (bacteria that do not normally cause disease or that serve a beneficial purpose and regularly inhabit the intestines). This sets the scene for the emergence of *C. difficile*, which may cause the patient a more serious health problem than the one the antibiotic was initially prescribed for. That is why physicians avoid routine prescription of broad-spectrum antibiotics, especially over the long term among the elderly. *C. difficile* can also become a problem in hospitals and nursing homes if hygiene standards fall short.

The CDC reported in 2005 that a new and more virulent (and more resistant to antibiotic therapy) strain of *C. difficile* had emerged in North America. Persons who contracted this strain included those not previously identified at risk for the infection, including non-hospitalized persons, children, persons not taking antibiotics, and one pregnant woman. Termed *C. difficile* 027, the organism was also responsible for three outbreaks and the deaths of 21 people in Quebec hospitals over a six-month period from October 2006 until March 2007. Researchers are working to develop new alternatives to antibiotic treatment for *C. difficile* 027 infection, including a substance that would bind to the toxin produced by the bacteria and neutralize it, along with a potential vaccine.

SEE ALSO *Nosocomial (Healthcare-Associated) Infections; Vancomycin-resistant Enterococci; Resistant Organisms.*

BIBLIOGRAPHY

Books

Wilks D., M. Farrington and D. Rubenstein. *The Infectious Disease Manual.* Malden: Blackwell, 2003.

Wilson, Walter R. and Merle A. Sande. *Current Diagnosis & Treatment in Infectious Diseases.* New York: McGraw Hill, 2001.

Web Sites

Centers for Disease Control and Prevention (CDC). "General Information about *Clostridium Difficile* Infections." Jul 22, 2005 <http://www.cdc.gov/ncidod/dhqp/id_CdiffFAQ_general.html> (accessed Jan 30, 2007).

Health Protection Agency. "*Clostridium Difficile.*" <http://www.hpa.org.uk/infections/topics_az/clostridium_difficile/default.htm> (accessed Jan 30, 2007).

CMV (Cytomegalovirus) Infection

■ Introduction

Cytomegalovirus (si-to-MEG-a-lo-vi-rus), or CMV, is one of the most common viruses infecting human beings. In healthy people, it rarely causes any symptoms. CMV infection is mainly of concern in persons who have weakened immunity, such as organ transplant recipients and those with HIV/AIDS. Some babies born with CMV infection, transmitted in the womb, may go on to suffer from severe health problems.

CMV belongs to the herpes family of viruses, all of which exist as viral particles of diameter around 200 nm, consisting of a protein exterior enclosing a molecule of double-stranded DNA. Other significant herpes viruses include the herpes simplex viruses, varicella-zoster virus (which causes chicken pox), and Epstein-Barr virus. CMV may lie dormant in white blood cells for many years, but the infection can be re-activated at any time. CMV cannot be eliminated, but symptoms of active infection can be treated with antiviral drugs, and there is also research on a preventive vaccine.

■ Disease History, Characteristics, and Transmission

CMV infects cells called fibroblasts, which are found in skin and connective tissue, and white blood cells. In most people, the infection lies dormant. Some people may experience symptoms similar to those of mononucleosis—fever, swollen glands, fatigue, and sore throat. These symptoms occur in many other conditions, however, so it is difficult to determine that CMV is responsible.

For people with weakened immunity, CMV can become a serious problem because the virus is no longer held in check. Those with HIV/AIDS may experience complications such as retinitis, an eye infection that can lead to blindness. CMV may also cause potentially fatal pneumonia among organ transplant recipients because

they take immunosuppressant drugs to protect the new organ. Another group at risk of CMV infection includes newborns, who may become infected in the womb. Congenital (present at birth) CMV infection can lead to many problems, including deafness and mental retardation, some of which may not become apparent until the child gets older.

Transmission of CMV is by contact with infected body fluids such as blood, semen, vaginal fluid, tears, urine, and saliva, although the infection is not spread by casual contact. A woman can transmit CMV to her baby through the placenta, while still in the womb, by exposure

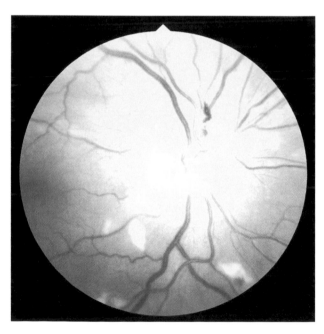

Retinitis, an inflammation of the retina, occurs due to an infection of cytomegalovirus (CMV). The disease usually begins as a white infiltrate within the retina and can progress rapidly to cause destruction of retinal tissue. Retinal damage can lead to detachment of the retina. © Mediscan/Corbis.

to cervical fluids during childbirth, or through breast milk. Infected children shed the virus in urine and other fluids for years and may transmit the infection horizontally to other children and adult caregivers in a nursery group setting.

■ Scope and Distribution

The prevalence of CMV worldwide is between 40% and 100% of all people infected, with those in less developed countries and of lower socioeconomic status being more at risk. In the United States, 50–80% of adults are infected with CMV by the time they are 40 years of age. One percent of newborns shed CMV in their urine, which indicates they have been infected, but 90% of them remain healthy. The rest may develop serious ongoing health problems.

CMV infection is widespread, but is generally contained by the immune system. If this begins to break down, then infection will take hold, which is why HIV/AIDS patients and organ transplant recipients are also at risk of infection, as they are from many other normally harmless microbes, such as *Candida*.

■ Treatment and Prevention

CMV does not respond to the antiviral drug acyclovir, but is sensitive to a closely related drug called ganciclovir, which has been shown to reduce the complications of CMV-induced mortality among immunosuppressed persons (persons with weakened immune systems, either through disease or deliberate medical treatment). Foscarnet is another antiviral drug that is used in the treatment of CMV retinitis in HIV/AIDS. Cidofovir, the other drug for CMV infection, can be used to protect people with HIV/AIDS and organ transplant recipients from episodes of infection.

Normal hygiene and precautions are currently the best way of preventing CMV infection; the drugs are too toxic to give to pregnant women. Vaccines for CMV are being developed and these could play a vital role in reducing infection among newborns.

■ Impacts and Issues

Congenital CMV infection is more common than other well-known congenital conditions such as Down syndrome, fetal alcohol syndrome, and neural tube defects. But only around 20% of those born with CMV will develop complications such as deafness, blindness, liver failure, and seizures. Those whose mothers become infected for the first time during pregnancy are most at risk of having babies with health problems. Scientists assume this is because there are no CMV antibodies present in the maternal blood supply to protect the fetus.

WORDS TO KNOW

ANTIBODY: Antibodies, or Y-shaped immunoglobulins, are proteins found in the blood that help to fight against foreign substances called antigens. Antigens, which are usually proteins or polysaccharides, stimulate the immune system to produce antibodies. The antibodies inactivate the antigen and help to remove it from the body. While antigens can be the source of infections from pathogenic bacteria and viruses, organic molecules detrimental to the body from internal or environmental sources also act as antigens. Genetic engineering and the use of various mutational mechanisms allow the construction of a vast array of antibodies (each with a unique genetic sequence).

CONGENITAL: Existing at the time of birth.

FIBROBLAST: A cell type that gives rise to connective tissue.

HORIZONTAL TRANSMISSION: Horizontal transmission refers to the transmission of a disease-causing microorganism from one person to another, unrelated person by direct or indirect contact.

IMMUNOSUPPRESSED: A reduction of the ability of the immune system to recognize and respond to the presence of foreign material.

SHED: To shed is to cast off or release. In medicine, the release of eggs or live organisms from an individual infected with parasites is often referred to as shedding.

In the United States, 1–4% of women develop such primary infections during pregnancy and one-third of these pass on the infection in the womb. Pregnant women and babies could benefit most from a vaccine against CMV.

SEE ALSO *Chickenpox (Varicella); Herpes Simplex 1 Virus; Herpes Simplex 2 Virus; Shingles (Herpes Zoster) Infection.*

BIBLIOGRAPHY
Books
Wilson, Walter R., and Merle A. Sande. *Current Diagnosis & Treatment in Infectious Diseases.* New York: McGraw Hill, 2001.

IN CONTEXT: EFFECTIVE RULES AND REGULATIONS

With regard to CMV infection, the Division of Viral and Rickettsial Diseases at Centers for Disease Control and Prevention (CDC), states the following:

- "CMV infection is very common in day care settings, but CMV usually does not harm the children who become infected. Adults who have not had CMV and who work with children in day care, especially children 1 to 2 years of age, are at high risk for CMV infection. Such adults face little risk of getting seriously sick from CMV infection. However, pregnant women who become infected with CMV are at high risk of passing the infection to their fetuses."

- "Pregnant mothers who have young children in day care or who work in day care centers can help prevent getting infected with CMV by practicing good hygiene (such as handwashing). They should also avoid direct contact with saliva through behaviors such as kissing young children on the lips."

- "Since CMV is spread through contact with infected body fluids, including urine and saliva, child care providers (meaning day care workers, special education teachers, therapists, and mothers) should be educated about the risks of CMV infection and the precautions they can take. Day care workers appear to be at a greater risk of becoming infected with CMV than

hospital and other health care providers, and this may be due in part to the increased emphasis on personal hygiene (such as handwashing) and the lower amount of personal contact in the health care setting."

- "Non-pregnant women of childbearing age who have never been infected with CMV and who are working with infants and children should not be routinely moved to other work situations to avoid CMV infection."

- "Pregnant women working with infants and children should be informed of the risk of getting CMV infection, the possible effects on the unborn child, and appropriate prevention strategies."

- "Routine laboratory testing for CMV antibody (immune protein) in female workers is not currently recommended. However, female workers who are pregnant or planning a pregnancy should be informed that a CMV antibody test can help them assess their risk. Whenever possible, CMV seronegative (without CMV antiobodies) pregnant women should consider working in a setting with less exposure to young children."

SOURCE: *Centers for Disease Control and Prevention, National Center for Infectious Diseases, Division of Viral and Rickettsial Diseases*

Tan, James S. *Expert Guide to Infectious Diseases.* Philadelphia: American College of Physicians, 2002.

Web Sites

Centers for Disease Control and Prevention (CDC). "Cytomegalovirus (CMV)." February 6, 2006 <http://www.cdc.gov/cmv/> (accessed May 1, 2007).

Coccidioidomycosis

■ Introduction

Coccidioidomycosis, also called valley fever, is a fungal disease caused by the spores (tiny seeds) of the fungus *Coccidioides immitis* (CI). The fungus is classified as dimorphic, meaning that it exists both as a mold and yeast. It is found in infected soil of the Sonoran climates of the southwestern United States, northwestern Mexico, and other isolated areas within the Western Hemisphere.

The disease causes several respiratory problems in humans. However, humans cannot acquire the disease from other people, only through inhalation of these airborne particles and contact with infected soil. Scientists assume that a person develops immunity to the disease once recovered from it.

Sixty percent of the time the disease causes no symptoms to the infected person. It is only recognized later by medical professionals when a coccidioidin skin test comes back positive from the laboratory. It is rarely fatal to humans, except to those with weakened immune systems.

■ Disease History, Characteristics, and Transmission

Coccidioidomycosis was first described in the late 1800s. Only severe cases were reported. Milder cases began to

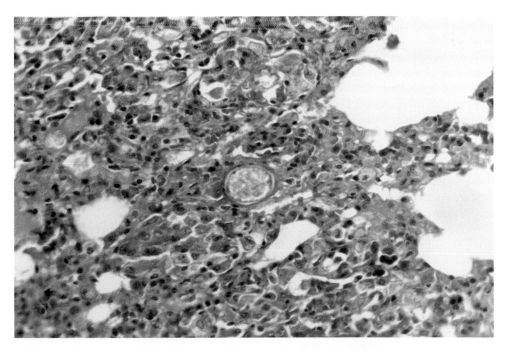

A light micrograph shows a section of human lung tissue infected with a spore (center) of the soil fungus *Coccidioides immitis*, which causes coccidioidomycosis, a pulmonary disease. This fungus, found in desert and semi-arid regions, is endemic to the southwestern United States as well as Mexico and South America.   *CNRI/Photo Researchers, Inc.*

WORDS TO KNOW

ACUTE: An acute infection is one of rapid onset and of short duration, which either resolves or becomes chronic.

CHRONIC: Chronic infections persist for prolonged periods of time—months or even years—in the host. This lengthy persistence is due to a number of factors including masking of the disease-causing agent (e.g, bacteria) from the immune system, invasion of host cells, and the establishment of an infection that is resistant to antibacterial agents.

DIMORPHIC: This refers to the occurrence of two different shapes or color forms within the species, usually occurring as sexual dimorphism between the males and females.

ENDEMIC: Present in a particular area or among a particular group of people.

IMMUNOCOMPROMISED: A reduction of the ability of the immune system to recognize and respond to the presence of foreign material.

be reported in the early 1900s. It is also called valley fever, San Joaquin Valley fever, desert fever, Posadas-Wernicke disease, and California valley fever.

No signs of symptoms occur in over half of reported cases. When symptoms are apparent, they range from mild to severe. Forty percent of the time, they are similar to influenza or the common cold. More serious cases result in pneumonia-like symptoms. Symptoms can initially include cough, headache, fever, skin rash (lower legs), and muscle and joint pain and stiffness. Other symptoms include chest pain, chills, night sweats, neck or shoulder stiffness, blood-tinged sputum, loss of appetite and weight loss, wheezing, change in behavior, joint swelling (ankles, feet, legs), arthritis, and light sensitivity. Most cases resolve on their own and are not treated medically.

The disease occurs in acute, chronic, and disseminated forms. Acute coccidioidomycosis is rare, with few or no symptoms. Some symptoms include cough, chest pain, breathing difficulties, fever, and fatigue. According to the National Institute of Health, only about 3% of people contract the acute form. Seven to 21 days is the usual incubation period. Almost all cases resolve themselves without medical help.

With chronic infection, the fungus enters internal tissues and organs, such as the meninges (protective covering of brain and spinal column), joints, heart, and bone.

It can also produce neurologic damage and tumors. People with compromised immune systems are especially affected by the chronic form of the disease. Coccidioidomycosis is not always recognized upon examination, but it does show up as nodules or cavities in the lungs. If diagnosis takes years, these lung abscesses can rupture. The chronic form occurs in 5–10% of infected patients.

Disseminated coccidioidomycosis is the most common form of the disease. It spreads to the lungs, bones (ankles, knees, feet, pelvis, wrists), organs (adrenal glands, gastrointestinal tract, liver, thyroid), meninges, brain, skin, and heart. Meningitis, the most serious complication, occurs in 30–50% of the cases.

Transmission occurs by inhalation of airborne dust containing the fungal spores. The fungus can also be contracted through the skin from infected soil. When they travel into lungs, the spores grow into spherical cells called spherules. The spherules enlarge, divide, and explode into numerous particles about 2–5 micrometers (one micrometer equals one millionth of a meter) in size.

Inhalation becomes more likely when soil is disturbed by artificial means (farming, excavation, construction) or by natural events (earthquakes, dust storms). Hispanic-, African-, and Asian-Americans are at higher risk than other ethnic groups. Pregnant women during the third trimester of pregnancy and immunocompromised individuals are also at higher risk.

■ Scope and Distribution

The disease is found in semiarid and desert regions of the southwestern United States (specifically, Arizona, California, Nevada, New Mexico, Texas, and Utah) and the northern part of Mexico. It is found in alkaline soils, climates with hot summers, and areas with annual rainfalls of 5–20 inches (13–50 cm). Between 1995 and 2005, California, New Mexico, and Arizona had the highest incidence of coccidioidomycosis, according to the NETSS (National Electronic Telecommunications System for Surveillance) of the Centers for Disease Control and Prevention (CDC). It is prevalent in California's San Joaquin Valley. It also occurs in parts of Central American and South America.

According to the CDC's Division of Bacterial and Mycotic Diseases, about 15 cases out of 100,000 occur in Arizona. Ten to fifty percent of people living in areas where the disease is common are found to be positive when tested. In the United States, about 100,000 people are infected with the fungus each year, but less than 10% of these people will develop the disease.

■ Treatment and Prevention

Diagnosis can be made in a variety of ways, including recovery of *Coccidioides immitis* from cultures and smears of sputum or other body fluid; blood tests showing the body's reaction to fungal presence; skin tests (such as Spherulin test); and chest x-ray. Their reliability, however, may vary depending on the disease's stage. Chest x rays are used to find lung abnormalities, however, the specific disease causing the abnormalities is difficult to identify from the x ray alone.

Coccidioidomycosis patients with flu-like symptoms are given antifungal medicines. In particular, amphotercin B (Abelcet®, Fungisome®) is used. However, this drug is toxic, especially when injected underneath the skull to treat meningitis. Thus, oral antifungal medicines are increasingly used, including ketoconazole (Nizoral®), fluconazole (Diflucan®), and itraconazole (Sporanox®). One-year treatments are common. Severe cases involving lung and bone damage may require surgery.

Patients with the acute form usually recover completely. Relapses can occur with chronic or severe forms. The highest death rates occur with the disseminated form of the disease. The most frequent complications are infectious relapses, accumulation of fluid between lung and chest cavity membranes, and drug complications.

■ Impacts and Issues

Coccidioidomycosis has plagued humans for many years. A cure has long been sought, but not yet attained. Currently, the disease is impossible to control and very difficult to treat. Researchers are trying to find an effective vaccine for the disease that would provide lifelong immunity. Although symptoms may subside, persons recovering from coccidioidomycosis often require repeated follow-up examinations from one to two years after symptoms disappear.

In the 1990s, one outbreak in California signaled a dramatic increase in the number of identified cases of coccidioidomycosis and illustrated the costs of an outbreak to the community. Even though most of the infections were self-limited, the cost of direct medical expenses and time lost from work was estimated to be more than $66 million during the outbreak in one California county alone. This particular outbreak was linked to heavy rainfall that ended a five-year drought in California. The rainfall enabled the *Coccidioides immitis* that had remained dormant throughout the drought to multiply to a higher density than usual, since many competing organisms were killed by the drought conditions. Scientists continue to study climate change and weather patterns to better understand their relationship to outbreaks of coccidioidomycosis.

According to the *Arizona Daily Star* newspaper, Arizona health officials have issued public information statements about the disease, since the state has been in the midst of an outbreak since 2005. A record 5,493 Arizonans were diagnosed with the disease in 2006, but as in years past, health officials say thousands of other cases

went unreported. An estimated 60% of all Arizonians have been infected with the fungus, and about 33% of persons diagnosed with pneumonia in Arizona actually have coccidioidomycosis. An ongoing campaign in Arizona is aimed at educating the medical community to consider coccidioidomycosis whenever anyone seeks medical treatment for flu or pneumonia symptoms in regions where coccidioidomycosis is endemic. The University of Arizona is also tracking the outbreak, and is studying the effectiveness of a new drug, nikkomycin Z, that has shown potential to cure the disease when tested in mice.

SEE ALSO *Airborne Precautions; Colds (Rhinitis); Influenza; Mycotic Disease; Pneumonia.*

BIBLIOGRAPHY

Books

Kumara, Vinay, Nelso Fausto, and Abul Abbas. *Robbins and Cotran Pathologic Basis of Disease.* 7th ed. Philadelphia: Saunders, 2004.

Ryan, K. J., and C. G. Ray. *Sherris Medical Microbiology: An Introduction to Infectious Diseases.* 4th ed. New York: McGraw Hill, 2003.

Periodicals

Hector, R., and R. Laniado-Laborin. "Coccidioidomycosis—A Fungal Disease of the Americas." *PloS Medicine*, January 25 2005. <http://medicine.plosjournals.org/perlserv/?request=get-document&doi=10.1371/journal.pmed.0020002> (accessed March 8, 2007).

Web Sites

Centers for Disease Control and Prevention. Division of Bacterial and Mycotic Diseases. "Coccidioidomycosis." <http://www.cdc.gov/ncidod/dbmd/diseaseinfo/coccidioidomycosis_t.htm> (accessed March 8, 2007).

Valley Fever Connections. "Valley Fever." <http://www.valley-fever.org> (accessed March 8, 2007).

IN CONTEXT: REAL-WORLD RISKS

Coccidioidomycosis is considered a re-emerging infectious disease. It has been difficult to determine the total number of cases each year, since many cases are unreported. Generally, it is estimated that about 7,500 new cases occur each year in the United States.

SOURCE: *Centers for Disease Control and Prevention (CDC)*

Cohorted Communities and Infectious Disease

■ Introduction

Living in close proximity to others is a strong risk factor for the transmission of many diseases, including tuberculosis, pneumonia, and influenza. That is why infections tend to spread among cohorted communities—that is, large groups of people occupying the same living space. Individuals tend to share, or come into contact with, items which could transmit infection. The types of diseases transmitted in cohorted communities vary,

depending on the characteristics of the group. However, three situations pose specific public health problems. College students living in dormitories may be more vulnerable to meningitis, an infection of the lining of the brain. People in prison, both inmates and staff, may be exposed to a number of infections, including HIV and tuberculosis. Finally, the elderly, frail residents of nursing homes run a high risk of urinary and gastrointestinal infections, as well as pneumonia.

■ History and Scientific Foundations

Close contact between individuals in overcrowded dwellings has always been a factor in the transmission of disease. In modern societies, people generally have more personal space, but there are still situations when they may be at risk of infection because they find themselves in close proximity to others. In recent years, college students have become a focus for concern.

At colleges and universities, thousands of students may live together in shared residence halls or dormitories. Although most students are young and healthy, these conditions put them at risk of two infections in particular—mononucleosis (sometimes known as glandular fever) and bacterial meningitis. Mononucleosis is spread through saliva (that is why it is sometimes known as the "kissing disease"), so close physical contact between individuals and sharing items such as drinking glasses will increase the risk. Mononucleosis is characterized by sore throat, fever, and extreme fatigue; there is no cure other than prolonged rest, which will interrupt studies.

Bacterial meningitis, an inflammation of the meninges, which are the membranes covering the brain and spinal cord, is a far more serious condition. In students, the cause of meningitis is usually *Neisseria meningitides* which is present in the normal flora—or natural bacterial community—of the nose and mouth. It has long been known that meningitis is transmitted more readily

WORDS TO KNOW

COHORT: A cohort is a group of people (or any species) sharing a common characteristic. Cohorts are identified and grouped in cohort studies to determine the frequency of diseases or the kinds of disease outcomes over time.

ISOLATION AND QUARANTINE: Public health authorities rely on isolation and quarantine as two important tools among the many they use to fight disease outbreaks. Isolation is the practice of keeping a disease victim away from other people, sometimes by treating them in their homes or by the use of elaborate isolation systems in hospitals. Quarantine separates people who have been exposed to a disease but have not yet developed symptoms from the general population. Both isolation and quarantine can be entered voluntarily by patients when public health authorities request it, or it can be compelled by state governments or by the federal Centers for Disease Control and Prevention.

among closed or crowded populations. Meningitis gives rise to high fever, severe headache, and stiff neck; it carries a mortality rate of around seven percent.

Prison inmates face a quite different spectrum of infection risk from overcrowding, with bloodborne viruses (BBVs) being the main concern. A high proportion of prison entrants have a history of drug use and so are likely to be infected with BBVs. Standards of hygiene within prison may be low, because of institutional failures combined with a lower standard of education among inmates, which encourages the spread of BBVs and also tuberculosis.

Finally, elderly residents of many nursing homes have been found to be at risk of several infections, including pneumonia, tuberculosis, diarrheal diseases; some of these infections are antibiotic resistant. Older people are more at risk of infection because they may have other chronic illnesses, and their immune systems tend to be weaker and less able to throw off an infection. Standards of hygiene may be lower in the presence of residents who are incontinent or who have dementia, thus increasing the likelihood of outbreaks of infectious disease.

■ Applications and Research

Research in prisons suggests that the rate of HIV infection ranges from 0.2% to over 10% and reveals case reports of transmission through sharing injecting equipment and sexual activity.

Meanwhile, research on nursing homes suggests influenza, which can be fatal in the elderly, is the most common cause of infectious outbreak. Reactivation of old tuberculosis (TB) infection is also common. Norwalk, rotavirus, and *Clostridium difficile* account for many outbreaks of gastrointestinal infection among nursing homes.

■ Impacts and Issues

There are many ways in which the spread of infection in cohorted communities can be prevented. Hygiene, both personal and institutional, should be paramount, whether the setting is a college dorm, a daycare center, a prison, or a nursing home. Programs that provide condoms and syringes have been found to decrease HIV transmission among at-risk populations. Screening of potential entrants to prisons and nursing homes for relevant infections such as HIV or TB can help identify those at risk and give treatment where appropriate. The CDC also recommends that freshmen entering dorms receive vaccination against meningitis.

Cohorting is also used to prevent the spread of infection under some conditions. Physicians, especially

those who specialize in treating children, often provide separate waiting areas in their offices to separate sick patients from those without symptoms. Hospitals often cohort patients with like infections into semi-private rooms. During a large-scale epidemic of infectious disease, community health officials have plans to both cohort infected persons (such as in the SARS outbreak in Singapore in 2003, where all suspected SARS cases were taken to one hospital for evaluation and care) and to suspend natural cohorting that could encourage disease spread (including temporarily closing schools).

SEE ALSO *Hepatitis B; Hepatitis C; HIV; Isolation and Quarantine; Meningitis, Bacterial.*

BIBLIOGRAPHY

Books

Mandell, G.L, J.E. Bennett, and R. Dolin. *Principles and Practice of Infectious Diseases.* 6th Ed. Philadelphia: Elsevier, 2005.

Periodicals

Hellard, M.E., and C.E. Aitken. "HIV in Prison: What are the Risks and What Can Be Done?." *Sexual Health.* 1 (2004): 107–113.

"Meningococcal Disease and College Students." *Morbidity and Mortality Weekly Reports.* 49 (June 30, 2000): 11–20.

Strausbaugh L.J., S.R. Sukumar, and C.L. Joseph. "Infectious Disease Outbreaks in Nursing Homes: An Unappreciated Hazard for Frail Elderly Persons." *Clinical Infectious Diseases.* 36 (2003): 870–876.

Susan Aldridge

IN CONTEXT: TRENDS AND STATISTICS

The Centers for Disease Control and Prevention (CDC) analyzed four studies of meningitis and concluded that American college students in dormitories, especially freshmen, had an increased risk of meningitis. Students in the United Kingdom run a similar risk. U.S. surveillance begun in 1998 suggested freshmen living in dormitories had a higher rate of meningitis (4.6 per 100,000) than any other group of the population, except for children under age two.

Cold Sores

■ Introduction

Cold sores, also commonly known as fever blisters, are caused by an infection with the herpes simplex 1 (HSV-1) virus. Almost everyone has been exposed to the HSV-1 virus (an estimated 95% of all people), and the infection causes one or more fluid-filled blisters in the tissues of the mouth or around the nose. After the initial outbreak, the virus lies dormant in the skin and surrounding nerve tissue, and is reactivated from time to time, most often due to colds, influenza, too much sun, or stress. Why the virus causes outbreaks at different times is not completely understood. At the time of outbreaks, the fluid within the blisters and the skin around the ulcer contain high levels of the HSV-1 virus, and so are highly contagious until the ulcer is healed. Frequent handwashing and avoiding direct contact with others will minimize the risk of spreading HSV-1. Some antiviral medications may shorten the course of the cold sore if given early in the outbreak.

Editor's note: Infrequently, HSV-1 is also responsible for eye infections and other skin infections. A small percentage of genital herpes cases are also caused by HSV-1. More information about cold sores is found in the article about their causative agent, the herpes simplex 1 virus.

SEE ALSO *Herpes Simplex 1 Virus.*

Colds (Rhinitis)

■ Introduction

The common cold, also called rhinitis, is a viral infection of the upper respiratory tract, which includes the linings of the sinuses (cavities in the head behind the nose and eyes), throat, and pharynx. The word "rhinitis" means inflammation of the nose. The common cold is indeed common, being the infectious disease most often caught by human beings. Cold symptoms include runny nose, sore throat, tiredness, and sometimes coughing or sneezing. The common cold is never fatal in people with normal immune systems. The viruses that cause colds exist in a great variety of slightly different forms, and although a person cannot catch the same cold—that is, be re-infected by exactly the same cold virus—twice, there are always plenty of other colds waiting to be caught. There is no vaccine for the common cold for the same reason. Because a cold is a viral infection, antibiotics do not affect it.

■ Disease History, Characteristics, and Transmission

History

Most colds are caused by an adenovirus or a coronavirus. The only other animals that can be infected by these viruses are the few primates most closely related to humans, including chimpanzees. Colds have been known throughout recorded history. Over two thousand years ago, the Egyptians represented a cold by a drawing of a nose followed by a symbol for something coming out. Pre-modern European doctors thought that colds were caused by an imbalance of the four "humors" (blood, yellow bile, black bile, and phlegm). The existence of disease-causing microorganisms was not known until the 1800s, and viruses were not known until the 1890s.

Even after the discovery of viruses, doctors mistakenly thought that colds were caused by bacteria for many years. The viral nature of colds was discovered in the early twentieth century, when Walter Kruse, a German researcher, showed that colds could be transmitted by

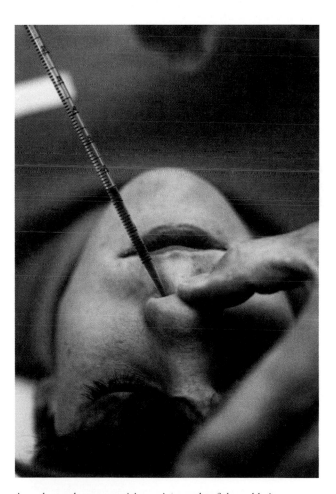

A student volunteer participates in a study of the cold virus conducted by the University of Virginia. The students were isolated in a hotel and infected with the virus through a pink solution introduced into the nose. © Karen Kasmauski/Corbis.

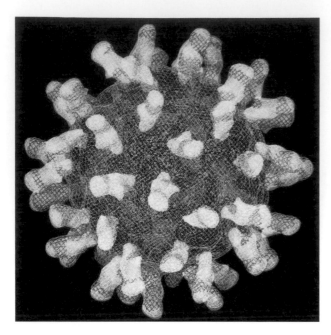

A computer-generated model of the human rhinovirus 16 is shown. Rhinoviruses cause more than half of all common colds in humans. *AP Images.*

nose secretions passed through a filter having holes too small for bacteria to pass. The actual viruses causing most colds were isolated and grown in culture in laboratories in the 1950s and 1960s.

Characteristics

Cold symptoms include stuffy nose, runny nose, mild fever and chills, tiredness, sore throat, cough, impairment of smell and taste, and hoarseness of voice. The average duration of a cold is 7.4 days; mild colds last only two to three days and about 25% of colds last about two weeks. Symptoms are not caused directly by the virus interfering with body functions, but by the body's defensive response to the virus. When cells in the respiratory tract are infected, substances called inflammatory mediators are released by the body. These cause small blood vessels to widen, which makes tissue swell. They also increase mucus secretion, stimulate pain-sensing nerve fibers, and activate cough and sneeze reflexes. The body eventually clears itself of a cold by learning to identify specific molecules, called antigens, which exist only on the surface of the particular cold virus causing that cold. Immune-system cells can then attack anything in the body that bears these antigens. The antigens on each cold virus are slightly different, which is why the body has to learn from scratch how to fight every new cold.

About 1–5% of colds are complicated by acute bacterial sinusitis, a bacterial infection of the sinuses that can have serious side effects, including eye infection and

meningitis. Unlike cold viruses, the bacteria that cause bacterial sinusitis can be killed using antibiotics.

Mild cases of influenza (also called flu) resemble colds; more severe cases cause the usual cold symptoms but also muscle aches, fever, and a more severe cough. However, influenza is a distinct disease from the common cold.

Transmission

Colds are usually contracted when cold-virus particles are picked up by touching a person with a cold or a surface contaminated with the cold virus. Cold-virus particles are then often transferred to the nostrils or eyes, again by touch. A virus can be inhaled into the nostrils and deposited in the back of the adenoid area (behind the soft palate at the back of the mouth). Virus particles in the eyes are transported down into the nasal passages and then to the adenoid area. There they colonize cells, which is why many colds begin with a sore throat. Some colds may be transmitted by airborne mucus particles ejected by sneezing. As few as one to 30 virus particles introduced into the nose can reliably produce an infection.

Cold viruses colonize cells by attaching to a molecular structure on the surface of the cell called a receptor (specifically, the ICAM-1 receptor). After attachment, the virus is absorbed into the cell, where it tricks the cell into manufacturing more of the virus. Eventually the cell produces so much virus that it ruptures, releasing many new virus particles. The cycle of virus reproduction takes about eight to 12 hours. Cold symptoms begin about 10 hours after infection and symptoms peak between 36 and 72 hours after infection.

■ Scope and Distribution

Colds afflict all nations, climates, and social classes about equally. Typically adults suffer one to four colds per year and children suffer six to ten colds annually.

Despite a widespread assumption that exposure to cold temperatures causes colds, populations living in colder climates do not get more colds. A 2005 experiment counting cold symptoms reported by groups who either underwent controlled chilling of the feet or did not showed a higher rate of symptoms among subjects whose feet had been chilled. However, the study has been criticized for not verifying whether experimental subjects who reported symptoms actually had colds. There is no scientific consensus that being chilled increases one's chance of catching a cold.

■ Treatment and Prevention

There is no effective treatment for the common cold. Contradictory evidence exists for the effectiveness of herbal treatments, zinc gluconate, and vitamin C, but there is no scientific agreement that any of these substances decrease one's chances of catching a cold, the length of a cold, or the severity of a cold. Cold treatment primarily targets the symptoms of the infection. Cold medicines often include antihistamines to reduce mucus production, pain relievers, cough suppressants, and alcohol and other drugs to induce sounder sleep.

Experimental antiviral drugs have shown some ability to combat the common cold, but scientists question whether the use of these drugs is appropriate, given the harmlessness of the common cold and the high cost and possible risks of antiviral drugs.

Colds can be prevented by following good hygiene practices. Four basic steps are recommended by disease-transmission specialists: washing hands, avoiding close contact with persons who have colds (or, if you have a cold, avoiding close contact with uninfected persons), covering up when sneezing or nose-blowing, and, for health-care professionals, wearing masks and clean gloves.

■ Impacts and Issues

There are at least 500 million colds per year in the U.S. population of about 300 million people, causing about 20 million lost workdays for adults and 21 million lost school days for children. The direct costs of colds, including purchase of cold remedies, are $17 billion per year in the U.S.; indirect costs, including lost productivity, are $22.5 billion. Lost workdays are a far more significant hardship for persons in nonprofessional, unskilled, or service-sector jobs that entitle the worker to few or no paid sick days.

In 2006, research at the Mayo Clinic indicated that some viruses that cause colds—picornaviruses—may damage the brain, causing cumulative loss of memory over a lifetime. "Our findings suggest that picornavirus infections throughout the lifetime of an individual may chip away at the cognitive [thinking ability] reserve, increasing the likelihood of detectable cognitive impairments as the individual ages," the researchers reported. There is no proof that picornavirus-caused colds do cause memory loss in human beings, but this is an active area of research.

SEE ALSO *Handwashing.*

BIBLIOGRAPHY

Books

Tyrrell, David, and Michael Fielder. *Cold Wars: The Fight Against the Common Cold.* New York: Oxford University Press, 2002.

Periodicals

Buenz, Eric J. "Disrupted Spatial Memory is a Consequence of Picornavirus Infection." *Neurobiology of Disease* 24 (2006): 266–273.

"Don't Catch Me If You Can." *Nature Structural and Molecular Biology* 11 (2004): 385.

Falsey, A.R., et al. "The Common Cold in Frail Older Persons: Impact of Rhinovirus and Coronavirus in a Senior Daycare Center." *Journal of the American Geriatrics Society* 45 (1997): 706–711.

Fendrick, A. Mark, et al. "The Economic Burden of Non-Influenza-Related Viral Respiratory Tract

WORDS TO KNOW

ANTIGEN: Antigens, which are usually proteins or polysaccharides, stimulate the immune system to produce antibodies. The antibodies inactivate the antigen and help to remove it from the body. While antigens can be the source of infections from pathogenic bacteria and viruses, organic molecules detrimental to the body from internal or environmental sources also act as antigens. Genetic engineering and the use of various mutational mechanisms allow the construction of a vast array of antibodies (each with a unique genetic sequence).

COLONIZATION: Colonization is the process of occupation and increase in number of microorganisms at a specific site.

RHINITIS: An inflammation of the mucous lining of the nose, rhinitis is a nonspecific term that covers infections, allergies, and other disorders whose common feature is the location of their symptoms. These symptoms include infected or irritated mucous membranes, producing a discharge, congestion, and swelling of the tissues of the nasal passages. The most widespread form of infectious rhinitis is the common cold.

IN CONTEXT: MANY VIRUSES CAN CAUSE COLDS

There are over 200 viruses that can cause colds. Most are rhinoviruses and coronaviruses, although several other types are known. The viruses that cause colds are RNA viruses; that is, they contain RNA (ribonucleic acid), a type of long, ribbonlike molecule that encodes information. RNA viruses reproduce by tricking body cells into producing proteins and RNA according to the instructions in the viral RNA. These proteins and pieces of viral RNA then self-assemble into new virus particles.

IN CONTEXT: REAL-WORLD RISKS

The National Institute of Allergy and Infectious Diseases (NIAID) asserts that research data does not support the popular linkage of colds to cold weather—or the development of the common cold from a person becoming either chilled or overheated. NIAID asserts that data developed by researchers find that "these conditions have little or no effect on the development or severity of a cold. Nor is susceptibility apparently related to factors such as exercise, diet, or enlarged tonsils or adenoids. On the other hand, research suggests that psychological stress, allergic disorders affecting the nasal passages or pharynx (throat), and menstrual cycles may have an impact on a person's susceptibility to colds."

SOURCE: *National Institutes of Health, National Institute of Allergy and Infectious Diseases*

Infection in the United States." *Archives of Internal Medicine* 163 (2003): 487–494.

Irwin, R.S., and J.M. Madison. "Primary Care: The Diagnosis and Treatment of Cough." *New England Journal of Medicine* 343 (2000): 1715–1721.

Squires, Sally. "Must You Be Such a Drip?" *Washington Post* (January 30, 2007).

Turner, Ronald B., et al. "An Evaluation of *Echinacea augustifolia* in Experimental Rhinovirus Infections." *New England Journal of Medicine* 353 (2005): 341–348.

Web Sites

Commoncold, Inc. "The Common Cold." 2005. <http://www.commoncold.org/> (accessed January 31, 2007).

Pan American Health Organization. "The Common Cold." <http://www.paho.org/English/AD/DPC/CD/AIEPI-1-3.9.pdf> (accessed January 31, 2007).

Contact Lenses and *Fusarium* Keratitis

Introduction

Fusarium is a type of fungus that is commonly found in the soil and on plants. In a 2005 outbreak of disease caused by *Fusarium*, the fungus was identified in contact lens cleaning solution, where it was transferred to the inner surface of a contact lens during the cleaning process. When the lens was worn, fungal growth caused an inflammation of the part of the eye called the cornea. Corneal inflammation is generally termed keratitis; in the case of this fungal infection, the inflammation is called *Fusarium* keratitis. Until recently, *Fusarium* keratitis was more common in agriculture-intensive regions, such as Florida, rather than in the general population.

The symptoms of *Fusarium* keratitis in contact lens wearers include blurred vision and a red and/or swollen eye. These symptoms do not improve when the contact lens is removed, since fungal growth is taking place in or on the cornea. Treatment typically involves antifungal drugs, such as natamycin and amphotericin B, which can be irritating and even toxic in high doses. In extreme cases, removal of the cornea and transplantation of another cornea is performed.

History and Scientific Foundations

Until 2005, *Fusarium* keratitis was a rare disease. This is because sources of the fungus, such as soil and plants, rarely come in contact with the solution used to clean contact lenses. However, in 2005, a case of *Fusarium* keratitis was diagnosed in the United States in a person who did not have a history of recent corneal damage. The infection was subsequently traced to contaminated contact lens cleaning solution. A wider investigation undertaken by the U.S. Centers for Disease Control and Prevention (CDC) uncovered 164 cases of *Fusarium* keratitis in 33 U.S. states and one U.S. territory by mid-2006.

Analysis of the data implicated a particular brand of contact lens solution (ReNu® with MoistureLoc). The source of the fungal contamination was not determined, since the fungus was not isolated from the production factory, storage warehouse, filtered samples of cleaning solutions, or unopened solution bottles from the same production runs. Nonetheless, sales of the product were stopped by Bausch & Lomb, who subsequently issued a recall of the product.

Applications and Research

Fusarium keratitis research is focused on understanding the scope of the problem. Whether *Fusarium* keratitis

---

WORDS TO KNOW

ANTIFUNGAL: Antifungals (also called antifungal drugs) are medicines used to fight fungal infections. They are of two kinds, systemic and topical. Systemic antifungal drugs are medicines taken by mouth or by injection to treat infections caused by a fungus. Topical antifungal drugs are medicines applied to the skin to treat skin infections caused by a fungus.

KERATITIS: Keratitis, sometimes called cornea ulcers, is an inflammation of the cornea, the transparent membrane that covers the colored part of the eye (iris) and pupil of the eye.

RESISTANT BACTERIA: Resistant bacteria are microbes that have lost their sensitivity to one or more antibiotic drugs through mutation.

IN CONTEXT: THE HUMAN EYE

The eye is the organ of sight in humans and animals. It transforms light waves into visual images and provides about 80% of all information received by the human brain. In humans, light enters the eye through the cornea (the transparent layer at the front of the eye), passes through the pupil (the opening in the center of the iris, the colored portion of the eye), and then through a clear lens behind the iris. The lens focuses light onto the retina, which functions like the film in a camera. Photoreceptor neurons in retinas, called rods and cones, convert light energy into electrical impulses, which are then carried to the brain via the optic nerves. At the visual cortex in the occipital lobe of the cerebrum of the brain, the electrical impulses are interpreted as images.

IN CONTEXT: REAL-WORLD RISKS

Eye infections can be caused by viral, bacterial, and fungal microorganisms. These organisms do not cause infections solely in the eye. In reality, eye infections tend to occur as infections disseminate, or spread, in the body. The cornea, the clear front part of the eye through which light passes, is subject to many infections and to injury from exposure and from foreign objects. Infection and injury cause inflammation of the cornea—a condition called keratitis. Tissue loss because of inflammation produces an ulcer. The ulcer can either be centrally located, thus greatly affecting vision, or peripherally located. There are about 30,000 cases of bacterial corneal ulcers in the United States each year.

is mainly due to an infrequent contamination of lens cleaning solution during manufacture, or is a more widespread problem involving improper hygiene on the part of the user is not clear. In addition, improved lens cleaners are being investigated, with the goal of developing a cleaner that is lethal to microbes but is safe for the user if cleaner residue remains on the lens.

The advent of molecular techniques of microorganism detection has aided the diagnosis of *Fusarium* keratitis. Advances in a technique that can quickly obtain many copies of a gene(s) of interest and the use of antibodies to *Fusarium* are being exploited to develop a rapid detection test for the fungus. Presently, the fungus is identified by culturing a scraping of cells from the

cornea, but this process can take up to a week to yield a result.

■ Impacts and Issues

In the United States, about one out of every 20 contact lens wearers develops a lens-related eye complication every year. Some of these complications can threaten vision permanently. As of early 2007, the source of the 2005–2006 fungal contamination outbreak is still being investigated by the CDC in collaboration with the Food and Drug Administration and Bausch & Lomb.

One factor that may play a role in the survival of the *Fusarium* fungus in the lens cleaning solution is the surface growth of the organism. It is now well established that some microorganisms, including fungi and bacteria, become very resistant to a variety of agents when the organisms grow attached to a nonliving or living surface. When unattached, the organisms are usually readily killed by antibiotic agents. The increased hardiness of the attached organisms involves changes in their growth following attachment. These changes can be the result of genetic adaptation, with the activity of some genes enhanced by attachment, while other genes becoming less active.

Until recently, contact lens keratitis usually involved bacterial infections, predominantly caused by bacteria common in the environment or on the surface of the skin. Fungal keratitis due to organisms such as *Fusarium* has typically been due to accidental contact of plant material with the eye, especially in people whose immune systems are functioning inefficiently as a consequence of illness or drug therapy. Common routes of transmission include rubbing an eye with soil-laden fingers, injury to the eye by a thorn, or contact of plant material with the eye during harvesting. The association of *Fusarium* keratitis with contact lenses is new, and may reflect the growing popularity of these lenses, particularly lenses that are non-disposable and repeatedly cleaned.

Fusarium keratitis is an example of how improper hygiene or contaminated lens cleaners can cause illness. Even a properly cleaned lens can become contaminated if, after handling soil or plant materials, hands have not been washed off. Also, repeated use of lens cleaning solution can cause contamination. Fresh solution should be used for each cleaning. According to the American Optometric Association, other useful precautions are wiping the lenses before storing them in the lens case and replacing the lens case every few months.

The problem of fungal keratitis is a growing concern, since extended wear contact lenses are becoming increasingly popular. These extended wear lenses remain in contact with the cornea for a longer period of time than conventional non-disposable lenses and they are cleaned less often. With the convenience of extended wear can come a relaxed vigilance concerning lens hygiene.

SEE ALSO *Contact Precautions; Mycotic Disease.*

BIBLIOGRAPHY

Books

Black, Jacquelyn. *Microbiology: Principles and Explorations.* New York: John Wiley & Sons, 2004.
Richardson, Malcolm, and Elizabeth Johnson. *Pocket Guide to Fungal Infection.* Boston: Blackwell, 2006.

Periodicals

Chang, Douglas C., et al. "Multistate Outbreak of *Fusarium* Keratitis Associated with Use of a Contact Lens Solution." *Journal of the American Medical Association* 296 (2006): 953–963.
Margolis, Todd P., and J. P. Whitcher. "Fusarium—A New Culprit in the Contact Lens Case." *Journal of the American Medical Association* 296 (2006): 985–987.

Brian Hoyle

Contact Precautions

Introduction

Contact precautions are a series of procedures designed to minimize the transmission of infectious organisms by direct or indirect contact with an infected patient or his environment. Along with standard precautions, which assume all body fluids and tissues are potentially infected with harmful microorganisms, contact precautions require the use of protective equipment such as disposable gowns, gloves, and masks when exposure to a patient's body fluids is anticipated. Contact precautions are often used with patients who have wound or skin infections.

A series of contact precautions has been formulated by the United States Centers for Disease Control and Prevention (CDC) and are intended to minimize the risk of the direct or indirect transfer of disease-causing (pathogenic) microorganisms. Direct-contact transmission involves person-to-person contact such as when a patient is touched by a healthcare provider. Indirect transfer involves contact with items that have been in contact with an infected person and which have become contaminated. These items, which are termed fomites, include clothing, towels, and utensils. A fomite may be only transiently contaminated by an infectious microbe, or the pathogen may actually colonize the object.

History and Scientific Foundations

It has been known for centuries that infection and hygiene are connected. More than 2,000 years ago, Hippocrates, who laid the groundwork for today's medical practices, observed that physicians' cleanliness affected their patients' health. Centuries later, Joseph Lister demonstrated in the mid-nineteenth century that spraying a disinfectant over a patient's wound during an operation reduced post-operative complications and death considerably. This was subsequently shown to be due to the protection of the wound from airborne microbes.

Microorganisms are readily transferred from one location to another via surfaces. The surface can be living, such as the skin of someone's hand, or non-living, such as a piece of equipment or clothing. Care must be taken to ensure that contact with a patient involves surfaces that are free of disease-causing (pathogenic) microorganisms.

The current CDC contact precautions have been in place since January 1996, as part of the overall *Guideline for Isolation Procedures in Hospitals.* Periodically, the guidelines are reviewed and, if necessary, revised.

Applications and Research

A fundamental contact precaution is handwashing. Proper washing with an anti-microbial soap will kill

---

WORDS TO KNOW

ANTIBIOTIC RESISTANCE: The ability of bacteria to resist the actions of antibiotic drugs.

FOMITE: A fomite is an object or a surface to which an infectious microorganism such as bacteria or viruses can adhere and be transmitted. Transmission is often by touch.

PATHOGENIC: Something causing or capable of causing disease.

STANDARD PRECAUTIONS: Standard precautions are the safety measures taken to prevent the transmission of disease-causing bacteria. These include proper handwashing, wearing gloves, goggles, and other protective clothing, proper handling of needles, and sterilization of equipment.

bacteria that are present on the surface of the skin, including normal residents of the skin such as *Staphylococcus aureus* and bacteria in the genus *Streptococcus*. Bacteria that are normally present on the skin will only be removed for a short time, but this will be long enough to protect patients. The physical act of washing, with the friction of skin rubbing against skin, helps remove viruses, provided it is done long enough. A few seconds of handwashing before surgery is dangerous, while a few minutes can save a life.

The CDC guidelines specify that handwashing be accomplished before and after contact with a patient and, if gloves are worn, as the final action after the gloves have been properly disposed of.

Fresh gloves need to be put on when contacting a patient for the first time. If various locations are to be touched on a patient, then the order should be from the least to the most contaminated, to minimize transfer of microbes to a relatively clean site. Gloves should be disposed of in a container designed for that purpose.

The high death rate following surgery that was the norm in the early decades of the nineteenth century was traced to the habit of physicians of wearing the same blood-soaked operating gowns during their rounds from patient to patient. Essentially, the physician was incubating each patient in turn with the collective microbial population that was adhering to the gown. To be an effective safety measure, disposable gloves, masks, and gowns are worn prior to seeing a patient and discarded in a designated container after seeing the patient. Containers should be available in each patient ward, so that the used protective clothing can be discarded in that room and not elsewhere on the hospital floor. This reduces the likelihood of transferring an infection from one room to another.

Another CDC-mandated contact precaution is to limit patient transport in the hospital as much as possible. A patient requiring contact precautions should only be moved when necessary, such as to an operating theater or X-ray room. Then, transport should be done to minimize contact with other patients. For example, a patient should not be moved into a hallway and kept there for a period of time before being transported to the final destination. Rather, transport should be direct and prompt. The more a patient is moved, the more the chance that an infection can be transferred from that patient to others.

When contact precautions are used, medical equipment such as blood pressure monitors, stethoscopes, or IV poles are dedicated solely to one patient, not shared. When contact precautions are discontinued, the equipment is cleaned and disinfected before use on another patient. Standards for the cleaning and disinfection of equipment, and for monitoring the success of these decontamination procedures, exist and must be followed. As well, records of equipment cleaning and maintenance must be kept, which makes it easier to investigate the source of a disease outbreak.

■ Impacts and Issues

Only 150 years ago, surgery was almost a death sentence. The cause of this dismal record was the inadvertent contamination of the patient by people whose task it was to ensure their care and recovery. Since then, precautions that minimize patient exposure to dangerous microbes has vastly improved the quality of health care.

Still, problems remain. The spread of antibiotic-resistant bacteria such as methicillin-resistant *S. aureus* (MRSA) in hospital wards shows that person-to-person transfer is still a reality. A big part of this problem remains the lack of proper handwashing by health care providers. Surveys done among health care providers in the United States, Canada, Europe, and elsewhere have revealed that nurses wash their hands correctly only about 50% of the time, with physicians being even less careful. The use of alcohol-based hand sanitizers, which are effective after only a few seconds exposure on the skin, is helping to encourage more compliance with handwashing by busy healthcare staff.

Contact precautions such as handwashing and wearing protective clothing are also important when dealing with a patient with diseases caused by antibiotic-resistant bacteria such as MRSA and bacteria that have developed resistance to the antibiotic vancomycin. Improper contact precautions can allow the bacteria to spread to both fellow patients and health care workers.

SEE ALSO *Airborne Precautions; Handwashing; Infection Control and Asepsis; Nosocomial (Healthcare-Associated) Infections; Standard Precautions.*

BIBLIOGRAPHY

Books

Black, Jacquelyn. *Microbiology: Principles and Explorations.* New York: John Wiley & Sons, 2004.

Tierno, Philip M. *The Secret Life of Germs: What They Are, Why We Need Them, and How We Can Protect Ourselves Against Them.* New York: Atria, 2004.

Websites

Yale-New Haven Hospital. "Contact Precautions." <http://www.med.yale.edu/ynhh/infection/contact/contact.html> (accessed May 27, 2007).

Brian Hoyle

Creutzfeldt-Jakob Disease-nv

■ Introduction

Creutzfeldt-Jakob Disease (CJD) is a rare, and invariably fatal brain disorder. It belongs to a group of diseases called the transmissible spongiform encephalopathies (TSEs), affecting both humans and animals and leading to the appearance of tiny holes within the brain tissue, giving it a "spongy" appearance. In 1996, several cases of a new form of CJD were reported in the United Kingdom. Because it differed in many ways from the so-called classical form of the disease, it was named variant CJD (vCJD, also known as new variant CJD, or CJD-nv). Since then, there have been around 200 cases of vCJD reported around the world. Exposure to bovine spongiform encephalopathy (also known as "mad cow" disease), a TSE of cattle, through consuming beef, appears to be the cause of vCJD. Control of BSE has led to a dramatic fall in the number of cases of vCJD. However, there is still a risk that the disease could be transmitted through blood donated by an infected, but asymptomatic, individual.

■ Disease History, Characteristics, and Transmission

The classical form of CJD has been known since the early years of the twentieth century. It is a rare disease, affecting around one in a million of the population around the world. About 15% of classical cases are inherited, while the rest are sporadic, arising for no obvious reason. The classical form usually affects people over 50 and is marked by ataxia (unsteadiness on the feet), dementia, (a sharp decline in mental performance), blurred vision, and slurred speech. The majority of patients with classical CJD die within six months of the onset of symptoms. vCJD, on the other hand, has been found largely among teenagers and young adults, although there have been cases in older people. It begins with psychiatric symptoms, such as anxiety and depression, and persistent pain and odd sensations in the face and limbs. Later, ataxia and sudden jerky movements set in, along with progres-

sive dementia. The time course of vCJD is longer, with death usually occurring around a year after the onset of symptoms. There are also significant differences in brain imaging, electroencephalogram, and pathology data between classical and vCJD.

The infective agent in all TSEs, including CJD, is neither a bacterium nor a virus, but an entity known as a

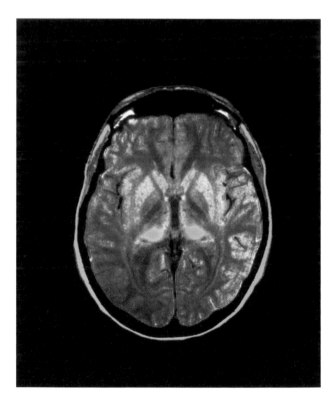

This colored magnetic resonance imaging (MRI) scan shows the brain of a 17-year-old male suffering from Creutzfeldt-Jakob Disease (CJD). In this axial "slice," the folded cerebrum is seen forming two hemispheres; the front of the head is at the top. The two green areas in the center show the thalamus diseased with CJD. *SPL/Photo Researchers, Inc.*

prion, which is best described as an infectious protein. A prion is an abnormally-shaped version of a protein that occurs naturally in the brain. When the normal prion protein comes into contact with the abnormal version, it is converted into the abnormal version and can go on to corrupt other normal prion protein molecules. This cascade of damage then spreads throughout the brain. In sporadic cases of CJD, there may be a spontaneous change of a normal prion protein molecule into the abnormal form; no risk factors for this are known, however. In inherited CJD, there are mutations in the gene for prion protein which may render a person more susceptible to prion infection. All reported cases of vCJD have involved individuals who have spent time in a country affected by BSE, which provides at least indirect evidence for the mode of transmission—consumption of BSE-contaminated beef. Meanwhile, there have been a few cases of so-called iatrogenic CJD where the disease has been transmitted from one person to another through contaminated human growth hormone (which used to be extracted from the pituitary glands of human cadavers) or instruments used in brain surgery. There have also been three cases of vCJD arising among recipients of blood from an asymptomatic donor who later developed the disease. However, there have been no cases of direct person-to-person transmission of vCJD.

■ Scope and Distribution

Most of the cases of vCJD have occurred in the United Kingdom. As of February 2007, there had been 162 primary cases (contracted, presumably, though contaminated beef) of which six are still alive. Recent research suggests that blood may be a very efficient carrier of vCJD. Prion infection in vCJD can be detected in tonsil tissue but not in blood. The U.K. Health Protection Agency is carrying out an anonymized survey of 100,000 tonsil samples that should reveal how many people are potentially incubating vCJD. As this is a new disease, little is known of its incubation time. However, kuru, a human TSE discovered in Papua New Guinea in the 1950s, can have an incubation period of up to 40 years. Without knowing more about the details of how vCJD is transmitted, it is impossible to say how many more cases of vCJD may occur.

■ Treatment and Prevention

There is no proven cure for any form of CJD at present. However, there are three potential drug treatments under investigation—quinacrine, pentosan polysulphate, and flupirtine. There is some evidence that pentosan polysulphate, given as an injection into the brain, could prolong survival, and the United Kingdom Medical Research Council (MRC) is analyzing data on a number

of patients who have received this treatment. One report suggests that flupirtine can improve cognition in CJD but it does not appear to prolong survival. The MRC is currently carrying out a clinical trial on flupirtine.

There are a number of drugs which can relieve symptoms and make the patient more comfortable, such as valproate and clonazepam for jerking movements. Eventually, all patients with CJD will require 24-hour nursing care, as they will lose the ability to do anything for themselves.

Prevention of vCJD depends upon elimination of exposure to BSE-contaminated beef. A number of measures have been adopted in Britain and elsewhere to this end. There remains the possibility that people could become infected through CJD-contaminated blood and blood products. The 20 remaining people who received blood from an infected donor in the United Kingdom have been banned from giving blood. In the United States, there are restrictions on people who have resided in the U.K. acting as blood donors, in case they are incubating vCJD.

■ Impacts and Issues

In 1986, bovine spongiform encephalopathy (BSE) appeared in cattle in the United Kingdom. Researchers identified cattle feed containing remnant parts of slaughtered cows, especially parts of the brain and nervous system, as the likely culprit spreading the disease. The U.K. government banned the use of cattle remnants in feed. In 1992, incidence of the BSE in U.K. cattle peaked in 1992 with 36,700 confirmed, about 1% of the U.K. cattle herd. Despite the epidemic of "mad cow disease," consumers were assured that British beef products were safe to eat. In 1996, researchers identified BSE-contaminated beef as the probable cause of vCJD in humans.

The link between BSE and vCJD had widespread social and economic effects. The United Kingdom cattle heard was culled of possibly infected animal, resulting in losses to herders. As the emergence of vCDJ received global media attention, consumption of beef within the U.K. dropped dramatically, some estimate as much as 40% in 1996-7. The meat slaughtering and packing industry was scrutinized, revealing slaughtering practices that carried the possibility of BSE-tainted nervous system tissue entering ground beef. Other European nations temporarily banned the import of U.K. beef products and began to evaluate their own herds for BSE. By 2005, BSE had been found in Europe, Asia, North America, and the Falkland Islands, a British territory off of the coast of Argentina. The vCJD epidemic peaked in Britain in 2000, with 28 cases. In 2006, there were five cases. After the U.K., France has had the highest number of vCJD cases. In the U.S., there have been three cases. Worldwide, there have been 201 cases of vCJD in 11 countries.

The vCJD epidemic also prompted fears about the safety of the international supply of human blood, plasma, tissues, and organs. Many nations excluded, or continue to exclude, donors who resided for several months in parts of Europe and the United Kingdom during 1980–2000. People who received transfusions or organ or tissue transplants in the U.K. are also excluded as potential donors in several countries. The three cases of transfusion-associated vCJD in the U.K. came from a pool of 23 recipients of blood from the infected donor. The latest case developed vCJD symptoms eight years after receiving a transfusion. Because the term of incubation for vCJD remains unknown, others who received the contaminated blood remain at risk. Tests that screen donated blood for vCJD are currently under development.

CJD, including vCJD, is still a very rare disease and one which is poorly understood. Although the U.S. researcher Stanley Prusiner was awarded the 1997 Nobel

Prize for Medicine or Physiology for his work on prions, there is still much to be learned about how these unconventional infective agents work. For example, the routes of transmission of prion diseases are not yet well established. There is no straightforward diagnostic test, such as a blood test, for CJD. Adding to the difficulty of making an unambiguous diagnosis, most neurologists never have seen a case of CJD even when symptoms are present. The disease, like other TSEs, may be present without symptoms for many years, putting people at risk of infection. However, current research aims to better understand all forms of CJD and other prion-transmitted diseases.

SEE ALSO *Blood Supply and Infectious Disease; Bovine Spongiform Encephalopathy ("Mad Cow" Disease); Kuru.*

BIBLIOGRAPHY

Books

Ridley, R.M, and H.F. Baker. *Fatal Protein: The Story of CJD, BSE and Other Prion Disease.* Oxford: Oxford University Press, 1998.

Web Sites

Centers for Disease Control and Prevention (CDC). "vCJD (Variant Creutzfeldt-Jakob disease)." January 4, 2007 <http://www.cdc.gov/ncidod/dvrd/cjd/> (accessed February 21, 2007).

U.K. Creutzfeldt-Jakob Disease Surveillance Unit. "National Creutzfeldt-Jakob Disease Surveillance Unit." February 5, 2007 <http://www.cjd.ed.ac.uk> (accessed February 21, 2007).

Susan Aldridge

Crimean-Congo Hemorrhagic Fever

■ Introduction

Crimean-Congo hemorrhagic fever (CCHF) is a viral disease caused by infection with a tick-borne virus. The virus that causes CCHF is contained within *Nairovirus*, a member of related pathogenic (disease-causing) viruses within the Bunyaviridae family.

All *Nairovirus* viruses are transmitted by the bite of argasid (soft) or isodid (hard) ticks. However, only a few of these ticks have shown to cause human infections. According to the World Health Organization (WHO) and the Centers for Disease Control and Prevention (CDC), the tick of the *Hyalomma* genus is most capable of serving as the vector for the disease, especially in small vertebrates on which immature ticks feed.

CCHF is an infectious disease that is capable of being transmitted by ticks between domesticated and wild animals; from animals to humans; and from humans to animals. Common animals infected are cattle, sheep, goats, and hares. Humans are infected through contact with infected animal blood or ticks.

■ Disease History, Characteristics, and Transmission

CCHF was documented in Russia in the twelfth century. However, the first accurate description came from the Crimea region of the former U.S.S.R. in 1944–1945. At that time, it was called Crimean hemorrhagic fever. In 1969, it was realized that the pathogen causing CCHF was also an illness identified in 1956 in Stanleyville (now Kisangani), Congo. Because of this, it was renamed Crimean-Congo hemorrhagic fever.

Small vertebrates on which the immature ticks feed seem to serve as the primary method that the virus spreads. Infected female ticks pass the disease into their eggs, which develop into infected immature ticks. Mature ticks carry the virus to larger animals, such as large vertebrates, who can become intermediate hosts.

CCHF transmission to humans occurs when people butcher or eat infected livestock, and when health workers became exposed to infected blood.

After a tick bite, the incubation period is about one to three days, but up to nine days. After contact with infected blood or tissue, the incubation period is usually five to six days, with a maximum of 13 days. Influenza-like symptoms occur suddenly. In most cases, they last for about one week. However, signs of bleeding appear 75% of the time in cases lasting longer than one week. Death occurs in 30–60% of cases.

Symptoms include high fever, aching muscles, dizziness, neck pain, backache, stomach pain, headache, sore eyes, and light sensitivity. Later, nosebleeds, red eyes, flushed face, red throat, bruising, bloody urine, vomiting, black stools, skin rash, and diarrhea occur. Still later, abdominal pain occurs, along with mental confusion and mood swings.

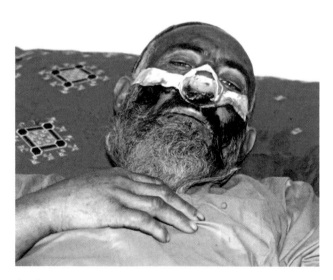

A Pakistani man with Crimean Congo hemorrhagic fever (CCHF) receives medical treatment at a local hospital. © *Fayyaz Ahmed/epa/Corbis.*

Unlike humans, most infected mammals do not show noticeable symptoms. Most cases occur in domesticated animals and wild animals. CCHF occurs less frequently in humans.

Scope and Distribution

The disease is found in over thirty countries around the world. It is reported in central Asia, northwestern China, the Middle East, eastern and southern Europe, the Indian subcontinent, across central and southern Africa (especially eastern and western parts) and Madagascar.

Small mammals carry the disease, especially the Middle-African hedgehog, multimammate rat, and European hare. Domestic animals, such as sheep, goats, and cattle, also carry the tick. Most birds do not become infected, except ostriches.

Groups most likely to become infected are slaughterhouse workers, veterinarians, surgeons and medical workers, animal herders, and agricultural workers. Widespread infections in medical facilities have occurred due to improperly sterilization of equipment, reuse of injection needles, and supply contamination. Travelers are at risk in countries where CCHF is present.

Treatment and Prevention

Diagnosis includes the following: serological test (to find antibodies in serum); immunohistochemical staining (to find viral antigen in tissue); microscopic examination (to find viral RNA [ribonucleic acid] sequence in blood or tissue); polymerase chain reaction (PCR) technique (to detect viral genome); and enzyme linked immunosorbent assay (ELISA) technique (to detect immunoglobulin-G and immunoglobulin-M antibodies in serum).

Oral and intravenous treatment involves the antiviral drug ribavirin (Copegus®, Ribasphere®, Virazole®). Ribavirin has been shown to be effective during actual outbreaks, although scientific studies have not supported that conclusion.

Treatment is generally supportive and based on the symptom's type and degree of severity. Fluid balance, electrolyte levels, and secondary infections are carefully monitored. Fatality rates in hospitalized patients range widely from 9% to 50%, depending on infection severity, care quality, and other variables.

CCHF is commonly prevented by governments that require de-ticking of farm animals. Insect repellents (containing DEET, N,N-diethy-m-toluamide), appropriate clothing (gloves and clothing treated with permethrin), and body inspections help prevent the disease. Persons are advised to avoid contact with blood and fluids of infected livestock and humans.

WORDS TO KNOW

ARTHROPOD: A member of the largest single animal phylum, consisting of organisms with segmented bodies, jointed legs or wings, and exoskeletons. Includes insects and spiders.

HEMORRHAGIC FEVER: A hemorrhagic fever is caused by viral infection and features a high fever and a high volume of (copious) bleeding. The bleeding is caused by the formation of tiny blood clots throughout the bloodstream. These blood clots—also called microthrombi—deplete platelets and fibrinogen in the bloodstream. When bleeding begins, the factors needed for the clotting of the blood are scarce. Thus, uncontrolled bleeding (hemorrhage) ensues.

INTERMEDIATE HOST: An organism infected by a parasite while the parasite is in a developmental form, not sexually mature.

VECTOR: Any agent, living or otherwise, that carries and transmits parasites and diseases. Also, an organism or chemical used to transport a gene into a new host cell.

IN CONTEXT: TRENDS AND STATISTICS

According to World Health Organization and the European Center for Disease Prevention and Control (ECDE), recent cases of Crimean hemorrhagic fever were reported in Albania (2001, 8 cases), Iran (1999–2004, 155 cases), Kosovo (2001, 18 cases), Mauritania (2003, 38 cases), Pakistan (2002, 3 cases), and Turkey (2001–2003, 83 cases). In Bulgaria and South Africa, between five and 25 cases are reported annually in each country. In July 2005, a major outbreak occurred in Turkey's Yozgat Province (one death out of 42 cases). Between January 1–4, 2006, 242 confirmed cases (20 deaths) were reported in Turkey.

SOURCE: *World Health Organization*

Impacts and Issues

Crimean-Congo hemorrhagic fever is one of the world's most severe arthropod-borne diseases. It has a mortality rate of up to 60%. CCHF remains a public health problem

IN CONTEXT: REAL-WORLD RISKS

As of May 2007, the World Health Organization states that "although an inactivated, mouse brain-derived vaccine against CCHF has been developed and used on a small scale in Eastern Europe, there is no safe and effective vaccine widely available for human use."

WHO also states that:

- The tick vectors are numerous and widespread and tick control with acaricides (chemicals intended to kill ticks) is only a realistic option for well-managed livestock production facilities. Persons living in endemic areas should use personal protective measures that include avoidance of areas where tick vectors are abundant and when they are active (spring to fall); regular examination of clothing and skin for ticks, and their removal; and use of repellents.

- Persons who work with livestock or other animals in the endemic areas can take practical measures to protect themselves. These include the use of repellents on the skin (e.g., DEET) and clothing (e.g., permethrin) and wearing gloves or other protective clothing to prevent skin contact with infected tissue or blood.

SOURCE: *World Health Organization*

in many parts of the world, including Africa, the Middle East, southern and eastern Europe, and western Asia.

Because of this, the CDC identifies the need for increased knowledge about CCHF. Currently, the prevalence of CCHF is not measured accurately. The CDC recommends: measurements to be performed on both animals and humans so accurate statistics are available; further CCHF research to be performed; effectiveness of treatments recorded; and a widespread, safe, and effective vaccine for CCHF developed. Currently, only a local vaccine developed in Eastern Europe, made from the brains of mice, is available.

Crimean-Congo hemorrhagic fever's causative agent, the *Nairovirus*, is classified as a biosafety level four

(BSL4) pathogen by the CDC. Scientists study biosafety level four pathogens, which are mostly viruses, in specialized facilities designed to contain them. All biosafety level four pathogens have the capacity to cause life-threatening diseases, and no effective vaccine is readily available to prevent them. Currently, there are eleven BSL4 facilities in the United States, and several more are planned or under construction. Access to BSL4 labs is usually restricted to essential personnel. Among the extensive safety measures used by scientists when conducting research with BSL4 pathogens are multi-containment areas, one-piece positive pressure personnel suits with separate ventilation systems, negative air pressure rooms, and a safe working area called a biological safety cabinet. Other viral hemorrhagic fevers such as Ebola, Lassa, and Marburg, are also considered BSL4 pathogens.

SEE ALSO *Arthropod-borne Disease; Hemorrhagic Fevers; Travel and Infectious Disease; Viral Disease.*

BIBLIOGRAPHY

Books

Ergonul, Onder, and Chris C. Whitehouse, eds. *Crimean-Congo Hemorrhagic Fever: A Global Perspective.* New York: Springer, 2007.

Farb, Daniel. *Bioterrorism Hemorrhagic Viruses.* Los Angeles: University of Health Care, 2004.

Web Sites

Centers for Disease Control and Prevention. "Crimean-Congo Hemorrhagic Fever." <http://dcd.gov/ncidod/dvrd/spb/mnpages/dispages/cchf.htm> (accessed March 8, 2007).

National Guideline Clearinghouse. "Hemorrhagic Fever Viruses as Biological Weapons: Medical and Public Health Management." March 5, 2007 <http://www.guideline.gov/summary/summary.aspx?ss=15&doc_id=3224&nbr=2450> (accessed March 11, 2007).

World Health Organization. "Crimean-Congo Hemorrhagic Fever." <http://who.int/mediacentre/factsheets/fs208/en/> (accessed March 8, 2007).

Cryptococcus neoformans Infection

■ Introduction

Cryptococcus neoformans is a yeast that is the sole species of the genus capable of causing mycotic (fungal) disease. There are three versions of *C. neoformans*, based on differences in the capsule that surrounds the yeast, in the use of various sugars as nutrients, and in the shape of the environmentally resilient structures called spores that can be produced by the yeast. *C. neoformans* variety *neoformans* causes most of the cryptococcal infections in humans.

■ Disease History, Characteristics, and Transmission

C. neoformans causes cryptococcosis. The infection begins in the lungs following the inhalation of the microorganism, particularly the small form of the organism called a basidiospore. These spores are smaller than the growing (vegetative) form of the yeast, and so can penetrate deeper into the very small air passages (alveoli) of the lung. In the warm and moist conditions of the lung, the basidiospores can increase in size and normal growth of the yeast can resume.

When the yeast begins to grow, a capsule that is usually only minimally produced by the spores is exuberantly produced. Like the capsule produced by some bacteria, the capsule of *C. neoformans* is made of sugars. The capsule helps shield the yeast from the immune response of the host, in particular the engulfing (phagocytosis) and breakdown of the yeast by a type of immune cell called a macrophage.

C. neoformans is equipped with enzymes known as proteases, which degrade proteins, as well as enzymes that destroy phospholipids. Both proteins and phospholipids are important components of the cell wall that surrounds cells. This causes the destruction of host cells, which makes it easier for *C. neoformans* to enter the host cells and to invade tissue.

Evidence from laboratory studies indicates that *C. neoformans* is not only capable of evading the host's immune response, but may also actively impair the response. This would explain the observation that people who survive a bout of cryptococcal meningitis can continue to have a malfunctioning immune system afterward.

Most commonly, *C. neoformans* causes the form of meningitis called cryptococcal meningitis. (Meningitis can also be caused by bacteria or viruses.) People who are immunocompromised—their immune system is not functioning properly due to infection with, for example, the human immunodeficiency virus (HIV) or deliberate suppression to lessen the rejection of a transplanted organ—can are at particular risk for a potentially fatal infection with *C. neoformans*. The yeast can become more widely distributed in the body. This can produce inflammation and damage of the nerves in the brain (meningitis); and infections of the eye (conjunctivitis), ear (otitis), heart (myocarditis), liver (hepatitis), and bone (arthritis). Prior to the explosion of the number of cases of AIDS and the more routine use of immunosuppressant drugs, *C. neoformans* infections were rare.

■ Scope and Distribution

C. neoformans is found all over the world. It is a natural inhabitant of some plants, fruits, and birds such as pigeons and chickens. The microbe is often transferred to humans via bird feces. As the feces dry, the yeast spores can be wafted into the air to be subsequently inhaled.

■ Treatment and Prevention

Treatment for cryptococcal meningitis usually includes anti-fungal drugs such as fluconazole. Often a compound called amphotericin B is also administered. It is usually given intravenously, which produces a higher concentration of the drug throughout the body. This is important since the infection can quickly become

WORDS TO KNOW

BASIDIOSPORE: A fungal spore of Basidomycetes. Basidomycetes are classified under the Fungi kingdom as belonging to the phylum Mycota (i.e., Basidomycota or Basidiomycota), class Mycetes (i.e., Basidomycetes). Fungi are frequently parasites that decompose organic material from their hosts, such as those growing on rotten wood, although some may cause serious plant diseases such as smuts (Ustomycetes) and rusts (Teliomycetes). Some live in a symbiotic relationship with plant roots (Mycorrhizae). A cell type termed basidium is responsible for sexual spore formation in Basidomycetes, through nuclear fusion followed by meiosis, thus forming haploid basidiospores.

IMMUNOCOMPROMISED: A reduction of the ability of the immune system to recognize and respond to the presence of foreign material.

MYCOTIC: Mycotic means having to do with or caused by a fungus. Any medical condition caused by a fungus is a mycotic condition, also called a mycosis.

widespread. The treatment has a variety of potential side effects, including fever, chills, headache, nausea with vomiting, diarrhea, kidney damage, and a decrease in the number of red blood cells due to the inhibition of bone marrow. Fewer red blood cells means less oxygen and iron is capable of being transported throughout the body, a condition called anemia. Also, some people can have an allergic reaction to the drug.

Amphotericin B is available as a liposome preparation; that is, the drug is packaged inside a sphere made of lipid. The liposomes can also contain proteins that recognize target proteins in the patient. This allows the drug to be more specifically targeted to a site within the body, rather than applying the drug generally.

Prospects for recovery are good if the infection is identified and treated while it is still confined to the lungs. However, spread of the infection beyond the lungs, especially to the central nervous system, is a serious complication, and can threaten the life of someone who is immunocompromised.

■ Impacts and Issues

Other the past several decades, the prevalence of cryptococcal illness on Vancouver Island on Canada's west coast has been increasing. Researchers from the United States Centers for Disease Control and Prevention and Health Canada who have been studying the illnesses have concluded that the increasingly temperate climate of the region is favoring the expansion of the yeast into a region that it formerly did not occupy. With regions of the world expected to warm over the next century, the geographic range of *C. neoformans* may increase.

As about 85% of cases of cryptococcosis in the United States occur among HIV-positive people, finding an affordable and readily available prevention strategy for persons whose immune system is already weakened is an important challenge for researchers. Globally, the increase in AIDS has made many more people vulnerable to *C. neoformans* infection.

SEE ALSO *AIDS (Acquired Immunodeficiency Syndrome); Mycotic Disease; Opportunistic Infection.*

BIBLIOGRAPHY

Books

Black, Jacquelyn G. *Pigeons: The Fascinating Saga of the World's Most Revered and Reviled Bird.* New York: Grove Press, 2006.

Blechman, Andrew D. *Microbiology: Principles and Explorations.* New York: John Wiley & Sons, 2004.

Web Sites

Centers for Disease Control and Prevention. "Cryptococcosis" <http://www.cdc.gov/ncidod/dbmd/diseaseinfo/cryptococcosis_t.htm> (accessed March 8, 2007).

Brian Hoyle

Cryptosporidiosis

■ Introduction

Cryptosporidiosis (KRIP-toe-spo-rid-ee-OH-sis) is a parasitic infection of the gastrointestinal tract that usually results in diarrhea. It occurs when the parasite *Cryptosporidium* is ingested due to contact between the mouth and fecal material containing the parasite. In addition to humans, more than 45 species of animals, including common farm animals, can become infected with *Cryptosporidium*.

There is often no treatment administered in otherwise healthy individuals following diagnosis, although fluid replacement may be necessary following severe diarrhea. Symptoms last around two weeks, and the disease is transmissible even in the absence of symptoms. Infection can be prevented through adhering to hygienic regimes including handwashing, washing or cooking food, boiling water, and avoiding contact with animals.

Outbreaks can occur, especially if drinking water becomes contaminated with the parasite. In this case, it is necessary to filter or boil water to prevent infection.

■ Disease History, Characteristics, and Transmission

Cryptosporidiosis was first diagnosed in humans in 1976 after a three-year-old girl suffering from vomiting and

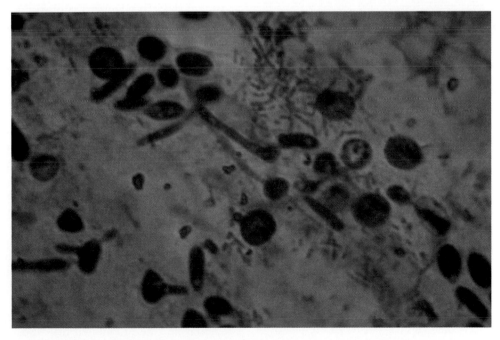

Cryptosporidium fungal cells, which cause cryptosporidiosis, are shown. Infection likely occurs via a fecal-oral transmission from kittens and puppies. © *Lester V. Bergman/Corbis.*

IN CONTEXT: PERSONAL RESPONSIBILITY AND PROTECTION

The Centers for Disease Control and Prevention, National Center for Infectious Diseases, Division of Parasitic Diseases recommends that states that "If you are unable to avoid using or drinking water that might be contaminated (with *Cryptosporidium parvum*), then you can make the water safe to drink by doing one of the following:

- Heat the water to a rolling boil for at least 1 minute OR use a filter that has an absolute pore size of 1 micron or smaller, or one that has been NSF rated for 'cyst removal.'
- Do not rely on chemicals to disinfect water and kill Cryptosporidium. Because it has a thick outer shell, this particular parasite is highly resistant to disinfectants such as chlorine and iodine."

SOURCE: *Centers for Disease Control and Prevention, National Center for Infectious Diseases, Division of Parasitic Diseases*

diarrhea was found to be infected with the parasite *Cryptosporidium*. The girl's digestive tract contained large amounts of gas in the colon, large amounts of fluid in the small and large bowel, and on further examination, the parasite was found within her digestive tract. Since the initial diagnosis, multiple outbreaks have occurred in the United States, including one significant outbreak transmitted through the Milwaukee, Wisconsin public water system occurred in 1993 during which 403,000 people became infected.

Cryptosporidiosis occurs after ingestion of the parasite *Cryptosporidium*. This parasite is a one-celled, ball-shaped organism that affects the digestive, biliary, and respiratory systems of other organisms. The parasite lays oocytes, which are egglike structures covered in a protective shell.

Oocytes leave an infected organism's body in fecal matter. Oocytes can remain viable for two to six months in a moist environment, and due to their protective outer covering, are highly resistant to chemical disinfectant. Therefore, these parasites are potentially highly infectious.

Ingestion of infected fecal matter results in transmission of the parasite to a new organism. Ingestion of fecal matter occurs when the mouth comes in either direct contact with fecal matter, or in contact with something that has touched fecal matter. The most common means are: not washing hands after using the toilet, handling infected animals, not washing food or cooking food thoroughly, and drinking contaminated water. In addition, swimming pools and spas are common places for infection to occur due to the moist environment, and the resistance of the parasite to chemicals, including pool chlorine. Swallowing pool water infected with the parasite can lead to infection.

■ Scope and Distribution

Cryptosporidiosis is widespread within the United States, and is also present worldwide. Outbreaks have occurred in over 50 countries worldwide on six continents. The U.S. Food and Drug Administration estimates that about 80% of the American population has had cryptosporidiosis, and its prevalence (the proportion of a population having a particular disease at a given time) is about 2% in North America.

The people most commonly infected by cryptosporidiosis are children younger than two years of age, animal handlers, health care workers, and travelers. While the people most at risk of suffering long term, or even fatal cases of cryptosporidiosis, are those with weak immune systems. Young children are at risk due to the likelihood of them placing infected objects into their mouth, or not washing their hands after using the toilet.

Animal handlers are required to come into contact with animals on a daily basis. If hygienic procedures such as handwashing and washing clothes are not undertaken, transmission can occur between the animals and humans. Animals that can be infected include a range of common farm animals such as cattle and sheep, as well as common pets such as cats, dogs, birds, and fish.

Health care workers usually come into contact with fecal matter on a daily basis, which could potentially result in them becoming infected, particularly if they are caring for patients infected with cryptosporidiosis. To avoid infection, healthcare workers use contact precautions, including handwashing and wearing gloves when anticipating contact with potentially infected feces. People taking care of children may also be exposed to infection during diaper changing, as they are likely to come into contact with fecal matter.

Travelers are at risk as they may travel through areas with differing levels of hygiene in terms of food preparation and water standards. Lower standards may result in food and water harboring the parasite. Therefore, their chances of infection are greater.

People with weak immune systems are most at risk of suffering prolonged or severe symptoms of cryptosporidiosis. Persons with AIDS, who have transplanted organs, or who were born with weakened immune systems are more likely to develop complications from cryptosporidiosis, including severe dehydration and lung infection (pulmonary cryptosporidiosis) that can lead to death.

■ Treatment and Prevention

The most common symptoms of cryptosporidiosis in humans are diarrhea, stomach cramps, nausea, vomiting, slight fever, and weight loss. These symptoms usually appear between two and 10 days after infection, and last up to two weeks, sometimes occurring sporadically during that time. Following recovery, relapses may occur. In some cases, symptoms are not present. However, the infection is still contagious and can be passed on to other humans.

There is no standard cure for cryptosporidiosis, and the symptoms usually disappear after about two weeks. One new drug approved for treating the disease, nitazoxanide, has shown effectiveness in treating the diarrhea associated with cryptosporidiosis in people that are otherwise healthy. Some people also receive relief from antibiotics and from common anti-diarrhea and anti-vomiting medicines. In order to prevent dehydration, fluid and electrolyte replacement may be necessary in some cases. Therefore, persons with *Cryptosporidium* are encouraged to increase their water intake, and to watch for signs of dehydration, such as dry mouth, headaches, fatigue, joint aches, and decreased skin elasticity.

In order to prevent contracting cryptosproidiosis, contact with fecal matter should be avoided. This may involve washing hands after handling soil, after toileting, or after handling animals. To avoid infection via food, washing with uninfected water, or cooking it thoroughly will remove or kill the parasite. Water is a major source of infection due to the parasite's protective covering against chemicals. Boiling infected water for at least one minute will kill the parasite, and filtering it through filters small enough to prevent the parasite passing will remove the parasite. This water can then be used for all water-related uses such as drinking, washing food, and making ice.

The Western Australian Health Department recommends that infected people remain away from public places, especially public swimming bodies, while exhibit-

IN CONTEXT: REAL-WORLD RISKS

Advertising on filters can be deceptive. The Centers for Disease Control and Prevention, National Center for Infectious Diseases, Division of Parasitic Diseases states that filters with any of the following messages on the package "should be able to remove Crypto" (*Cryptosporidium parvum*):

- Reverse-osmosis (with or without NSF testing)
- Absolute pore size of 1 micron or smaller (with or without NSF testing)
- Tested and certified by NSF Standard 53 for cyst removal
- Tested and certified by NSF Standard 53 for cyst reduction

"Filters labeled only with these words may not be designed to remove Crypto:"

- Nominal pore size of 1 micron or smaller
- 1-micron filter
- Effective against Giardia
- Effective against parasites
- Carbon filter
- Water purifier
- EPA approved - Caution: EPA does not approve or test filters.
- EPA registered - Caution: EPA does not register filters for Crypto removal
- Activated carbon
- Removes chlorine
- Ultraviolet light
- Pentiodide resins
- Water softener

SOURCE: *Centers for Disease Control and Prevention, National Center for Infectious Diseases, Division of Parasitic Diseases*

ing cryptosporidiosis symptoms to prevent possible infection of other people.

■ Impacts and Issues

Cryptosporidiosis has the potential to spread rapidly and affect many people in a short amount of time, and infection of a community's drinking source puts the whole community at risk. Before 2001, water treatment in many locations in the United States did not remove the parasite, as chemical treatment usually did not kill them, and filters were too large to prevent them passing. The outbreak in Milwaukee in 1993 resulted in over 400,000 reported cases and remains the single largest outbreak of waterborne disease reported in the United States. More than 100 people, mostly persons with AIDS or elderly persons, died during the outbreak. Estimated monetary costs of the outbreak spiraled to over 95 million dollars, including 30 million dollars of direct medical care costs and 60 million dollars attributed to lost productivity in the Milwaukee workplace. As a result of this outbreak, the U.S. Environmental Protection Agency (EPA) mandated that major U.S. water systems (those relying surface water sources, such as a rivers or lakes, and serving more than 10,000 people) implement new EPA standards by 2001 that strengthened control over microbial contaminants, including *Cryptosporidium*.

Another notable occurrence occurred in New York in 2005 at a popular water park. The Senaca Lake State Park was found to have two water storage tanks infected with *Cryptosporidium*. Over 3,800 people reported cryptosporidiosis symptoms.

Cryptosporidiosis disease is a major cause of diarrhea worldwide. Due to differing food and water quality controls over the world, this disease has a large impact on travelers who are unfamiliar with a region's water quality. Travelers are often advised to consider the following precautions to prevent infection: bringing water to a full boil for one minute, avoiding undercooked food, handling or peeling raw food such as fruit themselves, avoiding swimming in freshwater rivers and lakes, and carrying bottled water when unsure of an area's water quality.

Persons with compromised immune systems are often advised to take extra precautions with their drinking water to prevent *Cryptosporidium* infection, including boiling it, installing point-of-use filters that remove particles one micrometer or less in diameter, or drinking bottled water from protected well or protected spring water sources.

SEE ALSO *AIDS (Acquired Immunodeficiency Syndrome); Contact Precautions; Gastroenteritis (common causes); Handwashing; HIV; Parasitic Diseases; Travel and Infectious Disease; Water-borne Disease.*

BIBLIOGRAPHY

Books

Mandell, G.L., J.E. Bennett, and R. Dolin. *Principles and Practice of Infectious Diseases, vol. 2.* Philadelphia, PA: Elsevier, 2005.

Web Sites

Australian Government. "Cryptosporidiosis." April, 2006 <http://www.healthinsite.gov.au/topics/ Cryptosporidiosis> (accessed Jan. 29, 2007).
Centers for Disease Control and Prevention (CDC). "Cryptosporidium Infection Cryptosporidiosis." Aug. 19, 2005 <http://www.cdc.gov/ncidod/ dpd/parasites/cryptosporidiosis/factsht_ cryptosporidiosis.htm> (accessed Jan. 29, 2007).
Department of Health, Western Australia. "Cryptosporidiosis: Environmental Health Guide." 2006 <http://www.health.wa.gov.au/ envirohealth/water/docs/Cryptospordiosis_EH_ Guide.pdf> (accessed Jan. 29, 2007).
New York State Department of Health. "Cryptosporidiosis." June, 2004 <http://www.health. state.ny.us/diseases/communicable/cryptosporidiosis/ fact_sheet.htm> (accessed Jan. 29, 2007).

Culture and Sensitivity

■ Introduction

Culture and sensitivity in microbiology refers to laboratory techniques that allow a disease-causing microorganism to be identified, and that determine which antibiotics are sensitive to (effective against) the identified microorganism.

Physicians must take numerous important factors into account when deciding how to appropriately treat infectious disease. Broad patient-specific factors include the natural history of the infection and the strength of the patient's immune system. If antibiotic treatment of the disease is suitable, as in the case of bacterial, certain fungal, and some other microbial diseases, the type of antibiotics used may depend on ease of absorption, metabolism, ability to reach the infection site, and other factors. Microbe culturing and susceptibility testing offers information to help make appropriate decisions. The availability of such information from laboratory testing can be of life-saving assistance to doctors, but can also result in excessive reliance on testing when a simpler, broader approach to treatment may be more efficient.

■ History and Scientific Foundations

Most of the techniques of culturing microbes were developed in the mid- to late 1800s by Robert Koch, Paul Erlich, and Hans Christian Gram. Using some of these techniques, Louis Pasteur (1822–1895) developed the foundations of the modern science of infectious disease at that time.

The German physician Robert Koch (1843–1910) perfected a technique to distinguish different types of bacteria and grow pure cultures of these bacterial types, and in the process founded the science of bacteriology. He formalized the approach of determining whether a particular microbe caused a given disease in a set of rules now known as Koch's Postulates (1882), which supported the concept that a disease is caused by a specific microbe:

- The agent of an infectious disease must be present in every case of the disease.
- The agent must be isolated from the host and grown *in vitro* (pure culture) for several generations.
- The disease must be reproduced when a pure culture of the agent is inoculated into a healthy susceptible host.
- The same agent must be recovered once again from the experimentally infected host.

Koch developed a solid medium for bacterial growth using gelatin, later modified by other scientists to include a seaweed called agar to keep the medium solid at room temperature. The German bacteriologist Richard Julius Petri (1852–1921) developed a glass dish still used today that helps foster optimal bacterial growth.

In 1877, Koch also developed a technique for dry-fixing thin films of bacterial culture on glass slides, staining them with aniline dyes, and recording the microscopic images on film. Dry-fixing continues to be a standard procedure in identifying various bacterial cultures. Different types of media are optimal for specific types of bacteria, and identification of a specific pathogen can still be a matter of clinical experience and judgment.

Microbe staining techniques were developed in 1839 by the German scientist Christian Gottfried Ehrenberg (1795–1876). These staining techniques depended on two properties of stains: chromogenicity (inclusion of groups of atoms that are color-forming) and the ability to dissociate into positively charged ions (cations) and negatively charged ions (anions). For example, when the common methylene blue dye is added to water, it dissociates into a chloride anion and a methylene blue

WORDS TO KNOW

ANTIBIOTIC RESISTANCE: The ability of bacteria to resist the actions of antibiotic drugs.

ANTIBIOTIC SENSITIVITY: Antibiotic sensitivity refers to the susceptibility of a bacterium to an antibiotic. Bacteria can be killed by some types of antibiotics and not be affected by other types. Different types of bacteria exhibit different patterns of antibiotic sensitivity.

BROAD-SPECTRUM ANTIBIOTICS: Broad-spectrum antibiotics are drugs that kill a wide range of bacteria rather than just those from a specific family. For, example, amoxicillin is a broad-spectrum antibiotic that is used against many common illnesses such as ear infections.

COHORTING: Cohorting is the practice of grouping persons with like infections or symptoms together in order to reduce transmission to others.

CULTURE AND SENSITIVITY: Culture and sensitivity refer to laboratory tests that are used to identify the type of microorganism causing an infection and compounds that the identified organism is sensitive and resistant to. In the case of bacteria, this approach permits the selection of antibiotics that will be most effective in dealing with the infection.

GRAM-NEGATIVE BACTERIA: All types of bacteria identified and classified as a group that does not retain crystal-violet dye during Gram's method of staining.

GRAM-POSITIVE BACTERIA: All types of bacteria identified and classified as a group that retains crystal-violet dye during Gram's method of staining.

INPATIENT: A patient who is admitted to a hospital or clinic for treatment, typically requiring the patient to stay overnight.

OUTPATIENT: A person who receives health care services without being admitted to a hospital or clinic for an overnight stay.

MINIMAL INHIBITORY CONCENTRATION (MIC): The minimal inhibitory concentration (MIC) refers to the lowest level of an antibiotic that prevents growth of the particular type of bacteria in a liquid food source after a certain amount of time. Growth is detected by clouding of the food source. The MIC is the lowest concentration of the antibiotic at which the no cloudiness occurs.

SEPSIS: Sepsis refers to a bacterial infection in the bloodstream or body tissues. This is a very broad term covering the presence of many types of microscopic disease-causing organisms. Sepsis is also called bacteremia. Closely related terms include septicemia and septic syndrome. According to the Society of Critical Care Medicine, severe sepsis affects about 750,000 people in the United States each year. However, it is predicted to rapidly rise to one million people by 2010 due to the aging U.S. population. Over the decade of the 1990s, the incident rate of sepsis increased over 91%.

cation, which is visible in solution and makes methylene blue a "cation dye." Another common dye, eosin, dissociates into a sodium cation and a visible eosin anion and is an anion dye. Anionic dyes such as eosin interact with the cationic portions of the bacterial protein being identified, while the converse happens with cationic dyes.

The Gram stain, developed in 1884 and named after discoverer Hans Christian Gram (1853–1938) is in a different category from ionic stains. This technique involves first staining bacteria with gentian violet dye, then washing the stained bacteria with iodine solution, and then with ethyl alcohol. For "Gram-negative" bacteria, the second and third steps wash away the dye, while "Gram-positive" bacteria remain colored after washing with iodine and alcohol. The final step is to stain the Gram-negative bacteria with a reddish-pink dye that does not stain the Gram-positive bacteria. The Gram-positive bacteria will thus have violet structural features under the microscope, while the Gram-negative bacteria will have pinkish structural features. Whether a bacterium is Gram-positive or Gram-negative is often an indicator or whether the bacteria can be destroyed using a particular antibiotic.

Many antibiotics can kill Gram-positive bacteria, while Gram-negative bacteria resist common antibiotics. Gram-negative bacteria have an extra layer of polysaccharides, proteins, and phospholipids, which blocks many antibiotics from reaching the peptidoglycan cell wall. For example, penicillin works by attacking the cell wall, but is prevented from doing so by this extra layer, making the bacteria penicillin-resistant.

Antimicrobial Susceptibility Testing

The susceptibility methods used by clinical laboratories include the Kirby-Bauer disc diffusion susceptibility test, macrotube dilution susceptibility test, and the microtube dilution test. In the Kirby-Bauer test, disks containing antibiotics are placed over an agar plate inoculated with the organism. The size of the zone of inhibition indicates whether or not the organism is sensitive or resistant to the antibiotic at level normally used (doses). Laboratories report antibiotic sensitivities as "Susceptible," "Intermediate," or "Resistant" as defined by the National Committee on Clinical Laboratory Standards (NCCLS).

The minimal inhibitory concentration (MIC) is the lowest concentration of the antibiotic (mcg/ml) that will inhibit bacterial growth in vitro, and is correlated with the concentration of the antibiotic achievable in blood.

The MIC is traditionally determined using the macrotube dilution technique in which a standard inoculum is tested against serial dilutions of a particular antibiotic—a time-consuming process. A newer technique uses tiny wells in an automated plastic susceptibility card that are injected with standard dilutions of antimicrobial agents by the manufacturer. The laboratory adds a standard concentration of the organism to the card and the organism is automatically dispersed to all of the wells. After an incubation period of 12–24 hours, the card is machine-read for bacterial growth at hourly intervals and a growth curve for the isolate is calculated for each antibiotic on the plastic card. The antibiotics are grouped according to whether the organism being tested is Gram-positive or Gram-negative, and the antibiotics for the Gram-negative isolate are further grouped according to whether they can be used in an inpatient or outpatient setting depending on whether the patient is in the process of being admitted or discharged from the hospital.

Applications

Depending on MIC results, physicians may change the dosage of a particular antibiotic to be used in treatment, or choose a different antibiotic to treat the infection. For example, a blood-borne *Escherichia coli* infection tested with ampicillin may have a MIC of 2 mcg/ml (sensitive), multiplied by 2–4 times gives 4–8 mcg/ml as a potential peak level of the antibiotic in the blood, which is considerably less than an intravenous representative dose from the patient of 47 mcg/mg. Thus, ampicillin would be expected to provide adequate therapy for the patient.

In a different example of a leg wound tested with ampicillin, a higher MIC of, say, 16 mcg/ml would be correlated with a 32–64 mcg/ml peak blood concentration, which could fall over the range of the representa-

tive intravenous dose of 47 mcg/ml dose of bacteria from the patient. Furthermore, since the patient has a leg wound where the infection is in tissue rather than blood, the concentration of antibiotics in tissue will be lower than in blood. In this case, the physician would consider a higher ampicillin dose or a different antibiotic for treatment.

Impacts and Issues

Culturing and MIC testing are possible for most, but not all, types of bacteria-caused diseases. Infections for which cultures generally cannot be obtained include ear infections, sinusitis, and bronchitis, along with viral infections. For such infections there is a considerable risk of over-prescribing antibiotic treatments that are likely to be inappropriate and ineffective, and there are increasing calls for the distribution of procedures and new guidelines to address this issue.

The timing and choice of antibiotics can be important in treating older adults. For example, in sepsis (a generalized infection in the blood due to microorganisms or toxins) most research suggests that starting with broad-spectrum antibiotics without culturing is beneficial because deaths and long hospital stays are reduced if the initial antibiotic treatment attacks and reduces the infectious agent. Delaying therapy initiation by four or more hours after hospital admission, as could happen with long laboratory testing, is associated with higher mortality. On the other hand, up to 75% of antibiotic use in long-term care may be inappropriate, so strict minimum criteria for initiating antibiotic treatment should be set.

The emergence of resistant bacteria has led to the reliance on the newer class of antibiotics (fluoroquinolones) for relatively routine infections such as community-acquired pneumonia (CAP) in spite of the potential for adverse

IN CONTEXT: REAL-WORLD RISKS

The medical dangers and escalating health care costs associated with antimicrobial resistance led to the formation of a special interagency task force tasked with developing effective plans to combat the problem. Formed in 1999, the Interagency Task Force on Antimicrobial Resistance is co-chaired by the Centers for Disease Control and Prevention (CDC), the Food and Drug Administration (FDA), and the National Institutes of Health (NIH), and also includes the Agency for Healthcare Research and Quality (AHRQ), the Centers for Medicare and Medicaid Services (CMS, formerly the Health Care Financing Administration [HCFA]), the Department of Agriculture (USDA), the Department of Defense (DoD), the Department of Veterans Affairs (DVA), the Environmental Protection Agency (EPA), and the Health Resources and Services Administration (HRSA).

One of the top priorities of the task force is to "conduct a public health education campaign to promote appropriate antimicrobial use as a national health priority."

that show *in vitro* (in the body) potency against given infections when treatment with broad-spectrum antibiotics would provide faster treatment yet would not lead to resistance to the specialized antibiotics.

Furthermore, over-reliance on antibiotics in long-term care facilities and in hospitals can cause health care workers to disregard simple infection control activities such as handwashing, isolation, and cohorting (grouping) of infected patients, skin testing for tuberculosis, and immunization to prevent infection with resistant organisms in the first place.

SEE ALSO *Antibacterial Drugs; Bacterial Disease; Resistant Organisms; Vancomycin-resistant Enterococci.*

BIBLIOGRAPHY

Books

Ryan, Kenneth J. and C. George Ray. *Sherris Medical Microbiology: an Introduction to Infectious Disease.* New York: McGraw-Hill Medical, 2003.

Web Sites

National Center for Biotechnology Information. "Microbiologic Examination." in *Medical Microbiology*, 4th ed., Samuel Baron, ed. <http://www.ncbi.nlm.nih.gov/books/bv.fcgi?rid=mmed.section.5451> (accessed April 2, 2007).

University of Virginia Health Systems. "What is Microbiology?" <http://www.healthsystem.virginia.edu/uvahealth/adult_path/micro.cfm> (accessed April 2, 2007).

Kenneth T. LaPensee

effects. Over-utilization has, in turn, given rise to increasing fluoroquinolone resistance in some geographic regions. Current Infectious Disease Society of America guidelines advise keeping newer fluoroquinolones that are active against *S. pneumoniae* in reserve, while using other antibiotics such as an advanced generation cephalosporin (e.g., cefotaxime) as initial therapy.

This example demonstrates the vicious circle that arises from physicians' reliance upon specialized antibiotics

Cyclosporiasis

Introduction

Cyclosporiasis, (sigh-clo-spore-EYE-uh-sis) also called *Cyclospora*, is an infection caused by the pathogenic protozoan *Cyclospora cayetanensis*. The protozoan is a coccidium (causing disease in the gut) parasite that infects the gastrointestinal (GI) tract. It is spread when humans drink water or eat food that is contaminated with infected feces. The *Cyclospora* needs days or even a week after being passed in a bowel movement to become infectious.

Imported produce, especially raspberries, is most frequently associated with outbreaks of *Cyclospora* infection. *Cyclospora* often infect humans and other animals such as moles, myriapods (small, long arthropods such as centipedes), rodents, and vipers (poisonous snakes). Although still unproven, transmission between humans, and between animals and humans is unlikely. The primary source of the parasite is unknown. The infection sometimes causes diarrhea in travelers visiting foreign countries.

Disease History, Characteristics, and Transmission

According to the Division of Parasitic Diseases within the Centers for Disease Control and Prevention (CDC), the first human case of *Cyclospora* infection was documented in 1979, although it had been recognized as early as 1977. During the mid–1980s, cases frequently were reported. According to the Epidemiology and Disease Control Program (EDCP), large outbreaks were reported in the 1990s and 2000s within the United States and Canada. The first U.S. case occurred in Chicago, Illinois, inside a medical dormitory whose water source became infected. A U.S. epidemic occurred between 1996 and 1997 when basil, lettuce, and raspberries became contaminated. A Canadian epidemic occurred in 1999 when berries became contaminated.

In 2004, a Pennsylvania outbreak happened with basil and snow peas. After the AIDS (acquired immunodeficiency syndrome) epidemic bloomed, reported occurrences of Cyclosporiasis became more frequent.

The *Cyclospora cayetanensis* parasite is a one-celled organism and requires specialized microscopic inspection for identification, often from multiple stool samples. Transmission occurs when an oocyst (a fertilized sex cell) of *C. cayetanensis* is located within contaminated water that is ingested. It enters the small intestine (bowel) and travels to the mucous membrane (the moist lining inside body passages). The oocyst incubates for approximately one week (with a range from one to 14 days). After incubation is complete, the victim begins to experience symptoms of watery bloating, diarrhea, frequent and sometimes large bowel movements, low-grade fever, muscle aches, and stomach cramps. Other diarrhea-caused symptoms include fatigue, appetite and weight loss, and increased gas. However, some people show no symptoms. If not treated, the illness lasts from several days to about one month, sometimes longer. Relapses of the illness often occur.

All humans are susceptible to the infection worldwide. However, people in developing countries are most susceptible. Death rarely occurs, however, death can result in infected people with immunosuppressed systems, such as persons with AIDS. *Cyclospora* affect both sexes, and all ages and races equally, though children in developing countries are especially susceptible, as they are often the primary water carriers for their families.

Scope and Distribution

It is possible for the infection to occur anywhere in the world, although it is often found in underdeveloped or developing countries. It is frequently found (endemic) in Haiti, Nepal, and Peru. It has also been reported from people traveling within India, Indonesia, Mexico, Morocco, Pakistan, Puerto Rico, and Southeastern Asia. When it occurs in the United States, it happens mostly in the warmer months of late spring and summer.

WORDS TO KNOW

COCCIDIUM: Any single-celled animal (protozoan) belonging to the sub-class Coccidia. Some coccidia species can infest the digestive tract, causing coccidiosis.

ENDEMIC: Present in a particular area or among a particular group of people.

FOOD PRESERVATION: The term food preservation refers to any one of a number of techniques used to prevent food from spoiling. It includes methods such as canning, pickling, drying and freeze-drying, irradiation, pasteurization, smoking, and the addition of chemical additives. Food preservation has become an increasingly important component of the food industry as fewer people eat foods produced on their own lands, and as consumers expect to be able to purchase and consume foods that are out of season.

OOCYST: An oocyst is a spore phase of certain infectious organisms that can survive for a long time outside the organism and so continue to cause infection and resist treatment.

PROTOZOA: Single-celled animal-like microscopic organisms that live by taking in food rather than making it by photosynthesis and must live in the presence of water. (Singular: protozoan.) Protozoa are a diverse group of single-celled organisms, with more than 50,000 different types represented. The vast majority are microscopic, many measuring less than 5 one-thousandth of an inch (0.005 millimeters), but some, such as the freshwater Spirostomun, may reach 0.17 inches (3 millimeters) in length, large enough to enable it to be seen with the naked eye.

■ Treatment and Prevention

The diagnosis is oftentimes difficult because oocysts in feces and water are difficult to identify. Stool specimens are used; frequently, several specimens are taken over numerous days. The EDCP suggests that physicians specifically request a *Cyclospora* test in order to assure accurate laboratory results. The polymerase chain reaction-based DNA (deoxyribonucleic acid) test and acid-fast staining test are often used.

Treatment involves antibiotics, often in combinations such as trimethoprim and sulfamethoxazole. Traditional anti-protozoan drugs are usually not effective enough to stop the protozoan. People with compromised immune systems and severe diarrhea require additional supportive treatment.

To prevent its transmission through food, all fruits and vegetables should be washed before consuming. Handwashing before handling or eating food removes most of the parasites. Drinking water suspected to be contaminated, especially from rivers, streams, springs, and other untreated waters, should be avoided in order to prevent cyclosporiasis. Handwashing after using the toilet and changing diapers also prevents transmission of *Cyclospora*.

■ Impacts and Issues

Cyclosporiasis infection is part of a wider problem: emerging widespread foodborne outbreaks on a countrywide and international scale. Foodborne illnesses such as cyclosporiasis continue to increase in numbers and severity as the world rapidly moves toward a global food market. A contaminated food in one part of the world can now lead to an outbreak halfway across the globe in a matter of days.

According to the CDC, better recognition and management of outbreaks of foodborne infections such as those caused by *Cyclospora* are needed. Specifically, this would include: better coordination and action by federal, state, and local agencies; more comprehensive laboratory diagnostic training; structured development of epidemiologic studies; coordination between affected governments and the media; and early and effective involvement of companies involved in the growing, processing, exporting, importing, transporting, and wholesale and retail sales of foods.

Irradiation, the use of ionizing radiation for food pasteurization, is suggested as a way to reduce bacterial and parasitic causes of foodborne diseases. The CDC and World Health Organization and other international groups promote irradiation as a safe and effective method to reduce the risk of infection in globally distributed foods—but the use of ionizing radiation is opposed by some food advocacy groups and research continues.

SEE ALSO *Food-borne Disease and Food Safety; Microorganisms; Travel and Infectious Disease.*

BIBLIOGRAPHY

Books

Arguin, Paul M., Phyllis E. Kozarsky, and Ava W. Navin, eds. *Health Information for International Travel, 2005–2006*. Atlanta, GA: U.S. Department of Health and Human Services, Public Health Service, 2005.

U.S. Food and Drug Administration Center for Food Safety and Applied Nutrition. *Bad Bug Book:*

Foodborne Pathogenic Microorganisms and Natural Toxins Handbook. McLean, VA: International Medical Publishing, Inc., 2004.

Web Sites

Centers for Disease Control and Prevention. "Cyclospora Infection or Cyclosporiasis (sigh–clo–spore–EYE–uh–sis)." <http://www.cdc.gov/ncidod/dpd/parasites/cyclospora/factsht_cyclospora.htm> (accessed March 8, 2007).

Epidemiology and Disease Control Program (EDCP). "Cyclosporiasis Fact Sheet." <http://edcp.org/factsheets/cyclospor.html> (accessed March 8, 2007).

Demographics and Infectious Disease

■ Introduction

Demographic trends (trends in a population's vital statistics) within nations and across national boundaries have a profound effect on the distribution of infectious disease worldwide. Gender, age, the movement of populations due to economic opportunity or to escape conflict, and the sheer density of population relative to the capacity of local ecosystems, civic infrastructure, and public health resources all influence the infectivity and virulence (degree of ability to cause disease) of infectious diseases. Close quartering of a population such as in

refugee camps, prisons, or schools, can also affect the outbreak and spread of infectious disease.

■ History and Scientific Foundations

One clear example of how many of these factors came together at once was the mass exodus of more than a million Kurds from Iraq as they fled their villages under attack from the Iraqi army after the end of the first Gulf

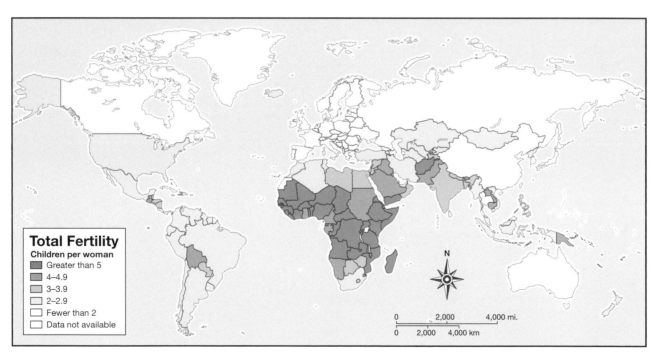

Map representing the average number of children born in each country per woman from 2000 to 2004. Many countries that already bear a high burden from AIDS and other infectious diseases due to a lack of immunization coverage and healthcare infrastructure, along with inadequate sanitation, are also among those with the highest fertility rates. The World Health Organization (WHO) estimates that by the year 2010, half of all deaths in children under age five will occur in Sub-Saharan Africa. *© Copyright World Health Organization (WHO). Reproduced by permission.*

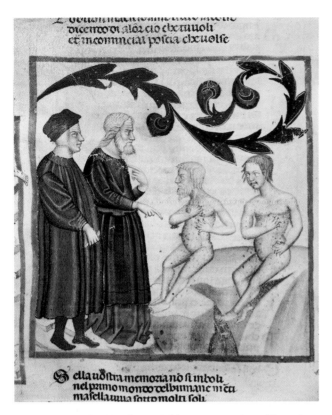

An anonymous drawing from a 16th-century version of Dante's *Divine Comedy* shows Dante (1265–1321) and Virgil (70 BC–19 BC) with people suffering from the plague in Europe. *Erich Lessing/ Art Resource, NY.*

War in 1991. With the absence of sanitary facilities and the crowding together of so many people in a weakened condition, contaminated water supplies from human waste quickly gave rise to an epidemic of cholera, as well as other communicable diseases. More recently, conflict in the Darfur region of Sudan has resulted in the movement of more than one million internally displaced persons who now live in crowded refugee camps where epidemics of typhoid, hepatitis E, cholera, and meningitis have taken hold.

Movement of populations such as migrants or refugees affects the population itself, the populations encountered, and the ecosystem. Each translocated person carries cultural practices, genetic vulnerabilities and resistances to infections, and organisms that have been held at bay by the individual's immunity, but lie dormant and are potentially dangerous to previously unexposed persons. In addition, the moving populations unwittingly transport microbes, animals that are disease vectors (transmitters), and other flora and fauna (plants and animals) that are foreign to the destination ecosystems.

Even when no mass population movements are taking place, the changing age and sex mix of stable populations over time will impact the spread of infectious disease. In other words, the population of potential dis-

ease hosts changes rather than remains stable. These changes affect the patterns of communicable diseases, particularly diseases that are sexually transmitted and that give rise to symptoms in one gender or the other (such as cervical cancer caused by human papilloma virus) or which attack people differentially in different age brackets, such as seasonal influenza, which usually infects older people more often than younger people.

Demographic factors in models of infectious disease

Demographics such as the population density of various age, sex, and ethnic subgroups, along with other statistics that affect patterns of disease can be made into mathematical models that help scientists map and predict infectious disease trends. These models involve various assumptions based on whether people can recover from infections, the rate of disease-related deaths, the development of immunity, and the duration of immunity (whether it is temporary or permanent). These models can also predict infectious disease catastrophes by location. For example, recent models have shown that the persistence (duration) of the AIDS epidemic in many rural African communities has reduced the population size to levels below those that are necessary to maintain the local population of the community. The models showed that AIDS was eliminating adults of reproducing age at a rapid rate.

The simplest models often assume that the total population size is constant. For short-term outbreaks of a disease, simple disease models used to predict the course of an epidemic assume that the population is fixed and closed, and depend only on the disease incidence and prevalence rates, disease duration (persistence), disease death rates, and occurrence of immunity. Models for an endemic disease (one that is naturally occurring in a region such as tuberculosis or malaria) usually assume that births and deaths balance each other so the population size remains unchanged. However, when the disease causes a significant number of deaths, as in the case of AIDS, this assumption is not realistic and more complicated models assuming variable population are needed to predict the course of the epidemic. These sophisticated models incorporate assumptions about both birth and death rates, which can be impacted by the incidence and prevalence of disease as well as other factors. By the same token, population size influences the rapidity with which a disease is spread, with large, dense populations promoting the rapid spread of disease, and small, dispersed populations inhibiting such spread.

■ Applications and Research

Demographics, seasonality, and infectious disease

Seasonality is an important factor in the in the spread of common infectious diseases that most affect the youngest

WORDS TO KNOW

CLUSTER: In epidemiology, cluster refers to a grouping of an infectious disease or foodborn illness that occurs very close in time or place.

DEMOGRAPHICS: The characteristics of human populations or specific parts of human populations, most often reported through statistics.

EPIDEMIOLOGY: Epidemiology is the study of various factors that influence the occurrence, distribution, prevention, and control of disease, injury, and other health-related events in a defined human population. By the application of various analytical techniques including mathematical analysis of the data, the probable cause of an infectious outbreak can be pinpointed.

HERD IMMUNITY: Herd immunity is a resistance to disease that occurs in a population when a proportion of them have been immunized against it. The theory is that it is less likely that an infectious disease will spread in a group where some individuals are less likely to contract it.

INCIDENCE: The number of new cases of a disease or injury that occur in a population during a specified period of time.

PERSISTENCE: Persistence is the length of time a disease remains in a patient. Disease persistence can vary from a few days to life-long.

PREVALENCE: The actual number of cases of disease (or injury) that exist in a population.

VIRULENCE: Virulence is the ability of a disease organism to cause disease: a more virulent organism is more infective and liable to produce more serious disease.

and oldest demographic groups (school children and the elderly). Illnesses such as influenza, measles, chickenpox, and pertussis (whooping cough) are all more prevalent at certain times of the year. Seasonality is a particularly important factor in models that predict whether these recurrent infectious diseases will occur in a given year or skip a year. Seasonal changes in disease transmission patterns and the susceptibility of a population susceptibility to a disease (such as attending school or staying inside in close quarters during the winter) can prevent late-peaking diseases (disease epidemics that take a long time to reach peak infectivity) from spreading widely. When this happens, the remaining population is more susceptible to future epidemics because of a lack of herd immunity (when the majority of immunized people in a group give some protection to those that are not immunized).

By analyzing seasonality and how much of the population remains susceptible to a disease, scientists can predict the course of newly emerging and re-emerging diseases, such as West Nile disease, that are brought on by seasonal vectors (transmitters) including mosquitoes or migratory birds.

Population clustering and disease spread

Of course, populations are not distributed uniformly even when they are stable and no significant migration is occurring. Infectious diseases spread in different patterns within a population that is divided into families or other groups, than in a population that consists mostly of people who are living alone. A household constitutes a small population cluster, which is in turn comprised of members that are resistant to the disease, along with members that are susceptible to the disease. An infectious disease spreads quickly and efficiently within the household, but the outbreak lasts longer if it spreads cluster by cluster, or from one household to another.

■ Impacts and Issues

Infectious disease in the elderly

As discussed above, the proportion of children and the elderly in a population is particularly important in the spread of communicable diseases, particularly because both age groups are more likely than the general population to be in very close quarters for extended periods in schools and in hospitals or nursing homes. In children, immune functioning is still developing and they are constantly being exposed to pathogens (disease-causing organisms) that are familiar to adults, but new to them. At the other end of the demographic scale, aging is associated with increased incidence and severity of many infectious diseases, including nosocomial infections (infections that originate in hospitals from contaminated equipment or close proximity to other infected people). This increased risk is due to an age-related decline in the body's immune system function. As the average age of the population increases in industrialized nations, the epidemiology (incidence and prevalence), morbidity (proportion of sick people), mortality (death rate), and needs for preventive action against nosocomial infections in the elderly also increase.

Impact of households on vaccination strategies

When an epidemic of a highly infectious disease is spreading in a community of households, the infection of any member of a household generally results in the infection of all susceptible members of that household. The rapidity of disease spread will thus depend on the household size and the variability of the number of susceptible people per household. If the rate of spread of infection from individual to individual within each household and the spread of infection from household to household are calculated, the rate and pattern of spread of the disease can be put into a mathematical model by public health scientists. This model can be used to calculate the levels of immunity that will be needed to prevent major epidemics in the community. It can also be used to evaluate alternative vaccination strategies that could immunize the same number of individuals.

For a community with households of approximately equal size (as seen in many suburban communities in the United States), random vaccination of individuals is better than immunizing all members of a fraction of households that would amount to the same total number of vaccinated people. On the other hand, when households vary widely in size (as seen in many U.S. urban areas) vaccinating all members of large households can slow down the spread of the epidemic more rapidly than would the vaccination of an equal number of randomly selected individuals. This is because disease transmission within these large households is easier than in the general community. Such epidemic spread models can also be used for a community of households with schools or day care centers. Immunizing every child within the school or day care center will be more effective than randomly immunizing an equal number of children in the community because the schools and day care centers are similar to very large households in which disease spread among many susceptible children is made easy by their close quarters.

Demographic characteristics of populations strongly determine the rate and extent of infectious disease distribution and spread. These demographic characteristics are in turn profoundly influenced by the processes of economic development, globalization, migration, and war. Although population demographics and patterns of infectious disease are in continual flux (change), they are rarely susceptible to policy-motivated human inter-

vention. Rather, they are all aspects of the evolution of human cultures, which are intimately interconnected with evolving technology and commerce. The tools of epidemiological models that use demographic factors to help forecast the spread of infectious disease will constantly need to be updated as population characteristics change with increasing velocity in the years and decades ahead.

SEE ALSO *Economic Development and Infectious Disease; Public Health and Infectious Disease.*

BIBLIOGRAPHY

Books

Connolly, M.A. *Communicable Disease Control in Emergencies: A Field Manual.* Geneva: World Health Organization, 2006.

Daly, D.J., and J. Gani. *Epidemic Modeling: An Introduction.* New York, Cambridge, 2001.

Jamison, Dean T., ed., et al. *Disease and Mortality in Sub-Saharan Africa.* New York: World Bank Publications, 2006.

Periodicals

Pramodh, Nathaniel. "Limiting the Spread of Communicable Diseases Caused by Human Population Movement." *Journal of Rural and Remote Environmental Health.* (2003): 2(1), 23–32.

Stone L., R. Olinky, A. Huppert. "Seasonal Dynamics of Recurrent Epidemics." *Nature.* (March 29, 2007): 533–6.

Web Sites

Science Blog. "Web Game Provides Breakthrough in Predicting Spread of Epidemics." <http://www.scienceblog.com/cms/web_game_provides_breakthrough_in_predicting_spread_of_epidemics_9874> (accessed May 30, 2007).

Kenneth T. LaPensee

Dengue and Dengue Hemorrhagic Fever

■ Introduction

If all of the infectious diseases of mankind were listed in order of incidence, dengue (DEN-gay) fever would clearly rank among the top ten—rivaling chickenpox, influenza, and urinary tract infection. Unfortunately, diseases that occur in tropical areas often acquire exotic names that are obscure and irrelevant to Western cultures. Thus, dengue is thought to derive from the Swahili *dinga*, meaning a seizure or cramp caused by evil spirits. Other diseases which bear such names are Chikungunya and O'nyong nyong.

■ Disease History, Characteristics, and Transmission

Historically, Dengue appears to have originated in the Old World. The disease was first reported in the Caribbean-Latin American region in 1827 (Virgin Islands), presumably imported with African slaves. A second pandemic during 1848–1850 involved Cuba and New Orleans; and a third pandemic struck the region during 1979–1980.

The fact that dengue is not exclusively a "tropical" phenomenon is well illustrated by the American experience with the disease. Dengue was first reported in the

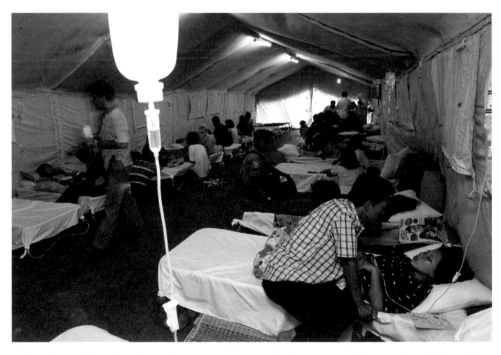

Indonesians suffering from dengue fever receive treatment in the tent of a military-run hospital in the West Java province in 2004. *Beawlharta/Reuters/Corbis.*

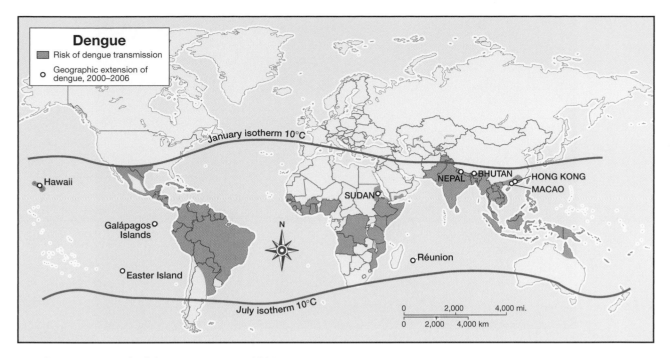

Map showing areas at risk of dengue transmission, 2006.   © *Copyright World Health Organization (WHO). Reproduced by permission.*

United States in 1827, and caused a number of massive outbreaks in Louisiana, Hawaii (50,000 cases in 1903) and Texas (500,000 cases in 1922).

Dengue virus was first isolated in Africa during 1964 to 1968, in Nigeria; however, surveys suggest that the disease is common in certain areas of West Africa, and probably East Africa as well. It is suggested that many cases are misdiagnosed as malaria. Although the disease had been relatively rare in Australia, as many as 800 cases per year are now reported in that country.

The virus that causes dengue is one of 19 Flaviviruses that infect humans. Flaviviruses account for 20 percent of all infectious virus species. Other Flaviviruses include the agents of Hepatitis C, West Nile fever, Japanese encephalitis, and yellow fever. Only 29 percent of virus diseases are acquired through the bites of mosquitoes; however, 53 percent of Flaviviruses are transmitted in this manner. A variety of mosquito species serve as vectors (transmitters) of Flaviviruses that cause dengue, most belonging to the species *Aedes*. Although dengue is almost exclusively a human disease, natural infection of monkeys has been reported in Asia.

In most cases, dengue is a self-limiting flulike illness. Two to fifteen days following the bite of a mosquito, patients experience fever with varying combinations of headache, retro-orbital (around the eyes) pain, myalgia (muscle aches), arthralgia (joint pain), rash, and leukopenia (low white cell count). Occasionally a "saddleback" fever pattern is evident, with a drop after a few days and rebounding within 24 hours. The pulse rate is often rela-

tively slow in relation to the degree of fever. Conjunctival redness (red eyes) and sore throat may occur, often with enlargement of regional lymph nodes. A rash appears in as many as 50 percent of persons with dengue, either early in the illness with flushing or mottling, or between the second and sixth day as a florid red rash that spreads out from the center of the body. The rash fades after two to three days.

Symptoms generally resolve within 2 to 7 days, with no long term residual effects; however, significant depression may occur and persist for several months.

In a small percentage of persons, dengue fever may evolve into a severe and even life-threatening illness: dengue hemorrhagic fever (DHF) or dengue shock syndrome (DSS). Over 700,000 cases of DHF and 21,345 deaths were reported worldwide during 1956 to 1980; and over 1.2 million cases of DHF and 15,940 deaths during the five-year span from 1986 to 1990.

DHF is characterized by initial symptoms of dengue fever, in addition to bleeding tendencies such as petechiae (tiny reddish skin lesions associated with blood vessel injury) or ecchymoses (spontaneous bruises related to blood leakage). In some cases, overt bleeding occurs from the nose, mouth, stomach, colon, or other sites. The blood platelet count is low (less than 100,000 per cubic millimeter) and the red blood cell concentration increases as a result of fluid leakage from the circulatory system. DSS is characterized by the findings of DHF, in addition to signs of shock: low blood pressure, cold clammy skin, and mental obtundation (dullness).

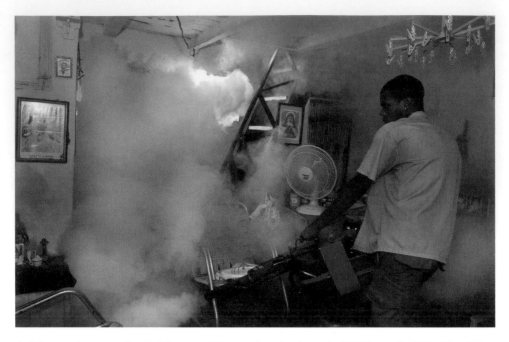

A Cuban worker sprays chemical fogger to kill mosquitoes in a house in Old Havana in 2005. After Cuban authorities initially denied dengue fever was a problem in Cuba, they began a campaign to control and prevent the spread of the disease by mosquitoes. *© Alejandro Ernesto/EFE/epa/Corbis.*

Scope and Distribution

Dengue is endemic (occurs naturally) in at least 115 countries, with over 2.5 billion persons at risk. Each year, an estimated 50 million to 100 million people are infected, most in Southeast Asia and Latin America. Approximately 30,000 to 50,000 persons die of dengue in any given year.

In recent years, most of the 100 or so cases reported annually in the U.S. have been acquired overseas; however, an outbreak of 122 cases was reported in Hawaii during 2001–2002, and 10–40 cases of local infection are reported in the southern border area of Texas each year.

Treatment and Prevention

Although few laboratories are equipped to cultivate the virus of dengue, a variety of rapid tests are available for diagnosis through identification of antibodies which appear during the course of illness. There is no specific drug therapy for dengue, and the development of effective vaccines has been hampered by the need to include all four viral types in any preparation, with a theoretical risk that the body might recognize the vaccine as dengue fever, and react with DHF/DSS when the person is later exposed to the native viruses.

Because the major damage in DHF/DSS is related to fluid loss, persons with these complications generally respond to intravenous fluid replacement of blood vol-ume. Isolation precautions are not necessary; however, steps should be taken to exclude mosquitoes from patient treatment areas in endemic areas.

Impacts and Issues

In recent years, *Aedes albopictus* (the Asian tiger mosquito) has gained prominence as a dengue vector in many parts of the world, largely as the result of dissemination of these insects in pools of water which accumulate in automobile tires transported on commercial ships. In addition, the spread of dengue fever is attributed to a rapid rise in the populations of cities in the developing world where dengue vectors thrive due to inadequate water storage and inadequate access to sanitation.

DHF and DSS appear to be related to immunological "over-reaction" in a person who develops dengue more than once in their lifetime. There are four serotypes (strains, or types) of Dengue virus, and sequential outbreaks in any given country may involve more than one serotype. Thus, if a person is infected with dengue type-1, and infected later in life (or during a later trip to a tropical area) with dengue type-2, his immunological experience from the first attack may prime him for a severe systemic (throughout the body) response to the new infection. As such, anyone who anticipates travel to an endemic country, or presents with signs suggestive of DHF/DSS, should be questioned regarding previous travel and experience with dengue.

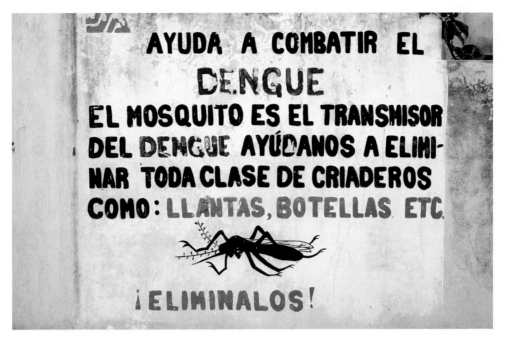

A sign posted in Mexico warns people of an outbreak of dengue fever. The posting calls on residents to help fight dengue by eliminating water sources where mosquitoes breed. © *BIOS Gunther Michel/Peter Arnold, Inc.*

■ Primary Source Connection

In tropical cities, crowded conditions with little sanitation infrastructure can lead to an outbreak of dengue fever during the rainy season. In the following newspaper article, the author Adisti Sukma Sawitri describes the conditions of one neighborhood in west Jakarta, Indonesia, as it was in the midst of a dengue outbreak in early 2007 that eventually resulted in over 13,000 cases of dengue fever and 45 deaths. Sawitri is a journalist for the *Jakarta Post*.

Officials Blame Poor Hygiene on Dengue Rise

Rusmiyati, a matron at Tarakan Hospital in Central Jakarta, has routinely requested leave in the first quarter of the year, after most of her friends go on holiday.

It is a wish that has never been granted because the children's ward she supervises is always full at that time with dengue fever patients from low-income families, who are treated for free at city-run hospitals like Tarakan.

"Dengue patients come and go so fast from January to March every year. I can hardly remember the names of the patients who died in my ward last week," she told *The Jakarta Post* on Thursday in her office as she leafed through the patient record book.

This month, the number of dengue cases escalated by the dozen—even by the hundred—each day, reaching 1,240 with six fatalities as of Tuesday, three of whom died in Tarakan.

The rapid increase in cases does not say much for the administration's fumigation and cleanup efforts.

There is still a high prevalence of dengue infection in many districts of the city, particularly those in South and East Jakarta.

Rosanti, a resident of Rawa Lele subdistrict in West Jakarta, who was admitted to the hospital with dengue three days ago, was surprised to find four of her neighbors in the same ward.

"We live in neighboring units," she said.

Rosanti said they had chosen the hospital, despite it being a long way from home, because it offered free treatment and quality medicines.

The administration offers free dengue treatment at 17 hospitals in the city.

However, many of them—including Tarakan, Koja in North Jakarta and Fatmawati in South Jakarta, receive more than their fair share of patients due to their location.

Jakarta Health Agency deputy head Salimar Salim said the constant stream of dengue cases was the result of longer transition periods between the rainy and dry seasons in the past four years.

WORDS TO KNOW

ENDEMIC: Present in a particular area or among a particular group of people.

SEROTYPE: A serotype is a sub-group of microorganisms that have a common set of antigen proteins on their cell surfaces.

VECTOR: Any agent, living or otherwise, that carries and transmits parasites and diseases. Also, an organism or chemical used to transport a gene into a new host cell.

of dengue cases and the resurgence of bird flu in the city exposed the low hygiene standards that many residents had as disease outbreaks tended to be associated with slum areas.

He said the time was ripe for the administration to make a bylaw on environmental standards in the city.

"We have to be more disciplined about hygiene. It is time to punish those who have filthy houses or pollute the environment."

Adisti Sukma Sawitri

SAWITRI, ADISTI SUKMA. "OFFICIALS BLAME POOR HYGIENE ON DENGUE RISE." *JAKARTA POST* (JANUARY 26, 2007).

See Also *Climate Change and Infectious Disease; Host and Vector; Mosquito-borne Diseases; Tropical Infectious Diseases.*

BIBLIOGRAPHY

Books

Speilman, Andrew, and Michael D'Antonio. *Mosquito: A Natural History of Our Most Persistent and Deadly Foe.* New York: Hyperion, 2001.

Web Sites

Centers for Disease Control and Prevention. "Dengue Fever." <http://www.cdc.gov/ncidod/dvbid/dengue/index.htm> (accessed May 25, 2007).

World Health Organization. "Dengue and Dengue Hemorrhagic Fever." <http://www.who.int/mediacentre/factsheets/fs117/en/> (accessed May 25, 2007).

Stephen A. Berger

She said that as a result, mosquito breeding was almost continuous.

People's poor living conditions, she added, also contributed to the mounting number of cases.

"People may clean up their houses and their gutters but there's a mound of garbage only meters away from their house. This too can potentially be a nesting place for mosquitoes after it rains."

The *Aedes aegypti* mosquito can fly 100 meters away from where it breeds and spread the fever, she added.

Efforts to curb dengue, Salimar said, required commitment from all levels of the community as well as the administration.

The head of City Council Commission E for social welfare, Dani Anwar, said the rapid growth in the number

Developing Nations and Drug Delivery

■ Introduction

In the developed world, access to medicines is taken for granted, despite ongoing debate over the price of certain drugs. However, around one-third of the world's population lacks access to essential medicines, such as antibiotics, painkillers, and drugs for HIV/AIDS, malaria, and leishmaniasis. In parts of Africa and Asia, this figure can rise to 50% of the population. Even if the drugs are available, people may be unable to afford to pay for them, or they may be of substandard or counterfeit quality, or improperly stored.

There have been some concerted efforts in recent years to improve the delivery of drugs to developing countries, led by the international humanitarian aid organization Médecins sans Frontières (MSF) and the World Health Organization (WHO). Not only do developing countries need access to essential medicines, they also need to know how to use them to gain maximum benefit.

■ History and Scientific Foundations

An early example of how to improve drug delivery in developing countries involved the treatment of river blindness (oncocerciasis) from 1989. The African Program for

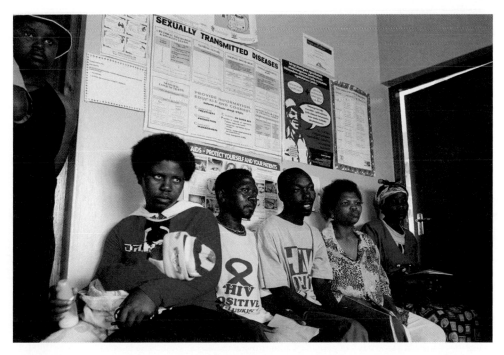

HIV-positive patients wait to see a nurse at an AIDS clinic in South Africa. © *Gideon Mendel/Corbis.*

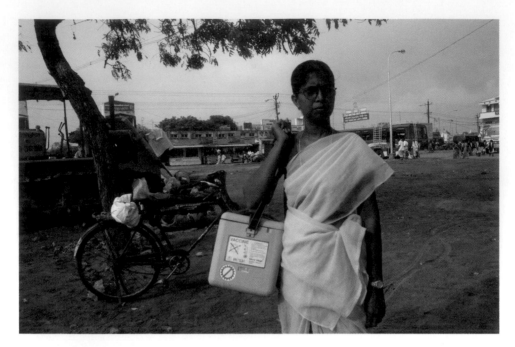

A village nurse carries a "vaccine bag," a suitcase that keeps vaccines cold, near Tamil Nadu in India.   © *Pallava Bagla/Corbis.*

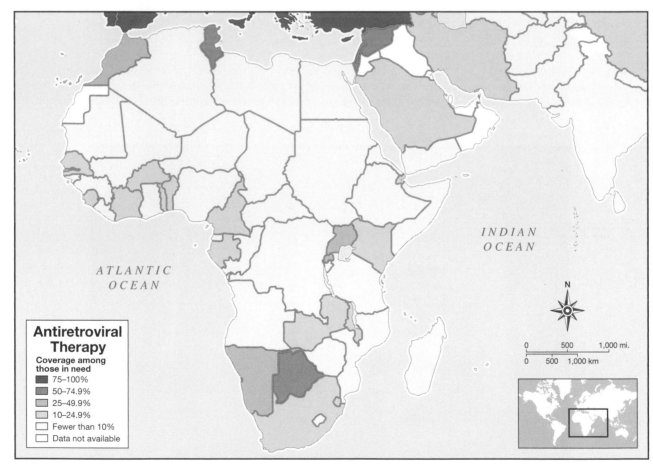

Map of Africa showing the estimated percentage of people on antiretroviral therapy among those in need as of June 2005.   © *Copyright World Health Organization (WHO). Reproduced by permission.*

Oncocerciasis (APOC) grew out of this and was focused upon distribution of the drug ivermectin, which is known to be effective against the disease. The drug is donated by Merck & Co., the company which discovered it. To date, the APOC has protected more than 600,000 people from blindness and reclaimed more than 62 million acres (25 million hectares) of previously infested land for resettlement and agricultural cultivation.

One major guidance document for drug delivery in developing countries is the WHO's List of Essential Medicines, which was first established in 1977. This helps countries to select the appropriate medicines for their public health priorities, according to the best scientific evidence on quality, safety, and efficacy. It also provides guidance to the pharmaceutical industry on the global need for medicines.

■ Applications and Research

The WHO also has guidelines on donation of medicines, to try to ensure these are of good enough quality to be used. Some pharmaceutical companies donate medicines in accordance with these guidelines. They may also have other arrangements to try to improve access to, for example, HIV/AIDS drugs. For instance, they may choose not to take out patent protection in less developed countries, or not to take action against competitors making generic versions of their drugs.

Two organizations which make major contributions to the delivery of drugs in developing countries are MSF and the International Network for the Rational Use of Drugs (INRUD). In 1999, MSF launched its Campaign for Access to Essential Medicines with the aim of improving the global availability of drugs for the treatment of infectious diseases like malaria and tuberculosis (TB). The campaign aims to find ways of lowering the price of essential medicines and bring certain cheap and effective drugs back into production. MSF is also pushing for more research into malaria, TB, sleeping sickness, and leishmaniasis.

INRUD was established in 1989 to develop strategies to improve the way drugs are prescribed, dispensed, and used, trying to therefore address the misuse of scarce resources in developing countries. The network comprises 23 groups, 18 from Africa, Asia, and Latin America, and others from the WHO, Harvard Medical School, and various other academic groups.

Most of the effort in improving drug delivery in developing countries has been focused on the major infectious diseases. In malaria, for instance, MSF has been persuading governments to consider funding the artemisinin-based combination therapy favored by the WHO. This will help address the growing problem of chloroquine resistance. Although chloroquine is relatively cheap, it will not be effective in the areas where the malaria parasites are resistant—therefore, there is a need for alternative drugs to be made available.

WORDS TO KNOW

ANTIRETROVIRAL (ARV) THERAPY: Treatment with antiretroviral (ARV) drugs prevents the reproduction of a type of virus called a retrovirus. The human immunodefiency virus (HIV), which causes acquired immunodeficiency syndrome (AIDS, also cited as acquired immune deficiency syndrome), is a retrovirus. These ARV drugs are therefore used to treat HIV infections. These medicines cannot prevent or cure HIV infection, but they help to keep the virus in check.

PARASITE: An organism that lives in or on a host organism and that gets its nourishment from that host. The parasite usually gains all the benefits of this relationship, while the host may suffer from various diseases and discomforts, or show no signs of the infection. The life cycle of a typical parasite usually includes several developmental stages and morphological changes as the parasite lives and moves through the environment and one or more hosts. Parasites that remain on a host's body surface to feed are called ectoparasites, while those that live inside a host's body are called endoparasites. Parasitism is a highly successful biological adaptation. There are more known parasitic species than nonparasitic ones, and parasites affect just about every form of life, including most all animals, plants, and even bacteria.

RESISTANT ORGANISM: Resistant organisms are bacteria, viruses, parasites, or other disease-causing agents that have stopped responding to drugs that once killed them.

Leishmaniasis, a group of parasitic diseases which is spread by sandflies, can reach epidemic proportions in countries like Sudan and Bangladesh. It can be very difficult to treat and resistance is developing to existing drugs. Therefore, research efforts need to be focused upon developing new and more effective drugs. Sleeping sickness, another parasitic disease, is common in many parts of Africa and is often fatal if not treated. Melarsoprol, the standard treatment for sleeping sickness, appears to be losing its effectiveness, according to clinical trials carried out by WHO. Alternatives now preferable include eflornithine and nifurtimox.

IN CONTEXT: DISEASE IN DEVELOPING NATIONS

According to the World Health Organization (WHO), more than fourteen million people die in developing countries each year due to curable diseases (such as diarrheal diseases, tuberculosis, and malaria). The HIV/AIDS epidemic is one example of how access to affordable drugs in impoverished nations, a key component in disease intervention, is complicated by trade restrictions, policy, and the interests of the pharmaceutical industry.

Brazil's National AIDS Program (NAP) is regarded as a successful model of combating the HIV/AIDS epidemic. Since its inception, HIV death rates in Brazil have dropped fifty percent. Despite spending $232 million by 2001 to implement this national health initiative, Brazil has estimated a savings of more than $1.1 billion in healthcare costs. Many researchers urge immediate action using this model of intervention in other developing nations in Asia and Sub-Saharan Africa. However, others are more cautious and argue that a methodical approach (slower to enact) is necessary to implement a system that is sustainable and effective for the long term. Often, developing countries lack the resources and infrastructure to assure adequate delivery of the drugs to the population targeted for prevention and treatment. Factors such as intellectual property rights and trade policy further cloud the issue. With a market worth more than $65 billion per year, some human rights organizations ask why drug companies aren't investing more research and development dollars where it's needed most, on diseases that primarily affect poor nations.

Health disparities are exacerbated as this disease continues to thrive in marginalized populations (i.e. developing countries, drug users, the poor, rural areas, and minorities). HIV infection in American infants has nearly vanished due to prophylactic (preventative) therapy with antiretroviral (ARV) drugs. In North America and Europe, death rates within ten years of diagnosis for those with HIV have dropped almost eighty percent with ARV use. However, in developing countries, of the six million in need of treatment, only 400,000 actually received ARV therapy in 2003. Fifty percent of the population requiring treatment is located in sub-Saharan Africa and India. Moreover, most of the fourteen million HIV/AIDS orphans in the world reside in Africa. Without timely intervention, this figure is estimated to climb as high as twenty-five million by the year 2010. According to the WHO, "immense advances in human well-being co-exist with extreme deprivation. In global health, we are witnessing the benefits of new medicines and technologies. But there are unprecedented reversals. Life expectancies have collapsed in some of the poorest countries to half the level of the richest—attributable to the ravages of HIV/AIDS in parts of sub-Saharan Africa and to more than a dozen 'failed states.'"

In 2003, UNAIDS established a Global Reference Group on HIV/AIDS and Human Rights. The result is that access to HIV/AIDS therapy is now a human rights issue (as well as a financially sound strategy). In the end, an integrated approach is needed using medical, structural, and cultural interventions, with the cooperation of politicians, governments, private industry, and others.

■ Impacts and Issues

It is now well established that antiretroviral (ARV) therapy for HIV/AIDS is effective treatment, enabling people to live with the condition rather than almost inevitably dying from it. Therefore, improving access to ARV for patients in developing countries has become a top priority.

A program begun by MSF in 2003 showed that giving ARV therapy in even the poorest countries of the world was feasible; people adhered to the complex treatment regimes and benefited from them, just as HIV/AIDS patients in the West did. Therefore, the UN World Summit in 2005 made a pledge to achieve universal access to ARV therapy by 2010. However, there is some way to go before this is achieved. As of December 2006, only two million out of seven million people in need of treatment were actually receiving ARV drugs.

Fortunately, the price of ARV drugs has fallen sharply in developing countries—from several thousand dollars for a year of treatment, to just a few hundred dollars at most and possibly as low as 150 dollars. One of the main reasons for this has been the relaxing of patent rules in certain places to allow for the production of cheap, generic ARV drugs. Funding to support the infrastructure needed to provide the drugs and monitor their

use has come from organizations such as the Global Fund for AIDS, TB and Malaria, the U.S. President's Emergency Fund for AIDS Relief, the World Bank, governments in developed countries, and various nongovernmental organizations.

There have been many challenges involved in trying to get ARVs to those who need them. For instance, there must be a reliable supply chain from the factory where the drug is manufactured to the patient, as the drugs must be taken every day. In many developing countries, transport and communication systems are chronically weak. The funding organizations have been trying to address this by commissioning experts in supply chain management to work in this area. Efforts are also being made to increase the number of health workers in areas severely affected by HIV/AIDS—both by recruiting trained volunteers from developed countries and by training local people.

Today, many developing countries have their own policies that are intended to make essential medicines available to their populations—an approach strongly encouraged by the WHO. These policies also focus on how to distribute drugs to where they are needed and how the safety of medicines can be guaranteed. Pharmaceutical pricing is a complex issue. Companies cannot necessarily be expected to follow the Merck ivermectin example and distribute drugs free, when they have to take their shareholders' interests into account. One way around this is for developing countries to establish their own pharmaceutical industries, focusing upon making cheaper generic copies of essential drugs.

Supplying drugs to developing countries is just one aspect of ensuring universal access to medicine. Education is also needed in the best way of using these medicines and the local infrastructure must be improved to ensure a reliable supply chain. Standardizing the quality of the medicines and their secure storage are also current challenges.

SEE ALSO *African Sleeping Sickness (Trypanosomiasis); AIDS (Acquired Immunodeficiency Syndrome); Leishmaniasis; Malaria; Médecins Sans Frontières (Doctors Without Borders).*

BIBLIOGRAPHY

Web Sites

Avert: Averting HIV and AIDS. "Providing Drug Treatment for Millions." April 19, 2007. <http://www.avert.org/drugtreatment.htm> (accessed May 26, 2007).

INRUD. "International Network for the Rational Use of Drugs." <http://www.inrud.org> (accessed May 26, 2007).

Médicins sans Frontières. "Campaign for Access to Essential Medicines." <http://www.accessmedmsf.org> (accessed May 26, 2007).

World Health Organization. "WHO Model List of Essential Medicines." April 2007. <http://www.who.int/medicines/publications/EML15.pdf> (accessed May 26, 2007).

Susan Aldridge

Diphtheria

■ Introduction

Diphtheria is an acute infectious illness affecting the throat and tonsils. In severe cases, suffocation may result and there may be complications involving the heart and nervous system. Diphtheria is caused by the bacterium *Corynebacterium diphtheriae*. In the past, diphtheria was a major killer, with children being especially susceptible. The introduction of mass immunization has made the disease rare in the industrialized world. However, immunity to diphtheria is lost over time. Those living in stable countries with high standards of public hygiene are unlikely to be at risk. The same cannot be said when health and political systems break down, or when childhood immunization is not universal. The re-emergence of diphtheria in the former Soviet Union in the 1990s resulted from a combination of these factors. The re-introduction of mass immunization eventually brought this epidemic under control. However, diphtheria remains a threat in countries where overcrowding, unsanitary conditions, and low levels of immunization are a fact of everyday life.

■ Disease History, Characteristics, and Transmission

C. diphtheriae is a Gram-positive bacillus. Bacilli are a group of bacteria characterized by their rodlike shape; Gram-positive refers to the way certain bacteria absorb

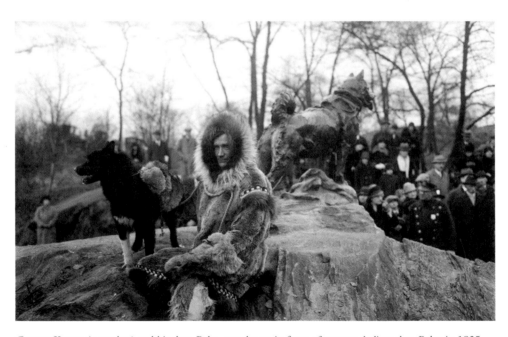

Gunnar Kasson (a musher) and his dog, Balto, are shown in front of a statue dedicated to Balto in 1925. Kasson and his team of dogs, led by Balto, braved blizzard conditions to bring serum to Nome, Alaska, by sled to help townspeople who were suffering from diphtheria. Their efforts saved many lives. © *Bettmann/Corbis.*

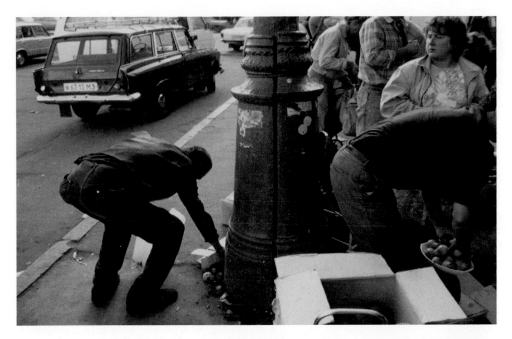

A man picks up discarded fruit in Moscow during a diphtheria epidemic in 1993. Peaking in 1995, the outbreak led to over 140,000 cases and 4,000 deaths in the former Soviet Republics. The epidemic was contained by the late 1990s due to widespread vaccination campaigns and improved economic conditions that allowed for better sanitation and public health measures. *© Keerle Georges De/Corbis SYGMA.*

stains applied for microscopic study of the organism. Most strains of *C. diphtheriae* produce a potent toxin that is responsible for the complications of diphtheria. There are two forms of the disease—respiratory diphtheria, which is the more common, and cutaneous diphtheria. The symptoms of respiratory diphtheria include painful tonsillitis and/or pharyngitis—inflammation of tonsils and/or throat. The voice may be hoarse and fever is often present. What distinguishes diphtheria from other throat infections is the presence of a pseudomembrane, a thick, bluish white or gray covering on the throat or tonsils that may develop greenish black patches. The pseudomembrane develops when the *C. diphtheriae* toxin kills cells within the mucous membrane lining the throat and tonsils. The membrane may spread downwards and can interfere with breathing, causing suffocation. At the same time, the neck tends to swell, giving the patient a characteristic "bull neck" appearance.

In 10 to 20% of cases, the toxin spreads to the heart and the peripheral nervous system. It can cause myocarditis, an inflammation of the heart muscle and heart valves, which may lead to heart failure in later life. In the nervous system, diphtheria toxin can cause paralysis, which could lead to respiratory failure. Even with prompt treatment, the death rate of respiratory diphtheria is 5 to 10%. Diphtheria tends to be more severe in children under five and in adults over 40.

Cutaneous diphtheria occurs when the bacterium infects bites or rashes and is more common in tropical regions. Again, a pseudomembrane forms at the site of the infection, and ulcers usually develop on the skin. However, the complications associated with respiratory diphtheria are far less common in the cutaneous form of the disease.

Diphtheria usually is transmitted by contact with droplets from the upper respiratory tract that are propelled into the air by the coughs and sneezes of infected individuals. It is highly infectious. People who are untreated remain infectious for two to three weeks. *C. diphtheriae* can also be spread by contaminated objects or food.

■ Scope and Distribution

Diphtheria was a major child killer in the eighteenth and nineteenth centuries. Now, thanks to mass immunization, it is rare in the United States and Western Europe. Before immunization there were 100 to 200 cases of diphtheria per 100,000 of the U.S. population; now there are only 0.001 cases per 100,000 of the population. In 1942, the year when immunization was introduced in the United Kingdom, there were 60,000 cases of diphtheria a year, of which around 4,000 proved fatal. Between 1937 and 1938 diphtheria was second only to pneumonia as a cause of death in childhood. With levels of immunization in the U.K. now reaching 94%, presently there are only very occasional cases. Several European countries have not seen a single case of diphtheria for many years.

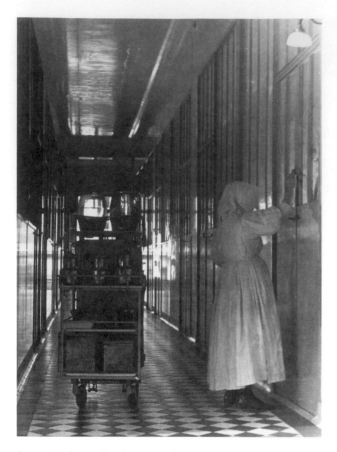

A nurse is shown distributing meals in the diphtheria section of the contagious disease hospital at the Pasteur Institute in Paris, France, in 1937. *Time Life Pictures/Getty Images.*

Before the discovery of the vaccine, children were most at risk from diphtheria. Now all ages seem to be at risk and, although the risk is higher among those who have not been vaccinated, cases occur among those who have had the vaccine too, because immunity appears to decline over time. In the United States, Canada, and many countries in Western Europe, childhood vaccination beginning in the 1930s and 1940s led to a rapid reduction in cases. Where diphtheria does occur, it tends to be in an incompletely vaccinated, or unvaccinated person, of low socioeconomic status.

Diphtheria is found in temperate climates. As with any highly infectious disease, diphtheria is more commonly found in areas with poor sanitation and overcrowding. The disease is endemic in the former Soviet Union, the Indian subcontinent, Southeast Asia, and Latin America. In temperate regions, diphtheria is more common in the colder months of the year. In 2000, the World Health Organization (WHO) reported 30,000 cases of diphtheria worldwide, of which 3,000 were fatal.

■ Treatment and Prevention

Since diphtheria is so rare in developed countries, it may be difficult for physicians to recognize when it does occur.

However, the presence of the pseudomembrane, together with heart rhythm abnormalities linked to the toxin, should alert a physician to the possibility of diphtheria. Ideally, the presence of *C. diphtheriae* should be confirmed in the laboratory (it requires special methods for its identification), but this should not delay the start of treatment. Diphtheria is treated with antitoxin, which neutralizes the toxin before it can do too much damage, and antibiotics. The antitoxin, which was discovered in 1888, has saved the lives of many children, since it causes the pseudomembrane to recede dramatically. Diphtheria antitoxin is prepared from the serum of horses that have been immunized against the disease, and it needs to be given within four days of the onset of symptoms. Erythromycin and penicillin are the two most commonly prescribed antibiotics for diphtheria. Hospitalization and isolation are essential when dealing with diphtheria—the latter to prevent others from being exposed to the infection. If breathing is obstructed by the pseudomembrane, a tracheostomy may be needed. This procedure involves cutting an artificial opening in the trachea, or windpipe, and inserting a tube so that the patient can breathe.

Immunization has been shown to be the best way of preventing the spread of diphtheria. A toxoid is an inactivated version of a bacterial toxin. It has been found to give an excellent immune response in diseases where bacterial toxins play an important role, such as diphtheria and tetanus.

Most countries use diphtheria toxoid in combination with tetanus toxoid and pertussis (whooping cough) vaccine (DTP vaccine) to protect children. DTP is given by injection. WHO recommends children receive three separate doses of DTP. One vaccination schedule administers the three primary doses as the age of six, ten, and 14 weeks, with a booster between 18 months and six years of age. However, there is considerable variation between countries as to the vaccine and vaccination schedule used. For example, in the United States the Centers for Disease Control (CDC) recommends the use of DTaP, rather than DTP, as the safer version offering lessened side effects. Some countries have been using a combination vaccine that includes vaccines against diphtheria, tetanus, pertussis, hepatitis B, and pneumonia.

Parents often worry that a vaccine may harm their child, and this is one reason that vaccine coverage is never universal (some parents always opt out). DTP can cause fever shortly after the child receives an injection and some complain of pain, redness, and swelling at the injection site. More severe reactions, such as convulsions or shock, occur occasionally. However, for the vast majority of children, the benefits of DTP far outweigh the risk. DTP is not usually given after six years of age. Older children and adults are offered a tetanus-diphtheria toxoid vaccine (Td) and, in 2005, a combination tetanus, diphtheria, and pertussis vaccine (Tdap) was approved for adolescents and adults in the United States. Booster injections may be needed every ten years

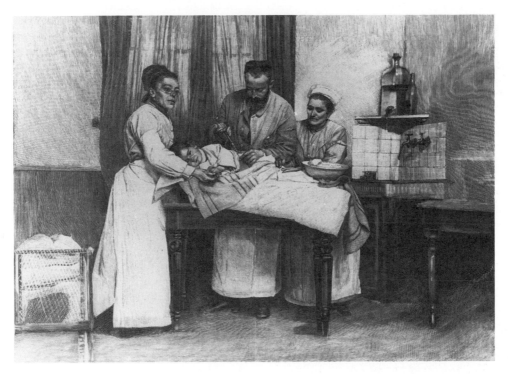

Engraving of a child being inoculated with the diphtheria vaccine in the 1890s. *Snark/Art Resource, NY.*

to maintain immunity, where this might be important (for instance, if traveling to an area where diphtheria is endemic). There is evidence that immunity to diphtheria tends to wane over time.

■ Impacts and Issues

Like cholera, diphtheria has a long history. The disease was first described by the Greek physician Hippocrates (ca. 460–357 BC), and it was also mentioned in ancient Syrian and Egyptian texts. In seventeenth century Spain, epidemic diphtheria was known as "El Garatillo" or "The Strangler." There were also significant epidemics in England in the 1730s and in Western Europe in the second half of the nineteenth century. Diphtheria was known in America from the eighteenth century and reached epidemic proportions in 1735, often killing whole families. At the start of the twentieth century, diphtheria was still one of the leading causes of death among infants and children. When the first data on the disease were gathered, in the 1920s, there were around 150,000 cases and 13,000 deaths each year.

Today, most physicians in the United States will never see a case of diphtheria. Though diphtheria, like tuberculosis, is highly infectious, it is likely to be endemic in less developed countries where there is poverty, overcrowding, malnutrition, and poor sanitation. Mass immunization is known to be an essential tool in the prevention of diphtheria. However, less developed countries tend not to have

the access to vaccine supplies or the health infrastructure to achieve WHO's goal of a 95% immunization rate.

Moreover, diphtheria still has the ability to spread and cause significant illness and death, even in a modern society where it had previously been all but eradicated. This was demonstrated clearly by the outbreaks and epidemics of the disease that occurred in the former Soviet Union in the 1990s. During the first half of the twentieth century, diphtheria rates were high in the Soviet Union; in the 1950s there were around 750,000 cases in Russia alone, but, after this time, the Communist regime of the former Soviet Union developed an excellent record on immunization. By 1976, rates of the disease were practically zero and eradication was thought to be within reach. However, in 1977, the disease began to make a comeback, with rates increasing in all age groups rather than just among children. Rates peaked in 1984 and then began to decline thereafter, although they never returned to the low of 1976. Researchers for the Centers for Disease Control and Prevention (CDC) argue that the military may have contributed to the spread of diphtheria in the 1980s. Military service was universal and led to the housing of recruits, many of whom had not been immunized, in overcrowded conditions. Adult immunity, among those immunized many years earlier, appeared to be declining, accounting for adult cases of diphtheria. The immunization schedule among children was also less intense than previously, in part due to a campaign against immunization that found favor in a population increasingly distrustful of its government.

The breakup of the Soviet Union in the late 1980s and early 1990s was the final event that set the stage for a new wave of diphtheria in the former Soviet Union. In 1990, diphtheria returned to Russia in force. There were over 1,000 cases reported from St Petersburg, Kaliningrad, Orlovskaya, and Moscow. The epidemic grew over the next few years and deaths occurred because of failures in a health care system facing economic crisis. Epidemic diphtheria became established in urban Russia, Ukraine, and Belarus. In 1993, 19,462 cases were reported of which 15,211 were in Russia, an increase of nearly 300% from the previous year. Many of these cases were, again, among adults. This was the first large-scale diphtheria epidemic in a developed country for over three decades. At the peak of the epidemic, in 1995, there were over 50,000 cases reported in the region, compared to only 24 cases in the rest of Europe.

In 1994 and 1995, WHO, the United Nations Children's Fund, other agencies, and governments in the affected countries undertook massive efforts to vaccinate both children and adults. These efforts soon began to bring the epidemic under control, resulting in a 60% drop in cases by 1996. According to WHO data, gathered in 2000, incidence rates of diphtheria in Armenia, Estonia, Lithuania, and Uzbekistan were 0.5 to 1 per 100,000 of the population. In Russia and Tajikistan, rates were as high as 27 to 32 per 100,000 of the population. Fatality rates were 2 to 3% in Russia and Ukraine and 6 to 10% in Armenia, Kazakhstan, Moldova, and Latvia. In Azerbaijan, Georgia, and Turkmenistan the death rate from diphtheria was 17 to 23%. By 2004, the number of cases reported to the WHO European region, which includes the former Soviet Union, was down to 176.

The CDC says that the outbreak of diphtheria in the former Soviet Union shows that adults can become vulnerable to childhood diseases again when immunization does not confer lifelong immunity. This condition applies in any other country where there is mass immunization against diphtheria. However, there have been no similar epidemics anywhere else in the Western world. It was probably the combination of factors in the Soviet Union at the time that set the scene for the epidemic. Added to the decline in both childhood and adult immunity was the political breakup of the Soviet Union and the formation of several new states. Economic pressures led to mass migrations of people from rural areas into the cities in Russia; many failed to find work and ended up sleeping in primitive or crowded conditions. Many diphtheria cases occurred in this group. Refugees fleeing from fighting in Georgia, Armenia, Azerbaijan, and Tajikistan were also at risk. People were on the move in the region on a scale never seen before. This powerful factor—not seen in neighboring nations—probably encouraged the spread of the disease. The success of mass vaccination in controlling the epidemic in the former Soviet Union reconfirms the importance of this primary tool for fighting diphtheria.

A WHO report of a diphtheria outbreak in Afghanistan illustrates the factors that increase the risk of the disease. Between June and August 2003, there were 50 cases of diphtheria, including three deaths, in a resettlement camp for internally displaced people in Kandahar. About 75% of the patients were ages five to 14. A mass immunization campaign for the 40,000 residents of the camp was launched in August 2003. The Ministry of Health was assisted by WHO and several other organizations, such as Médecins sans Frontières-Holland and the Red Cross, in provision of drugs, antitoxin, and vaccine supplies to help bring the outbreak under control.

Lessons learned from Russia and Afghanistan can be applied to other diseases and other countries. Improving living conditions, mass immunization, and establishing a health infrastructure within a stable political system are the ways in which highly infectious diseases can best be controlled.

■ Primary Source Connection

Advances in the treatment of diphtheria and many other infectious diseases (along with advances in the treatment of illnesses such as diabetes) have significantly changed the expectations of parents and communities in countries with advanced health care and public health capacity.

Russell Baker is a Pulitzer Prize-winning writer. The excerpt below is republished from his autobiography and allows readers some insights into the resignation and thinking of a time, less than a century ago in America, when disease "mostly with prayer, and early death was commonplace."

Memoir of a Small-Town Boyhood

As I was growing up, my mother loved to tell me about the happiness of her childhood days and I loved to listen, for I knew only the ruined and colorless landscapes of the Depression, and her talk evoked beautiful pictures of a world that was bright and sunny. But when she got to the part about her father and the inevitable, "Now Papa was a real gentleman," my interest faded. Though he was my grandfather, I couldn't abide his being such a splendid man. I took my revenge by shutting him out of my mind.

It was years before I cared enough to look into the Papa matter. A delightful surprise awaited. The fact was, Papa had not made anything at all of himself, though not for want of trying. When he died at 53, debt-ridden from timber speculation and uninsured out of respect for God, he left his family destitute. My mother had to quit college and go to work. Her education qualified her to teach school, but not for choice assignments. In her middle 20's she came to the Arlington School in the northernmost reaches of Loudoun County, Virginia. A few miles west lay the Blue Ridge, a few miles north, the Potomac River and 400 yards away lay one of the most popular landmarks in the region, a bootleg-whisky still operated by the celebrated anti-Prohibition guerrilla Sam Reever. The dirt road past the school carried a steady traffic of pilgrims in quest of moonshine.

One day, my mother was outside during recess when an old Model T sputtered and died right beside the schoolyard. A lanky, dark-haired young man stepped out and inspected the engine. He opened the tool chest on the fender and took out a wrench and a Mason jar recently filled by Sam Reever. My mother hated whisky and admired men who could leave it alone. What a shame, she thought, for such a nice looking man to be ruining his life with whisky. He looked like a man who might be able to make something of himself if a good woman took him in hand.

When presently my mother had her chance, her first goal was to stop his drinking. But as months passed and the courtship became complicated, her program went awry. And then there was a crisis. She was pregnant.

Out-of-wedlock pregnancies were fairly commonplace in that part of Virginia. They occasioned mild scandal when the news spread, but there was no taint or disgrace if the man "did the right thing" and a marriage ensued. When his mother, Ida Rebecca,

---

IN CONTEXT: REAL-WORLD RISKS

The Coordinating Center for Infectious Diseases/Division of Bacterial and Mycotic Diseases states that diphtheria "circulation appears to continue in some settings even in populations with 80% childhood immunization rates. An asymptomatic carrier state exists even among immune individuals."

Because immunity lessens over time "decennial booster doses are required to maintain protective antibody levels. Large populations of adults are susceptible to diphtheria in developed countries—[and] appear to be increasing in developing countries as well."

SOURCE: *Coordinating Center for Infectious Diseases/Division of Bacterial and Mycotic Diseases, Centers for Disease Control and Prevention (CDC)*

learned of the pregnancy, however, she declared violently against marriage.

Ida Rebecca Baker was a domineering woman, and her 13 sons were trained to obey her. In a normal crisis of this sort, her opposition would have closed the case against the mother-to-be. This time, though, she was pitted against a woman as fierce as she.

In March of 1925, her 11th son, Benjamin, and his schoolteacher, Lucy Elizabeth Robinson, went discreetly down to Washington to be married. I was born uneventfully six months later into the governance of Calvin Coolidge.

My father's decision to defy Ida Rebecca may have been the bravest act of his life. With enough money, he probably would have moved away, put distance between bride and mother. Well, there wasn't enough money. There was almost no money at all. He was a stonemason by trade, but in a region where stone was plentiful, stonemasons were also plentiful and earnings were small. And he was a man who liked a good time. What little he earned went into repairs for the Model T, flings in nearby urban sinks like Lovettsville and Brunswick and the moonshine Sam Reever ladled into Mason jars. During all these years, my father was under a sentence of death. In 1918, he had been drafted by the Army and discharged after five days with papers stating he had "a physical disability." From his childhood, it had been Morrisonville's common knowledge that Benny had "trouble with his kidneys." What the Army doctors found is not clear from the records. Maybe they told him the truth—that he had diabetes—but if so he kept their terrible diagnosis a secret. In 1918, insulin was still unknown. As a 21-year-old diabetic, whether he knew it or not, he was doomed to early death.

The discovery of insulin in 1921 would have lifted that sentence and offered him a long and reasonably healthy life. If he ever learned about insulin, though, he certainly never used it, for the needle required for daily injections was not part of our household goods. Perhaps he didn't know how seriously ill he was, but the state of medicine in Morrisonville must also be allowed for. New medical wonders were slow to reach up the dirt roads of back-country America. Around Morrisonville, grave illness was treated mostly with prayer, and early death was commonplace. Children were carried off by diphtheria, scarlet fever and measles. I heard constantly of people laid low by typhoid or mortally ill with "blood poisoning." Remote from hospitals, people with ruptured appendixes died at home waiting for the doctor to make a house call.

Since antibiotics lay far in the future, tuberculosis, which we called "TB" or "consumption," was almost always fatal. Pneumonia, only slightly less dreaded, took its steady crop for the cemetery each winter. Like croup and whooping cough, it was treated with remedies Ida Rebecca compounded from ancient folk-medicine recipes: reeking mustard plasters, herbal broths, dosings of onion syrup mixed with sugar.

Russell Baker

BAKER, RUSSELL, "MEMOIR OF A SMALL-TOWN BOYHOOD"
THE NEW YORK TIMES. SEPTEMBER 12, 1982.

SEE ALSO *Cholera; Médecins Sans Frontières (Doctors Without Borders).*

BIBLIOGRAPHY

Books

Garrett, Laurie. *The Coming Plague: Newly Emerging Diseases in a World out of Balance.* London: Virago Press, 1995.

Wilson, Walter R., and Merle A. Sande. *Current Diagnosis & Treatment in Infectious Diseases.* New York: McGraw Hill, 2001.

Periodicals

Vitek, C.R., and M. Wharton. "Diphtheria in the Former Soviet Union: Reemergence of a Pandemic Disease." *Emerging Infectious Diseases* 4 (October-December 1998). This article is available online <http://www.cdc.gov/ncidod/eid/vol4no4/vitek.htm>

Web Sites

Health Protection Agency. "Diphtheria." February 2, 2006. <http://www.hpa.org.uk/infections/topics_az/diphtheria/gen_info.htm> (accessed February 16, 2007).

Todar's Online Textbook of Bacteriology. "Diphtheria." <http://textbookofbacteriology.net/diphtheria.html> (accessed February 16, 2007).

World Health Organization. "Diphtheria." <http://www.who.int/topics/diphtheria/en/> (accessed February 16, 2007).

Susan Aldridge

Disinfection

■ Introduction

Disinfection refers to treatments that reduce the numbers of living microorganisms and viruses (which are not considered to be alive, but which can cause disease when they infect a host cell) to a safe level. Disinfection is not intended to kill all the microbes present, which is the process that is called sterilization. Nonetheless, disinfection is a key component in infection control.

Health care facilities maintain three different levels of disinfection, based upon patient care levels and the purpose for which equipment and surfaces are used. High-level disinfection destroys all microorganisms on a surface, with the exception of high numbers of bacte-

rial spores. Intermediate-level disinfection kills *Mycobacterium tuberculosis*, most viruses and fungi, and bacteria, but it does not kill bacterial spores. Low-level disinfection kills most bacteria, certain viruses and fungi, but does not reliably kill bacterial spores or the bacteria that causes tuberculosis.

■ History and Scientific Foundations

Until the middle of the nineteenth century, surgeries and hospitalization frequently resulting in infections.

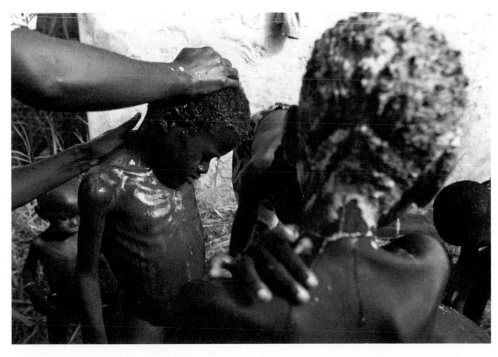

Hutu refugees are bathed with disinfectant soap at a transit camp outside of Kigali, Rwanda, in May 1997. *AP Images.*

WORDS TO KNOW

BIOFILM: Biofilms are populations of microorganisms that form following the adhesion of bacteria, algae, yeast, or fungi to a surface. These surface growths can be found in natural settings such as on rocks in streams, and in infections such as can occur on catheters. Microorganisms can colonize living and inert natural and synthetic surfaces.

HIGH-LEVEL DISINFECTION: High-level disinfection is a process that uses a chemical solution to kill all bacteria, viruses, and all other disease-causing agents except for bacterial endospores and prions. High-level disinfection should be distinguished from sterilization, which removes endospores (a bacterial structure that is resistant to radiation, drying, lack of food, and other things that would be lethal to the bacteria) and prions (misshapen proteins that can cause disease) as well.

INTERMEDIATE-LEVEL DISINFECTION: Intermediate-level disinfection is a form of disinfection that kills bacteria, most viruses, and mycobacteria.

LOW-LEVEL DISINFECTION: Low-level disinfection is a form of disinfection that is capable of killing some viruses and some bacteria.

STERILIZATION: Sterilization is a term that refers to the complete killing or elimination of living organisms in the sample being treated. Sterilization is absolute. After the treatment the sample is either devoid of life, or the possibility of life (as from the subsequent germination and growth of bacterial spores), or it is not.

The importance of personal hygiene and clean clothing had yet to be realized by health care providers. As a result, microbial infections easily spread from patient to patient. The French chemist Louis Pasteur (1822–1895) proposed that infections were connected with the presence of microorganisms. This idea prompted an English surgeon named Joseph Lister (1827–1912) to study this suggestion. Lister became convinced that infections following surgery often did involve microorganisms infecting the incision. To minimize this risk, Lister sprayed a film of carbolic acid over the patient during surgery. The treatment effectively disinfected the wound and helped reduce post-surgical infections. As Lister's findings became accepted, the importance of disinfection to medicine was recognized.

■ Applications and Research

Disinfection uses a chemical or other type of agent (typically ultraviolet light) to kill microorganisms. All of these agents are termed disinfectants.

Ultraviolet light disinfects because of the high energy of the waves of light. The energy is sufficient to break the strands of genetic material of the microbes. When many breaks occur in the deoxyribonucleic acid (DNA) or ribonucleic acid (RNA) the damage is lethal, as it cannot be repaired by the microorganism. Ultraviolet light can be used to disinfect liquids of small volume, surfaces, and some types of equipment.

Alcohol is a liquid disinfectant that tends to be used on the skin to achieve short-term disinfection. It kills microbes, such as bacteria, by dissolving the membrane around the organisms. It can be sprayed on surfaces; the droplets of alcohol will kill microbes on contact. The spray needs to be fairly heavily applied to a surface to ensure disinfection because the alcohol evaporates quickly. If it evaporates within a few seconds, the microorganisms may not be exposed long enough to be killed. Alcohol-based hand washes are also available, and are becoming more widely used in hospitals because a busy doctor or nurse need only rub their hands for 10–15 seconds with an alcohol-based solution to adequately disinfect their hands between seeing patients. Typical disinfectant soaps such as those used in the home require skin contact of 30 seconds or more to be effective disinfectants.

The compound iodine is another disinfectant. In hospitals, surgical scrubbing is often accomplished using an iodine-containing soap. As with alcohol-based handwashing, the intent is to lower the number of living bacteria on the surface of the skin, although iodine is a more efficient disinfectant than alcohol.

Another liquid disinfectant that remains on a surface much longer is sodium hypochlorite. The active component of the disinfectant is chlorine, and it is also the disinfectant agent in household bleach. Water can also be treated using chlorine, and this is the basis of drinking water chlorination. The concentration of sodium hypochlorite used is important—too much chlorine can dissolve metal surfaces and can irritate the cells in the eye and the nose. A sodium hypochlorite solution (bleach) is used by medical personnel in the field when investigating outbreaks of diseases that can be spread by contact with infected body fluids, droplets, or contaminated surfaces, and when local infrastructure will not support high-tech disinfection methods. For example, the Centers for Disease Control and Prevention (CDC) recommended household bleach diluted with water in a 1:100 ratio to disinfect areas contaminated with blood and body fluids in a makeshift isolation ward hospital during a 2003 outbreak of Ebola in the Cuvette West region of the Democratic Republic of Congo.

Surfaces can also be disinfected using compounds that contain a phenol group. A popular example is Lysol®. In a hospital, phenol-based disinfectants are not used in certain cases, such as in an operating theater. This is because some disease-causing bacteria and viruses are resistant to phenol.

Chlorhexidine is a chemical disinfectant that kills fungi and yeast much more effectively than bacteria and viruses. Formaldehyde and glutaraldehyde possess a chemical group called an aldehyde, which is a very potent disinfectant. Glutaraldehyde is a general disinfectant, which means it is effective against a wide array of microbes after only a few minutes of contact. Another effective general disinfectant is quaternary ammonium.

The disinfection strategy that is selected depends on a number of factors. These include the surface being disinfected and the intended use of that surface (a doctor's hands should be disinfected rigorously, for example). A smooth crack- or crevasse-free surface is easier to disinfect, and so typically requires less time to disinfect than does a rougher surface. A rough surface, which has niches that microorganisms can fit into, is not an appropriate surface to disinfect with a rapidly evaporating spray of alcohol. The surface material is also important. For example, a wooden surface may soak up liquids and reduce the concentration of the disinfectant that acts on the microorganisms.

The number of microorganisms present can determine the type of disinfectant used and how long it should be used for. Higher numbers of microbes usually require a lengthier exposure time to reduce the number of living organisms to a level that is considered safe. How the organisms grow is also important. For example, many disease-causing bacteria can grow in a slime-encased community known as a biofilm. Biofilm bacteria are much more resistant to disinfectants than they are when dispersed from the biofilm. As another example, bacteria such as *Bacillus anthracis*, the organism that causes anthrax, and *Clostridium botulinum*, a neurotoxin-producing bacterium that can contaminate foods, can form a hardy structure called a spore, which often survives exposure to disinfectants.

Many disinfectants act against a variety of microbes; they are known as broad-spectrum disinfectants. Glutaraldehyde, sodium hypochlorite, and hydrogen peroxide are broad-spectrum disinfectants. Other disinfectants act on specific microorganisms, while the activity of other disinfectants is in between these extremes. An example of the latter is alcohol. It dissolves cell membranes that are made of lipids, and so is effective against many bacteria and viruses. Spores or viruses that do not have a lipid membrane, however, are not as affected by alcohol as bacteria.

■ Impacts and Issues

Disinfectants are a vital defense against infectious disease, especially in the health care, cosmetic, and food service industries. Still, the full benefits of disinfection have yet to be realized. Surveys conducted in North America and Europe have shown that health care providers do not wash their hands between patient visits as often as they should. Transfer of infection from patient to patient via the hands of medical personnel and their equipment (such as a stethoscope) still occurs, even though it could be avoided in many cases. Alternatively, overuse of disinfectants can cause microorganisms to develop resistance to disinfectants, if, for example, the compound is not applied for an adequate amount of time. This resistance can make it more difficult to eliminate sources of infection, which allows for their spread.

On a broader scale, wide-scale disinfection of drinking water supplies was one of the most significant public health accomplishments of the twentieth century. Outbreaks of waterborne diseases such as typhus and cholera were common in both the United States and abroad before modern disinfection methods were put into place. In the 1990s, researchers recognized that while disinfectants neutralized many pathogens (disease-causing organisms) in water, some disinfectants also reacted with naturally occurring organic and inorganic matter in water sources and municipal water delivery systems. These reactions produced potentially harmful compounds called disinfection byproducts (DBPs). After DBPs were found to cause cancer and adverse reproductive effects in laboratory mice, the Environmental Protection Agency (EPA) set in place in 2001 new regulations to maximize disinfection of drinking water supplies while minimizing public exposure to DBPs.

SEE ALSO *Antimicrobial Soaps; Infection Control and Asepsis.*

BIBLIOGRAPHY

Books

Gladwin, Mark, and Bill Trattler. *Clinical Microbiology Made Ridiculously Simple.* 3rd ed. Miami: Medmaster, 2003.

Prescott, Lansing M., John P. Harley, and Donald A. Klein. *Microbiology.* New York: McGraw-Hill, 2004.

Tortora, Gerard J., Berell R. Funke, and Christine L. Case. *Microbiology: An Introduction.* New York: Benjamin Cummings, 2006.

Brian Hoyle

Dracunculiasis

Introduction

Dracunculiasis, (dra-KUNK-you-LIE-uh-sis) or guinea worm disease, is a preventable helminth (parasitic worm) infection caused by the large female roundworm *Dracunculus medinensis*. It is endemic in some African countries (including Sudan, Ghana, and Nigeria) within rural communities without safe drinking water

This disease occurs when people drink water contaminated with *Dracunculus medinensis* larvae. However, symptoms do not usually manifest until about a year after infection. It is at that stage that the female worm ruptures the skin to release larvae, causing severe pain and discomfort to the infected person. There is no treatment for the infection itself except to manually remove the worm.

Disease History, Characteristics, and Transmission

The mode of infection of dracunculiasis was recognized in 1870 when a Russian naturalist noticed the release of larvae from the female worm into a freshwater source. In the 1980s, it was found to be endemic throughout Africa and an eradication initiative was launched.

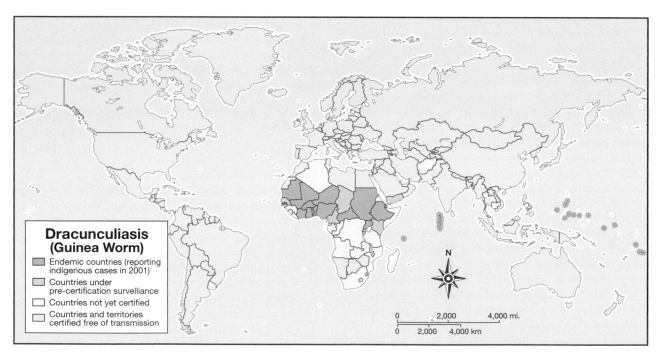

Dracunculiasis (Guinea Worm)

- Endemic countries (reporting indigenous cases in 2001)
- Countries under pre-certification survelliance
- Countries not yet certified
- Countries and territories certified free of transmission

Map showing Dracunculiasis (Guinea worm disease) eradication status as of 2002. *© Copyright World Health Organization (WHO). Reproduced by permission.*

Symptoms of dracunculiasis do not usually present until around one year after infection, at which time a blister will form at a distal (away from the center) site of the body, such as the lower leg or foot. Some persons may experience allergic-type symptoms such as wheezing, fever, swelling around the eyes, and burning sensations of the skin just prior to lesion formation. After a few days, this blister will burst and the female worm emerges.

Upon making contact with water, the female worm releases millions of larvae that are subsequently ingested by copepods called "water fleas," where they develop into the infective stage. Human infection occurs by drinking contaminated water. The water flea is digested, but the larvae survive, migrate to the small intestine, mate, and the females mature to adult size of up to 39 inches (100 cm). The female then migrates to the distal site and the process repeats.

Scope and Distribution

The people most commonly affected by dracunculiasis are those living in rural communities without established water treatment facilities. Due to the mode of transmission, males and females of all ages are vulnerable to infection if exposed to a contaminated water source. In some endemic areas, over half of the infected individuals are children, as they are they main water carriers.

Following eradication efforts, by 2006, the occurrence of dracunculiasis was mostly restricted to remote rural villages in only 12 countries of sub-Saharan Africa. Over half of these cases had been reported from Sudan, where ongoing war conditions made it difficult to successfully eradicate the disease.

Sporadic cases of dracunculiasis have been noted in America and Australia among African immigrants.

Treatment and Prevention

Treatment for dracunculiasis is limited and there is no definitive medication available to eliminate or prevent infection. The most common method for removing the worm once it has immerged is to gently pull it out a few inches each day. This slow process allows for the complete removal of the worm. This process may only take a few days, but generally takes weeks. Analgesics may also be used to reduce swelling and help with pain management.

As dracunculiasis is transmitted only by drinking contaminated water, disease prevention is possible by implementing simple measures. Ensuring the maintenance of a water source free from contamination is vital and the filtration of water prior to drinking would be further beneficial. Prevention is most often accomplished by either treating ponds with insecticide that kills the copepods that host the larvae while still leaving the

---

> ## WORDS TO KNOW
>
> **DISTAL:** Distal comes from the same root word as "distant," and is the medical word for distant from some agreed-on point of reference. For example, the hand is at the distal end of the arm from the trunk.
>
> **HELMINTH:** A representative of various phyla of worm-like animals.
>
> **POTABLE:** Water that can is clean enough to drink safely is potable water.

---

water potable, or by filtering untreated water before it is consumed. Both methods break the chain of transmission. It is also essential to prevent people with open guinea worm wounds from swimming or bathing in shared water facilities used for drinking.

Impacts and Issues

Although the mortality rate for dracunculiasis is very low, morbidity is a major concern as the disease often affects entire communities and proves to be a heavy social and economic burden. Persons are often bedridden for some time during and following the emergence of the worm and as such, are unable to contribute to the work within the community. The seasonality of out breaks further highlights the impact of disease whereby emergence often occurs during the peak of the agricultural year, often at harvest time, when the loss of labor is most damaging.

Children of parents infected with dracunculiasis are more likely to suffer from malnutrition than children of uninfected families. With an incapacitated parent, children are often required to assume adult roles within the family that, as a result, may also affect their chances of gaining an education. It is the culmination of these nutritional, social, economic, and educational factors, along with the practicality of possible prevention measures, that has made world health authorities identify dracunculiasis a candidate for eradication.

Former United States President Jimmy Carter has led a campaign to eliminate guinea worm disease for more than twenty years. Working in conjunction with the Centers for Disease Control and Prevention (CDC) and others, if successful, the Carter campaign will result in the first eradication of an infectious disease since smallpox. Before the campaign, there were between three and five million cases occurring per year and the disease was endemic throughout Africa and areas of Asia.

IN CONTEXT: ERADICATION PROGRAM EFFECTIVENESS

Since the implementation of the eradication program in the 1980s, the global prevalence of dracunculiasis has drastically decreased. While in 1986, an estimated 3.5 million people were suffering from the disease worldwide, only 32,193 cases were reported in 2003, a decrease of over ninety percent.

SOURCE: *World Health Organization (WHO)*

By 1996, the number of worldwide cases had been reduced to around 150,000. By 2006, cases of reported guinea worm disease decreased to about 12,000, the disease was eliminated from Asia, and remained endemic in only about nine African countries.

SEE ALSO *Helminth Disease; Roundworm (Ascariasis) Infection; Sanitation; Vector-borne Disease; War and Infectious Disease; Water-borne Disease.*

BIBLIOGRAPHY

Books

Mandell, G.L., Bennett, J.E., and Dolin, R. *Principles and Practice of Infectious Diseases.* Vol. 2. Philadelphia, PA: Elsevier, 2005.

Periodicals

Cairncross, S., Muller, R., and Zagaria, N. "Dracunculiasis (Guinea Worm Disease) and the Eradication Initiative." *Clinical Microbiology Reviews.* 15, 2 (2002): 223–246.

Hopkins, D.R., Ruiz-Tiben, E., Downs, P., Withers, P.C., and Maguire, J.H. "Dracunculiasis Eradication: The Final Inch." *The American Journal of Tropical Medicine and Hygiene.* 73, 4 (2005): 669–675.

Web Sites

Directors of Health Promotion and Education. "Guinea Worm Disease." 2005 <http://www.dhpe.org/infect/guinea.html> (accessed Feb. 22, 2007).

World Health Organization (WHO). "Dracunculiasis eradication." 2007 <http://www.who.int/dracunculiasis/en/> (accessed Feb. 22, 2007).

Droplet Precautions

■ Introduction

Droplet precautions are measures that have been developed to limit the airborne spread of microorganisms in droplets that are larger than 5 microns in diameter (a micron is 10^{-6} of a meter or one millionth of a meter). These droplets are typically expelled into the air by coughing, sneezing, and even by talking.

Droplets that are smaller in diameter are considered to be aerosols and, since they may travel greater distances, are governed by the airborne precautions category of infection control.

■ History and Scientific Foundations

The droplet precautions developed by agencies including the U.S. Centers for Disease Control and Prevention (CDC) and issued as guidelines in 1996 are designed to limit the spread of droplets with the cells of the eyes, nose, and mouth. This is important in a hospital, where droplets expelled by someone with an infection could spread the disease to someone else.

Because the droplets are relatively large, they are heavier and tend not to travel as far (less than three feet) as aerosolized microorganisms. Thus, droplet precautions are designed to prevent the movement of microorganisms from one person to someone else who is within about three feet or less.

Viral diseases for which droplet precautions are necessary include chickenpox, influenza, measles, German measles, mumps, smallpox, and severe acute respiratory syndrome (SARS). Bacterial diseases requiring these precautions include whooping cough, a form of meningitis, psittacosis, Legionnaire's disease, diphtheria, and pneumonia. Finally, the inhalation of fungi-laden droplets can cause allergic alveolitis, aspergillosis, histoplasmosis, and coccidiodomycosis.

■ Applications and Research

Droplet precautions are a necessary part of a hospital's infection control strategy. Without such precautions, the airborne spread of disease would occur more frequently. These precautions can be initiated by the attending health care providers, including the physician and the nursing staff, and by the person in charge of infection control. The latter usually has the final say in whether precautions will be observed or not. The use of droplet precautions must be documented in the patient records. This information that can be important in tracing the effectiveness of the precautions in controlling the infection and minimizing its spread.

Placing the infected patient in a separate room can be sufficient to prevent the spread of droplet-borne microbes. Specially ventilated rooms are not required, nor does the door to the room need to be closed. If a separate room is not available, then the infected patient should be housed with a patient who has an infection with the same microorganism and no other condition. That way, if the microbe is transferred between the

---

WORDS TO KNOW

AEROSOL: Particles of liquid or solid dispersed as a suspension in gas.

CONTACT PRECAUTIONS: Contact precautions are actions developed to minimize the transfer of microorganisms by direct physical contact and indirectly by touching a contaminated surface.

DROPLETS: A drop of water or other fluid that is less than 5 microns (a millionth of a meter) in diameter.

patients via droplets, it will have a negligible influence on either patient's health. The patients's beds should be physically separated by a minimum of three feet, and visitors should not be allowed within three feet of the patient they are visiting.

A face mask should be worn when either a health care provider or a visitor comes in close contact with the infected patient. Standard masks, similar to the type worn by carpenters to prevent inhalation of dust and other construction debris, are sufficient. Ideally, the mask should be put on as a person enters the patient's room and should be discarded in a hazardous waste container as the person is leaving.

The infected patient should be moved to other areas of the hospital only as is necessary, and should wear a mask during the transport. In addition, any visitors who have not been previously exposed to the infection that the patient has should not be allowed to enter the patient's room. Droplet precautions are often used in conjunction with contact precautions (infection control procedures designed to minimize the spread of disease by direct or indirect contact) in hospitals.

Droplet precautions can be discontinued when a patient's symptoms, such as coughing, have disappeared.

■ Impacts and Issues

Droplet precautions are intended to benefit the patient and medical personnel and to control and contain a disease outbreak. However, these measures come not only with a financial cost, but with a psychic cost when images of masked patients, cargivers, and even members of the general public are given wide circulation by the media. A recent example occurred in Toronto, Canada, in March 2003, when several hundred people were affected by a SARS outbreak. Unsettling images of masked citizens in China (where the SARS outbreak originated) engaging in everyday activities, and of masked healthcare workers in Toronto were shown around the world. The precautions observed during the Toronto outbreak were subsequently cited as key in containing the infection. Yet, this success came at a cost. A report released in 2005 documented that infection control procedures, including droplet precautions, lost revenue, and additional labor costs, for one of the several affected Toronto hospitals totaled $12 million.

SEE ALSO *Airborne Precautions; Contact Precautions; Infection Control and Asepsis; Isolation and Quarantine; Nosocomial (Healthcare-Associated) Infections.*

BIBLIOGRAPHY

Books

Drexler, Madeline. *Secret Agents: The Menace of Emerging Infections.* New York: Penguin, 2003.

Tierno, Philip M. *The Secret Life of Germs: What They Are, Why We Need Them, and How We Can Protect Ourselves Against Them.* New York: Atria, 2004.

Wenzel, Richard P. *Prevention and Control of Nosocomial Infections.* New York: Lippincott Williams & Wilkins, 2002.

Web Sites

Centers for Disease Control and Prevention. "Droplet Precautions." April 1, 2005. <http://www.cdc.gov/ncidod/dhqp/gl_isolation_droplet.html> (accessed April 3, 2007).

Brian Hoyle

Dysentery

Introduction

Dysentery is the name given to an inflammation of the intestines, and especially the colon, that leads to abdominal pain and frequent stools which contain blood and mucus. Dysentery can be caused by bacteria, protozoa, worms, or even non-infectious agents. *Shigella* species are the causative agent in most cases of bacterial dysentery. *Entamoeba histolytica*, a protozoa, is the main cause of amebic dysentery.

Overcrowding and poor hygiene are major risk factors for dysentery. It occurs all around the world, among people of all ages. Dysentery is sometimes known as "travelers' diarrhea" because it often affects those who visit developing countries. Although the disease normally clears up without treatment, antibiotics and drugs to get rid of amebic parasites might be necessary. Prior to the advent of antibiotics and improved sanitation, dysentery could be fatal and indeed, claimed the lives of many famous figures, including King Henry V of England (1387–1422) and the Spanish explorer Hernando Cortes (1485–1547).

Disease History, Characteristics, and Transmission

The four main *Shigella* species responsible for bacterial dysentery are *S. sonnei*, *S. flexneri*, *S.boydii* and *S. dysenteriae* and this disease is sometimes known as shigellosis. The *Shigellae* are rod-shaped bacteria of one to two millimeters in diameter, Gram-negative, and closely related to the *Escherichia* genus. Infection with *Shigella* is sometimes known as shigellosis. Gram-negative refers to the way bacteria interact with the Gram stain when being prepared for microscopic examination. Meanwhile, amebic dysentery—also called amebiasis—is caused by a single-celled protozoan parasite called *Entamoeba histolytica*.

The incubation period of shigellosis is usually one to three days. For amebic dysentery, the incubation time is much longer—maybe up to one year. Therefore, returning travelers who have acquired amebic dysentery abroad

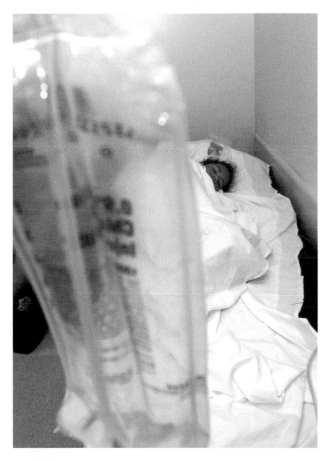

A child rests after receiving treatment for symptoms of dysentery at a regional medical center in Biloxi, Mississippi, in 2005. An outbreak of dysentery occurred at a shelter in Biloxi in the wake of Hurricane Katrina. *Barry Williams/Getty Images.*

WORDS TO KNOW

GRAM-NEGATIVE: A method of identifying bacteria based on whether crystal-violet dye is retained or not retained after being stained and decolorized with alcohol in a process called Gram's method.

INCUBATION PERIOD: Incubation period refers to the time between exposure to disease causing virus or bacteria and the appearance of symptoms of the infection. Depending on the microorganism, the incubation time can range from a few hours (an example is food poisoning due to *Salmonella*) to a decade or more (an example is acquired immunodeficiency syndrome, or AIDS).

MORTALITY: Mortality is the condition of being susceptible to death. The term "mortality" comes from the Latin word *mors,* which means "death." Mortality can also refer to the rate of deaths caused by an illness or injury, i.e., "Rabies has a high mortality."

PROTOZOA: Single-celled animal-like microscopic organisms that live by taking in food rather than making it by photosynthesis and must live in the presence of water. (Singular: protozoan.) Protozoa are a diverse group of single-celled organisms, with more than 50,000 different types

represented. The vast majority are microscopic, many measuring less than 5 one-thousandth of an inch (0.005 millimeters) but some, such as the freshwater Spirostomun, may reach 0.17 inches (3 millimeters) in length, large enough to enable it to be seen with the naked eye.

RELAPSE: Relapse is a return of symptoms after the patient has apparently recovered from a disease.

SENTINEL: Sentinel surveillance is a method in epidemiology where a subset of the population is surveyed for the presence of communicable diseases. Also, a sentinel is an animal used to indicate the presence of disease within an area.

SEPSIS: Sepsis refers to a bacterial infection in the bloodstream or body tissues. This is a very broad term covering the presence of many types of microscopic disease-causing organisms. Sepsis is also called bacteremia. Closely related terms include septicemia and septic syndrome. According to the Society of Critical Care Medicine, severe sepsis affects about 750,000 people in the United States each year. However, it is predicted to rapidly rise to one million people by 2010 due to the aging U.S. population. Over the decade of the 1990s, the incident rate of sepsis increased over 91%.

may not immediately make the connection between infection and symptoms, which may delay diagnosis.

The symptoms of shigellosis and amebic dysentery are similar, the chief one being diarrhea containing blood and mucus. Amebic dysentery is more likely to produce blood. There may also be severe pain in the abdomen, fever, nausea and vomiting. Shigellosis tends to produce a watery diarrhea that progresses to dysentery, especially when *S. dysenteriae* and *S. flexneri* are involved.

Symptoms of dysentery, including the frequency of attacks of diarrhea, can range from mild to severe. Complications are more likely with *S. dysenteriae* and include sepsis (blood poisoning) and kidney failure. Blood clots may also be seen in the liver and the spleen. Dysentery with severe complications can have a mortality (death) rate of 5–20%. However, the symptoms of most cases of dysentery last for only a few days, although relapse and chronic infection can also occur.

The fecal-oral route is important in the transmission of *Shigella*—that is, eating or drinking contaminated food or water. Cases in Europe have been linked to

infected milk and food. Houseflies also carry the disease. Dysentery is highly infectious and can also be transmitted just by contact with infected individuals. *Shigella* species enter through the mouth and progress to the colon where they multiply producing the severe inflammation which causes the symptoms of the disease. A person with shigellosis may remain infectious for up to four weeks after the onset of symptoms.

Amebic dysentery is transmitted in a similar way. In part of its life cycle, the amebae can exist as a cyst—a group of cells surrounded by a wall that can survive the acid of the stomach and progress to the intestines. The cysts can stick to the walls of the colon, causing bleeding ulcers, loss of appetite, and weight loss. The cysts are passed in the feces and can infect others under conditions of poor sanitation.

■ Scope and Distribution

Dysentery has long had an impact on human health, but it was not until the nineteenth century that the cause was realized to be either bacterial or amoebic. The *Shigella* get their name from Kiyoshi Shiga (1871–1951) who discovered them in 1898. Dysentery has caused massive casualties in conflicts ranging from the Peloponnesian War in 431 BC to World War II (1939–1945). In the American Civil War (1861–1865), there were nearly two million cases of diarrhea, most of which was probably dysentery, resulting in over 44,000 deaths. It has only been with the advent of antibiotics that dysentery has ceased to be such a major problem in military campaigns.

S. dysenteri causes most outbreaks of dysentery in developing countries, in the tropics and subtropics and under conditions of overcrowding or war. Epidemic dysentery in the tropics is more common in the rainy season, perhaps because people tend to spend more time indoors together and sanitation suffers from the abundance of surface water. *S. sonnei* and *S. flexneri* are the most common causes of shigellosis in the United States, England, Europe, Egypt, the Middle East, and Asia. *S. boydii* is found mainly in India and Egypt, although strains of all four species have been found in the U.S. as well.

Shigellosis is endemic throughout the world, but is more common in less developed countries. In Europe, the United States, and other developed regions, shigellosis tends to be a disease of institutions—nursery schools, mental institutions, prisons, and military barracks. In the U.S. and the United Kingdom, shigellosis is a notifiable disease.

Around 10% of the world's population is infected with *Entamoeba histolytica*, but fewer than 10% of those infected exhibit any signs of disease. Infection is prevalent in Central and South America, southern and western Africa, the Southeast Asia, India, and China. Amebic dysentery is relatively rare in Australia, New Zealand, Canada, the United States and Europe. However, travelers may become infected abroad. Pregnant women, children, and people in developing nations are most at risk to contract amebic dysentery.

Treatment and Prevention

Most cases of bacterial and amebic dysentery resolve with rest and drinking plenty of fluids to replace that which is lost from the diarrhea. This is especially important for babies with dysentery as they can become rapidly dehydrated. Sometimes antibiotic treatment, including hospitalization for intravenous therapy is needed. Trimethoprim-sulfamethoxazole or ampicillin are often used.

A good standard of personal hygiene will prevent the transmission of dysentery. This means frequent handwashing, especially after using the toilet or after contact with someone who is infected with *Shigella*. Hands should also be washed before handling and cook-

ing food, eating, handling babies, and feeding the young or elderly. To avoid spreading infection, personal items like towels or face cloths should not be shared.

Travelers should avoid drinking tap water in countries known to have poor sanitation. Ice cubes, salad, and uncooked vegetables should also be avoided, because these could have been washed in contaminated water. A child who has had dysentery should stay away from school or nursery care for at least 48 hours after symptoms have ceased. An adult with dysentery should not return to work in a food or healthcare environment without first consulting their employer.

Impacts and Issues

There are approximately 165 million cases of shigellosis worldwide each year. Shigellosis disproportionately affects developing nations. The United Nations World Health Organization (WHO) reports 163.2 million annual cases in developing countries, compared to 1.5 million cases in industrialized countries.

Among residents of industrialized nations, the increased popularity of international travel accounts for a significant percentage of dysentery cases. The WHO estimates that there are approximately 580,000 reported cases of tourism-related shigellosis annually. The Centers for Disease Control (CDC) and several international health organizations publish infectious disease warnings and vaccination and medication advisories for travelers. Many travelers' warnings also contain information on the quality and safety of local water. Individuals should consult these publications before traveling and follow their recommendations.

Dysentery is common wherever sanitation is inadequate or lacking, as with so many other water-borne infections. Therefore, development of adequate sewage disposal and access to clean drinking water should be a priority in helping prevent this globally important disease.

The WHO estimates that over one billion people worldwide do not have daily access to clean water. A greater number of people live in areas that lack basic sanitation systems. In 2005, the United Nations announced an initiative to halve by 2015 the number of people worldwide who lack potable water. The International Decade for Action, "Water for Life" project involves several U.N. and government agencies, as well as private charitable and health organizations.

■ Primary source connection

In this online news article, author Heidi Ledford discusses how travelers returning home inadvertently served as sentinels (lookouts) for an outbreak of *Shigella* in Africa in the 1990s, and how similar cases could alert health authorities in developing countries to future outbreaks if networks for sharing data are improved. Ledford has a PhD in plant biology and is a science journalist based in Boston, Massachusetts.

Jetsetters are Key Clues to Epidemics

TRAVELLERS WHO BRING ILLNESS HOME ACT AS SENTINELS OF DISEASE

When the first patients with dysentery started trickling into health clinics in Sierra Leone in early 1999, Philippe Guerin wasn't sure what to think. Guerin, a medical epidemiologist, knew that the symptoms he was seeing could be produced by several different pathogens, but resources were slim in the war-torn country, and healthcare workers did not have the facilities to pinpoint the source of the outbreak. As the flow of patients began to swell, healthcare workers collected samples and shipped them to Paris for testing.

About six months later, after three thousand cases of dysentery, and more than a hundred deaths, the results were in. Sierra Leone was in the midst of an outbreak of *Shigella*, a bacterium that causes bloody diarrhoea and kills more than a million people a year. The strain of Shigella in Sierra Leone, called "Sd1," was known for its exceptional mobility and aptitude for causing epidemics in tropical regions. But although the strain had been working its way through other developing nations, it

hadn't yet been reported in West African countries like Sierra Leone.

"Because of the harsh conditions and the civil war, everything was in place to nest this outbreak," says Guerin, a Paris-based scientific director at Epicentre, a non-profit public-health organization created by Médecins san Frontières. "But we lost at least six months waiting on a diagnosis."

Now Guerin says that West African healthcare workers could have been warned of the Sd1 outbreak if industrialized nations had better disease-surveillance networks to pass on information about their travelers' symptoms.

FROM NORWAY TO AFRICA

Guerin first had this realization when he was trawling through a Norwegian database of diseases. There, he noticed that in the late 1990s, two travellers to West Africa had been diagnosed with *Shigella* after they had returned to Norway. The evidence of the epidemic's cause was already there, he realized, years before healthcare workers in West Africa even knew they had a problem.

Guerin and his colleagues then searched systematically through published papers from 1940 to 2002 and surveillance data from 16 European countries for reports of Sd1 from 1990 to 2002. Their results, published in BMC Public Health this month[1], showed that surveillance data had picked up the presence of Sd1 in West Africa in 1992—seven years before the outbreak in Sierra Leone.

The added warning time could have been valuable, says Guerin. Clinics in West African could have prepared to treat cases of dysentery aggressively using the class of antibiotics that would fend off Sd1. "Instead, there was no plan," he says.

BUGS IN THE SYSTEM

The World Health Organization estimates that every year, about 580,000 travellers from industrialized nations pick up *Shigella* during their journeys. Some of those travellers carry it home with them, where they are then diagnosed and treated.

Wealthy travelers wandering through poor nations make an excellent sentinel for disease, notes Kevin Kain, an epidemiologist at the Toronto General Research Institute in Ontario. "Immunologically, they're like a one-year old," he says. "They're a canary in the coal mine."

But although the disease might then be entered into a surveillance network like the Program for Monitoring Emerging Diseases (ProMed) or GeoSentinel, that information is not systematically shared with the developing nations where the disease came from, says Stephen Morse, an epidemiologist at Columbia University in New York.

An added difficulty, notes Morse, is that not all travellers who get a nasty disease are diagnosed properly. Some never turn up at a clinic at all. Kain admits to having treated himself after coming down with a case of dysentery in Tanzania in 1991. He didn't report anything to Tanzanian officials, and returned home healthy. "I was part of the problem," he says.

But Guerin suggests that a single report is enough to sound an alarm, which would trigger a better inspection of travel surveillance networks and data sharing with the country concerned (hopefully without too many false alarms from isolated incidents). There will still be problems, of course, if the source country doesn't have the resources to tackle the outbreak.

Heidi Ledford

LEDFORD, HEIDI. "JETSETTERS ARE KEY CLUES TO EPIDEMICS." *NATURE.COM* JANUARY 29, 2007 <HTTP:// WWW.NATURE.COM/NEWS/2007/070129/FULL/070129-5. HTML> (ACCESSED MAY 18, 2007).

SEE ALSO *Amebiasis; Shigellosis; War and Infectious Disease.*

BIBLIOGRAPHY

Books

Ericsson, Charles D. *Traveler's Diarrhea* Hamilton, ON, Canada: BC Decker, 2003.

Web Sites

Centers for Disease Control and Prevention (CDC). "Amebiasis." Jan 21, 2004 <http://www.cdc.gov/ ncidod/dpd/parasites/amebiasis/factsht_ amebiasis.htm> (accessed May 12, 2007).

Tropical Medicine Central Resource. "Shigellosis." <http://tmcr.usuhs.mil/tmcr/chapter19/ intro.htm> (accessed).

Susan Aldridge

Ear Infections (Otitis Media)

■ Introduction

Otitis media is a recurring bacterial or, occasionally, viral, infection of the middle ear. The bacteria most commonly involved are *Streptococcus pneumoniae*, a type of *Haemophilus influenzae*, and *Moraxella catarrhalis*.

■ Disease History, Characteristics, and Transmission

The human ear is composed of three parts—the external or outer ear, the middle ear, and the inner ear. The outer ear is the visible portion that lies outside of the skull. It functions as a sound trap to route sound waves via a canal to the middle ear. Separating the outer and middle ear is the tympanic membrane or eardrum. In the middle ear, an arrangement of three bones passes the sound vibrations to nerve cells that form the inner ear. The eustachian tube connects the middle portion of the ear to the nasal cavity and throat. Normally the eustachian tube acts to equalize the pressure on the two sides of the eardrum. However, when the inflammation associated with otitis media affects the eardrum, the pressure difference on either side of the eardrum can become so great that the eardrum ruptures, a painful complication.

There are several different kinds of otitis media. One type, called acute otitis media, tends to be associated with a runny or stuffy nose, and is triggered when the eustachian tube becomes blocked during the upper respiratory infection. In addition to inflammation, pus and fluid accumulate in the middle ear. The infection can also be associated with fever and irritable behavior. Other symptoms include interrupted sleep, tugging at the effected ear, and loss of balance due to the ear blockage. The acute infection tends to be of short duration.

An ear infection that does not display symptoms, including fever and irritable behavior, is known as otitis media with effusion (the infection was known as serous or secretory otitis media). Often, after the acute version of the infection, otitis media with effusion can last longer.

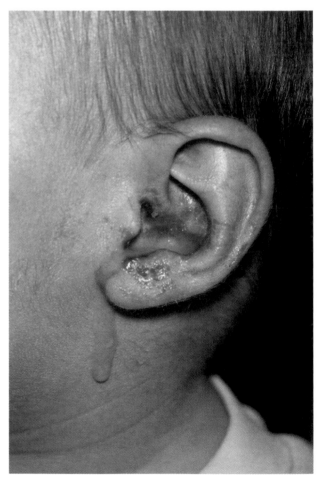

Close-up of pus (yellow) in the ear of a five-month-old boy with secretory otitis media, a middle ear infection. This chronic accumulation of fluid in the middle ear may cause hearing loss. *Dr. P. Marazzi/Photo Researchers, Inc.*

If the infection lasts longer than several weeks, it is referred to as chronic otitis media. The chronic form can involve bacteria growths that have become colonized, or well established in the ear. These growths are often present as surface-adherent, polysaccharide (slime)-enclosed communities called biofilms. Antibiotic treatment will kill some of the bacteria and lessen the infection. However, bacteria deeper within the biofilm survive and can be the cause of a future infection. This is the reason that chronic otitis media can persist for years.

■ Scope and Distribution

In humans, episodes of otitis media typically can begin as early as a few months of age. It is a common childhood ailment. Less frequently, the infection occurs in adults. More than 10 million children visit a doctor for treatment of ear infections each year in the United States. As children grow older and the structure of the ear changes, the frequency and incidence of ear infections usually drop. Specifically, as children mature, the eustachian tube becomes more slanted from inside to outside, which allows fluid to drain more easily. In the earlier years of childhood, the eustachian tube can have a more horizontal orientation or can even slant more towards the inside of the ear, which impedes fluid drainage and encourages the development of frequent infections.

■ Treatment and Prevention

Treatment of otitis media can involve decongestants or antihistamines to help clear the blocked eustachian tube and antibiotics if the bacteria are the cause of the infection (antibiotics are not effective against viruses). Even with antibiotic treatment an infection may take weeks or months to completely clear, as bacteria within the biofilm are progressively killed. For this reason, the full course of antibiotic therapy must be followed. Stopping treatment early, because symptoms diminish or disappear, may allow bacteria to survive. These survivors may develop resistance to the antibiotic that was used, making treatment of the next infection more difficult.

When a chronic infection does not respond to treatment, more drastic action may be necessary. Surgery to install a plastic drainage tube—a procedure called myringotomy—may be performed. Less frequently, surgical removal of infected, swollen adenoids or tonsils may be done. Myringotomy is a common childhood surgery in the United States. The tube is removed later, as the maturing eustachian tube more naturally drains fluid from the middle ear.

Research concerning the nature of the biofilms formed by bacteria in otitis media is underway. It is unclear whether there are some distinguishing features about the bacteria that make them more likely to cause an infection. If so, identification of the genetic factors

involved is important, since it could lead to better strategies to deal with an infection or, perhaps, help in the development of preventive measures. Current research also aims to discover why some children are more prone to ear infections than other children and to develop more accurate and rapid means of diagnosing otitis media.

■ Impacts and Issues

Otitis media is the number one reason that parents bring a sick child to a physician. Medical costs and lost wages due to otitis media in the United States alone are estimated to be almost $5 billion per year. The ultimate challenge for researchers in otitis media is to create a vaccine for infants that would prevent the first acute otitis media infection. Several vaccine candidates are at different stages in the testing and approval process, from animal testing to first-phase clinical trials.

OTITIS MEDIA VS. SWIMMER'S EAR

The The Centers for Disease Control and Prevention (CDC), Division of Parasitic Diseases is careful to warn the public that middle ear infection is not the same as Swimmer's Ear. The CDC states, "If you can wiggle the outer ear without pain or discomfort then your ear infection is probably not Swimmer's Ear."

SOURCE: *The Centers for Disease Control and Prevention (CDC), Division of Parasitic Diseases*

Otitis media can be a serious infection, producing chronic diminished hearing ability or permanent hearing loss. Hearing impairment in a child during the years of language acquisition can result in learning and socialization delays, and speech disabilities.

As with other chronic bacterial infections, the symptoms associated with chronic ear infections can be less severe and uncomfortable than those of the acute form of the infection. Chronic infections may thus escape detection for long periods of time, potentially leading to serious complications, including permanent damage to the ear and hearing loss.

SEE ALSO *Antibiotic Resistance; Swimmer's Ear and Swimmer's Itch (Cercarial Dermatitis).*

BIBLIOGRAPHY

Books

Friedman, Ellen M., and James P. Barassi. *My Ear Hurts!: A Complete Guide to Understanding and Treating Your Child's Ear Infections.* Darby, PA: Diane Publishing Company, 2004.

Schmidt, Michael A. *Childhood Ear Infections: A Parent's Guide to Alternative Treatments.* Berkeley, CA: North Atlantic Books, 2004.

Periodicals

Jackson, Patricia L. "Healthy People 2010 Objective: Reduce Number and Frequency of Courses of Antibiotics for Ear Infections in Young Children." *Pediatric Nursing* 27 (2000): 591–595.

Web Sites

National Institute on Deafness and Other Communication Disorders. "Otitis Media (Ear Infection)." July 2002. <http://www.nidcd.nih.gov/health/hearing/otitism.asp> (accessed April 10, 2007).

Brian Hoyle

Eastern Equine Encephalitis

■ Introduction

Eastern equine encephalitis (EEE) is a mosquito-borne virus that infects birds and mammals, including horses and humans. It is a rare disease—an average of five human cases of EEE occur in the United States each year. However, its high mortality rate makes it one of the country's most serious mosquito-borne diseases.

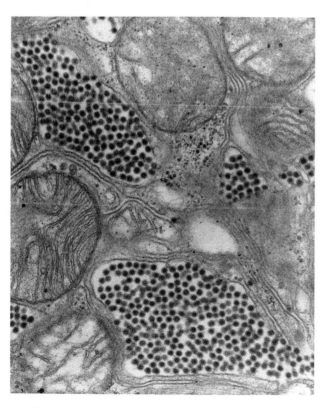

This transmission electron micrograph (TEM) shows a salivary gland of a mosquito that was infected by the eastern equine encephalitis (EEE) virus. The EEE virus occurs mainly in the eastern half of the United States. Due to the high fatality rate, it is regarded as one of the more serious mosquito borne diseases in the nation. © CDC/PHIL/Corbis.

Transmission of EEE to humans usually occurs from bird hosts via mosquitoes from the *Aedes* and *Coquillettidia* species. While some cases are asymptomatic, some people experience mild to severe symptoms such as fevers, headache, and seizures. Severe infections occur when the disease spreads to the central nervous system, which results in permanent neurological damage, or death. No vaccine is available for humans, and no drug treatment for the infection is known. Prevention of infection is best achieved by avoiding mosquitoes, either by reducing mosquito populations or wearing protective clothing.

EEE is distributed in North America, Central and South America, and the Caribbean. Increased migration of humans into areas more likely to contain EEE infection raises the potential for exposure to infected mosquitoes, and thus increases the risk of infection in humans.

■ Disease History, Characteristics, and Transmission

Eastern equine encephalitis (EEE) was first recognized in humans in 1938, although it had been diagnosed in horses since 1831. Transmission occurs via mosquitoes, and infection can cause a range of symptoms.

EEE is transmitted by the bite of an infected mosquito. Generally, the virus lifecycle is composed of passerine birds acting as hosts and the mosquito, *Culiseta melanura*, acting as the vector. However, other mosquitoes—including the *Aedes* and *Coquillettidia* species—which more commonly feed on mammals, such as horses and humans, are also capable of becoming infected and transmitting the disease. Horses and humans have a low level of the virus in their blood, making them ineffective as hosts for transmission. However, birds retain a high level of the virus and act as reservoirs for continued mosquito infection. Therefore, infection is more likely to occur from a mosquito that has fed on an infected bird, rather than via a mosquito that has fed on an infected

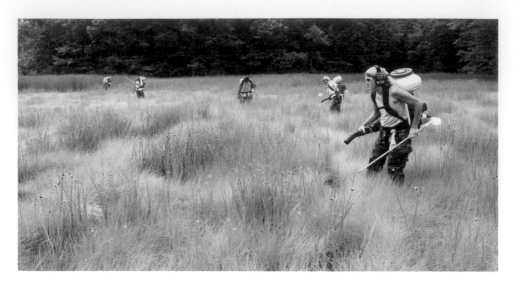

Workers spray a marsh to kill millions of mosquito larvae in New Hampshire in June 2006. They are trying to prevent a seasonal outbreak of eastern equine encephalitis (EEE), a mosquito-borne disease that affects humans and horses. *AP Images.*

mammal. Furthermore, infection in humans by blood transfusions is unlikely to occur. EEE tends to disappear during the winter months because low temperatures kill the vector populations. However, the infection tends to break out again when the weather becomes warm.

In some cases, EEE infection does not result in illness, but, in other cases, it can cause mild to severe symptoms. Mild symptoms include a flulike illness characterized by fever, headache, and sore throat. Severe symptoms arise when the infection enters the central nervous system. Severe symptoms include sudden fever and headache, followed by seizures and coma. The outcome of a severe infection of EEE is mild to severe permanent neurological damage, or death. The CDC reports that a third of severe cases of EEE are fatal, while half of those who surviving a severe EEE infection will have mild to severe permanent neurological damage. Symptoms generally appear 3 to 10 days after being bitten by an infected mosquito, and, in severe cases, rapid deterioration or death occurs soon after symptoms arise.

■ Scope and Distribution

The primary transmission cycle of the EEE virus, which involves the mosquito *Culiseta melanura* and passerine birds, occurs in freshwater, hardwood swamp environments. Therefore, EEE infections generally occur in these regions. Globally, EEE is found in North America, Central and South America, and the Caribbean. Within the United States, the disease is most prevalent in the Atlantic and Gulf Coast states and the Great Lakes region.

EEE is a serious disease as it has significant mortality rates in horses and humans. However, it is a rare disease, with the CDC reporting an average of five human cases occurring in most years. With increased migration of people in the United States into previously undeveloped areas, especially previously uninhabited swampland, the risk of infection has increased, making EEE an emerging infectious disease. During 2006, three people were reported infected with EEE in the state of Massachusetts with one fatal case. In 2005, four cases of infection were reported. In the four years prior to 2006, four people died from EEE.

While human cases of EEE are uncommon, outbreaks are more common among horses. In 2006, an epidemic of 26 equine cases was reported in North Carolina. The scope of equine cases is argued to be under-reported because owners may not consult a veterinarian when horses exhibit signs of EEE and thus no record is made of the infection.

■ Treatment and Prevention

There is no treatment for EEE. A vaccine is available for horses and for laboratory personnel working with the virus. As of 2007, there is no vaccine available for the general public. Infection with the EEE virus is thought to confer lifelong immunity against reinfection with this virus. However, this immunity is limited to the EEE virus and does not confer protection against other viruses.

When EEE is symptomatic, treatment is given for the symptoms of the infection. This involves hospitalization, supportive care, prevention of secondary infections, and physical therapy. There are no antiviral drugs against EEE, and antibiotic drugs do not fight viral infections.

EEE infections can be prevented by avoiding mosquitoes. In the United States, large-scale actions, such as the spraying of insecticides across regions known to be infected, may take place. This mosquito-control action reduces the likelihood that humans will come into contact with infected mosquitoes. Smaller scale methods to avoid mosquitoes include wearing protective clothing, using insect repellent, avoiding outdoor activities while mosquitoes are active, and removing standing bodies of water that may be used as breeding sites by mosquitoes.

■ Impacts and Issues

Since EEE infection has a 30% fatality rate and survivors of severe infection may suffer permanent neurological damage, it is considered a major health concern in the United States despite its low incidence. However, there are some challenges associated with the control of this disease. No vaccination or drug treatment is available for humans as of 2007. Therefore, prevention of infection relies on avoidance of mosquitoes and recovery depends on the extent of infection. Prevention and control methods of EEE infection are expensive and controversial, since the most common control method is large-scale use of insecticides to reduce mosquito populations. A conflict of interest arises between laws mandating wetland protection and the need to apply toxic insecticides for mosquito control.

Another emerging issue is associated with the increased migration of humans into previously uninhabited swamplands. The transmission cycle of the EEE virus occurs naturally within these habitats, since *Culiseta melanura*, the mosquito that transmits this virus among birds, breeds there. Therefore, exposure to the virus increases as humans move into these areas.

The extent to which this disease is present among bird and horse populations is also uncertain. The prevalence of infection in horses is likely to be understated as owners fail to report cases of EEE. This may impact the extent to which a region prepares itself for the possibility of transmission of the EEE virus into the human population.

SEE ALSO *Arthropod-borne Disease; Emerging Infectious Diseases; Encephalitis; Host and Vector; Japanese encephalitis; Mosquito-borne Diseases; St. Louis Encephalitis; Vaccines and Vaccine Development; Vector-borne Disease; Viral Disease.*

WORDS TO KNOW

ENCEPHALITIS: A type of acute brain inflammation, most often due to infection by a virus.

HOST: Organism that serves as the habitat for a parasite, or possibly for a symbiont. A host may provide nutrition to the parasite or symbiont, or simply a place in which to live.

VECTOR: Any agent, living or otherwise, that carries and transmits parasites and diseases. Also, an organism or chemical used to transport a gene into a new host cell.

IN CONTEXT: TRENDS AND STATISTICS

With regard to the incidence of Eastern equine encephalitis (EEE) the Division of Vector-Borne Infectious Diseases, Centers for Disease Control and Prevention (CDC) offers the following statistics regarding human cases:

- Approximately 220 confirmed cases in the U.S. 1964–2004
- Average of 5 cases/year, with a range from 0–15 cases
- States with largest number of cases are Florida, Georgia, Massachusetts, and New Jersey.
- EEEV transmission is most common in and around freshwater hardwood swamps in the Atlantic and Gulf Coast states and the Great Lakes region.
- Human cases occur relatively infrequently, largely because the primary transmission cycle takes place in and around swampy areas where human populations tend to be limited.

SOURCE: *Centers for Disease Control and Prevention, National Center for Infectious Diseases, Division of Vector-Borne Infectious Diseases*

BIBLIOGRAPHY

Books

Mandell, G.L., J.E. Bennett, and R. Dolin. *Principles and Practice of Infectious Diseases.* Vol. 2. Philadelphia: Elsevier, 2005.

Web Sites

Centers for Disease Control and Prevention. "Eastern Equine Encephalitis Fact Sheet." July 12, 2006. <http://www.cdc.gov/ncidod/dvbid/arbor/eeefact.htm> (accessed February 22, 2007).

Directors of Health Promotion and Education.
"Eastern Equine Encephalitis." <http://
www.dhpe.org/infect/equine.html> (accessed
February 22, 2007).

Boston Globe. "Middleborough Boy with EEE Dies."
August 31, 2006. <http://www.boston.com/
news/globe/city_region/breaking_news/2006/
08/middleborough_b.html> (accessed February
22, 2007).

Ebola

■ Introduction

Ebola is a type of hemorrhagic fever that is caused by four subtypes of a virus called the Ebola virus. The virus is one of two members of Filoviridae, a family of RNA viruses. The name of the virus comes from a river located in the Democratic Republic of the Congo, formerly called Zaire, where the virus was first discovered during an outbreak of the disease.

Ebola is a terrifying disease that can progress steadily towards death. The destruction of internal organs caused by the infecting virus produces a great deal of internal bleeding and can cause bleeding from various parts of the body such as the eyes, gums, and nose. The disease caused by Ebola-Zaire, the first of the four types of the virus yet discovered, is fatal over 90% of the time.

The progression from health to death within a few weeks for those unlucky enough to contract the infection is one terrifying aspect of Ebola. The other is, essentially, a fear of the unknown. Even though the disease has been known since the late 1980s, the origin of Ebola, its reservoir, and how the disease can be prevented are still largely mysterious. The main reason for this is the infrequency of outbreaks and the speed of their appearance

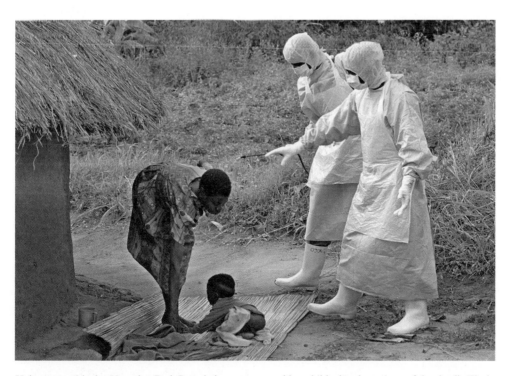

Volunteers with the Ugandan Red Cross help a woman and her child who show signs of the deadly Ebola virus. The two were taken from their village to a hospital in the Gulu region of northern Uganda to have their blood tested for the virus. *Tyler Hicks/Getty Images.*

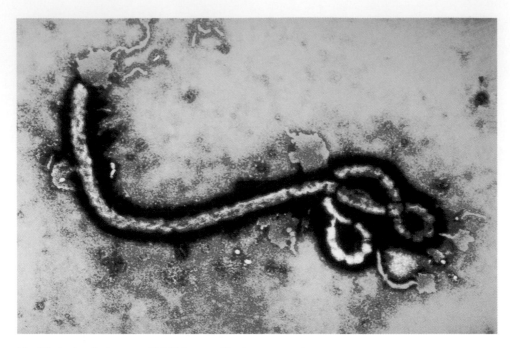

The Ebola virus is shown at 108,000x magnification. © *Royalty-Free/Corbis.*

and disappearance. The infection quickly spreads from person to person through a local population and, because of the high death rate, soon disappears after running out of new hosts to infect. This pattern has made the study of Ebola difficult.

It is thought that Ebola is transmitted to humans from a natural host by a vector. This route of transmission occurs in some other diseases. One example is malaria, which is transferred to a susceptible person from an infected animal or person via mosquitoes. Ebola may be naturally present in chimpanzees. At least two outbreaks of Ebola-Zaire were determined to be due to contact between humans and infected chimpanzees. However, it may be that chimpanzees are not the natural host, but are themselves infected by the virus, which is transmitted to them from another host. As discussed below, the natural host may be bats, although this has not been proven. Likewise, studies by the World Health Organization (WHO) and the U.S. Centers for Disease Control and Prevention (CDC) have not yet identified the vector that carries the virus from that host to humans. What is clear from the ferocity of past outbreaks is that once someone has been infected with Ebola, the virus is easily transferred from person to person.

■ Disease History, Characteristics, and Transmission

As of 2007, four subtypes of Ebola virus have been identified. Three of the subtypes cause disease in humans. The four subtypes of Ebola are slightly different

in the sequence of their genetic material and in the composition of the proteins that are present on their surfaces. Analysis of blood obtained from people infected by one of the four viral subtypes has revealed slightly different antibody patterns. (An antibody is a protein produced by the immune system in response to the presence of a specific protein, which is termed an antigen.) The four subtypes of virus may have originated from a single virus that mutated to create the four slightly different subtypes over time, but this hypothesis has not yet been confirmed.

The first Ebola virus to be discovered was Ebola-Zaire. It was isolated near the Ebola River in the Democratic Republic of the Congo during an outbreak in 1976. There were 318 reported cases. Of these, 280 people died, a mortality rate of 88%. Other known occurrences of Ebola due to Ebola-Zaire include:

- Democratic Republic of the Congo, 1977 (one case, one death)
- Gabon, 1994 (52 cases, 31 deaths)
- Democratic Republic of the Congo, 1995 (315 cases, 250 deaths)
- Gabon, January to April 1996 (37 cases, 21 deaths)
- Gabon, July 1996 to January 1997 (60 cases, 45 deaths)
- South Africa, 1996 (two cases, one death; the disease was contracted in the Democratic Republic of the Congo)
- Gabon and the Democratic Republic of the Congo, October 2001 to March 2002 (53 cases, 53 deaths

WORDS TO KNOW

AMPLIFICATION: A process by which something is made larger, or the quantity increased.

ANTIBODY: Antibodies, or Y-shaped immunoglobulins, are proteins found in the blood that help to fight against foreign substances called antigens. Antigens, which are usually proteins or polysaccharides, stimulate the immune system to produce antibodies. The antibodies inactivate the antigen and help to remove it from the body. While antigens can be the source of infections from pathogenic bacteria and viruses, organic molecules detrimental to the body from internal or environmental sources also act as antigens. Genetic engineering and the use of various mutational mechanisms allow the construction of a vast array of antibodies (each with a unique genetic sequence).

ANTIGEN: Antigens, which are usually proteins or polysaccharides, stimulate the immune system to produce antibodies. The antibodies inactivate the antigen and help to remove it from the body. While antigens can be the source of infections from pathogenic bacteria and viruses, organic molecules detrimental to the body from internal or environmental sources also act as antigens. Genetic engineering and the use of various mutational mechanisms allow the construction of a vast array of antibodies (each with a unique genetic sequence).

ANTISENSE DRUG: An antisense drug binds to mRNA, thereby blocking gene activity. Some viruses have mRNA as their genetic material, so an antisense drug could inhibit their replication

BUSH MEAT: The meat of terrestrial wild and exotic animals, typically those that live in parts of Africa, Asia, and the Americas; also known as wild meat.

HEMORRHAGIC FEVER: A hemorrhagic fever is caused by viral infection and features a high fever and a high volume of (copious) bleeding. The bleeding is caused by the formation of tiny blood clots throughout the bloodstream. These blood clots—also called microthrombi—deplete platelets and fibrinogen in the bloodstream. When bleeding begins, the factors needed for the clotting of the blood are scarce. Thus, uncontrolled bleeding (hemorrhage) ensues.

HOST: Organism that serves as the habitat for a parasite, or possibly for a symbiont. A host may provide nutrition to the parasite or symbiont, or simply a place in which to live.

RESERVOIR: The animal or organism in which the virus or parasite normally resides.

VECTOR: Any agent, living or otherwise, that carries and transmits parasites and diseases. Also, an organism or chemical used to transport a gene into a new host cell.

---

in the Gabon outbreak; 57 cases, 43 deaths in the Congo outbreak)

- Democratic Republic of Congo, December 2002 to April 2003 (143 cases, 128 deaths)

- Democratic Republic of Congo, 2003 (35 cases, 29 deaths).

The second type of Ebola virus to be discovered was Ebola-Sudan. It was discovered in 1976 during an outbreak that occurred in Sudan (284 cases, 151 deaths). Other outbreaks involving Ebola-Sudan include:

- England, 1976 (one case; when a lab technician studying the virus accidentally contracted the virus from a needle puncture)

- Sudan, 1979 (34 cases, 22 deaths)

- Uganda, 2000–2001 (425 cases, 224 deaths)

- Sudan, 2004 (17 cases, 7 deaths)

The third type of Ebola virus to be discovered was Ebola-Reston. Outbreaks of Ebola occurred simultaneously in 1989 in three animal facilities in the United States that had received monkeys imported from the Philippines. One of the facilities was in Reston, Virginia, and the virus took its name from the outbreak among the primates at this facility. No humans died in the outbreak, although four people were infected, as shown by the antibodies that they developed to the virus. This outbreak formed the basis for a best-selling book by Richard Preston called *The Hot Zone* and a motion picture called *Outbreak* Other outbreaks of Ebola-Reston in 1990, 1992, and 1996 involved deaths among other primates, but no human fatalities (although some people had produced antibodies to the virus). Thus far, Ebola-Reston has not caused human illness.

The final subtype of Ebola virus, as of 2007, is Ebola-Ivory Coast, which was discovered in 1994 in Ivory Coast. It caused one non-lethal case involving a scientist who contracted the infection after conducting an autopsy on a chimpanzee.

IN CONTEXT: DISEASE IN DEVELOPING NATIONS

As of May 2007, the natural reservoir of the Ebola virus remained unknown. The World Health Organization (WHO) states that "the natural reservoir of the Ebola virus is unknown despite extensive studies, but seems to reside in the rain forests on the African continent and in the Western Pacific."

"Although non-human primates have been a source of infection for humans, they are not thought to be the reservoir. They, like humans, are argued to be infected directly from the natural reservoir or through a chain of transmission from the natural reservoir. On the African continent, Ebola infections of human cases have been linked to direct contact with gorillas, chimpanzees, monkeys, forest antelope and porcupines found dead in the rainforest. So far, the Ebola virus has been detected in the wild in carcasses of chimpanzees (in Côte-d'Ivoire and Republic of Congo), gorillas (Gabon and Republic of Congo) and duikers (Republic of Congo)."

"Because bats deliberated infected with Ebola do not die there is continued scientific speculation that bats or mammals may play a role in harboring the virus in the wild."

SOURCE: *World Health Organization*

The various types of Ebola virus are all filoviruses. One characteristic of filoviruses is their long, stringlike shape. When observed using the high magnification power of the electron microscope, the viruses can be coiled, circular, U-shaped, or even shaped like a cane (or a shepherd's crook). The different shapes may not be natural, but rather may be formed artificially during purification of the virus.

The molecular details of the Ebola infection have been clarified. This work can only be done in a few laboratories in the world that are designed for research involving highly dangerous and infectious microorganisms. The infection begins when a protein on the surface of the virus recognizes a host molecule. It is not known whether the host molecule is another protein, lipid, or carbohydrate. Following the linkage between the viral protein and the host receptor, the viral genetic material enters the host cell. It is not known how this occurs. Increased understanding of these early steps is vital, since by blocking the viral attachment to the host cell and/or the transfer of the genetic material into the host cell, the subsequent infection could be stopped. Efforts to develop a vaccine are focusing on these steps. For example, blocking the adherence of a microbe to a host cell has proven successful in the development of a preliminary vaccine for cattle against a bacterium called *Escherichia coli* O157:H7, which can cause a lethal infection in humans, popularly known as "hamburger disease."

Ebola viruses contain RNA. For the manufacture of a new virus, the infecting virus must use the host cell's genetic machinery to read the viral payload of RNA and to manufacture one of the viral proteins. Once this so-called nonstructural protein is made, it can decode the remaining viral genetic material to manufacture seven other proteins. These proteins are described as being structural—they are used to form the new virus. The new virus particles are eventually released from the host cell when the cell bursts, and another cycle of infection begins as new cells are infected. How the virus, with just eight proteins, manages to make new copies of itself and evade the attempts by the hosts' immune system to stop the infection is unclear.

In their natural host, the Ebola virus presumably does not cause a serious infection. If it did, it would not persist, since the host would be killed. However, in humans the resulting infection can be devastating. Within days, Ebola-Zaire and Ebola-Sudan produce a high fever, headache, generalized muscle aches (myalgia), abdominal pain, tiredness, and diarrhea. Cells lining the intestinal tract and stomach can be damaged, causing bloody diarrhea and vomiting of blood. At this stage some people do recover. But, for many, the infection worsens. Massive internal bleeding sends a person into shock and can cause heart damage. Death soon follows.

One of the challenges of combating an Ebola outbreak is the fact that the early symptoms of the infection are similar to those of the flu, malaria, typhoid fever, and several bacterial infections, which occur more often and are not as serious. By the time the true nature of the infection becomes known, many people in a community could have been infected.

The swiftness of the infection has been noted by some authors. Others feel, however, that the two-week course of the infection is not unusually quick. The latter view is true when a patient is near medical care in a developed country. However, in rural regions of Africa where Ebola is most common, medical care may be days in coming and even then may not be capable of dealing with a severe infection. In that situation, even a disease that develops within a week is swift and serious.

In some Ebola outbreaks, the initial infection has been traced to contact between humans and an animal (usually a primate) that harbors the virus. However, it is still unclear whether the primate is the natural host or becomes infected through contact with another animal. What is now clear is that the contagious person-to-person transmission of the virus subsequently occurs via infected blood or body fluids. This transfer can occur directly, with someone coming into contract with blood or body fluids during handling and care of a patient. Accidental infection during study of the virus also has occurred.

The rapid spread of Ebola is also aided by the location of most of the outbreaks. The areas in Africa where Ebola appears are poor, rural, and do not have medical facilities close by. The health care facilities that are available are not likely to have space available to isolate the infected patient from other patients, which can contribute to the spread of the infection.

The pattern of the Ebola-Reston outbreak that occurred in Virginia in 1989 indicates that the virus may be capable of airborne spread. In that outbreak, at least one of the primates who became ill was never in contact or even in the same room as the other sick primates. Lab studies have demonstrated that aerosols of the virus can infect test animals. Whether this route plays a major role in Ebola is unclear, but the general feeling is that airborne transmission is not as important as transmission by body fluids.

■ Scope and Distribution

Almost all confirmed cases of Ebola through 2007 have been in Africa. However, the infection may also occur in the Western Pacific because the Reston, Virginia, outbreaks were caused by monkeys imported from the Philippines.

The rapid deterioration of a person following the appearance of symptoms and the fact that the affected villages can be difficult to reach has meant that response to infections by disease control officials from organizations such as the WHO and the CDC occurs long after the disease has begun. This has made the discovery of Ebola's origin difficult. As of 2007, the source of the Ebola viruses is still unknown. The general agreement among scientists who study Ebola is that, because other filoviruses can infect African monkeys, macaques, and chimpanzees without causing harm to these hosts, the host for the Ebola viruses may be similar. However, Ebola does harm some primates. Furthermore, an intensive 12-year-long sampling of tens of thousands of amphibians, mammals, birds, reptiles, and insects failed to detect the viruses.

Bats have also been considered as Ebola's natural host. The people who first became ill in two of the outbreaks worked in buildings where bats lived and may have come into contact with the bats. Furthermore, in a study that deliberately introduced Ebola virus into a number of vertebrates, the virus persisted only in bats. More evidence supporting the involvement of bats was published in *Nature* in 2006. The study reported on a survey of over 1,000 animals from Gabon and Republic of the Congo, including over 650 bats. Of these, Ebola virus RNA was found in 13 fruit bats. Bats also can harbor several other viruses that are related to Ebola. This evidence for the involvement of bats as the natural host of Ebola is still circumstantial. To date, there is no evidence that an infected bat is capable of infecting another animal, such as a primate.

■ Treatment and Prevention

Currently, there is no cure for Ebola. Treatment consists of keeping the patient as comfortable and pain-free as possible and minimizing the spread of infection. Additional treatment measures include restoring lost fluids,

---

IN CONTEXT: CULTURAL CONNECTIONS

Because the Ebola virus is transmitted by direct contact with the body fluids (blood, secretions, etc.) of infected persons, living or dead, various cultural practices can facilitate Ebola transmission. The World Health Organization (WHO) states "Burial ceremonies where mourners have direct contact with the body of the deceased person can play a significant role in the transmission of Ebola."

WHO also reports that "the infection of human cases with Ebola virus has been documented through the handling of infected chimpanzees, gorillas, and forest antelopes—both dead and alive—as was documented in Côte d'Ivoire, the Republic of Congo and Gabon."

SOURCE: *World Health Organization*

---

trying to minimize bleeding, and dealing with any secondary infections that might occur.

As of 2007, prevention of Ebola is impossible, but research is underway on several fronts. Antisense drugs have been used successfully in a small number of infected Rhesus monkeys. Antisense therapy uses genetic material that is complimentary to the region of interest in the virus. Because the added stretch of genetic material is complimentary, it binds with the target region. This prevents the target region from being used in the viral replication process. Put another way, antisense drugs can shut down the infectious process. Whether this approach will prove successful as a prevention strategy for Ebola is unclear, and much research still remains to be done.

Vaccines are another preventative strategy that is being actively explored. In the case of Ebola, several other viruses have been engineered to contain one of the Ebola proteins that is present on the surface of the virus. This bioengineered virus is then administered to monkeys, and the monkeys produce antibodies to the Ebola surface protein. When an intact Ebola virus is given to the monkeys, the anti-Ebola antibody can block the attachment of the Ebola surface protein to the host cell. This approach has shown enough promise to warrant giving the vaccine to humans to see if they produce the anti-Ebola antibody. As of 2007, this vaccine is still being studied.

■ Impacts and Issues

Ebola affects people in the most basic way. It strikes with little warning and can sweep through a village in a short time. In the rural settings where the disease usually occurs, medical care is minimal and health care providers are stretched to their limits to contain the infection and provide basic comforts to those who are ill.

Though the best selling book *The Hot Zone* and the movie *Outbreak* were somewhat sensational, they address the lethality of Ebola. These popular depictions of Ebola served a useful purpose in making the average person more aware of Ebola specifically and infectious diseases in general.

Ebola is a striking example of how human encroachment on regions that were previously uninhabited can bring people into contact with microorganisms to which they had not been previously exposed. Another example of this phenomenon is the emergence of avian influenza in humans. Long a disease transferred between some species of poultry, closer human contact with poultry has enabled the avian flu virus to adapt so that it is capable of, initially, bird-to-human transmission and, within the past several years, human-to-human transmission.

In the case of Ebola, human encroachment on previously uninhabited areas includes increased contact with the natural host of the disease. The blurring of the boundaries between the human and the natural world has brought people into closer contact with primates, who are either the natural reservoir of the virus or who acquire the infection from the natural reservoir, possibly a fruit bat. The virus can spread to humans who kill and eat apes or chimpanzees. Bush meat, including the meat of primates, has long been eaten by rural Africans, and its sale is still an important part of the rural economy. In addition, bush meat has become increasingly popular as a delicacy in the western world.

The link between the consumption of bush meat and the spread of Ebola has spurred efforts to restrict poaching. A 2005 meeting involving 23 African nations and representatives of the United Nations addressed the problem of the declining great ape population and urged stricter controls on poaching and deforestation (which increases the access of people to ape territory). While admirable, the effectiveness of the campaign is debatable. Ape meat is still available for sale in many local markets in regions of Africa and is sought by buyers in western countries.

While some species may naturally harbor the Ebola virus without harm, other species are being decimated. Beginning in 2002, conservationists in some regions of Africa began to note a die-off of western gorillas and common chimpanzees. The great ape population in the African nation of Gabon has declined by half since the 1990s, with Ebola and poaching cited as the most likely causes. Without a concerted effort, these near-human creatures may become extinct within decades.

Part of the reason for the ferocity of an Ebola outbreak is a lack of understanding of the disease among those who are most affected by it. More education targeting those who are at risk of acquiring the infection is still needed. For example, burial customs in many African cultures include an open viewing of the deceased, which potentially exposes the mourners to the virus.

This practice can amplify the spread of the virus—that is, the virus can affect more people than it otherwise would. Amplification is an important means by which a variety of viral and bacterial diseases can spread. In the case of Ebola and mourning customs, learning to pay respect to the deceased person without touching or even seeing them would help reduce the spread of Ebola.

During some initial outbreaks, well-meaning medical personnel helped spread the virus. The infection of health care workers is, unfortunately, a common aspect of Ebola outbreaks. The use of protective measures, such as masks and gloves, lessens the risk of passing the infection to caregivers. In some rural clinics, however, such measures—commonplace in medical clinics in developed countries—are a luxury.

Development of a vaccine is a primary goal of those concerned with the control of Ebola. In 2003, researchers at the Dale and Betty Bumpers Vaccine Research Center and the U.S. Army Medical Research Institute reported the development of a vaccine that protects monkeys from injected Ebola virus. The vaccine involves a two-stage process in which immunity results from the injection of non-infectious genetic material from the Ebola virus followed a few weeks later by the introduction of another virus that carries genes of the Ebola virus, which are vital to the establishment of an infection. The resulting immune response can stop the Ebola infection.

As of 2007, the DNA vaccine is still undergoing evaluation. Small-scale human trials have been done. However, one stumbling block in its development concerns the ethical issue of testing the vaccine in humans on the large scale required for approval processes, since this would involve exposing people to the virus. In addition, it is not clear whether a vaccine will work in people whose immune systems are not functioning normally. This is an important consideration, since Africa is also home to millions of people who suffer from acquired immunodeficiency syndrome (AIDS, also cited as acquired immune deficiency syndrome), a disease whose hallmark is the deterioration in immune system function.

Another issue concerning serious infections, including Ebola, is the potential of the microbe to be used as a weapon. Indeed, Ebola has been considered for development as a biological weapon by both the United States and Russia (then the Soviet Union). More recently, members of the Japanese cult Aum Shinrikyo—who released sarin gas in the Tokyo subway system in 1995, killing 12 people and injuring almost 1,000—visited Zaire in 1992. Under the guise of offering medical aid to victims of an Ebola outbreak, cult members instead tried to acquire some virus to use as a terrorist weapon.

■ Primary Source Connection

The following press release from the World Health Organization details its field response to a 2004 Ebola outbreak in southern Sudan. Along with mobilizing supplies and health workers, education of local villagers at the center of the outbreak was crucial in containing the spread of the disease.

WHO Announces End of Ebola Outbreak in Southern Sudan

Geneva—Today marks the 42nd day since the last person identified as infected with Ebola haemorrhagic fever died on 26 June 2004 in Yambio Hospital, southern Sudan. As 42 days is twice the maximum incubation period for Ebola, and as no further cases have been identified, WHO declares today that the outbreak in southern Sudan is over.

"The rapid containment of this outbreak was a tremendous success for the health authorities, WHO, and the international community involved in the control operations," said Dr Abdullah Ahmed, head of WHO, southern Sudan, and coordinator of the response.

As of today, the health authorities of Yambio County have reported a total of 17 cases, including seven deaths from Ebola. Ebola haemorrhagic fever is a febrile illness which causes death in 50–90% of all clinically ill cases. It is transmitted by direct contact with the blood, secretions, organs or bodily fluids of infected persons.

"In Yambio, WHO and our partners were able to apply lessons learned during responses to the five Ebola outbreaks that have occurred since 2000," said Dr. Pierre Formenty, who worked as part of WHO's response team. Ebola outbreaks have been detected more frequently in recent years, making local and international collaboration essential.

During this outbreak, Ebola virus (sub-type Sudan) was confirmed by laboratory tests at the Kenya Medical Research Institute and the Centers for Disease Control and Prevention in the United States. When the outbreak was first reported in late May, a response team including members from WHO southern Sudan Early Warning and Response Network (EWARN), and WHO headquarters was formed to work with local health authorities in creating a Crisis Committee to control the outbreak.

The committee included UNICEF, Médecins Sans Frontières-France and other non-governmental organizations and churches working in public health. The international response to the outbreak also included partners from WHO's Regional Office for the Eastern Mediterranean, the Global Outbreak Alert and Response Network (GOARN) as well as experts from the CDC, the European Programme for Intervention Epidemiology Training, Field Epidemiology Training Programme, Egypt and the Health Protection Agency in the United Kingdom.

Intensive social mobilization for Ebola was essential to the outbreak's containment. Key messages about the disease and behaviour-specific precautionary advice were passed on to the people in and around Yambio by local community advocates.

"Once the people of Yambio were convinced of the very real risks Ebola posed and they understood what they could do to protect themselves and their families the outbreak response was greatly accelerated," said Ms. Asiya Odugleh from the WHO Mediterranean Centre for Vulnerability Reduction, Tunis, who assisted the county social mobilization team.

The control efforts included, for example, an isolation ward at Yambio Hospital with a low fence so that patients were effectively isolated, yet still able to see and talk to their family and friends over the fence at a safe distance. Such simple adaptations of disease control measures made it easier for families to accept the case management of patients in the isolation unit, while ensuring maximum protection for the medical team and patients.

"The lessons we learned in Yambio from this outbreak will strengthen our responses to future outbreaks," said Dr. Hassan El Bushra from the WHO Regional Office for the Eastern Mediterranean in Cairo. The Yambio experience has proven the value of rapid outbreak detection, local response capacities, active community involvement, and the coordination of specialized international assistance to the outbreak's containment.

"WHO cannot predict where or when the next Ebola outbreak will happen," said Dr. El Bushra, "But we can continue laying the groundwork by building on what we have learned in Yambio."

World Health Organization. Epidemic and Pandemic Alert and Response.

WORLD HEALTH ORGANIZATION. "WHO ANNOUNCES END OF EBOLA OUTBREAK IN SOUTHERN SUDAN." PRESS RELEASE, AUGUST 7, 2004. AVAILABLE ONLINE AT <HTTP://WWW.WHO.INT/CSR/DON/2004_08_07/EN/INDEX.HTML>

SEE ALSO *Antiviral Drugs; Emerging Infectious Diseases; Hemorrhagic Fevers; Vector-borne Disease.*

BIBLIOGRAPHY

Books

Hirschmann, Kris. *The Ebola Virus.* San Diego: Lucent Books, 2006.

Regis, Ed. *Virus Ground Zero: Stalking the Killer Viruses with the Centers for Disease Control.* New York: Pocket Books, 2003.

Smith, Tara. *Ebola.* London: Chelsea House Publications, 2005.

Periodicals

Leroy, E.M., et al. "Fruits Bats as Reservoirs of Ebola Virus." *Nature* 438 (December 1, 2005): 575–576.

Brian Hoyle

Economic Development and Infectious Disease

■ Introduction

Across the nations of the world, there is a relationship between income and health. Developed nations often have lower average morbidity (illness) and mortality (death) rates than developing nations. Mortality rates drop over time as countries increase in wealth. Within countries, wealthier people typically live longer than poorer people.

■ History and Scientific Foundations

The impact of economic conditions on health status has long been recognized, based on studies of the effects of food scarcity, shelter, and living space. Although economic conditions have been de-emphasized as factors in mortality and morbidity because of the dissemination of medical technologies, there is increasing evidence that this diffusion of health knowledge and technology has had differential effects in developed and underdeveloped nations. Studies of this topic typically focus on national income (the value of all goods and services produced in a given period). Secondly, per capita income (income per person) is the leading indicator of economic development and motivates many health policy decisions. Thus, many observers are calling for greater global economic development. Critics assail the emphasis on economic development over public health, but others assert that

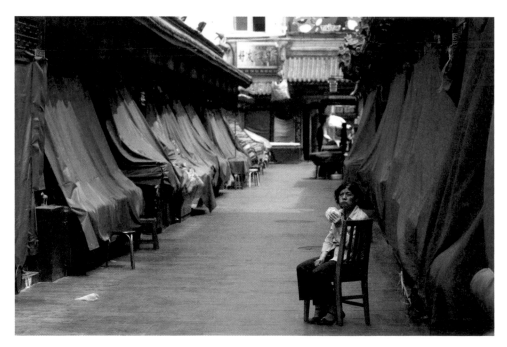

A Chinese vendor is shown having lunch on a closed street in a tourist district in Beijing in spring 2003. The government estimates Beijing's tourism industry lost $7 billion because of SARS.   © *Reuters/Corbis.*

276

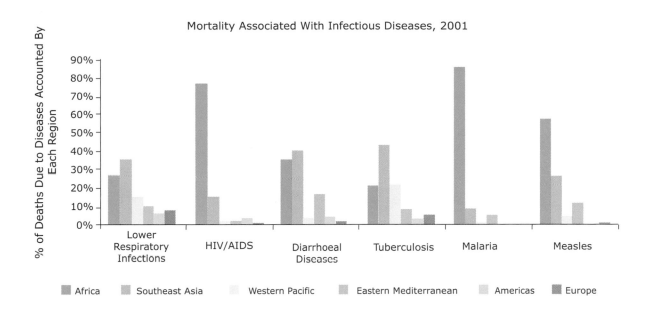

This 2001 chart illustrates that the deaths resulting from five types of infectious diseases that occur more frequently in developing countries. © *World Health Organization (WHO).*

public health initiatives are too often thwarted by political and economic instability and food scarcity.

Studies have found a significant positive correlation between income and health status in both developed and developing economies. In more developed countries, the causal path typically goes from health status to income, with feedback from income to health. Healthier people are wealthy, but wealthy people may have increased access to healthcare and wellness resources. However, whether income "buys" better health and just how this may occur has proven difficult for economists to quantify, especially for adults in the work force. In developed countries, the most documented connection between income and health is based on studies of infant mortality rates, the scope of which cannot support a robust analysis of the feedback from health to income.

The mechanisms producing a relationship between money and health are complex. Variables such as race, education, and urban or rural status may also influence income or health for many individuals. The causes of poor health status in less developed countries may be different from the factors that undermine health in industrialized countries. In developing countries, infectious disease, lack of clean drinking water, and inadequate diet may present the greatest public health risks. In developed nations, lifestyle-related chronic diseases and reduced physical activity may present the greatest public health threats.

The connecting mechanisms underlying the relationship between health and income are sometimes not specific to the level of industrialization. This relationship in

"middle income" or transition economies may be particularly hard to analyze because persons in the same communities, and even in the same households, can be disproportionately affected by problems common to both developed and less-developed regions. For example, obese women may be neighbors or even housemates of malnourished children. Thus the scientific underpinnings of the relationship between development, income and health are best served by focusing on universal mechanisms—such as psychosocial stress (stress caused by social, psychological, and environmental factors)—that are likely to be found in every society and community.

A study of data sponsored by the World Health Organization (WHO) summarized below that confirms a link between income and health casts light on the interplay between wealth and health. In particular, the study focused on how income improves health apart from the availability of medical services. The study results indicate that increased earnings capacity, along with policies that provide for income transfers to those less wealthy, may be as important for health outcomes as additional funds for service provision. Within countries, income is strongly correlated with health outcomes, especially in settings where the health services delivery is weak. This correlation exists apart from the presence of vital public health campaigns to provide clean water, eradicate malaria, vaccinate children, or deliver AIDS treatment drugs in developing countries.

In view of the possible independence of income as a factor in improving health, a question arises regarding the efficiency of public and private funds aimed at health

WORDS TO KNOW

MORBIDITY: The term "morbidity" comes from the Latin word "morbus," which means sick. In medicine it refers not just to the state of being ill, but also to the severity of the illness. A serious disease is said to have a high morbidity.

MORTALITY: Mortality is the condition of being susceptible to death. The term "mortality" comes from the Latin word *mors*, which means "death." Mortality can also refer to the rate of deaths caused by an illness or injury, i.e., "Rabies has a high mortality."

PATHOGEN: A disease causing agent, such as a bacteria, virus, fungus, etc.

promotion. For example, investment in economic development, employment opportunities and income support for the poor might have equal or greater impact on health than would public expenditures on health services availability. People with more income may spend income on goods and services associated with better health—more nutritious food, better housing, exercise, or leisure activities.

■ Applications and Research

The impact of improved pensions on health in South Africa

A "natural experiment" reported by Princeton University that illuminated the relationship between income and health dealt with the institution of larger pension payments to all elderly South Africans. To determine whether income has a causal effect on health, WHO-sponsored investigators identified state old-age pension payments as a source of income that is not determined by a respondent's health status. According to the report, in South Africa, women aged 60 and older and men aged 65 and older are eligible for a monthly cash transfer, if they do not have an employer-based pension, and over 80% of eligible people take up this source of income, which in many communities, where unemployment reaches up to 40%, is the only stable and considerable source of income.

The health survey showed that pension income had a protective effect on the self-reported health of all adults in which the pension income was pooled with that of other household members. For pensioners living in households in which income was not pooled, the beneficial health effects of the pension accrued only to the pensioners, after they started receiving the pension.

These effects persisted regardless of geographic location, race, educational level, and income level.

The researchers investigated whether higher income tended to have an impact on four major areas of daily life: medical care, water and sanitation, nutrition, and psychosocial stress. They found no evidence from the survey data suggesting that higher incomes enabled respondents to spend more time and money seeking out better health services such as private physicians and better equipped clinics. Also, access to cleaner water was apparently not improved, although higher and pooled income families were more likely to have a flush toilet. However, higher and pooled income families were more likely to report improved nutrition and fewer skipped meals, which were correlated with better health status. Finally, income was correlated with reduced self-reported depression symptoms connected to psychosocial stress. Depression has been associated with increased all-cause medical symptoms in many studies. Thus the researchers concluded that income has a causal effect on health status, which is mediated by a combination of improved sanitation, nutrition, and the reduction of psychosocial stress.

■ Impacts and Issues

Social inequality and infectious disease

Evidence is mounting that social inequalities contribute significantly to disease emergence. These inequalities have impacted not only the distribution of infectious diseases, but also the severity and outcome of disease in affected persons. Analyses of outbreaks of Ebola, AIDS, and tuberculosis indicate that disease emergence is influenced by specific events and processes, subject to local variation. Close examination of mutations in microorganisms often shows that human actions have been key factors in increasing the spread of disease and resistance to antibiotics. For example, tropical diseases such as malaria generally affect people in lower socioeconomic brackets, while people with higher incomes may purchase mosquito nets, insect repellants, or live in areas with better drainage and fewer mosquitoes.

The distribution of Ebola outbreaks affect (apart from researchers) people living in poverty and health care workers who serve the poor, but often not others in close physical proximity. For example, the 1976 outbreak in Zaire affected 318 persons. The cases could be traced to failure to follow contact precautions and improper sterilization of syringes and other equipment and supplies. Once these measures were taken, the outbreak was terminated. This explanation suggests that Ebola does not always emerge randomly. Rather, the likelihood of coming into contact with unsterile syringes in, for example, health clinics, is inversely proportional to social status. Population groups with access to high-quality medical services are thus unlikely to contract Ebola even in Ebola affected regions.

The reemergence of tuberculosis is another powerful example of the impact of social inequality on the epidemiology of infections. For decades the disease was largely absent Western Europe and North America, but remained endemic in many developing and underdeveloped nations worldwide. World trade, increased migration, and international travel have reintroduced tuberculosis to regions where the disease had once been eliminated.

Thus, socioeconomic (social and economic factors considered) inequality within nations may have helped foster the virulence of old and new infectious diseases. Economic inequality between nations may also accentuate differences in the distribution of infectious diseases. National borders cannot keep out all pathogens (disease-causing organisms), but can be substantial boundaries to infectious disease response and the provision of healthcare.

Economic development's impact on tuberculosis in India

Approximately a half-million people in India die of tuberculosis annually. Until recently, fewer than 50% of people with tuberculosis received an accurate diagnosis. Less than half of these people received effective treatment. A study by the Ministry of Health and Family Welfare analyzed the impact of health policies promulgated in 1993 that devoted increased resources such as improved diagnosis, case management of treatment, and the use of uniform anti-tuberculosis treatments as well as improved case reporting methods. The program trained more than 200,000 health workers and improved access to services for 436 million people (more than 40 percent of India's population). Under the program's auspices, about 3.4 million patients were evaluated for tuberculosis, and nearly 800,000 had received treatment by late 2001, with a success rate greater than 80 percent. Thus India's tuberculosis control program has succeeded in improving access to care, the quality of diagnosis, and the probability of successful treatment. This has translated into the prevention of 200,000 deaths and the alleviation of indirect medical costs (e.g., productivity and caregiving costs) of more than $400 million—an order of magnitude greater than the cost of program implementation.

In spite of the program's success, ministry officials observe that it will be a challenging to sustain and expand the program due to the country's current limited primary health care system and large—but mainly unregulated—private health care system. Furthermore, India struggling with an increase in incidence of HIV and multi-drug-resistant tuberculosis.

The advance of public health systems and spread of advanced medical knowledge and technology has certainly resulted in improvements in the health status worldwide. However, lack of economic development and vast income inequalities across and within national boundaries continue to present major obstacles to public health. Poverty has prevented equality in healthcare among nations. Infectious diseases continue to be the major cause of death worldwide, with 25% of all deaths and 30% of the global disease burden attributed to communicable diseases. More than 95% of these deaths, the majority of which are preventable, occur in the poorest areas of the developing nations. HIV/AIDS, tuberculosis, and malaria are the three most lethal infectious diseases in these regions.

Health assistance to developing countries, especially for these three diseases, has been based on advocacy for the principles of social justice and the human right to health in the developing world. Given the increasing integration of the global economy, economic development in lower income countries will increase profitable investment opportunities for wealthier countries in the developing world. Improved public health in developing countries also has political and international security benefits for developed nations.

■ Primary Source Connection

The following press release from the World Health Organization (WHO) outlines the economic impacts of malaria, including the costs on present generations for past failures to more significantly control the disease.

Economic Costs Of Malaria Are Many Times Higher Than Previously Estimated

AFRICA'S GDP WOULD BE UP TO $100 BILLION GREATER THIS YEAR IF MALARIA HAD BEEN ELIMINATED YEARS AGO, ACCORDING TO NEW RESEARCH BY HARVARD, LONDON SCHOOL AND WHO.

Abuja, Nigeria—The control of malaria in Africa would significantly increase the continent's economic productivity and the income of African families, according to the findings of a new report released today by the World Health Organization, Harvard University and the London School of Hygiene and Tropical Medicine.

"The evidence strongly suggests that malaria obstructs overall economic development in Africa," said Dr. Jeffrey Sachs, Director of the Center for International Development at Harvard University. "Since 1990, the per person GDP in many sub-Saharan African countries has declined, and malaria is an important reason for this poor economic performance."

According to statistical estimates in the report, sub-Saharan Africa's GDP would be up to 32% greater this year if malaria had been eliminated 35 years ago. This would represent up to $100 billion added to sub-Saharan Africa's current GDP of $300 billion. This extra $100 billion would be, by comparison, nearly five times greater than all development aid provided to Africa last year.

According to the report, malaria slows economic growth in Africa by up to 1.3% each year. This slowdown in economic growth due to malaria is over and above the more readily observed short run costs of the disease. Since sub-Saharan Africa's GDP is around $300 billion, the short-term benefits of malaria control can reasonably be estimated at between $3 billion and $12 billion per year. "Malaria is hurting the living standards of Africans today and is also preventing the improvement of living standards for future generations," said Dr. Gro Harlem Brundtland, Director General of the World Health Organization. "This is an unnecessary and preventable handicap on the continent's economic development."

The report also finds that:

- Malaria-free countries average three times higher GDP per person than malarious countries, even after controlling for government policy, geographical location, and other factors which impact on economic well-being.

- One healthy year of life is gained for every $1 to $8 spent on effectively treating malaria cases, which makes the malaria treatment as cost-effective a public health investment as measles vaccinations. This analysis, carried out by Dr. Ann Mills, LSHTM, demonstrates that malaria control tools and intervention strategies provide good value for money.

"Malaria is taking costly bites out of Africa," said Dr. David Nabarro, executive director at WHO. "It is feasting on the health and development of African children and it is draining the life out of African economies."

The report recommends that $1 billion annually be devoted to malaria prevention and control and that most of this expenditure be focused in Africa. This is many times greater than the amount which is currently being spent. It argues that spending this amount is economically justifiable as the short-term benefits of malaria control can reasonably be estimated at between $3 billion and $12 billion per year.

"The benefits of committing substantial new economic resources to malaria will greatly exceed the costs," said Sachs.

The findings of the report will be presented today at the first ever summit to focus on malaria. The heads of state of twenty African nations and the executive directors of the African Development Bank, World Bank, UNDP, UNICEF, UNESCO and WHO are expected to be present to hear the findings. The Summit is being hosted in Abuja, Nigeria by the country's president, His Excellency Olusegun Obasanjo, and is co-sponsored by WHO.

Malaria accounts for nearly one million deaths each year in Africa; an estimated 700,000 of these deaths are among children. Research has found that the wider availability and use of insecticide treated bednets would result in 50 percent less malaria illness among children. Yet presently, only 2% of African children are protected at night with a treated bednet.

"Roll Back Malaria aims to help African families create a mosquito free zone in the home through the use of nets, drapes, or bednets treated with insecticide," said Dr. Awash Teklehaimanot, acting project manager for Roll Back Malaria. "Our goal is to ensure that every person at risk of malaria in Africa is protected with an insecticide-treated bednet within the next five years."

In addition to ensuring wider availability of treated nets, Roll Back Malaria is also working to provide greater access to rapid diagnosis and quick treatment with the appropriate therapies—ideally in the home; preventing malaria illness during pregnancy; and detecting and responding to epidemics quickly.

"Halving the burden of malaria is realistic and achievable," said Dr. Gro Harlem Brundtland, Director-General of WHO. "We have the tools. We have the economic justification. We now need leaders from both the public and private sectors stepping forward to make this happen."

World Health Organization

WORLD HEALTH ORGANIZATION (WHO). "ECONOMIC COSTS OF MALARIA ARE MANY TIMES HIGHER THAN PREVIOUSLY ESTIMATED" PRESS RELEASE. APRIL 25, 2000.

SEE ALSO *Developing Nations and Drug Delivery; Public Health and Infectious Disease; World Trade and Infectious Disease.*

BIBLIOGRAPHY

Books

Lopez, Alan, Colin Mathers, and Majid Ezzati. *Global Burden of Disease and Risk Factors.* World Bank Group, 2006.

Periodicals

Adler, Nancy E., and Joan M. Ostrove. "Socioeconomic Status and Health: What We Know and What We Don't," *Ann N Y Acad Sci.* (1999): 3-15.

Farmer, P. "Social Inequalities and Emerging Infectious Diseases." *Emerging Infectious Diseases* Vol. 2, No. 4 (October-December, 1996).

Smith, J.P. "Healthy Bodies and Thick Wallets: The Dual Relationship between Health and Economic Status." *Journal of Economic Perspectives*, 13 (2) (1999): 145-66.

Web Sites

United Nations. "UN Millennium Development Goals." <http://www.un.org/millenniumgoals/> (accessed June 8, 2007).

Other Resources

Case, Anne, and Francis Wilson. "Health and Wellbeing in South Africa: Evidence from the Langeberg Survey," mimeo. Princeton University, 2001.

Kenneth T. LaPensee

Emerging Infectious Diseases

■ Introduction

Emerging infectious diseases are human diseases caused by pathogens (disease-causing organisms) that have increased in prevalence over the past several decades (since the 1970s), or microbial diseases that are becoming more widespread. These diseases can be new, previously unrec-

ognized, or re-emergent (diseases that were once under control but which have reappeared and again become a concern).

Acquired Immunodeficiency Syndrome (AIDS, also cited as acquired immune deficiency syndrome) is an example of a disease that has truly emerged. Another example of a newly emerging infectious disease is avian

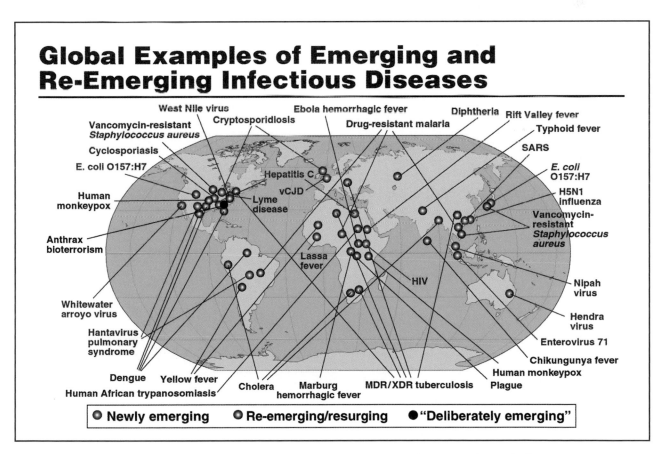

Map showing newly emerging and re-emerging infectious diseases by color in 2007: newly emerging diseases (red); re-emerging/resurging diseases (blue); and "deliberately emerging" diseases (black). *Courtesy of Anthony S. Fauci, M.D., National Institute of Allergy and Infectious Diseases.*

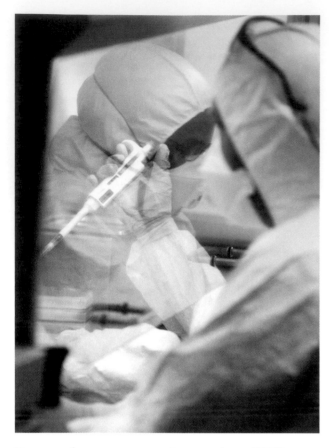

Doctors perform severe acute respiratory syndrome (SARS) research in a laboratory in Rotterdam, The Netherlands, in April 2003. Their experiments on monkeys confirmed the identity of the emerging coronavirus that causes SARS. *AP Images.*

influenza, a viral disease originally a problem in poultry that has evolved to be capable of infecting humans. Tuberculosis (TB) is an example of a re-emergent disease. Incidence of TB has increased in many regions and developed several drug-resistant strains.

■ History and Scientific Foundations

A microbial disease can appear and spread in a population for several reasons. Emergence may be genuine—that is, a microbe changes in some way that makes it capable of causing disease or of being transmitted. An example is *Escherichia coli* O157:H7, which emerged as a serious pathogen when a toxin-coding gene was passed to a non-pathogenic version of *E. coli* by a related organism, *Shigella*. Other changes can occur that alter the surface structure of a bacterium or virus that makes the organism more capable of infecting a host, environmentally hardy, or resistant to antibacterial agents.

Alternatively, a disease may be present but remain undetected in a population until the occurrence of an outbreak. An example is Hantavirus, which was first recognized in the early 1950s in Korea, but which sprang to prominence in 1993 when an outbreak in the southwestern United States. Ebola, which likely existed in its natural reservoir (an unaffected host that may be several species of fruit bat) for a long time, was not recognized as a human pathogen until a large human outbreak occurred in Uganda in 2000–2001.

Emerging infectious disease can also involve once-problematic diseases that were controlled but which have re-emerged as a problem. In addition to tuberculosis, other examples of reemerging infectious diseases include malaria, influenza, and gonorrhea.

Approximately 75% of all emerging infectious diseases are zoonotic in nature, meaning they are transmitted from animals to people. As humans increasingly encroach on wild habitats, the opportunity to contract such infectious organisms increases. This is the main reason for the increased prevalence in the United States of the infections caused by the water-borne protozoa of the genera *Cryptosporidium* and *Giardia* and of the appearance and spread of Lyme disease, which is caused by a tick-borne bacterium.

At some point in time, all infectious diseases were emerging diseases. Polio and smallpox are two examples. Today, smallpox has been eradicated and polio remains endemic (occurs naturally) in only four countries: Afghanistan, India, Nigeria, and Pakistan. More recent examples of emerging diseases include AIDS and variant Creutzfeld-Jakob (nv-CJD or v-CJD) disease.

The first report of AIDS in the science literature was in 1981. Even then, the disease was already spreading. By 2004, an estimated 40 million people were infected with the Human Immunodeficiency Virus (HIV), the virus linked to AIDS. Efforts to combat HIV/AIDS include an international consortium called the Global HIV/AIDS Vaccine Enterprise and, as of February 2007, the Canadian HIV Vaccine Initiative, a $139 million initiative funded by the government of Canada and the Bill & Melinda Gates Foundation.

Malaria is considered to be a reemerging disease because of its increasing prevalence. Malaria disproportionately affects pregnant women and young children in underdeveloped and developing countries. From one million to 2.7 million people die of the disease each year.

An estimated two million people die of tuberculosis each year and 30% of the world's population is infected with *Mycobacterium tuberculosis*. The appearance of *M. tuberculosis* that is resistant to multiple antibiotics is a great concern to agencies such as the World Health Organization (WHO). In May 2007, two cases of tuberculosis that were resistant to every drug available to treat the disease were reported; there is concern that extremely drug-resistant tuberculosis (XDR-TB) will become a growing global problem.

Applications and Research

The ability to isolate the genetic material from a variety of infectious microorganisms and determine the genetic sequence of the material—a process that can now be completed in just a few days—is allowing researchers to identify the sequences that are important in disease. The discipline of proteomics, in which the structure and function of proteins are determined, is helping to identify targets for antimicrobial drugs and to design vaccines and other antimicrobial agents that prevent or treat infections.

Disease surveillance is important in monitoring the appearance and spread of emerging infectious diseases. As of 2007, organizations including WHO and CDC are closely tracking the spread of H5N1 avian influenza, especially the few, but geographically diverse, cases involving person-to-person transmission. Scientists are studying how the flight patterns of migratory birds interact with outbreaks of this strain of influenza. Researchers from the University of Georgia reported in 2006 that wood ducks and laughing gulls are highly susceptible to the H5N1 strain of avian influenza, and that these two species could serve as sentinels (indicators, or lookouts) for the presence of the H5N1 virus in wild birds in North America.

Impacts and Issues

The emergence or re-emergence of infectious diseases is influenced by a number of factors. A nation's economy affects the type and availability of health care; inadequate vaccination programs and a lack of general health care can make it easier for a disease to become established. As well, the overall heath and nutritional status of citizens in developing nations can be compromised, which makes them more susceptible to infectious disease.

Of the nearly 40 million people infected with HIV, two-thirds live in sub-Saharan Africa. Widespread poverty exacerbates the HIV/AIDS crisis in Africa as drug treatments are typically expensive. Efforts by organizations such as the WHO, UNICEF, CDC and some pharmaceutical companies are helping make HIV/AIDS drugs less expensive and more widely available in Africa.

One well-known agent of emerging infectious diseases is the increased resistance of a variety of bacteria to antibiotics. The resistance has been driven by the overuse and misuse of antibiotics—such as when used to combat a viral infection or when antibiotic therapy is stopped too soon. This selective pressure encourages the development of changes in bacteria that confers resistance and aids the proliferation of the newly-resistant bacteria.

Political change or conflict can favor the proliferation of an existing disease or the spread of an emerging

> ## WORDS TO KNOW
>
> **ENDEMIC:** Present in a particular area or among a particular group of people.
>
> **PATHOGEN:** A disease causing agent, such as a bacteria, virus, fungus, etc.
>
> **RESERVOIR:** The animal or organism in which the virus or parasite normally resides.
>
> **RESISTANT ORGANISM:** Resistant organisms are bacteria, viruses, parasites, or other disease-causing agents that have stopped responding to drugs that once killed them.
>
> **SELECTIVE PRESSURE:** Selective pressure refers to the tendency of an organism that has a certain characteristic to be eliminated from an environment or to increase in numbers. An example is the increased prevalence of bacteria that are resistant to multiple kinds of antibiotics.
>
> **SENTINEL:** Sentinel surveillance is a method in epidemiology where a subset of the population is surveyed for the presence of communicable diseases. Also, a sentinel is an animal used to indicate the presence of disease within an area.
>
> **STRAIN:** A subclass or a specific genetic variation of an organism.
>
> **ZOONOSES:** Zoonoses are diseases of microbiological origin that can be transmitted from animals to people. The causes of the diseases can be bacteria, viruses, parasites, and fungi.

one. Military conflict disables access to food, water, and adequate health care, as well as results in the mass movement people. Malnutrition and densely populated refugee or displaced person camps, many lacking proper sanitation, can exacerbate disease outbreaks. A vivid example is the influenza epidemic that occurred in the aftermath of World War I (1914–1918). Troops returning home from the battlefield spread influenza across Europe, to Russia, the United States, Australia, and New Zealand. The pandemic eventually spread worldwide. From 1918–1919, influenza claimed at least 20 million people, more than had been killed in the just-ended war.

The delivery of health services that lead to the emergence of a disease can be interrupted by changes other than war. For example, the global effort to completely eradicate polio suffered a setback in 2003 when vaccination of people in rural regions of the African country of Nigeria were halted by the government as a rumor circulated that the vaccine could cause sterility or AIDS. By the time these fears had been quelled and vaccination resumed in 2004, nearly 700 children had become infected with polio, representing almost 75% of the total number of cases around the world for the year. In 2005, WHO re-initiated the polio vaccination campaign in Nigeria. On National Immunization Day in May 2005, approximately 140,000 WHO-sanctioned volunteers went door-to-door in an attempt to inoculate every Nigerian child under five years of age.

WHO's Department of Communicable Disease Surveillance and Response is responsible for the global coordination of efforts to eradicate emerging infectious diseases such as avian influenza. Their global scope is necessary, as in the era of rapid travel diseases can quickly spread around the globe. This was exemplified by the 2003 emergence of Severe Acute Respiratory Syndrome (SARS), which spread within days from Taiwan to North America, and eventually caused 229 deaths on four continents.

SEE ALSO *AIDS (Acquired Immunodeficiency Syndrome); Avian Influenza; Bioterrorism; Climate Change and Infectious Disease; Globalization and Infectious Disease; Pandemic Preparedness; Re-emerging Infectious Diseases; Virus Hunters.*

BIBLIOGRAPHY

Books

DiClaudio, Dennis. *The Hypochondriac's Pocket Guide to Horrible Diseases You Probably Already Have.* New York: Bloomsbury, 2005.

Fong, I.W., and Karl Drlica, eds. *Reemergence of Establish Pathogens in the 21st Century.* New York: Springer, 2003.

Palladino, Michael A., and Stuart Hill. *Emerging Infectious Diseases.* New York: Benjamin Cummings, 2005.

Web Sites

National Institute of Allergy and Infectious Diseases. "Emerging Infectious Diseases." <http://www.niaid.nih.gov/dmid/eid/> (accessed May 25, 2007).

Brian Hoyle

Encephalitis

■ Introduction

Encephalitis is a type of acute brain inflammation, most often due to infection by a virus. When the inflammation occurs in the spinal cord, the condition is called myelitis, and when inflammation is in both the spinal cord and the brain, the condition is called encephalomyelitis. However, in reality, an infection in both areas is often referred to as encephalitis. The swelling in the brain that occurs in encephalitis can be serious and even life-threatening; brain damage, strokes, seizures, coma, and death can result. Encephalitis often accompanies bacterial meningitis (an infection of the lining of the brain known as the meninges).

■ Disease History, Characteristics, and Transmission

There are two types of encephalitis—a primary form and a secondary form. Primary encephalitis is directly due to a new viral infection. This form of encephalitis can be localized in just one region of the brain or spinal cord (focal infection) or can be more widely distributed (diffuse infection).

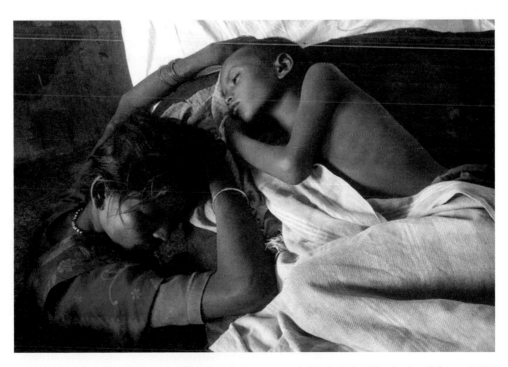

A mother comforts her child, who suffers from Japanese encephalitis in India. The death toll from a 2005 Japanese encephalitis outbreak in northern India crossed the 1,000 mark, making it the most fatal outbreak of the illness in nearly two decades. Nearly all the dead were children. *STR/AFP/Getty Images.*

WORDS TO KNOW

ACUTE: An acute infection is one of rapid onset and of short duration, which either resolves or becomes chronic.

ARTHROPOD-BORNE DISEASE: A disease caused by one of a phylum of organisms characterized by exoskeletons and segmented bodies.

LATENT: A condition that is potential or dormant, not yet manifest or active, is latent.

MENINGITIS: Meningitis is an inflammation of the meninges—the three layers of protective membranes that line the spinal cord and the brain. Meningitis can occur when there is an infection near the brain or spinal cord, such as a respiratory infection in the sinuses, the mastoids, or the cavities around the ear. Disease organisms can also travel to the meninges through the bloodstream. The first signs may be a severe headache and neck stiffness followed by fever, vomiting, a rash, and, then, convulsions leading to loss of consciousness. Meningitis generally involves two types: nonbacterial meningitis, which is often called aseptic meningitis, and bacterial meningitis, which is referred to as purulent meningitis.

VECTOR: Any agent, living or otherwise, that carries and transmits parasites and diseases. Also, an organism or chemical used to transport a gene into a new host cell.

Secondary encephalitis, or post-infective encephalitis, arises as a consequence of an ongoing viral infection or from an immunization procedure that utilizes a virus. The latter uses a virus that has been altered to be incapable of causing harm. However, in rare cases, the vaccine itself becomes harmful. Secondary encephalitis, which is also termed acute disseminated encephalitis, typically appears 2–3 weeks following the first infection or the immunization injection.

Worldwide, encephalitis due to infections by the herpes simplex viruses causes only about 10% of all cases of the disease. However, over half of these cases result in death. Many of the cases involve the reactivation of an earlier infection by a herpes simplex virus that became latent (this occurs when the viral genetic material is incorporated into the host's genetic material). Upon reactivation, production of new copies of the virus resumes, and the symptoms associated with the infection appear.

The original infection may be with herpes simplex type 1, which commonly causes cold sores and facial blistering. Encephalitis related to this virus can occur in anyone, but is most prevalent in people under 20 years of age and older than 40. The disease is contagious, being spread most often by inhalation of water droplets expelled by a cough or sneeze. The person who contracts the infection develops a headache and fever that can last almost a week. Subsequently, changes in personality and behavior, seizures, and delusions may appear, and severe brain damage may result. Encephalitis due to herpes simplex type 2 is typically spread through sexual contact or, less commonly, a newborn can contract the virus from his or her infected mother during birth.

In the United States and Canada, Powassan encephalititis is transmitted to humans by ticks, which have previously acquired the virus from infected deer. The symptoms of Powassan encephalitis—headache, fever, nausea, and disorientation—begin within two weeks following the tick bite. Paralysis and coma also can occur. About 50% of those who contract Powassan encephalitis will have permanent brain damage and more than 15% of those who become infected die of the infection.

In the United States, there are four types of mosquito-borne viral encephalitis. These are: equine encephalitis, LaCrosse encephalitis, St. Louis encephalitis, and West Nile encephalitis.

Rarely, a form of the disease known as limbic system encephalitis occurs. The primary symptom of this form of encephalitis is memory impairment similar to what is seen in individuals suffering from Alzheimer's disease or Creutzfeldt-Jacob disease. A variation of limbic encephalitis called paraneoplastic limbic encephalitis is linked to the development of cancer.

■ Scope and Distribution

In the United States, there are several thousand reported cases of encephalitis every year. However, according to the U.S. National Institute of Neurological Disorders and Stroke, the actual tally is likely much higher, since many people do not seek medical help for cases that produce mild symptoms or no symptoms at all.

Encephalitis occurs in many regions of the world. For example, mosquito-borne forms of encephalitis are present in North and South America, Europe, Russia, Asia, India, northern Africa, and even Australia.

In the United States, encephalitis is usually caused by an enterovirus, by the herpes simplex virus types 1 and 2, by an arbovirus that is transmitted from an infected animal to humans via a vector such as a mosquito (an example is West Nile disease) or tick, or by the bite of a rabid animal such as a raccoon that is infected with the rabies virus. Lyme disease, which is caused by the bacterium *Borrelia burdorferi*, can also cause encephalitis.

One factor that has contributed to the global distribution of encephalitis is the fact that it is contagious, and can be passed from person to person by coughing or sneezing, releasing contaminated droplets into the air. In addition, the microorganisms that cause encephalitis can contaminate food and water.

Herpes simplex-mediated encephalitis is rare in the United States, occurring in about 1 person per 250,000–500,000 population per year. The other forms of the disease can occur more frequently. For instance, children can develop encephalitis after a bout of measles, mumps, or rubella.

Viral encephalitis that is transmitted to humans via a vector, like a mosquito or tick, is more common in the United States. One such vector-borne encephalitis is equine encephalitis. As its name implies, equine encephalitis can affect horses. This disease in horses can be serious, and often comes before the detection of the disease in humans. A form called eastern equine encephalitis (EEE) is prevalent along the eastern coastal region of the United States and the coast of the Gulf of Mexico. Fever, muscles aches, and headache develop 3–10 days after being bitten by a virus-carrying mosquito. The headache becomes progressively worse, and, in severe cases, a person can lapse into a coma and die. The disease is still rare, despite having been known to occur in the United States since the 1930s. Only an average of five cases of eastern equine encephalitis appear in the United States each year; for these people, however, the consequences can be dire, as up to 50% may die.

The natural host of the EEE virus is still not precisely known, but the virus tends to infect birds that live near freshwater swamps. Whether the virus can survive the winter in northern climates is also unknown. Surveys of birds that live year-round in the northern climates have not detected the virus, and scientists suspect that returning migratory birds in the spring bring the virus back to these areas.

Western equine encephalitis is distributed in the western and central states of the United States. The virus was isolated in the United States in 1930 from an infected horse. Both horses and humans can be affected by this disease. The virus normally resides in a number of species of animals and birds, and is transmitted by mosquitoes. Symptoms begin about a week following infection. Children are particularly at risk of developing a severe form of the disease that can produce permanent brain damage.

The prevalence of western equine encephalitis has been influenced by agricultural practices. For example, the increasing irrigation of land has created more regions of stagnant water, which become breeding grounds for mosquitoes. In addition, the land becomes populated by bird species that naturally carry the virus.

Another form of equine encephalitis called Venezuelan equine encephalitis has killed thousands of people

---

IN CONTEXT: INFLAMMATION AS A NON-SPECIFIC DEFENSE

Inflammation is a localized, defensive response of the body to injury, usually characterized by pain, redness, heat, swelling, and, depending on the extent of trauma, loss of function. The process of inflammation, called the inflammatory response, is a series of events, or stages, that the body performs to attain homeostasis (the body's effort to maintain stability). The body's inflammatory response mechanism serves to confine, weaken, destroy, and remove bacteria, toxins, and foreign material at the site of trauma or injury. As a result, the spread of invading substances is halted, and the injured area is prepared for regeneration or repair. Inflammation is a nonspecific defense mechanism; the body's physiological response to a superficial cut is much the same as with a burn or a bacterial infection. The inflammatory response protects the body against a variety of invading pathogens and foreign matter, and should not be confused with an immune response.

SOURCE: *Centers for Disease Control and Prevention*

---

in epidemics in Central and South America. Survivors can have permanent brain damage.

LaCrosse encephalitis is another form of vector-borne encephalitis found in the United States. It is named for LaCrosse, Wisconsin, where the disease was first detected in 1963. It is typically distributed in midwestern states including Illinois, Indiana, Ohio, Iowa, and Wisconsin, but also has occurred in more eastern states. The virus is passed to mosquitoes from infected chipmunks and squirrels. Children and adolescents under 16 years of age are most at risk. Headache, fever, vomiting, and fatigue develop about one week following the mosquito bite. In more severe cases, a person can experience seizures. About 100 cases occur in the United States each year.

St. Louis encephalitis has been among the most common encephalitis diseases reported in the United States. Typically, there are around 130 cases reported to the U.S. Centers for Disease Control and Prevention (CDC) each year, although outbreaks can make thousands of people ill. There have been approximately 4,500 reported cases since 1964, with an average of almost 200 cases each year. The disease is transferred to mosquitoes from infected birds. In contrast to other forms of encephalitis, adults are affected more severely than are children. Symptoms include headache, fever, and, in more serious cases, mental disorientation, muscles tremors, convulsions, and unconsciousness.

The final mosquito-borne encephalitis is West Nile disease. Its geographical distribution in the United States has expanded since it was first detected in 1999. The disease is also found in Canada, Africa, the Middle East, Russia,

India, and Indonesia. People whose immune systems are impaired are most at risk. In addition to transmission by mosquito, the virus can be present in transplanted organs or transfused blood and blood products.

Japanese encephalitis is the most common cause of encephalitis worldwide. Approximately 50,000 cases and 15,000 deaths occur each year, according to the World Health Organization (WHO). This form of encephalitis is common in certain regions of Asia, including China, Korea, Japan, Taiwan, Sri Lanka, and the south of India. It also occurs on some Pacific islands. The disease is especially prevalent where rice production and pig rearing occur. This is because the mosquitoes that spread the disease can breed in the rice paddies and pigs are a host of the virus. The mosquitoes acquire the virus when taking a blood meal from a pig and then can spread the virus to humans.

■ Treatment and Prevention

The diagnosis of encephalitis involves an assessment of nerve function, hearing, speech, vision, balance and coordination, mental capability, and changes in behavior. The examination of body fluids, such as urine and blood, and a swab from the throat can be useful in revealing a bacterial or viral infection.

Tests that rely on growth of bacteria or the appearance of clear zones in a layer of bacterial growth (the clear zones are places where virus production has destroyed the bacteria) take 2–3 days. Antibody-based tests to detect protein components of the target bacteria or viruses and the use of polymerase chain reaction to amplify and detect specific regions of the viral or bacterial genetic material can produce results in as little as a day.

Other diagnostic procedures rely on imaging the brain or spinal cord. The two most widely used imaging procedures are computed tomography (CT) and magnetic resonance imaging (MRI). These techniques can be sensitive enough to detect inflammation of the meninges. These examinations need to be done promptly, since the inflammation associated with encephalitis can cause damage rapidly.

If viral encephalitis is suspected, treatment usually involves the antiviral drugs acyclovir and ganciclovir. Both drugs are similar in their three-dimensional structure to certain building blocks of the viral genetic material. Incorporation of the drug into the replicating genetic material instead of the normal building block inhibits the activity of an enzyme that is vital for the continued replication of the virus.

Milder cases of encephalitis are treated with bed rest and over-the-counter medications to relieve headache and make the person feel as comfortable as possible. In more severe cases, hospitalization may be necessary, and drugs may be given to control or prevent seizures. The swelling of the meninges can be reduced using corticosteroids, which are usually administered intravenously (into a vein) to get the drug to the site of swelling quickly and to maintain an effective concentration of the drug.

The best way to prevent encephalitis is to minimize contact with the vectors of the disease. Examples of preventative measures include the use of mosquito repellent, wearing protective clothing when outdoors, and eliminating sources of stagnant water (which can become breeding grounds for mosquitoes). In reality, however, these and other preventative measures are difficult to consistently maintain.

As of 2007, no vaccine for the forms of encephalitis that are prevalent in the United States is available, although development is underway. A vaccine for Japanese encephalitis is available in the United States. In Europe, a vaccine for tick-borne encephalitis is available. In addition, vaccines to protect horses from various forms of the disease are available.

■ Impacts and Issues

Encephalitis can be a devastating disease when it causes lasting effects, such as brain damage. A person can be incapable of resuming work or study, and can require assistance to perform routine daily tasks. This can place a burden on caregivers and can affect the person's capabilities as a family member and worker.

Sizeable outbreaks of encephalitis can occur. For example, a 1995 outbreak of Venezuelan equine encephalitis in Venezuela and Colombia sickened an estimated 90,000 people. The size of such an outbreak imposes yet another burden on developing countries, particularly those where acquired immunodeficiency syndrome (AIDS, also cited as acquired immune deficiency syndrome) is prevalent. The impaired immune system function that is a characteristic of AIDS makes individuals with the disease more susceptible to a wide range of other maladies, including encephalitis.

Even in a developed country with a relatively high access to medical care, like the United States, the costs of encephalitis are considerable. The CDC has estimated the cost of medical care, disease detection, and efforts such as spraying programs that are intended to control mosquito and other vector populations, at approximately $150 million a year. In addition, developed countries are becoming increasingly affected as the population ages and immune-compromising diseases, such as AIDS, become more prevalent. It is also likely that encephalitis will become more common in the more northerly regions of the United States, Canada, and Europe as global warming continues, since the warmer temperatures will be more favorable for the breeding of vectors, such as mosquitoes.

West Nile encephalitis is an emerging health hazard in the United States. The disease was first detected in the United States in 1999, and, in the following year, 284 Americans are known to have died of the disease. Since then, West Nile has increased in its geographical range and in the number of people affected. It has replaced St. Louis encephalitis as the most prevalent form of the disease in the United States. The CDC reported almost 1,300 cases of West Nile encephalitis in 2005, more than double the number of cases in 2002.

While vaccines are available for some forms of encephalitis, such as Japanese equine encephalitis, the high cost of the vaccines can make them prohibitively expensive for poorer nations. A number of agencies, such as WHO, are working to make encephalitis vaccines more widely available. For example, one of the priorities of the World Health Organization's Programme for Immunization Preventable Diseases in cooperation with the government of Nepal is the control of Japanese encephalitis. Over 8,000 cases, mainly involving children, have been reported in Nepal from 1998–2003.

Efforts also are underway to control encephalitis in North America. The CDC's Division of Vector-Borne Infectious Diseases conducts surveillance programs that monitor the occurrence of the disease and manages programs that try to control the disease in these hotspots.

■ Primary Source Connection

This newspaper article details the temporary closing of an elementary school in Rhode Island in early 2007 after a student at the school died from an unusual form of encephalitis that was caused by a common bacteria. Two other students contracted the disease during the outbreak, prompting the school district to close all its schools for almost a week, and the CDC to investigate the outbreak.

School is Shut After Outbreak of Encephalitis Kills a Pupil

State and federal health officials are investigating an extremely rare outbreak of encephalitis here that killed a second-grader last month and led officials to close his elementary school this week.

Health officials said the cases of encephalitis, which is usually brought on by a virus and causes the brain to swell, are unusual because they appear to be caused by a common bacteria, *Mycoplasma pneumoniae*, or walking pneumonia.

"It's very rare for someone to be hospitalized with mycoplasma, and it's even more rare to see such a severe complication as encephalitis," said Cynthia Whitney, acting branch chief for the respiratory diseases branch of the Centers for Disease Control and Prevention. "What makes this so unusual is that more than one case has been linked to this outbreak of mycoplasma."

The second-grader, Dylan Gleavey of Warwick, died of encephalitis on Dec. 21. A classmate of Dylan's at Greenwood Elementary School became ill with menin-

IN CONTEXT: SCIENTIFIC, POLITICAL, AND ETHICAL ISSUES

Centers for Disease Control and Prevention, National Center for Infectious Diseases, Division of Vector-Borne Infectious Diseases argues that "Mosquito-borne encephalitis offers a rare opportunity in public health to detect the risk of a disease before it occurs and to intervene to reduce that risk substantially. The surveillance required to detect risk is being increasingly refined by the potential utilization of these new technologies which allows for rapid identification of dangerous viruses in mosquito populations. These rapid diagnostic techniques used in threat recognition can shorten public health response time and reduce the geographic spread of infected vectors and thereby the cost of containing them."

SOURCE: *Centers for Disease Control and Prevention, National Center for Infectious Diseases, Division of Vector-Borne Infectious Diseases*

gitis that progressed to a mild form of encephalitis, said Dr. David R. Gifford, Rhode Island's director of health.

The classmate and a West Warwick middle school student who had encephalitis and walking pneumonia were recovering at home, Dr. Gifford said.

Health officials also are investigating higher-than-normal absentee rates among students in two Coventry schools who were reported to have had symptoms of walking pneumonia.

Over the weekend, Warwick officials turned Greenwood Elementary School into a makeshift clinic, swabbing throats and drawing blood from all but 3 of the 275 students, their families, teachers and staff members. Antibiotics were given to everyone who showed up.

The school was closed after five students tested positive for walking pneumonia. Mayor Scott Avedisian said officials were keeping it closed for an extra week after Christmas break so the students would be apart for two weeks, well into the incubation time of one to three weeks.

State officials said it was the first time a school had been closed for such an outbreak, and federal officials said they rarely intervened in cases of walking pneumonia.

"I've been here for 13 years, and we have not shut down a school due to mycoplasma," Ms. Whitney said.

Mayor Avedisian said more than 1,400 rounds of antibiotics were dispensed and nine informational sessions were held for concerned parents. Parents were notified of the illness by computerized phone calls.

Parents were upset, Mr. Avedisian said, but he said he believed they had been given enough information and the chance to ask questions.

Rather than close additional schools, officials were stressing the importance of handwashing and advising people to sneeze into their arms rather than their hands. Lisa Freeman, 41, whose three children attend Greenwood Elementary, said her entire family was taking antibiotics. Her son, Stone, was in the same class as Dylan's brother.

"It was scary, definitely scary," she said. "But I feel it was handled in a very professional way."

Ms. Freeman, her husband and children spent New Year's Day getting throat cultures, and came back the next day for blood work. Doctors discovered that Stone had an ear infection, causing neighbors and concerned parents to call and see if he was feeling all right.

"It's very close-knit here," Ms. Freeman said as a gaggle of neighborhood children played in her backyard. "I think it was the right decision to close school and put us all on antibiotics."

Katie Zezima

ZEZIMA, KATIE. "SCHOOL IS SHUT AFTER OUTBREAK OF ENCEPHALITIS KILLS A PUPIL." *NEW YORK TIMES* (JANUARY 4, 2007): A14(L)

SEE ALSO *Arthropod-borne Disease; Climate Change and Infectious Disease; Climate Change and Infectious Disease; Eastern Equine Encephalitis; Emerging Infectious Diseases; Encephalitis; Japanese Encephalitis; Meningitis, Viral; Mosquito-borne Diseases; Vector-borne Disease; West Nile.*

BIBLIOGRAPHY

Books

Bloom, Ona, and Jennifer Morgan. *Encephalitis.* London: Chelsea House Publications, 2005.

Booss, John, and Margaret M. Esiri. *Viral Encephalitis in Humans.* Washington, DC: ASM Press, 2003.

Web Sites

Medline Plus. "Encephalitis." <http://www.nlm.nih.gov/medlineplus/encephalitis.html> (accessed March 20, 2007).

Brian Hoyle

Endemicity

■ Introduction

An endemic disease is one that occurs naturally in a community. This is opposed to an epidemic disease, in which the rate of infection suddenly increases in a community. Endemicity can be measured by determining how common an infection is, or by determining the change in rates of infection over time.

The endemicity of a disease may be altered by a number of factors. Human intervention has led to many previously endemic diseases being eradicated from specific regions. This has been achieved by vaccination, as well as by the elimination of the cause of the disease, such as a vector (the organism that aids in the transmission of the disease).

However, endemic diseases can also develop in previously non-endemic regions, or can develop into epidemics. This often occurs when infections are introduced, undergo mutation, or when conditions within a community change due to events such as wars or natural disasters. The extent to which the change persists influences whether the change in endemicity will be long term.

■ History and Scientific Foundations

An endemic disease is one with a constant rate of infection in a community. When new individuals are born into that community, they become infected, cured, and eventually recover and retain the infection for life, or obtain immunity. Conversely, an epidemic occurs when a disease is introduced to a community and it multiplies, or when the rate of infection of an existing disease increases and causes an excess of cases in a community.

Endemicity can be measured by examining the prevalence rate or incident rate of a disease. (Prevalence refers to how common the disease is within a given community.) Some communities may have higher levels of ende-micity, which indicates a higher prevalence of infection. The incident rate refers to the change in the level of infection over time. Many infections tend to show seasonal incident rates, in which the level of infection increases during certain periods. When the incident rate increases above a certain threshold, the disease becomes an epidemic, that is, the rate of infection causes an excess of cases.

Within a community, there can be "foci," or areas of increased prevalence. Host focality refers to areas in which hosts have more severe infections than other hosts. For example, the infection schistosomiasis is characterized by infection with parasite eggs. Some hosts suffer heavier parasite loads due to more severe infections. When these heavier infections occur in specific areas, they form host foci. Geographic focality refers to a higher prevalence rate of the disease in certain regions. For example, malaria tends to show varying prevalence rates in urban versus rural regions.

The foci of a disease affect the treatment and eventual containment of the disease. If treatment methods aim to treat the entire community to the same extent, foci will maintain the infection. On the other hand, targeting foci will ensure that the infection is contained.

■ Applications and Research

Endemic diseases may not always remain endemic. In some cases, transmission of the disease may increase, causing the disease to become an epidemic. On the other hand, transmission of the disease may decrease, causing the number of cases in the community to go below an endemicity threshold. Many factors can influence the endemicity of a disease. Eradication techniques have played a major role in decreasing the endemicity of certain diseases in the world. Within the United States, measles, which was endemic prior to 1997, is no longer considered an endemic disease due to vaccination efforts. Similarly, malaria, which is still endemic in some regions

WORDS TO KNOW

EPIDEMIC: From the Greek *epidemic*, meaning "prevalent among the people," is most commonly used to describe an outbreak of an illness or disease in which the number of individual cases significantly exceeds the usual or expected number of cases in any given population.

FOCI: In medicine, a focus is a primary center of some disease process (for example, a cluster of abnormal cells). Foci is pleural for focus (more than one focus).

GEOGRAPHIC FOCALITY: The physical location of a disease pattern, epidemic, or outbreak; the characteristics of a location created by interconnections with other places.

HOST FOCALITY: Host focality refers to the tendency of some animal hosts, such as rodents carrying hantavirus and other viruses, to exist in groups in specific geographical locations, acting as a local reservoir of infection.

INCIDENCE: The number of new cases of a disease or injury that occur in a population during a specified period of time.

PREVALENCE: The actual number of cases of disease (or injury) that exist in a population.

of the world, has been eradicated from the United States and some western European countries following large scale eradication efforts.

The viral disease measles is highly communicable among humans. As a result, it is endemic in many regions of the world. In the United States, measles was once a common childhood disease with over 90% of children under the age of 12 infected. However, following the introduction of a measles vaccine in 1963, measles outbreaks have decreased. Aside from outbreaks occurring following introduction of the disease from other countries, measles no longer circulates in the United States. Vaccination is an effective way of increasing the immunity of a population and causing a decrease in the transmissibility of an infection. As a result, when most or all of a population is vaccinated against a certain disease, that disease does not retain its endemic state.

Vaccination is one eradication technique employed against infectious diseases. However, vaccinations have not been developed for all infectious diseases. As a result, other methods must be used to control some endemic diseases. Malaria is an example of an endemic infectious

disease that cannot be controlled by vaccination. This disease is transmitted via mosquitoes, which infect new hosts when they feed on them. Eradication efforts involved spraying human living spaces with dichloro-diphenyl-trichloroethane (DDT), a toxic insecticide that kills mosquitoes (DDT was banned from use in most developing countries in the 1980s). This technique was designed to remove the mode of transmission for the disease (in this case, the mosquito vector), with the expectation that this would prevent the spread of the disease.

Malaria was once a major endemic infectious disease worldwide. However, since the late 1940s, malaria is no longer endemic in the United States nor in many countries of Western Europe. However, worldwide efforts to completely eradicate malaria have not been as successful. A variety of problems, such as mosquito tolerance to DDT, banning of DDT use, outbreaks of war, lack of funding, and population movements, have hindered efforts to eradicate malaria worldwide. Health authorities now attempt to control outbreaks of malaria, rather than to eradicate it completely.

■ Impacts and Issues

Endemicity can develop in countries in which the disease did not previously exist or only existed in low numbers. A disease may be introduced to countries with no history of the disease, and thus no immunity against it. Endemicity may develop as the disease spreads unchecked throughout the community. If transmission continues to infect an increasing number of people, the endemic disease may develop into an epidemic.

Endemicity may also develop when a disease that is usually only transmitted from animal to human, begins to be transmitted between humans, causing an increased rate of human infection. For example, avian influenza, or bird flu, tends to be predominantly spread between birds, and occasionally from bird to human. However, the virus that causes this disease may mutate, allowing it to be transmitted more easily between birds and humans, and, perhaps, between human hosts. Therefore, avian influenza is being closely monitored in order to keep it from becoming an endemic—and possibly—epidemic.

Not only can certain conditions cause a disease to become endemic, but some conditions may prompt an endemic disease to develop into an epidemic. Climate change and disasters, such as floods or wars, may cause changes that favor disease transmission. Some diseases, such as malaria, are dependent upon an arthropod vector to spread among hosts. A change in the climate, such as increased temperature or moisture, may be favorable to the vector, causing an increased number of vectors in a region. This increases the chance that a human will become infected. If a disease is already endemic in the region, an increase in the number of cases may result in an epidemic.

Disasters, such as war or floods, may also cause other more favorable conditions for a disease. For example, during war, or following a flood or earthquake, a large number of people are often required to live together in close quarters, often with only very basic sanitation. As a result, diseases are more easily transmitted. Airborne diseases benefit from the close proximity of people, orally transmitted diseases benefit from the poor sanitation conditions, and vector-borne diseases benefit from conditions that promote vector breeding. Therefore, diseases may erupt during these times. However, when people are allowed to return to their homes, conditions change again and may no longer favor the transmission of infectious diseases. This can cause the transmission rate to decrease and thus a disease may no longer be endemic or epidemic.

SEE ALSO *Arthropod-borne Disease; Avian Influenza; Bilharzia (Schistosomiasis); Climate Change and Infectious Disease; Epidemiology; Host and Vector; Immigration and Infectious Disease; Influenza; Influenza Pandemic of 1918; Influenza, Tracking Seasonal Influences and Virus Mutation; Malaria; Measles (Rubeola); Mosquito-borne Diseases; Pandemic Preparedness; Sanitation; Travel and Infectious Disease; United Nations Millennium Goals and Infectious Disease; Vector-borne Disease; War and Infectious Disease.*

BIBLIOGRAPHY

Books

Arguin, P.M., P.E. Kozarsky, and A.W. Navin. *Health Information for International Travel 2005–2006.* Washington, DC: U.S. Department of Health and Human Services, 2005.

Nelson, Kenrad E., and Carolyn F. Masters Williams. *Infectious Disease Epidemiology: Theory and Practice.* 2nd ed. Sudbury, MA: Jones & Bartlett, 2007.

Webber, R. *Communicable Disease Epidemiology and Control.* New York: CABI Publishing, 2005.

Web Sites

Centers for Disease Control and Prevention. "Avian Influenza (Bird Flu)." June 30, 2006. <http://www.cdc.gov/flu/avian/gen-info/pdf/avian_facts.pdf> (accessed April 10, 2007).

Centers for Disease Control and Prevention. "Malaria." April 23, 2004. <http://www.cdc.gov/malaria/index.htm> (accessed April 10, 2007).

Tony Hawas

IN CONTEXT: ENDEMIC DISEASE AND THE PANAMA CANAL

Endemic diseases such as yellow fever, plague, and malaria had frustrated earlier French attempts to build a canal through the Isthmus of Panama by disabling and killing thousands of project workers and managers. Dr. William Crawford Gorgas (1854–1920), chief of sanitary affairs for the American project, made the canal possible by organizing public health and sanitation efforts. It was not ignorance of public health principles that had doomed earlier efforts to build the canal, but a lack of effective public health organization and the thorough implementation of disease control measures.

Epidemiology

■ Introduction

Epidemiology is the study of the causes and distribution of illness and injury. It constitutes the scientific underpinning of public health practice. According to noted British epidemiologist Sir Richard Doll (1912–2005), "Epidemiology is the simplest and most direct method of studying the causes of disease in humans, and many major contributions have been made by studies that have demanded nothing more than an ability to count, to think logically and to have an imaginative idea." In practice, epidemiology is applied in the three main areas of public health: safety and injuries, chronic disease, and infectious disease. This article will emphasize examples and applications in infectious disease epidemiology.

■ History and Scientific Foundations

The first physician known to consider the fundamental concepts of disease causation was the ancient Greek Hippocrates (c.460—c.377 BC), when he wrote that medical thinkers should consider the climate and

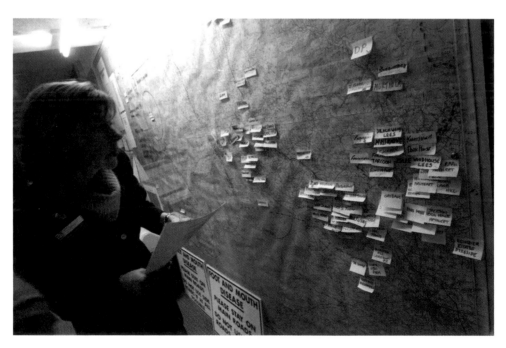

An epidemiologist updates a map of affected farms in Scotland during a foot and mouth disease outbreak affecting cattle and sheep in the United Kingdom in 2001. Veterinary epidemiologists fought the spread of the disease for almost a year by tracking the proliferation of the disease; culling infected and exposed animals; restricting people from traveling to infected farms and inadvertently spreading the disease via their shoes and the tires of their cars; and placing a ban on transporting animals. © The Scotsman/Corbis Sygma.

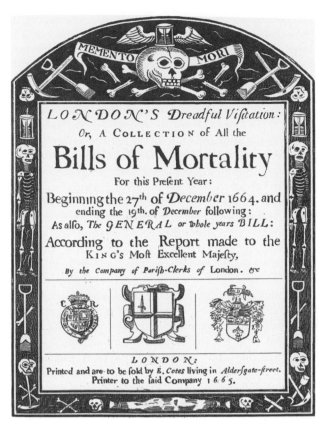

Bills of Mortality contained a listing of people who died during a given year. This bill lists London's dead from 1664–1665, covering part of the period of the Great Plague. John Graunt (1620–1674), considered by many to have founded the science of demography, based his statistical analysis on these weekly and yearly tables.
HIP/Art Resource, NY.

seasons, the air, the water that people use, the soil and people's eating, drinking and exercise habits in a region. Subsequently and until recent times, these causes of diseases were often considered, but not quantitatively measured. In 1662, John Graunt (1620–1674), a London haberdasher, published an analysis of the weekly reports of births and deaths in London, the first statistical description of population disease patterns. Among his findings, he noted a higher death rate for men than women, a high infant mortality rate, and seasonal variations in mortality. Graunt's study, with its meticulous counting and disease pattern description, set the foundation for modern public health practice.

Graunt's data collection and analytical methodology was furthered by the physician William Farr, who assumed responsibility for medical statistics for England and Wales in 1839 and set up a system for the routine collection of the numbers and causes of deaths. In analyzing statistical relationships between disease and such circumstances as marital status, occupations such as mining and working with earthenware, elevation above sea

level and imprisonment, he addressed many of the basic methodological issues that contemporary epidemiologists deal with. These issues include defining populations at risk for disease and the relative disease risk between population groups, and considering whether associations between disease and the factors mentioned above might be caused by other factors, such as age, length of exposure to a condition, or overall health.

A generation later public health research came into its own as a practical tool when another British physician, John Snow (1813–1858), tested the hypothesis that a cholera epidemic in London was being transmitted by contaminated water. By examining death rates from cholera, he realized that they were significantly higher in areas supplied with water by the Lambeth and the Southwark and Vauxhall companies, which drew their water from a part of the Thames River that was grossly polluted with sewage. When the Lambeth Company changed the location of its water source to another part of the river that was relatively less polluted, rates of cholera in the areas served by that company declined, while no change occurred among the areas served by the Southwark and Vauxhall. Areas of London served by both companies experienced a cholera death rate that was intermediate between the death rates in the areas supplied by just one of the companies. The geographic pattern of infections was carefully recorded and plotted on a map of London. In recognizing the grand but simple natural experiment posed by the change in the Lambeth Company water source, Snow was able to make a uniquely valuable contribution to epidemiology and public health practice.

After Snow's seminal work, investigations by epidemiologists have come to include many chronic diseases with complex and often still unknown causal agents, and the methods of epidemiology have become similarly complex. Today researchers use genetics, molecular biology, and microbiology as investigative tools, and the methods used to establish relative disease risk make use of the most advanced statistical techniques available. Yet, reliance on meticulous counting and categorizing of cases and the imperative to think logically and avoid the pitfalls in mathematical relationships in medical data remain at the heart of all of the research used to show elevated disease risk in population subgroups and to prove that medical treatments are safe and effective.

Basic Epidemiological Concepts and Terms

The most basic concepts in epidemiology are the measures used to discover whether a statistical association exists between various factors and disease. These measures include various kinds of rates, proportions, and ratios. Mortality (death) and morbidity (disease) rates are the raw material that researchers use in establishing disease causation. Morbidity rates are most usefully expressed in terms of disease incidence (the rate with

WORDS TO KNOW

INCIDENCE: The number of new cases of a disease or injury that occur in a population during a specified period of time.

MORBIDITY: The term "morbidity" comes from the Latin word *morbus*, which means sick. In medicine it refers not just to the state of being ill, but also to the severity of the illness. A serious disease is said to have a high morbidity.

MORTALITY: Mortality is the condition of being susceptible to death. The term "mortality" comes from the Latin word *mors*, which means "death." Mortality can also refer to the rate of deaths caused by an illness or injury, i.e., "Rabies has a high mortality."

NOTIFIABLE DISEASES: Diseases that the law requires must be reported to health officials when diagnosed, including active tuberculosis and several sexually transmitted diseases; also called reportable diseases.

PREVALENCE: The actual number of cases of disease (or injury) that exist in a population.

SURVEILLANCE: The systematic analysis, collection, evaluation, interpretation, and dissemination of data. In public health, it assists in the identification of health threats and the planning, implementation, and evaluation of responses to those threats.

which members of a population or research sample contract a disease) and prevalence (the proportion of the group that has a disease over a given period of time).

The most important task in epidemiology is the assessment or measurement of disease risk. The population at risk is the group of people that could potentially contract a disease, which can range from the entire world population (e.g., at risk for the flu) to a small group of people within a remote and isolated community (e.g., at risk for contracting a particular, ecologically restricted parasite). The most basic measure of a population group's risk for a disease is relative risk—the ratio of the prevalence of a disease in one group with particular biological, demographic, or behavioral characteristics to the prevalence in another group with different characteristics.

The simplest measure of relative risk is the odds ratio, which is the ratio of the odds that a person in one group has a disease to the odds that a person in a second, comparator group has the disease. The odds for contracting a disease are the ratio between the proportion of people in a population group that share particular characteristics that put them at risk for a disease to the proportion of people in a reference or control population (often the general population in a certain region or jurisdiction). For example, patients with chronic obstructive pulmonary disease (COPD), an inflammatory condition of the lungs associated with smoking and long exposure to air pollution, are at significantly greater risk of contracting community-acquired pneumonia (CAP) compared to a general population group matched on age and gender. Thus in a sample of subjects that includes both COPD patients and subjects who do not have COPD, epidemiologists expect that the odds ratio for the COPD patients contracting CAP would be significantly greater than 1.0.

The mortality rate is the ratio of the number of deaths in a population, either in total or disease-specific, to the total number of members of that population, and is usually given in terms of a large population denominator, so that the numerator can be expressed as a whole number. Thus, in 1982, the number of deaths from all causes was 1,973,000 and number of people in the United States was 231,534,000, yielding a death rate from all causes of 852.1 per 100,000 per year. That same year there were 1,807 deaths from tuberculosis yielding a disease-specific mortality rate of 7.8 per million per year.

Assessing disease frequency is more complex because of the factors of time and disease duration. For example, disease prevalence can be assessed at a point in time (point prevalence) or over a period of time, usually a year (period prevalence, annual prevalence). This is the prevalence that is usually measured in illness surveys that are reported to the public in the news. Researchers can also measure prevalence over an indefinite time period, as in the case of lifetime prevalence, which is the prevalence of a disease over the course of the entire lives of the people in the population under study up to the point in time when the researchers make the assessment. Researchers calculate this by determining for every person in the study sample whether or not he or she has ever had the disease, or by checking lifetime health records for everybody in the population for the occurrence of the disease, counting the occurrences, and then dividing by the number of people in the population.

The other basic measure of disease frequency is incidence, the number of cases of a disease that occur in a given period of time. Incidence is a critical statistic in describing the course of a fast-moving epidemic, in which medical decision-makers must know how quickly a disease is spreading. The incidence rate is the key to public health planning because it enables officials to understand what the prevalence of a disease is likely to be in the future. Prevalence is mathematically related to the cumulative incidence of a disease over a period of time as well as the expected duration of a disease, which can be a week in

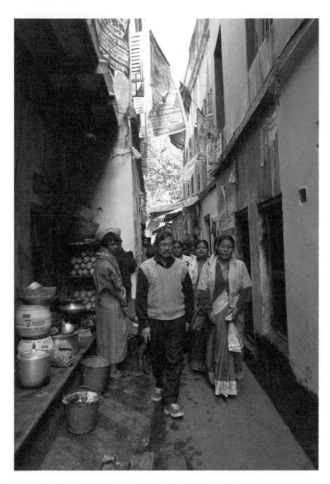

Epidemiologist Smarajit Jana walks through the narrow streets of the sex-trade area of Calcutta, India, where the Sonagachi social project he initiated has dramatically reduced the incidence of sexually transmitted diseases such as syphilis and gonorrhea. The program has also held the rate of HIV infection steady. © *Kapoor Baldev/Sygma/Corbis.*

the case of the flu or a lifetime in the case of juvenile onset diabetes. Therefore, incidence not only indicates the rate of new disease cases, but is the basis of the rate of change of disease prevalence.

Epidemiologists use statistical analysis to discover associations between death and disease in populations and various factors—including environmental (e.g., pollution), demographic (age and gender), biological (e.g., body mass index or "BMI" and genetics), social (e.g., educational level), and behavioral (e.g., tobacco smoking, diet or type of medical treatment)—that could be implicated in causing disease.

Familiarity with basic concepts of probability and statistics is essential in understanding health care and epidemiological research. Statistical associations take into account the role of chance in contracting disease. Researchers compare disease rates for two or more population groups that vary in their environmental, genetic, pathogen

exposure, or behavioral characteristics and observe whether a particular group characteristic is associated with a difference in rates that is unlikely to have occurred by chance alone.

■ Applications and Research

Applications in Public Health Practice

Certain concepts are basic to infectious disease epidemiology. These include the *infectious agent*, which is the organism that can develop within a human host and be passed along to other people via a particular *mode of transmission*, for example by air, food, or sexual intercourse. Infectious diseases have geographic scope or *occurrence*, and take a certain length of time to result in disease symptoms called the *incubation period*. After this incubation period, there is a period during which the individual can pass the infection along to others, called the *period of communicability* of the disease. The *infectivity* of a disease is the probability that an infected individual can pass the infection to an uninfected person, and the *virulence* of an infectious agent is the relative power and pathogenicity possessed by the organism. Populations of animals or human groups that harbor the infectious agent constitute a *reservoir* of the disease, and an organism such as a tick or insect that carries the infectious agent from such a reservoir to vulnerable individuals is called a *vector*.

Once the epidemic is underway, public health officials must begin attempts to control it even as they continue to gather epidemiological information about its cause and distribution. These control efforts consist of preventive measures for individuals and groups, which are measures designed to prevent further spread of the disease, and treatment in order to minimize the period of communicability of the infection, as well as reduce morbidity and mortality. Control of patient contacts and the immediate environment are foremost among such preventive measures, which can extend to patient isolation and observance of universal precautions, including handwashing, wearing of gloves and masks, and sterilization in dangerous instances. Epidemic measures, including the necessary abrogation of civil rights as in quarantines, are sometimes necessary to contain a communicable disease that has spread within an area, state, or nation. The epidemic may have disaster implications if effective preventive actions are not initiated, and the scope of actions can be international, requiring the coordination of disparate public health capabilities across national boundaries.

Screening Programs

Screening a community using relatively simple diagnostic tests is one of the most powerful tools that healthcare professionals and public health authorities have in preventing or combating disease. Familiar examples of screening include HIV testing to help prevent AIDS, tuberculin testing to screen for tuberculosis, and hepatitis C testing by insurers to detect subclinical infection that could result in liver cirrhosis over the long term. In undertaking a screening program, authorities must always judge whether the benefits of preventing the illness in question outweigh the costs and the number of cases that have been mistakenly identified, called false positives.

The ability of the test to identify true positives (sensitivity) and true negatives (specificity) makes screening a valuable prevention tool. However, the usefulness of the screening test is proportional to the disease prevalence in the population at risk. If the disease prevalence is very low, there are likely to be more false positives than true positives, which would cast doubt on the usefulness and the cost-effectiveness of the test. For example, if the prevalence of a disease in the population is only 2% and a test with a false positive rate of 4% is given to everyone (normally a good rate for a screening test), then individuals falsely identified as having the disease would be twice as frequent as individuals accurately identified with the disease. This would render the test results virtually useless. Public health officials deal with this situation by screening only population subgroups that have a high risk of contracting the disease. In infectious disease, screening tests are valuable for infections with a long latency period, which is the period of time during which an infected individual does not show disease symptoms, or which have a lengthy and ambiguous symptomatic period.

Clinical Trials

Clinical trials are the experimental branch of epidemiology in which scientific sampling with randomized selection of research subjects is combined with prospective study design and experimental controls involving a placebo or comparator active treatment control group. The statistical analysis used in clinical trials is similar to what is used in other types of epidemiological studies, usually simple counting of cases that improve or deteriorate and comparisons of morbidity and mortality rates between the trial treatment groups.

Clinical trials in infectious disease are most common when a significant follow-up period is available. One such trial was a rigorous test of the effectiveness of condoms in HIV/AIDS prevention. This experiment was reported in 1994 in the *New England Journal of Medicine*. Although in the United States and Western Europe the transmission of AIDS has been largely within certain high-risk groups, including drug users and homosexual males, worldwide the predominant mode of HIV transmission is heterosexual intercourse. The effectiveness of condoms to prevent HIV transmission is generally acknowledged, but even after more than 25 years of the growth of the epidemic, many people remain ignorant of the scientific support for their preventive value.

A group of European scientists conducted a prospective study of HIV negative subjects that had no risk factor for AIDS other than having a stable heterosexual relationship with an HIV infected partner. A sample of 304 HIV negative subjects (196 women and 108 men) was followed for an average of 20 months. During the trial 130 couples (42.8%) ended sexual relations, usually due to the illness or death of the HIV-infected partner. Of the remaining 256 couples that continued having exclusive sexual relationships, 124 couples (48.4%) consistently used condoms. None of the seronegative partners among these couples became infected with HIV. On the other hand, among the 121 couples that inconsistently used condoms, the seroconversion rate was 4.8 per 100 person-years.

Because none of the seronegative partners among the consistent condom-using couples became infected, this trial presents extremely powerful evidence of the effectiveness of condom use in preventing AIDS. On the other hand, there appear to be several main reasons why some of the couples did not use condoms consistently. Therefore, the main issue in the journal article shifts from the question of whether or not condoms prevent HIV infection—they clearly do—to the issue of why so many couples do not use condoms in view of the obvious risk. Couples with infected partners that got their infection through drug use were much less likely to use condoms than when the seropositive partner got infected through sexual relations. Couples with more seriously ill partners at the beginning of the study were significantly more likely to use condoms consistently. Finally, the longer the couple had been together before the start of the trial was positively associated with condom use.

■ Impacts and Issues

The control of infectious disease is an urgent mission for epidemiologists employed in various state and federal public health agencies and their partners in private industry and research foundations. The American Public Health Association (APHA) provides guidance for the epidemiology and control of more than 100 communicable diseases that confront public health practitioners at present.

Infectious disease epidemiology requires accurate and timely incidence and prevalence data such as is provided with comprehensive disease surveillance of usual and emerging diseases. Although the development of an organized surveillance system is critical to the provision of these data, the system's effectiveness depends on the willingness and ability of health care providers to detect, diagnose, and report the incidence of cases that the system is supposed to track. A reporting system functions at four levels: 1) the basic data is collected in the local community where the disease occurs; 2) the data are assembled at the district, state, or provincial levels; 3) information is aggregated under national auspices (e.g., the Centers for Disease Control and Prevention (CDC) in the United States); and 4) for certain prescribed diseases, the national health authority reports the disease information to the World Health Organization (WHO).

The reporting of cases at the local level is mandated for *notifiable* illnesses that come to the attention of healthcare providers. Case reports provide patient information, suspect organisms, and dates of onset with basis for diagnosis, consistent with patient privacy rights. Collective case reports are compiled at the district level by diagnosis stipulating the number of cases occurring within a prescribed time. Any unusual or group expression of illness that may be of public concern should be reported as an epidemic, whether the illness is included in the list of notifiable diseases and whether it is a well-known identified disease or an unknown clinical entity.

Because of the emergence or re-emergence of HIV/AIDS and resistant strains of tuberculosis, malaria, gonorrhea, and *E. coli* among others, infectious disease epidemiology, once thought to be waning in importance due to significant advances in public sanitation and immunization programs, has re-emerged as an urgent challenge. Infectious diseases currently threaten to destroy social order in some developing nations and pose extremely difficult public health problems even in the wealthiest societies. Hantavirus infections, thought to be a serious problem primarily in Asia, have emerged as an epidemic in the southwestern United States. Lyme disease continues to afflict ever larger populations in the Northeast United States; Ebola virus has jumped from monkeys to humans in Africa and pneumococci are becoming resistant to the antibiotics used to treat infections.

Air travel has created the situation in which travelers can return home from areas where particular pathogens are endemic within the incubation period of every infectious disease, which can potentially precipitate an epidemic.

■ Primary Source Connection

John Snow (1813–1858) was an English physician who made great advances in the understanding of both anesthetics and the spread of disease, especially cholera.

The first pandemic, which reached Great Britain in 1831, caused as much fear and panic as tuberculosis did in the early twentieth century and HIV/AIDS does today. The death rate from cholera was over 50 percent and medical opinion was sharply divided as to the cause. At the time, John Snow was a doctor's apprentice gaining his first experience with the disease, noting its symptoms of diarrhea and extreme dehydration.

The germ theory of disease, which holds that viruses and bacteria are the causative infectious agents of diseases such as yellow fever, smallpox, typhoid, cholera, and others, was in its infancy at this time. Some doctors accepted the hypothesis of *contagion* in which disease spreads from one person to another. Others assumed that "miasmata" or toxins in the air, spread disease.

Snow first began a serious scientific investigation of cholera transmission during the 1848 London epidemic. In his classic essay, *On the Mode of Communication of Cholera*, published on August 29, 1849, he postulated that polluted water was a source of cholera—especially water contaminated by the waste of an infected person, a not-uncommon occurrence at the time. When an outbreak erupted a few years later in central London at the end of August 1854, close to where Snow himself lived, he resumed his research.

The historical claim that Snow removed the pump handle himself—which would, of course, have stopped exposure to the contaminated water—has little evidence and may be a myth. Snow recommended its removal, but the actual removal was probably done by the local curate, Henry Whitehead, several days after the outbreak began.

It is partially thanks to John Snow's work in the Broad Street area that Britain suffered fewer major outbreaks of cholera after this time. An influential figure in medical circles, he had been elected president of the Medical Society of London in 1855. Fortunately for British public health, the successful proof of his theory on the transmission of cholera—from person to person via contaminated water—took hold, and the "environmental" theory eventually died away. Although the actual causative agent, the bacterium *Vibrio cholerae*, would not be identified until 1883, Snow's preventive methods worked. Indeed, they are still effective today, for despite the advent of vaccination and antibiotics, handwashing and the avoidance of contaminated food and water are still fundamental ways of preventing infection.

Because Snow based his investigation on the idea of germ theory, which French microbiologist Louis Pasteur (1822–1895) would later prove, he used a scientific approach and epidemiological study of cholera victims to validate his hypothesis. As his case notes amply demonstrate, much of his research was driven by his patients' visible suffering.

SEE ALSO *Demographics and Infectious Disease; Public Health and Infectious Disease; Notifiable Diseases.*

BIBLIOGRAPHY
Books

Bennenson, A.S., ed. *Control of Communicable Diseases Manual.* 16th ed. Washington, DC: American Public Health Association, 1995.

Centers for Disease Control. *Tuberculosis Statistics: States and Cities, 1984.* Atlanta: Centers for Disease Control, 1985.

Graunt, J. *Natural and Political Observations Made upon the Bills of Mortality.* London, 1662. Reprinted by Johns Hopkins Press, 1939.

Hennekens, C.H., and J.E. Buring. *Epidemiology in Medicine.* Boston: Little, Brown, 1987.

Hippocrates. *On Airs, Waters and Places.*

Shephard, David A.E. *John Snow: Anaesthetist to a Queen and Epidemiologist to a Nation.* Cornwall, Prince Edward Island, Canada: York Point, 1995.

Epidemiological Investigation Solves London Epidemic

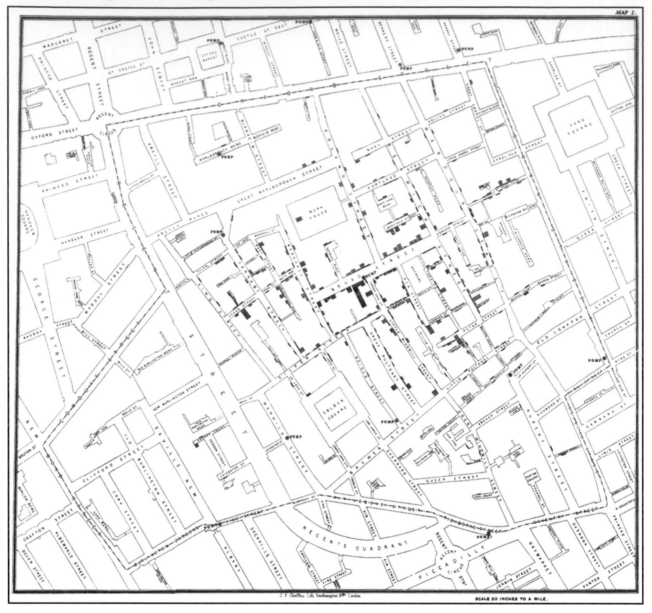

Map showing the area of central London where British physician John Snow (1813–1858) documented cholera cases in 1854 (shown by dark bars) and linked them with contaminated water from a public pump in Broad Street. Snow's work was among the first examples of investigating a disease outbreak using principles of epidemiology.   *Courtesy, Dr. Ralph R. Frerichs, http://www.ph.ucla.edu/epi/snow.htmlr.*

Periodicals

De Vincenzi, I. "A Longitudinal Study of Human Immunodeficiency Virus Transmission by Heterosexual Partners." *New England Journal of Medicine* 331 (August 11, 1994): 341–346.

UCLA. Department of Epidemiology. School of Public Health. "John Snow." <http://www.ph.ucla.edu/epi/snow.html> (accessed March 30, 2007).

Kenneth LaPensee

Epstein-Barr Virus

■ Introduction

Epstein-Barr Virus (EBV) is also known as the Human Herpesvirus 4 (HHV-4). It is one of the most common viruses present in humans. The Centers for Disease Control and Prevention (CDC) estimates that 95% of all adults aged 35–40 in the United States have been infected by EBV. Most people infected with EBV during childhood either show no symptoms or suffer a brief illness with symptoms indistinguishable from other mild, common illnesses.

In teenagers and young adults, EBV can result in mononucleosis, commonly called mono, with prolonged and more severe symptoms. Teenagers and young adults typically acquire EBV from infected cells in the mouth. EBV is present in saliva, also earning mononucleosis the nickname "the kissing disease."

■ Disease History, Characteristics, and Transmission

Epstein-Barr virus was first discovered in 1964 by Michael Epstein and Yvonne Barr while they were studying Burkett's lymphoma, a form of cancer that is relatively common in Africa. The virus was named after these

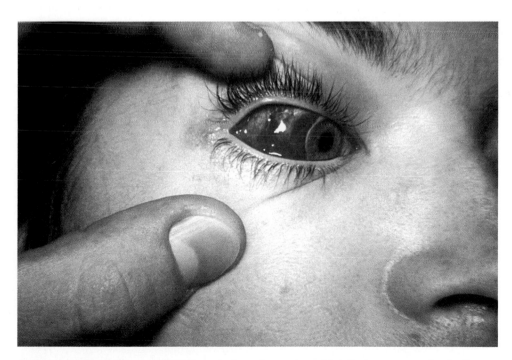

A conjunctival hemorrhage of the right eye is shown in a patient with infectious mononucleosis. On occasion, non-infectious conjunctivitis may occur in people suffering from infectious mononucleosis or Epstein-Barr Virus because of the body's systemic response to viral infections. *Science Source.*

discoverers. Its role as the cause of infectious mononucleosis was later identified.

The virus is extremely prevalent in humans. The infection can persist, as the virus may remain latent for years. In response to triggers that are still not fully known, EBV can reinitiate an active infection. Latency and recurrence occur most often in individuals with compromised immune systems.

Initially, an EBV infection begins when the virus infects and then makes new copies of the virus in the thin layer of epithelial cells that line the mouth, throat, and cervix. The infection then expands to include B cells—cells that are components of the immune system. It is within the B cells that the virus becomes latent by integrating its DNA into the DNA of the host cells. As the host DNA duplicates by cell division, so does the viral DNA. Virus particles that are made in the B cells can escape to other cells in the body. Virus production in these other cells affects the functioning of the tissue, producing some of the symptoms of infection.

EBV is contagious—it can be spread from person to person. Transmission of EBV typically occurs through contact with saliva. Contact with infected cervical cells through sexual activity may transmit EBV. Transmission via blood transfusions is possible but rare.

■ Scope and Distribution

Epstein-Barr virus can be present in almost any person, in any country. However, studies that have examined the prevalence of antibodies against the virus have shown that EBV is almost universally present in adults in developing countries. Worldwide, most people are exposed to EBV early in life, when infection is most likely to cause only mild illness. In the United States, 50% of the population is positive for antibodies to the virus by the age of five.

■ Treatment and Prevention

Infection is determined by detecting the presence of the antibodies that have been produced by the immune system in response to the presence of the virus. The level of a particular antibody in the blood called the heterophile antibody is a reliable indicator of the intensity of the infection. Even though the virus is common in the cells of the mouth and throat, samples of cells taken from the areas are not a reliable means of detecting the virus.

Treatment of Epstein-Barr virus infection is difficult, as the virus can become latent for months or years. There are no available vaccines or antiviral drugs to prevent or treat EBV. Teenagers and young adults suffering from infectious mononucleosis are typically given medications to ease symptoms such as fever, aches, and fatigue that can persist for up to four weeks.

■ Impacts and Issues

Epstein-Barr virus affects just about everyone at some time. In most people, the infection is brief and may either produce no symptoms or brief, mild illness. The most severe symptoms associated with EBV occur in people aged 10–21 who were not previously exposed to EBV in early childhood and who develop mononucleosis. Infectious mononucleosis can have more serious impacts on people living in underdeveloped regions because the condition can leave persons more susceptible to other infections.

From the mid–1980s through the early 1990s, researchers identified EBV as a possible cause of chronic fatigue syndrome (CFS) in adults. Many persons who displayed the symptoms of CFS—headaches, memory loss, and severe, prolonged exhaustion—also carried EBV. The CDC embarked on a four-year study of CFS, eventually finding no link between EBV and CFS. The scientific community now disregards EBV as a direct cause of chronic fatigue syndrome.

EBV has also been linked to the formation of certain types of cancer. EBV is linked to a cancer of the upper respiratory tract, nasopharyngeal carcinoma. This type of cancer occurs most commonly in Africa and parts of China, however, researcher have noted that the increase of nasopharyngeal carcinoma in China could also be influenced by environmental factors and diet. In equatorial Africa, malaria infections can reduce the body's ability to respond to chronic EBV infection. The two diseases in tandem have been linked to Burkitt's lymphoma, a cancer that often forms large tumors on the jaw.

SEE ALSO *Mononucleosis; Viral Disease.*

BIBLIOGRAPHY

Books

Hoffman, Gretchen. *Mononucleosis.* New York: Benchmark Books, 2006.

Powell, Michael, and Oliver Fischer. *101 Diseases You Don't Want to Get.* New York: Thunder's Mouth Press, 2005.

Tselis, Alex, and Hal B. Jenson. *Epstein-Barr Virus.* London: Informa Healthcare, 2006.

Web Sites

Centers for Disease Control and Prevention. "Epstein-Barr Virus and Infectious Mononucleosis." <http://www.cdc.gov/ncidod/diseases/ebv.htm> (accessed April 10, 2007).

Brian Hoyle

IN CONTEXT: TRENDS AND STATISTICS

The National Center for Infectious Diseases, Centers for Disease Control and Prevention (CDC) states the Epstein-Barr virus (EBV) is "one of the most common human viruses. The virus occurs worldwide, and most people become infected with EBV sometime during their lives. In the United States, as many as 95% of adults between 35 and 40 years of age have been infected. Infants become susceptible to EBV as soon as maternal antibody protection (present at birth) disappears. Many children become infected with EBV, and these infections usually cause no symptoms or are indistinguishable from the other mild, brief illnesses of childhood. In the United States and in other developed countries, many persons are not infected with EBV in their childhood years. When infection with EBV occurs during adolescence or young adulthood, it causes infectious mononucleosis 35% to 50% of the time."

SOURCE: *National Center for Infectious Diseases, Centers for Disease Control and Prevention*

Escherichia coli O157:H7

■ Introduction

Escherichia coli is a Gram-negative bacterium (a bacterium that has a cell wall that contains two membranes sandwiching a thin, but strong supporting layer) that normally inhibits the intestinal tracts of humans and other warm-blooded animals.

There are hundreds of different types (strains) of *E. coli* that differ from one another only slightly in their composition. Most of these strains are harmless and many are beneficial, as they can manufacture some vitamins that are needed for proper functioning of the body. Strain O157:H7 is an exception; in contrast to many of the other strains, *E. coli* O157:H7 does not normally reside in the human intestinal tract of humans. It normally lives in the intestinal tract of cattle. While harmless in the cattle, it can be dangerous to people. Ingesting food or water that is contaminated with O157:H7—typically by exposure of the food or water to cattle feces or handling by someone whose hands are soiled—can produce a severe, even life-threatening infection.

The descriptor O157 is a code that refers to a structure called lipopolysaccharide that is located on the outer surface of the bacterium. Different configurations of lipopolysaccharide are possible, which can affect the disease-causing ability of the bacterium. The other descriptor, H7, refers to a form of the bacteria's locomotive structure called the flagellum.

Since its first description in the early 1980s, the illness due to *E. coli* O157:H7 has sickened thousands, and over one thousand people have died as a result of the infection that can destroy intestinal and kidney cells.

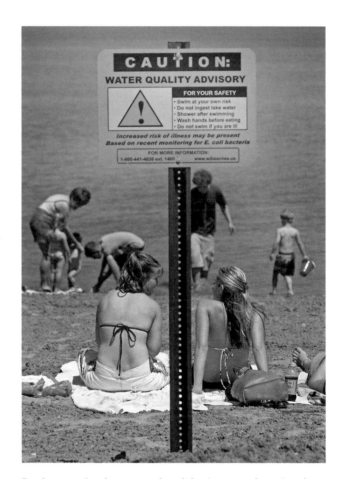

Beachgoers enjoy the water and sand despite a posted warning about the potential of dangerous *E. coli* bacteria in the water. *AP Images.*

■ Disease History, Characteristics, and Transmission

E. coli O157:H7 is one of four types of the bacterium that can infect the gastrointestinal tract, causing a disease called gastroenteritis. Additionally, O157:H7 is described as being enterohemorrhagic—this means it is able to destroy the cells lining the intestinal tract, which causes copious bleeding.

The severe intestinal damage that occurs during an infection by *E. coli* O157:H7 is due to the production of powerful toxins. These toxins, which are called verotoxin and shiga-like toxin, are similar to the destructive toxin

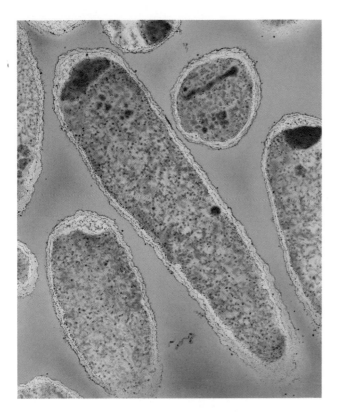

A color transmission electron micrograph (TEM) shows *Escherichia coli* O157:H7 bacteria, a cause of food-borne illness. *K. Lounatamaa/Photo Researchers, Inc.*

WORDS TO KNOW

GRAM-NEGATIVE BACTERIUM: Any type of bacterium that is identified and classified by its property of not retaining crystal-violet dye during Gram's method of staining.

STRAIN: A subclass or a specific genetic variation of an organism.

TOXIN: A poison that is produced by a living organism.

produced by another disease-causing bacterium, *Shigella dysenteriae.*

Indeed, the similarity of the toxins in the two different bacteria reflects how strain O157:H7 came into existence. The strain was discovered in Argentina in 1977. Studies of the sequences of the genetic material in O157:H7 and *S. dysenteriae* support the idea that, likely in the intestinal tract of a cow, a typical *E. coli* acquired genetic material from a neighboring *S. dysenteriae.* The acquired genetic material included the gene that coded for the destructive *Shigella* toxins. The genetically altered *E. coli,* O157:H7, now was capable of producing the toxins.

In 1982, strain O157:H7 was first identified as a cause of illness, when an outbreak of severe diarrhea in several states in the United States was found to be due to undercooked hamburgers. The disease became known as "hamburger disease." This is unfortunate, since subsequently it became clear that other foods including various kinds of produce, fruits, unpasteurized juices and milk, and cheese products can be contaminated with strain O157:H7. Produce and fruits can become contaminated when sprayed with sewage-containing water during their growth. If the food is not washed prior to eating, the bacteria can be ingested. In 2006, for example, a multi state illness outbreak due to O157:H7 was traced to organically grown lettuce. Some consumers had eaten the lettuce without first washing it.

The U.S. Centers for Disease Control and Prevention (CDC) estimates that up to 85% of all O157:H7 infections are food-borne infections.

When cattle are slaughtered, intestinal contents can splatter on the carcass. In whole cuts of meat such as a T-bone steak, the bacterial-contaminated surface can be made safe to eat by proper cooking of the cut of meat. However, when surface-contaminated meat is ground up, bacteria including O157:H7 can be distributed throughout the meat. The only way to kill all these bacteria is to adequately cook the meat. This is why undercooked meat can still contain living O157:H7 that are capable of causing the infection.

O157:H7 can also contaminate drinking water. This occurs when O157:H7-containing feces mixes with the drinking water. If the water is not properly treated to remove or kill the bacteria, drinking the water can sicken a person. For example, in the summer of 2000, one of the wells in the community of Walkerton, Ontario, Canada was contaminated by storm run-off from a cattle field. Improper treatment of the water caused thousands of people to become ill and seven people died. Some of the survivors had permanent kidney damage due to the destruction of the kidney caused by the O157:H7 toxins.

In a few instances in the U.S. and Canada, O157:H7 infection has been traced to childrens' petting zoos; stroking fur that is soiled by feces can be dangerous if the child puts the hand in their mouth.

The toxins are so destructive because they not only damage the host cells they contact, but, because they shut down the manufacture of host cell proteins, they prevent repair of the damage. The toxins can damage the cells because the bacteria bind very tightly to the cells. In fact, the association of O157:H7 with a host cell causes the cell to change its shape, forming a pedestal on which the bacterium anchors. This strong association enables the bacteria to remain in position and establish the infection.

An early symptom of the infection, which occurs as the intestinal cells become damaged, is watery diarrhea.

IN CONTEXT: PERSONAL RESPONSIBILITY AND PREVENTION

The U.S. Department of Agriculture's Food Safety and Inspection Service and Centers for Disease Control and Prevention (CDC) recommend to avoid *E. coli* O157:H7 infection that people:

- Cook all ground beef and hamburger thoroughly. Because ground beef can turn brown before disease-causing bacteria are killed, use a digital instant-read meat thermometer to ensure thorough cooking. Ground beef should be cooked until a thermometer inserted into several parts of the patty, including the thickest part, reads at least 160° F (71.1° C). Persons who cook ground beef without using a thermometer can decrease their risk of illness by not eating ground beef patties that are still pink in the middle.
- If you are served an undercooked hamburger or other ground beef product in a restaurant, send it back for further cooking. You may want to ask for a new bun and a clean plate, too.
- Avoid spreading harmful bacteria in your kitchen. Keep raw meat separate from ready-to-eat foods. Wash hands, counters, and utensils with hot soapy water after they touch raw meat. Never place cooked hamburgers or ground beef on the unwashed plate that held raw patties. Wash meat thermometers in between tests of patties that require further cooking.
- Drink only pasteurized milk, juice, or cider. Commercial juice with an extended shelf-life that is sold at room temperature (e.g. juice in cardboard boxes, vacuum sealed juice in glass containers) has been pasteurized, although this is generally not indicated on the label. Juice concentrates are also heated sufficiently to kill pathogens.
- Wash fruits and vegetables under running water, especially those that will not be cooked. Be aware that bacteria are sticky, so even thorough washing may not remove all contamination. Remove the outer leaves of leafy vegetables. Children under 5 years of age, immunocompromised persons, and the elderly should avoid eating alfalfa sprouts until their safety can be assured. Persons at high risk of complications from foodborne illness may choose to consume cooked vegetables and peeled fruits.
- Drink municipal water that has been treated with chlorine or another effective disinfectant.
- Avoid swallowing lake or pool water while swimming. (For more information, see the CDC Healthy Swimming website.)
- Make sure that persons with diarrhea, especially children, wash their hands carefully with soap after bowel movements to reduce the risk of spreading infection, and that persons wash hands after changing soiled diapers. Anyone with a diarrheal illness should avoid swimming in public pools or lakes, sharing baths with others, and preparing food for others.

SOURCE: *Centers for Disease Control and Prevention (CDC)*

Destruction of intestinal cells causes the diarrhea to become bloody. A person can also experience nausea and vomiting. The fluid loss and pain can be debilitating and intake of fluids is important to prevent more serious problems. In most people, these symptoms fade within several weeks, as the body's immune system is able to successfully deal with the infection. People whose immune systems are immature or malfunctioning can develop a more widespread infection. The kidney damage that can occur can be so extensive that the kidney stops functioning. This occurs in 10–15% of those who contract the infection. The infection can also affect the pancreas, brain, and other organs; this assault can be overwhelming and can cause death.

Approximately 10–15% of those infected with strain O157:H7 develop hemolytic uremic syndrome. The syndrome is the leading cause of sudden-onset kidney failure in children in the world. As well, the elderly can develop a condition known as thrombocytopenic purpura, which consists of fever and nerve damage. In the elderly, this complication of *E. coli* O157:H7 infection can kill almost half of those who become infected.

Scope and Distribution

E. coli O157:H7 is worldwide in distribution and occurrence. The prevalence of the illness is higher in countries where agriculture is more prominent and where standards of infection control in food sources are not as stringent as other countries.

There is no evidence that race or gender makes any difference in the susceptibility to infection. However, those with immune systems that are relatively inefficient can be at increased risk; this includes children, the elderly, and those whose immune systems have been impaired by surgery or during the course of caring for another illness.

Treatment and Prevention

Treatment of *E. coli* O157:H7 infection is supportive, including blood replacement and kidney dialysis in persons with hemolytic uremic syndrome.

E. coli O157:H7 infections can be lessened by properly preparing food (such as by adequate cooking until the center of a hamburger is no longer red), washing preparation surfaces that have been in contact with raw ground meat, and handwashing. O157:H7 is readily killed by heat; boiling drinking water will kill the bacteria and destroy the toxins.

Impacts and Issues

The CDC has estimated that the illness afflicts over 70,000 Americans each year. Of these, over 2,000 require hospitalization and approximately 60 people die. For those who become infected, the best that can be expected is a bout of severe diarrhea. Fortunately, for many, recovery is complete and the misery of the infection becomes a memory. For others, the infection can damage the kidney or completely destroy kidney function. For the latter, dialysis or a kidney transplant becomes a fact of life.

Aside from these human costs, the economic consequences of O157:H7 are important. The costs of medical care and lost productivity related to O157:H7 exceed $400 million annually in the United States.

E. coli O157:H7 highlights the necessity of proper hygiene, particularly proper handwashing after using the bathroom. Many food-borne cases of the illness could be prevented if food preparation was accomplished with clean hands. Furthermore, the infection can be easily prevented by cooking ground meat thoroughly. Since the initial outbreak in 1982, many restaurants no longer serve hamburgers that are not cooked to an internal temperature of 160°F (71.1°C), or are not considered "well done."

In 2007, a Canadian bio-pharmaceutical company announced the successful development and testing of a vaccine for cattle. The vaccine operates by blocking the formation of the bacteria to the intestinal epithelial cells. The stranded bacteria are washed out of the intestinal tract. By vaccination of cattle herds, the reservoir of O157:H7 could gradually be eliminated, and outbreaks from beef would be a thing of the past. In the meantime, food safety scientists are studying other methods to decrease contamination of meat on the farm and in the slaughterhouse, and encourage the use of irradiation to keep the ground beef supply safe.

SEE ALSO *Food-borne Disease and Food Safety; Vaccines and Vaccine Development; Water-borne Disease.*

BIBLIOGRAPHY

Books

Drexler, Madeline. *Secret Agents: The Menace of Emerging Infections.* New York: Penguin, 2003.

Nestle, Marion. *What to Eat.* New York: North Point Press, 2006.

Periodicals

Davies. M., et al. "Outbreaks of *Escherichia coli* O157: H7 associated with petting zoos—North Carolina, Florida, and Arizona, 2004 and 2005." *Morbidity and Mortality Weekly.* 54: 1277–1281 (2005).

Brian Hoyle

IN CONTEXT: REAL-WORLD FACTORS IN REPORTING DISEASE

Public health inspectors and scientists use variations of DNA fingerprinting on bacteria to determine the source of an *E. coli* infection. By comparing samples from patients exposed and potential sources, investigators can often identify a common source of an outbreak.

There are always delays between infection and source identification, typically two to three weeks. The Centers for Disease Control and Prevention (CDC) publishes the following the timeline of identification procedures so that, in part, the number of cases possible during an outbreak may be more accurately estimated:

1. Incubation time: The time from eating the contaminated food to the beginning of symptoms. For *E. coli* O157, this is typically 3-4 days.

2. Time to treatment: The time from the first symptom until the person seeks medical care, when a diarrhea sample is collected for laboratory testing. This time lag may be 1 to 5 days.

3. Time to diagnosis: The time from when a person gives a sample to when *E. coli* O157 is obtained from it in a laboratory. This may be 1 to 3 days from the time the sample is received in the laboratory.

4. Sample shipping time: The time required to ship the *E. coli* O157 bacteria from the laboratory to the state public health authorities that will perform "DNA fingerprinting." This may take 0 to 7 days depending on transportation arrangements within a state and the distance between the clinical laboratory and public health department.

5. Time to "DNA fingerprinting": The time required for the state public health authorities to perform "DNA fingerprinting" on the *E. coli* O157 and compare it with the outbreak pattern. Ideally this can be accomplished in 1 day. However, many public health laboratories have limited staff and space, and experience multiple emergencies at the same time. Thus, the process may take 1 to 4 days.

SOURCE: *Centers for Disease Control and Prevention (CDC)*

Exposed: Scientists Who Risked Disease for Discovery

■ Introduction

Most physicians would not find much commonality between yellow fever and stomach ulcers. Yellow fever is a viral illness spread by the bite of an infected mosquito, and spiral-shaped bacteria living in the extremely acidic environment of the stomach cause the majority of stomach ulcers. The common thread lies in the stories of the medical researchers who solved the mysteries presented by these otherwise distinct ailments.

■ History and Scientific Foundations

Yellow fever is a viral disease now preventable by vaccination, but until the early twentieth century, this virus caused epidemics of severe disease and death. Called "yellow jack," yellow fever caused yearly summer epidemics in American coastal cities, and the disease struck year round in the tropics. The initial attempt by French engineers to build the Panama Canal in the 1880s failed in large part due to yellow fever and malaria putting a majority of canal workers in either the hospital or the grave. The United States Army lost more troops to yellow fever during the Spanish American War than to any other single cause. Some regiments lost over 50% of their men to yellow fever. When the United States began to plan resuming construction of the canal in the 1890s, medical officials realized the need to deal with yellow fever.

In 1900, United States Army Surgeon General George Sternberg (1838–1915) appointed four United States Army physicians to serve on the fourth Yellow Fever Commission. The physicians—Walter Reed (1851–1902), James Carroll (1854–1907), Aristides Agramonte (1868–1931), and Jesse Lazear (1866–1900)—received orders to travel to Cuba and initiate experiments to discover the cause of yellow fever. The prevailing medical wisdom asserted that yellow fever infected people when they came in contact with clothing or bedding contaminated by those afflicted with yellow fever. A competing theory taught that the bite of infected mosquitoes spread yellow fever. In 1897, physicians Ronald Ross and Patrick Manson showed that the *Anopheles* mosquito carried malaria, and Carlos Finley, a Cuban physician, had long-championed the belief that yellow fever was also carried by a mosquito.

The four physicians of the Yellow Fever Commission quickly found evidence refuting the contaminated bedding

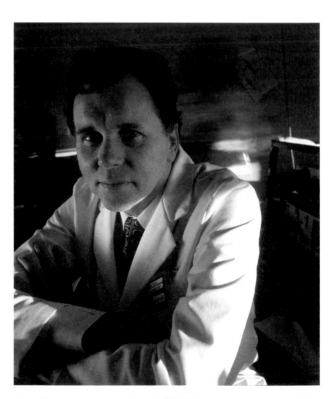

Australian scientist Barry Marshall (1951–) was co-recipient of the 2005 Nobel Prize in physiology or medicine. He and fellow Australian J. Robin Warren (1937–) won the award for their work detailing how *Helicobacter pylori* plays a role in gastritis and peptic ulcer disease. © *Tony McDonough/epa/Corbis.*

theory, but they soon discovered providing evidence for the mosquito transmission theory would require dramatic actions. Yellow fever affected only humans. Animals are not susceptible. In order to show the bite of infected mosquitoes caused yellow fever, human volunteers needed to allow themselves to be bitten. The physicians agreed to experiment on themselves before requesting human volunteers. Agramonte was immune to yellow fever since he had acquired the disease years earlier, and Reed traveled back to Washington to complete a report to Surgeon General Sternberg. As the only physicians available, Lazear and Carroll, began the experiments with humans.

The doctors obtained mosquitoes that had fed on those suffering from yellow fever, and in late August 1900, James Carroll allowed these mosquitoes to feast on his blood. He fell sick a few days later. Two days later a second human volunteer, Private William Dean of the Seventh Calvary, also contracted yellow fever after a deliberate exposure to infected mosquitoes. Both Carroll and Dean recovered; however, Carroll's co-worker, the physician Jesse Lezear, developed a fatal case of yellow fever. Lezear's exposure was officially ruled accidental, but many historians argue Lezear also allowed himself to be a human guinea pig. The determination of accidental exposure allowed life insurance payments to his family. Reed, Carroll, and Agramonte went on to carry out a series of experiments, which conclusively showed the mosquito, *Aedes aegypti*, transmitted yellow fever.

The research did not provide the cause of yellow fever. Many years would pass before research determined yellow fever to be due to a virus, but showing that mosquitoes spread the disease provided a means to control yellow fever. American public health physicians rapidly declared war on the mosquito populations in American cities, and the summer epidemics of yellow fever along the southern and gulf coasts soon became a memory. The building of the Panama Canal in the early twentieth century proceeded without the horrific death toll of malaria and yellow fever due to aggressive control of the mosquito population.

Fast-forwarding nearly a century, stomach ulcers presented a serious problem as these ulcers frequently caused life-threatening bleeding. Stomach ulcers could be treated, but not cured. Few physicians investigated stomach ulcers since the cause of these ulcers was not in dispute; most physicians assumed and taught that stress together with dietary indiscretion caused stomach ulcers. Excessive acid in the stomach due to stress, diet, or smoking corroded the stomach lining and produced an ulcer.

Treating patients with acid-lowering drugs seemed to confirm this thinking as the ulcers did respond to the treatment; however, when patients stopped the drugs, the ulcers recurred. Pathologist J. Robin Warren (1937–) found odd bacteria present in the stomachs of many patients with stomach ulcers and gastritis (inflammation

WORDS TO KNOW

BIOSAFETY LABORATORY: A place for scientific study of infectious agents. A biosafety laboratory is specially equipped to contain infectious agents, prevent their dissemination, and protect researchers from exposure.

COLONIZATION: Colonization is the process of occupation and increase in number of microorganisms at a specific site.

HELSINKI DECLARATION: A set of ethical principles governing medical and scientific experimentation on human subjects; it was drafted by the World Medical Association and originally adopted in 1964.

INFORMED CONSENT: An ethical and informational process in which a person learns about a procedure or clinical trial, including potential risks or benefits, before deciding to voluntarily participate in a study or undergo a particular procedure.

of the stomach lining). These bacteria presented a difficulty to explain because conventional medical wisdom thought bacteria could not survive in the highly acidic environment of the stomach. Another Australian physician, Barry Marshall (1951–), became interested in these novel bacteria, which eventually received the name *Helicobacter pylori*.

Marshall, collaborating with Warren, began to collect evidence that the spiral-shaped bacteria caused stomach ulcers. Since medical establishment already "knew" the cause of ulcers, Marshall's ideas resulted in considerable skepticism. The medical community derided Marshall's ideas and provided him little funding for research. Despite the obstacles from 1981 to 1984, Barry Marshall gathered considerable evidence implicating *H. pylori* as a cause of stomach ulcers and gastritis. The bacteria were present in biopsy specimens taken from ulcer patients, and grown in pure culture from these specimens. However, like the case with yellow fever, no animal model existed to study stomach ulcers. Marshall could not inoculate an ulcer-free animal with the *H. pylori* bacteria and show that ulcers or gastritis developed. This experiment was essential to show that *H. pylori* did indeed cause stomach ulcers, and the bacteria were not just colonizing (maintaining a population without causing disease) in the human stomach.

By 1984, Marshall and Warren had a good circumstantial case implicating *H. pylori* as the causative agent of most stomach ulcers. They also developed a treatment strategy, which clearly both destroyed the bacteria in the stomach and healed the ulcers and gastritis. What they still lacked was definitive proof that when *H. pylori* infected someone, ulcers or gastritis developed. Marshall knew he would not likely be able to get permission to experiment on humans, so he decided to swallow a pure culture of *H. pylori*. He would be the animal model to see if ulcers developed. He had already determined that his stomach did not harbor *H. pylori*. Within a week of ingesting the bacteria, Barry Marshall had classic symptoms of gastritis. Biopsies from his stomach showed bacteria and infection where previously there had been a healthy stomach lining.

Soon after Marshall published the result of his self-experimentation, he was able to obtain funding for a more detailed experiment to determine the role of *H. pylori* in stomach disease. Marshall and Warren went on to work out the way the bacteria cause infections and disease. They also determined why many people harbor the bacteria in their stomachs, but never develop disease. Other researchers confirmed their findings, and by the early 1990s, the role *H. pylori* played in stomach ulcers and chronic gastritis was well established. For their research, Marshall and Warren shared the Nobel Prize for medicine in 1995.

These stories dramatically illustrate medical research using human volunteers. At the time James Carroll and Jesse Lezear contracted yellow fever, medical research using the scientific method was scarcely a few decades old. No guidelines on using human volunteers existed when Carroll exposed himself to a deadly disease in the name of science. Many decades would elapse before guidelines established what truly constitutes informed consent.

The physicians of the Yellow Fever Commission knew they would need to obtain consent of the volunteers. When approached, both U.S. Army soldiers and Spanish immigrants consented to be part of the yellow fever experiments. The consent documents established a contract between individual volunteers and the Yellow Fever Commission, represented by Reed.

Each volunteer was at least 25 years old and each explicitly volunteered to participate in the research. The documents discussed the near certainty of contracting yellow fever while being in Cuba versus the risks of developing the disease as part of the experiment. The volunteers received promises of expert and timely medical care, and the volunteers had to remain at Camp Lazear, the site of the experiments, for the duration of the studies. The volunteers received $100 "in American gold," with an additional $100 if they developed yellow fever. This money represented a near fortune for a poor Spanish immigrant or an underpaid Army private. A family member could receive the money in case of death, but if the volunteer deserted prior to completion of the experiment, they forfeited all payments.

This consent is quite coercive by the standards of today. Essentially, the volunteers heard that they would likely get yellow fever anyway, so if they volunteered they would receive both money and better medical care than the average soldier or immigrant would likely obtain. No organization overseeing human research would allow such a means of obtaining volunteers for research today. This "informed consent" has elements of coercion, forceful persuasion, and manipulation, particularly in the military situation with officers asking enlisted personnel to participate. However, the involved physicians truly put themselves first in line, and at that time, obtaining any consent was remarkable.

The modern practice of informed consent in human research did not come into being until after the revelations of the horrific abuse of human subjects the middle of the twentieth century. The well-documented atrocities committed by German and Japanese physicians during World War II (1939–1945) have made the names Josef Mengele and Shiro Ishii synonymous with torture in the name of medical science. Perhaps less well documented are the experiments during World War II by American physician Stafford Warren. In attempts to learn of radiation effects, researchers injected plutonium into humans without their consent. Experiments on American troops using mustard gas were conducted with the "volunteers" not knowing what they were volunteering for. Unlike the example of Carroll, none of the physicians involved in these experiments stepped forward to experiment first on themselves.

Knowledge of the abuse of human subjects in the Nazi concentration camps resulted in the drafting of the Nuremburg Code. Perhaps one of the most important of the ten principles in the Nuremburg Code is the assertion that consent to participate in medical research must be given free of coercive influence. Also directed in the codes is the assertion that the benefits of the research should exceed the risk to the human volunteers.

■ Issue and Impacts

In 1964, medical leaders drafted another somewhat more thorough set of guidelines known as the Declaration of Helsinki. This document sets forth ethical principles for medical research involving human subjects. The declaration—amended several times and most recently in 2004—together with the Nuremburg Code sets forth the ethical principles to which medical research using human beings must adhere.

Marshall discussed the ethics of his decision to experiment on himself in his Nobel Lecture. Marshall stated, "I had to be my own guinea pig." He felt that he was the only one who could make truly informed consent to his own experiment, and this thinking confirmed his approach to the problem of using human subjects to prove the role of *H. pylori* in stomach disease. He clearly felt the benefits outweighed the risks.

Modern medical researchers delve into diseases involving very deadly bacteria and viruses. Experimental designs minimize the risks of exposure to these pathogens. Special containment facilities (biosafety laboratories) ensure that accidental exposures do not occur easily. Special animal models are built by genetic techniques, negating the need for experiments such as those used by Carroll. Still, a need will certainly always exist for courageous individuals to take great risks in order to solve serious medical problems.

SEE ALSO Helicobacter pylori; *Malaria; Public Health and Infectious Disease; Yellow Fever.*

BIBLIOGRAPHY

Books

Pierce, John R., and James V. Writer. *Yellow Jack: How Yellow Fever Ravaged America and Walter Reed Discovered Its Deadly Secrets.* Hoboken, N.J.: John Wiley & Sons, 2005.

Web Sites

Marshall, Barry J. *Nobelprize.org.* "Nobel Lecture: Helicobacter Connections." 1995. <http://nobelprize.org/nobel_prizes/medicine/laureates/2005/marshall-lecture.html/b> (accessed June 3, 2007).

National Institutes of Health. "Guidelines for the Conduct of Research Involving Human Subjects at NIH." <http://ohsr.od.nih.gov/guidelines/guidelines.html> (accessed June 1, 2007).

University of Virginia Health System. "Yellow Fever and the Walter Reed Commission." <http://www.healthsystem.virginia.edu/internet/library/historical/medical_history/yellow_fever/index.cfm> (accessed June 1, 2007).

Lloyd Scott Clements

Fifth Disease

■ Introduction

Fifth disease, or erythema infectiosum (infectious redness) refers to a common childhood viral infection that is characterized by a mild rash. The infection lasts less than two weeks, and is also known as slapped cheek syndrome, because of the characteristic redness of the face that develops.

The illness can also occur in adults, where it can also involve the joints. In people with some forms of anemia or immune system malfunction, fifth disease can become a more serious condition.

■ Disease History, Characteristics, and Transmission

While fifth disease is likely ancient in origin, its cause has been known only since 1975. Fifth disease is caused by a type of virus called human Parvovirus B19. Only humans can be infected by this virus, although other types of Parvovirus infect dogs and cats. Parvovirus B19 cannot be spread from humans to dogs and cats, nor can the parvoviruses that infect dogs and cats be passed to humans.

The designation fifth disease arose because, when the prevalence of childhood rash-producing illnesses were determined, it was fifth in occurrence behind scarlet fever and three forms of measles.

A hallmark feature of fifth disease is the presence of a bright red rash on the cheeks of the face. A duller rash can also be present on the arms, legs, stomach, and back. The rash sometimes fades, only to be re-activated by stresses like sunlight, exercise, and heat.

A child with fifth disease may also develop a mild fever and coldlike symptoms, and become tired in the few days before the appearance of the rash. Other symptoms can include swollen glands, red eyes, sore throat, and diarrhea.

Some adults who are infected with Parvovirus B19 may not develop symptoms. Others can develop the characteristic rash. In others, joints can become swollen and painful in a way that is similar to arthritis. Still other adults will develop both the rash and the joint discomfort.

Fifth disease is contagious, at least until the rash appears. This can occur as early as four days after infection with the parvovirus, but some people can be symptom-free for almost three weeks. Person to person transmission is likely during this time, especially among children who may be in close contact with each other in a day care or other facility, since both the child and the caregiver are usually unaware that an infection is present and so no special precautions are yet being taken. By the time the rash has appeared a child or adult is no longer contagious.

The incubation period for the disease is 4–20 days from the time of exposure. Transmission of the virus occurs via contaminated droplets, by the passage of saliva, sputum, or mucous from the nose from one person to another. Likely routes also include sharing eating utensils or drink containers.

■ Scope and Distribution

Fifth disease occurs worldwide and is a common childhood illness. It tends to be seasonal, occurring more frequently late in the winter and in early spring. However, cases can occur anytime of the year. During outbreaks in schools, from 10–60% of students acquire the disease.

Fifth disease occurs more commonly among children ages 5 to 14, but also occurs in preschool-age children and their parents. About 50% of tested adults show antibodies in their blood to the disease, meaning they have already contracted it and are immune.

■ Treatment and Prevention

Treatment is usually not necessary, as the infection passes within a week or two. In some adults with fifth disease, joint swelling and pain can last for several months. Over-the-counter medications can be helpful in easing joint discomfort. In those with more serious symptoms, treatment with Parvovirus B19 antibodies can be useful. As of 2007, there is no vaccine for fifth disease.

Options for infected women who are pregnant and their unborn children should be discussed with a personal physician. As of 2007 the CDC asserted that there was "no universally recommended approach to monitor a pregnant woman who has a documented parvovirus B19 infection. Some physicians treat a parvovirus B19 infection in a pregnant woman as a low-risk condition and continue to provide routine prenatal care. Other physicians may increase the frequency of doctor visits and perform blood tests and ultrasound examinations to monitor the health of the unborn baby."

A bout of fifth disease protects a person from a further illness, as the immunity that is built up to the parvovirus last for a person's life.

■ Impacts and Issues

Fifth disease is an almost-universal aspect of childhood. Fortunately for the millions of children around the world who contract the infection every year, the illness is not severe and resolves on its own. A woman who contracts fifth disease during pregnancy is at risk for more serious complications that include development of anemia by the fetus or, if the anemia is especially severe, spontaneous abortion.

Children with fifth disease are sometimes excluded from school when the characteristic rash appears on the face, in an effort to reduce the chance of spreading the disease. In fact, the contagious period is earlier, when cold or flulike symptoms are present. Once the rash appears, the children are no longer able to spread the disease.

For people with anemia (a condition where the transport of oxygen by the blood is impaired), fifth disease can cause the anemia to become more severe. People whose immune system is not functioning efficiently due to illness (such as acquired immunodeficiency syndrome, [AIDS]) or deliberate immunosuppression, as occurs to lessen the rejection of a transplanted organ, can develop anemia with fifth disease that is more long-lasting.

See Also *Childhood Infectious Diseases, Immunization Impacts; Viral Disease.*

IN CONTEXT: EFFECTIVE RULES AND REGULATIONS

The National Center for Infectious Diseases, Respiratory and Enteric Viruses Branch states, "Excluding persons with fifth disease from work, child care centers, or schools is not likely to prevent the spread of the virus, since people are contagious before they develop the rash."

SOURCE: *Centers for Disease Control and Prevention (CDC)*

IN CONTEXT: EFFECTIVE RULES AND REGULATIONS.

The CDC does not recommend that "pregnant women should routinely be excluded from a workplace where a fifth disease outbreak is occurring."

The CDC "considers that the decision to stay away from a workplace where there are cases of fifth disease is an personal decision for a woman to make, after discussions with her family, physician, and employer."

SOURCE: *Centers for Disease Control and Prevention (CDC)*

BIBLIOGRAPHY

Books

Black, Jacquelyn. *Microbiology: Principles and Explorations.* New York: John Wiley & Sons, 2004.

Douglas, Ann. *The Mother of All Toddler Books.* New York: John Wiley & Sons, 2004.

Web Sites

Centers for Disease Control and Prevention. "Parvovirus B19 (Fifth Disease)" <http://www.cdc.gov/ncidod/dvrd/revb/respiratory/parvo_b19.htm> (accessed on April 1, 2007).

Brian Hoyle

Filariasis

■ Introduction

Filariasis is a preventable parasitic disease caused by the threadworms *Wuchereria bancrofti*, *Brugia malayi*, and *Brugia timori*. It is endemic in over 80 countries and is considered to be the main cause of permanent disability worldwide.

When symptomatic, patients may present with severe lymphatic and limb swelling, commonly referred to as elephantiasis. The disfigurations resulting from elephantiasis and lymphodema raise issues among some communities and add to the socioeconomic impacts of this debilitating disease.

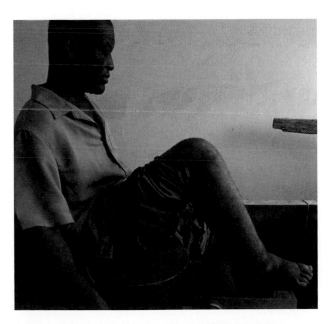

A Haitian man waits in a clinic to be treated for lymphatic filariasis, a disfiguring disease. Also known as elephantiasis, the mosquito-borne parasitic disease invades the lymph system. © *Karen Kasmauski/Corbis.*

Infection is transmitted through mosquito bites, where both the vector (disease carrier) and the human host are necessary in the successful completion of the parasitic life cycle. Anti-parasitic treatment is available, but is expensive and can take around a year to eliminate the parasites. Filariasis infection has been successfully curtailed in countries such as China, which has given hope for the campaign of global eradication.

■ Disease History, Characteristics, and Transmission

Filariasis was first recognized in its infectious form in 1866 when filarial larvae were detected in urine and identified as the causative agent.

The infection is usually acquired in childhood, but takes years to manifest and usually remains asymptomatic until adulthood. Once developed, symptoms may include chronic swelling of the lymph nodes and swelling of the arms, legs, and genitals. Elephantiasis refers to the thickening of skin and underlying tissue and often accompanies symptoms. Without presentation of symptoms, internal damage to the kidneys and the lymphatic system may also develop.

Transmission of filariasis is through mosquito bites, whereby the larval form is drawn out of blood by mosquitos, develops to the infective stage, and is injected into a new host. Here the larvae develop into the adult form, migrate to the lymph nodes, mate, and release millions of larvae into the host's bloodstream. Adult worms may live up to six years, during which time the host will remain a source of infection for others.

■ Scope and Distribution

Filariasis is a disease largely associated with poverty with more than a billion people in over 80 countries at risk. Infection caused by *W. bancrofti* is endemic in tropical regions of Southeast Asia, Africa, India, and Central and

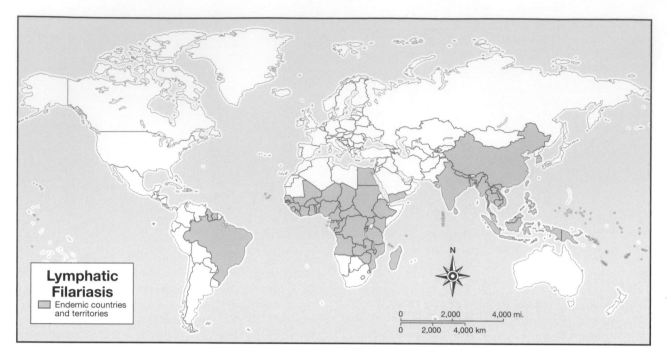

Map showing lymphatic filariasis endemic countries and territories, 2006. *© Copyright World Health Organization (WHO). Reproduced by permission.*

South America, while *B. malayi* and *B. timori* are generally limited to areas of Southeast Asia. This disease state is rare in western countries with no cases having been reported within the United States.

Filariasis has been recognized as the leading cause of permanent disability worldwide. Of the 120 million people affected, 40 million have been left disfigured and completely incapacitated. Chronic disease symptoms present more in men than women as seen in endemic areas where from 10 to 50% of men are infected versus up to 10% of women.

Disease distribution is also affected by habitat suitability for the various forms of mosquito responsible for transmission of the parasite.

■ Treatment and Prevention

Treatment of this disease consists of a multifaceted approach. Treatment of the infection itself may be achieved with a concurrent dosage of strong anti-parasitic drugs such as diethylcarbamazine citrate (DEC), DEC-fortified salt, and albendazole. This proves to be 99% effective in removing microfilaria from the blood after one year of treatment.

Lymphodema and elephantiasis are often exacerbated due to bacterial and fungal infections taking advantage of the patient's compromised lymphatic condition. Following rigorous hygiene routines as prevention against infection from opportunistic pathogens and completing exercises to improve lymph flow often helps

to reduce these causes of swelling. Surgery may be necessary for treatment of severe genital swelling in men.

Prevention of filariasis is achievable by reducing exposure to mosquito bites and treating endemic communities, in total, to remove the pool of infection. Some means of prevention are relatively simple and inexpensive. Using mosquito netting in sleeping areas, wearing clothing that covers the arms and legs, applying mosquito repellant on exposed skin, and remaining indoors during peak times of mosquito activity all reduce the risk of exposure to filariasis. These measures are the basis of a global campaign to eradicate filariasis.

■ Impacts and Issues

Filariasis causes permanent—and often painful—disability in over 40 million people worldwide. Most cases occur in developing or underdeveloped regions. Many disabled by filariasis cannot regularly farm, work, or attend school. Malnourishment rates are often higher among those affected by filariasis than in the surrounding non-affected population.

The social impacts of filariasis present not only in the loss of work labor due to incapacitation, but also in community relations. People disfigured by the disease are frequently shunned by society and chronic complications are often deemed shameful. Marriage is considered a near impossibility among those suffering genital manifestations, which then puts growth and development of the community at risk.

Filariasis is a disease with potential for eradication, but one that remains endemic in poor communities. The continued increase in infection may be attributed to the rapid growth of cities and the resultant spread of poverty-stricken housing areas. These regions provide breeding sites for the mosquitoes and aid in disease transmission. It is for these reasons that endemic areas are trapped in a vicious cycle of infection that has proven difficult to break.

SEE ALSO *Demographics and Infectious Disease; Economic Development and Disease; Helminth Disease; Host and Vector; Opportunistic Infection; Parasitic Diseases.*

BIBLIOGRAPHY

Books

Mandell, G.L., Bennett, J.E., and Dolin, R. *Principles and Practice of Infectious Diseases.* Volume 2. Philadelphia, PA: Elsevier, 2005.

Web Sites

Centers for Disease Control and Prevention (CDC). "Lymphatic Filariasis." February 16, 2007 <http://www.cdc.gov/ncidod/dpd/parasites/lymphaticfilariasis/index.htm> (accessed March 5, 2007).

Directors of Health Promotion and Education (DHPE). "Lymphatic Filariasis." 2005 <http://www.dhpe.org/infect/Lymphfil.html> (accessed March 5, 2007).

World Health Organization (WHO). "Lymphatic Filariasis." September 2000 <http://www.who.int/mediacentre/factsheets/fs102/en/> (accessed March 5, 2007).

WORDS TO KNOW

LYMPHATIC SYSTEM: The lymphatic system is the body's network of organs, ducts, and tissues that filter harmful substances out of the fluid that surrounds body tissues. Lymphatic organs include the bone marrow, thymus, spleen, appendix, tonsils, adenoids, lymph nodes, and Peyer's patches (in the small intestine). The thymus and bone marrow are called primary lymphatic organs, because lymphocytes are produced in them. The other lymphatic organs are called secondary lymphatic organs. The lymphatic system is a complex network of thin vessels, capillaries, valves, ducts, nodes, and organs that runs throughout the body, helping protect and maintain the internal fluids system of the entire body by both producing and filtering lymph, and by producing various blood cells. The three main purposes of the lymphatic system are to drain fluid back into the bloodstream from the tissues, to filter lymph, and to fight infections.

SOCIOECONOMIC: Concerning both social and economic factors.

VECTOR: Any agent, living or otherwise, that carries and transmits parasites and diseases. Also, an organism or chemical used to transport a gene into a new host cell.

IN CONTEXT: RELATED DISEASE GROUPS

Filariasis is a group of tropical diseases caused by thread like parasitic round worms (nematodes of the order Filaraiidae, commonly called filariae) and their larvae. The group affects humans and animals. The larvae transmit the disease to humans through a mosquito bite. Filariasis is characterized by fever, chills, headache, and skin lesions in the early stages and, if untreated, can progress to include gross enlargement of the limbs and genitalia in a condition called elephantiasis. There are hundreds of described filarial parasites, but only eight that cause infections in humans: *Brugia malayi, Wucheria bancrofti, Brugia timori, Onchocerca volvulus, Loa loa, Mansonella streptocerca, Mansonella ozzardi,* and *Mansonella perstans.*

Food-borne Disease and Food Safety

■ Introduction

Food is necessary for our growth and survival. The nutrients in many foods that are vital to humans, however, also provide a meal for microorganisms. The organic (carbon-containing) compounds and moisture content of many foods permit the growth of microbes. Sometimes this co-existence is beneficial. For example, bacteria in the genus *Lactobacillus* help produce yogurt. However, the presence of some microorganisms in foods threatens the food supply and the health of those who eat it.

Some bacteria that can form structures called spores can survive for extended periods of time in foods that are too acidic to permit growth of the bacteria. But, if the food is eaten, the spores can germinate and growth can resume in the more hospitable environment of the intestinal tract.

Bacteria, viruses, parasites, and the poisons (toxins) produced by some of the microbes cause more than 200 different food-borne diseases. This is a serious health threat worldwide. For example, in the United States, food-borne diseases occur an estimated 76 million times every year—affecting 30% of the population—and kills 7,000 to 9,000 people.

■ Disease History, Characteristics, and Transmission

Food-borne illnesses tend to be from microorganisms that usually live in the intestinal tract. Generally, the illnesses produce intestinal upset, often with nausea and vomiting. Food-borne illnesses are commonly called "food poisoning". However, the term food poisoning obscures the fact that there are several types of food-borne illnesses that vary in cause and severity. While mild to moderate illnesses tend to pass after a few days, more serious illnesses can cause kidney damage or failure, muscle paralysis, and death.

Death most often is due to the excessive loss of fluid that occurs in diarrhea. A person can lose fluid at a rate that is difficult to replace by drinking water. If they cannot get medical attention (such as the continual provision of fluids intravenously) they can go into shock and suffer organs failure.

In countries including the United States and Canada, *Campylobacter jejuni* is the leading cause of food-borne illness. The major source is poultry. The bacterium is a

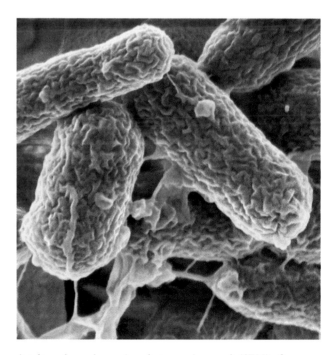

A color enhanced scanning electron micrograph (SEM) of *Escherichia coli* O157:H7 shows a strain of the bacteria that produces a powerful toxin, which causes abdominal cramps and bloody diarrhea, with kidney failure occurring in extreme cases. It can live in the intestines of healthy cattle; it is spread during the milking and slaughter processes. Another source of infection is sewage-contaminated water.   *Dr. Gary Gaugler/Photo Researchers, Inc.*

normal resident in the intestinal tract of poultry. When poultry such as chickens are slaughtered, the intestinal contents can be spread onto the skin. Even with washing of the carcasses, bacteria can remain stuck in crevasses and other areas on the surface. Indeed, monitoring studies have proven that 70–90% of the poultry that reaches the supermarket shelf is contaminated with *C. jejuni*.

Even with the hundreds of millions of poultry meals eaten in the United States each year, the number of illnesses produced by *C. jejuni* is relatively low. This is because the bacteria are very susceptible to heat, thorough cooking will kill the bacteria long before the meal is eaten. However, improper cooking and the re-contamination of cooked meat by, for example, laying the meat on a cutting board that has not been washed after use, sickens millions of American annually.

Another bacteria, Salmonella is the next leading cause of food-borne illness in the United States, with an estimated 1.3 million cases each year. The estimated medical cost of treating these illnesses is $260 million. There are hundreds of species of Salmonella, and dozens are capable of causing illness. For example, *S. enteritidis* is commonly associated with egg containing prepared salad dressing or custards that have been left for several hours at room temperature. This allows the contaminating bacteria to grow to numbers that cause disease when eaten.

The third leading cause of food-borne illness in the United States is *Escherichia coli* O157:H7 and related *E. coli* that cause severe intestinal illnesses (they are collectively known as enterohemorrhagic *E. coli*, or EHEC). Still other varieties of *E. coli* are normally found in the intestinal tract of humans and animals; these are usually harmless. However, strain O157:H7 arose in the 1970s when genetic material from another bacterium called Shigella was somehow transferred to *E. coli*. The genetic material coded for the production of a very potent toxin, and made the new *E. coli* extremely dangerous. The toxin damages intestinal cells, which causes bleeding, and can spread via the bloodstream to the kidneys, potentially causing permanent organ damage or failure.

O157:H7 can be a normally part of the bacterial community found in the intestinal tract of cattle. The illness is usually produced when cattle feces contaminate drinking water. As well, the bacterium can contaminate ground beef during slaughter and packaging. As with Campylobacter, inadequate cooking allows the bacteria to remain alive. Vegetables can also become contaminated by manure supplied as fertilizer. Raw vegetables should be thoroughly washed before consumption. In September, 2006, contamination of organically grown spinach with O157:H7 killed three people and sickened hundreds in the United States.

Some bacteria in the genus *Listeria* also cause food-borne illnesses. *Listeria monocytogenes*, causes listerosis, a rare but serious illness. *Listeria* especially threatens people with compromised immune systems, the elderly, and

WORDS TO KNOW

FOOD PRESERVATION: The term food preservation refers to any one of a number of techniques used to prevent food from spoiling. It includes methods such as canning, pickling, drying and freeze-drying, irradiation, pasteurization, smoking, and the addition of chemical additives. Food preservation has become an increasingly important component of the food industry as fewer people eat foods produced on their own lands, and as consumers expect to be able to purchase and consume foods that are out of season.

IONIZING RADIATION: Any electromagnetic or particulate radiation capable of direct or indirect ion production in its passage through matter. In general use: Radiation that can cause tissue damage or death.

IRRADIATION: A method of preservation that treats food with low doses of radiation to deactivate enzymes and to kill microorganisms and insects.

pregnant women. In addition to the usual symptoms associated with food poisoning, listerosis can cause a severe form of meningitis. *Listeria* bacteria flourish in temperatures between 39°F (4°C) and 98.6°F (37°C).

Another common source of food-borne illness is a virus known as the Norwalk-like virus. The virus normally lives in the human intestinal tract, and is usually spread to food when the food is handled by people who have not washed their hands properly after a bowel movement. Over nine million infections are estimated to occur each year in the United States alone. Most of these could be eliminated by proper handwashing.

■ Scope and Distribution

Food-borne infections can affect anyone, anywhere. The World Health Organization (WHO) estimates that over two million people around the world die each year from diarrhea caused by food-borne infections. Most deaths from food-borne illnesses occur in developing nations.

Because food-borne illnesses are mainly caused by microorganisms that are residents of the intestinal tract, most outbreaks are related to fecal contamination of food and water rather than to the time of year or particular aspect of a culture. Worldwide, poor hygiene is the culprit.

Although food irradiation is opposed by some advocacy groups and research continues, Centers for Disease Control and Prevention (CDC) states that "food irradiation is a promising new application of an established technology. It holds great potential for preventing many important food-borne diseases that are transmitted through meat, poultry, fresh produce and other foods. An overwhelming body of scientific evidence demonstrates that irradiation does not harm the nutritional value of food, nor does it make the food unsafe to eat. Just as for the pasteurization of milk, it will be most effective when irradiation is coupled to careful sanitation programs. Consumer confidence will depend on making food clean first, and then using irradiation or pasteurization to make it safe. Food irradiation is a logical next step to reducing the burden of food-borne disease in the United States."

SOURCE: *Centers for Disease Control and Prevention*

■ Treatment and Prevention

Prevention of food-borne illness must consider a number of factors. The type of disease-causing organism can be important. For example, Campylobacter can be effectively treated by the proper cooking of foods, whereas Clostridium, which can form an environmental hardy structure called a spore, may still be capable of causing an infection even after heating of the food. The environment is another factor; temperature and the amount of moisture in the food can influence the type of organisms that can thrive. Environment also includes the various places that the food passes through on its way to the dinner table; a food entering a processing plant may be safe only to become contaminated during processing. These factors are inter-related. For example, protecting a food from questionable environments, but failing to decontaminate the food does little to lessen the chance of a food-borne illness.

Treatment of foods prior to eating is absolutely important in preventing illness. Some treatments, such as drying or preserving food in salt prior to a sea voyage, were done centuries ago. Canning of foods as a means of preservation and protection from spoilage began in the eighteenth century. In the nineteenth century, the association of an unhygienic environment and disease was recognized. As food began to be shipped further to market, the problem of food deterioration during transit became apparent.

Food safety owes a great deal to Louis Pasteur, who developed the process of pasteurization. Pasteurization began in the 1890s. The process heats milk for a short time at temperatures high enough to be lethal to those microbes that would be expected to be contaminants without altering the taste or appearance of the milk. Milk is now routinely pasteurized before sale. Innovations in the pasteurization technique have increased the shelf-life of refrigerated milk and developed means of transporting and storing milk without the need for refrigeration.

Another prevention strategy is the development and legal enforcement of standards of food preparation, handling and inspection. In many places, food quality must be demonstrated or else the product can be pulled from the shelf and, if necessary, those responsible for its manufacture or distribution prosecuted. In the United States, the Food and Drug Administration (FDA) regulates processing and labeling of most foods. However, the Department of Agriculture (USDA) regulates and oversees the safety of all meat, poultry, and egg products. The two agencies work together to ensure the safety of food produced within and imported into the United States. Both agencies also provide assistance to international organizations and developing nations who wish to implement or strengthen food safety programs.

While government agencies monitor the safety of food as it is produced and sold, monitoring food preparation and hygienic practices in the home must be done by individuals. Improper storage of foods prepared with raw or undercooked eggs, can cause growth of microorganisms in the food. Improper cleaning of cutting boards and other preparation surfaces can cross-contaminate one food by another. Many cases of food poisoning due to *Clostidium botulium* are related to improper home-canning of foods; the spores of the bacterium can survive the food preparation steps and remain capable of causing illness when the food is eaten, even years later.

■ Impacts and Issues

The impact of food-borne illnesses on the individual is substantial. The 76 million food-borne illnesses that are thought to occur each year (likely an underestimate, since many people will suffer from an illness without seeking medical attention) hospitalizes 325,000 people and kills 7,000 to 9,000, according to the Centers for Disease Control and Prevention. Society suffers as well; medical costs, lost work days, travel costs to seek treatment, and the premature loss of people who would otherwise contribute wealth to the economy costs the United States almost seven billion dollars a year.

In February 2007, peanut butter was responsible for a nationwide Salmonella outbreak in the United States affecting over 300 people in approximately 40 states. The FDA warned consumers not to purchase or eat certain brands of peanut butter manufactured at a facility in Georgia. Soon afterwards, companies with brands associated with the salmonella outbreak recalled all potentially contaminated products. While Salmonella is typically associated with poultry products, the 2007 outbreak was not the first associated with peanut butter. A similar Salmonella event that occurred in Australia in the mid–1990s was traced to contaminated peanut butter.

In underdeveloped countries, where medical care is not as available or advanced, food-borne illnesses can be even more devastating. Diarrheal illnesses afflict millions of people every year, many of them are children. The illnesses are a major cause of the malnutrition that is a part of everyday life in many underdeveloped regions.

Prevention of food-borne illnesses does have some controversial aspects. Many food safety organizations advocate irradiation, or cold pasteurization, as method of preventing food-borne illnesses. Irradiation involves exposing food to extremely low levels of ionizing radiation to sterilize food. Proponents cite irradiation's ability to the causes of harmful bacteria such as *E. coli*, *Listeria*, and *S. enteritidis*. Irradiation can also destroy parasites and agricultural pests, as well as prolong the shelf-life of fruits and vegetables by preventing sprouting and delaying spoilage. Critics of irradiation cite the use of radioactive materials in some (mostly older) irradiation technology as a potential environmental and health threat. Others assert that irradiation forms new chemical compounds in treated foods and that the long-term effects of ingesting irradiated products have not been thoroughly studied. Furthermore, while irradiation is effective at killing the sources of many food-borne illnesses, food can still become contaminated after irradiation by improper storage or handling. Irradiation is approved to sterilize meat, egg, poultry, and other agricultural products in several countries, and most require labeling to indicate its use.

A food safety issue that has become more urgent since the 2001 terrorist attacks in the United States is the monitoring of foods to ensure their safety from deliberate tampering. The chain from the field to the supermarket leaves food vulnerable to the deliberate addition of microbiological agents that cause illness or death. While storage conditions, monitoring programs and even the design of packing that can detect contam-

ination is useful in protecting foods from accidental contamination, it is very difficult to protect food from deliberate harm.

SEE ALSO Escherichia coli *O157:H7*; Salmonella *Infection (Salmonellosis)*.

BIBLIOGRAPHY

Books

DeGregori, Thomas R. *Bountiful Harvest: Technology, Food Safety, and the Environment*. Washington, Cato Institute, 2002.

Nestle, Marion. *What to Eat*. New York: North Point Press, 2006.

United States Food & Drug Administration. *Bad Bug Book: food-borne Pathogenic Microorganisms and Natural Toxins Handbook*. McLean: International Medical Publishing, 2004.

Brian Hoyle

Gastroenteritis (Common Causes)

■ Introduction

Gastroenteritis is an inflammation of the stomach and the intestines that is produced by the immune system's response to an infection that can be caused by a number of bacteria or viruses. Gastroenteritis is sometimes referred to as the stomach flu, but is not caused by influenza viruses.

The symptoms of gastroenteritis include a stomach or intestinal upset, vomiting, and often the production of watery feces that is called diarrhea. In developing regions of the world, and especially among children, gastroenteritis-induced diarrhea is a killer. Millions of deaths of newborns and children due to gastroenteritis occur each year in Asia, Africa, parts of the Indian subcontinent, and Latin America.

■ Disease History, Characteristics, and Transmission

Gastroenteritis is caused mainly by viruses, but can also be caused by infection with bacteria and protozoa. The viruses that cause gastroenteritis include rotaviruses, enteroviruses, adenoviruses, caliciviruses, astroviruses, Norwalk virus, and a group of Norwalk-like viruses. Rotavirus infections are the most common.

The symptoms of viral gastroenteritis usually appear quickly, within a few days of ingesting the virus in contaminated water or food. The illness tends to pass quickly, usually being over within the same week. But, people whose immune system function is inefficient such as the young and the elderly, people who are ill with another ailment such as acquired immunodeficiency syndrome (AIDS, also cited as acquired immune deficiency syndrome), or someone whose immune system has been deliberately subdued (such as someone who has received an organ transplant, to reduce the chances of organ rejection) can be ill for a longer time.

Rotavirus is a member of the Reoviridae family of viruses, which contain ribonucleic acid (RNA) as the genetic material. When the virus infects a host cell, the host's genetic machinery is used to make deoxyribonucleic acid (DNA) from the viral RNA; the viral DNA can then be transcribed and translated with host DNA to produce the components that will make new virus particles. There are three main groups of rotavirus that differ from each other slightly in the composition of the protein shell that surrounds the genetic material. These differences mean that a host's immune system will produce different antibodies to the different viruses. Group A rotavirus causes over three million cases of gastroenteritis in the United States annually. Group B rotavirus causes diarrhea that is more prevalent in adults; it has caused several large outbreaks in China. Group C causes diarrhea in children and adults, but is less common than the other two types of rotaviral gastroenteritis.

Rotavirus gastroenteritis hospitalizes 70,000 children every year in the United States. The main reason that rotaviral gastroenteritis is so common is the contagious nature of the virus. Rotavirus easily is spread from person to person, usually when fecal material gets into the mouth. This is known as the fecal-oral route of transmission. Not surprisingly, this type of gastroenteritis occurs frequently in day care facilities, where touching of soiled diapers and hand-to-mouth contact are common. In older children and adults, improper hygiene, particularly washing of the hands, is the main reason for the spread of the virus. People who are infected can excrete (or shed) very high numbers of virus in the watery diarrhea, and spread the infection. Also, handling of utensils and preparation of food with hands that are soiled spreads the virus to the diner. Another route of transmission that is not related to hygiene is the consumption of shellfish. Shellfish are filter feeders—they filter water through an apparatus that traps small food particles. The filter can also trap rotavirus that is present in fecal-contaminated water. As the shellfish feeds, more and more virus can accumulate, until the shellfish becomes toxic to anyone eating it. The danger is especially pronounced in shellfish such as oysters, which some people prefer to eat raw.

Another virus that causes gastroenteritis is the Norwalk virus. This form of the illness tends to be more common in adults, although surveys of children using sophisticated molecular techniques of viral detection have revealed the presence of Norwalk antibodies in children, meaning they have been exposed to the virus, or to a protein that is very similar to the Norwalk viral protein.

Bacteria also cause gastroenteritis. Common examples include certain strains of *Escherichia coli*, *Salmonella*, *Shigella*, and *Vibrio cholerae*. Bacterial gastroenteritis occurs less in developed countries, as the treatment of drinking water, and treatment and disposal of sewage water tends to be much better than in underdeveloped regions. In developing nations, bacterial gastroenteritis due to contaminated water remains a significant concern. Bacterial gastroenteritis can also be caused by eating contaminated food. Examples include foods such as potato salad that has been left at room temperature for some time prior to the meal and contaminated with *Salmonella*, and the presence of a type of *E. coli* designated O157:H7 in undercooked meat; a toxin produced by O157:H7 damages the cells lining the intestinal tract, causing bloody diarrhea.

A protozoan called *Cryptosporidium parvum*, which resides in the intestinal tract of some animals, also causes gastroenteritis when it contaminates drinking water. This type of gastroenteritis is becoming more prevalent in the United States. One reason is the continuing expansion of urban areas into regions that were previously wild, which brings humans into closer contact with wildlife and the *C. parvum* they carry. Another reason is that the protozoans can form an environmentally hardy form called a cyst that allows the protozoan to persist through water treatments such as chlorination and, because of the small diameter of the cysts, to pass through filters used in water filtration. Once inside a person, the cyst can rejuvenate into the growing form that is the cause of the illness.

The symptoms of gastroenteritis always include diarrhea. Fever and vomiting are also common. Typically, these symptoms last only several days and progressively lessen over the next few days as the infection abates. The diarrhea in gastroenteritis is very loose and watery. Bowel movements occur frequently, even several times an hour, as fluid pours out of the cells lining the intestine as a consequence of the infection and as an attempt to flush out the infecting bacteria or virus. Dehydration is not usually a problem in an adult, who will instinctively drink water. If dehydration occurs very quickly or if the individual is so sick that they are unaware or unable to take care of themselves, then they can become very ill. Hospitalization of a child for diar-

WORDS TO KNOW

ANTIBODY: Antibodies, or Y-shaped immunoglobulins, are proteins found in the blood that help to fight against foreign substances called antigens. Antigens, which are usually proteins or polysaccharides, stimulate the immune system to produce antibodies. The antibodies inactivate the antigen and help to remove it from the body. While antigens can be the source of infections from pathogenic bacteria and viruses, organic molecules detrimental to the body from internal or environmental sources also act as antigens. Genetic engineering and the use of various mutational mechanisms allow the construction of a vast array of antibodies (each with a unique genetic sequence).

FECAL-ORAL ROUTE OF TRANSMISSION: The spread of disease through the transmission of minute particles of fecal material from one organism to the mouth of another organisms. This can occur by drinking contaminated water, eating food that was exposed to animal or human feces (perhaps by watering plants with unclean water), or by the poor hygiene practices of those preparing food.

ORAL REHYDRATION THERAPY: Patients who have lost excessive water from their tissues are said to be dehydrated. Restoring body water levels by giving the patient fluids through the mouth (orally) is oral rehydration therapy. Often, a special mixture of water, glucose, and electrolytes called oral rehydration solution is given.

VIRAL SHEDDING: Viral shedding refers to the movement of the herpes virus from the nerves to the surface of the skin. During shedding, the virus can be passed on through skin-to-skin contact.

rhea is usually because of complications of the excessive fluid loss rather than any direct effect of the stomach and intestinal infection.

■ Scope and Distribution

Gastroenteritis is global in distribution. However, it most affects people living in the developing world, and most of these are children. Estimates put the death toll of children due to gastroenteritis-related diarrhea at 1–2 million each year, and the great majority of these deaths occur in developing countries. Still, this is much less than the near five million deaths that occurred annually until the 1980s, and the introduction of what is called oral hydration therapy—drinking a solution containing salts and sugars that helps replenish the body's essential electrolytes (salts and sugars) and fluids that are lost due to diarrhea.

The differences in the severity of the infection and the death rates in the developed versus developing worlds highlight the influence of living conditions, hygiene, and cultural practices on the consequences of gastroenteritis. Age is another factor; the very young and the elderly are particularly susceptible as they may be physically unable to seek prompt relief from the dehydration of diarrhea.

■ Treatment and Prevention

In the treatment of gastroenteritis it is important to distinguish whether the infection is due to bacteria, virus, protozoan or some other non-biological factor. An example of the latter is lactose intolerance. It is important to know the cause, as antibiotics are effective against bacteria, but are not useful against viruses and can actually make the disease worse since antibiotics can remove normal intestinal bacteria that can help clear the viral infection.

Antibiotics such as fluroquinolone are useful in treating bacterial forms of gastroenteritis, and over-the-counter compounds that lessen diarrhea can also be beneficial. Making sure a person is receiving plenty of fluids is a very important part of the treatment.

A vaccine for rotaviral gastroenteritis was approved for use in 1998, however complications in some children who received the vaccine resulted in its withdrawal from the market a few years later. In 2006, two rotavirus vaccines were licensed for use by the European Medicines Agency and the U.S. Food and Drug Administration (FDA). Both are taken orally and consist of a weakened version of the virus—it is incapable of causing an infection, but stimulates the immune system to develop protective antibodies against rotavirus.

■ Impacts and Issues

The overwhelming impacts of gastroenteritis are its prevalence and the high death toll among children in under-

developed and developing countries due to the debilitating effects of diarrhea. Diarrheal diseases are the second most common cause of death each year in children aged five years or less, according to the World Health Organization (WHO), resulting in over two million child deaths. Earlier and larger death tolls have been reduced by the use of oral rehydration therapy, which is spearheaded by organizations such as UNICEF.

Despite the availability of vaccines against rotavirus, the diarrheal gastroenteritis that is caused by this virus still kills over 600,000 children each year and over two million children require hospitalization because of the severity of their infection. Overwhelmingly, the deaths are in developing countries, where the vaccines and treatment are not as readily available as in developed countries.

Beginning in 2003, a number of agencies including the WHO and the U.S. Centers for Disease Control and Prevention initiated the Rotavirus Vaccination Program, which has sought to make rotavirus vaccines more widely available. As well, beginning in 2005, the Pan American Health Organization commenced an annual campaign of immunization that includes the FDA-licensed rotavirus vaccine.

SEE ALSO *Bacterial Disease; Cholera;* Escherichia coli *O157:H7; Food-borne Disease and Food Safety; Norovirus Infection;* Salmonella *Infection (Salmonellosis); Sanitation; Shigellosis; Water-borne Disease.*

BIBLIOGRAPHY

Web Sites

Centers for Disease Control and Prevention (CDC). "Cholera." <http://www.cdc.gov/ncidod/dbmd/diseaseinfo/cholera_g.htm> (accessed May 25, 2007).

World Health Organization. "International Network to Promote Household Water Treatment and Safe Storage." <http://www.who.int/household_water/en/> (accessed May 25, 2007).

Centers for Disease Control and Prevention (CDC). "Viral Gastroenteritis." <http://www.cdc.gov/ncidod/dvrd/revb/gastro/faq.htm> (accessed May 25, 2007).

Brian Hoyle

Genetic Identification of Microorganisms

Introduction

Genetic identification of microorganisms utilizes molecular technologies to evaluate specific regions of a microbial genome and uniquely determine to which genus, species, or strain that microorganism belongs. The techniques used were adapted from the DNA fingerprinting technology originally developed for human identification, which has led some individuals to refer to the genetic identification of microorganisms as a "microbial fingerprinting." Having these technologies available has resulted in a great improvement in the ability of clinical and forensic microbiology laboratories to detect and specifically identify an organism quickly and accurately.

History and Scientific Foundations

The process of genetic identification of microorganisms is basically a comparison study. In order to identify an unknown organism, its key DNA sequences (the order of structural units, called nucleotides, that make up a strand of DNA) are compared to DNA sequences from known organisms. An exact match will occur when the DNA sequences from the two organisms are the same. Related individuals have genetic material that is identical for some regions and dissimilar for others. Unrelated individuals will have significant differences in the DNA regions being evaluated. Developing a database of key sequences that are unique to and characteristic of a series of known organisms facilitates this type of analysis.

Applications and Research

Depending on the level of specificity required, an assay can provide information on the genus, species, and/or strain of a microorganism. The most basic type of iden-

tification is classification to a genus. Although this general identification does not discriminate between the related species that comprise the genus, it can be useful in a variety of situations. For example, if a person is thought to have tuberculosis, a test to determine if *Mycobacterium* cells (the genus that includes the tuberculosis causing organism) are present in a sputum sample will most likely confirm the diagnosis. However, if there are several species within a genus that cause similar diseases but that respond to different drug therapy, it would then be critical to know exactly which species is present for proper treatment. A more specific test using genomic sequences unique to each species would be needed for this type of discrimination.

In some instances, it is important to take the analysis one step further to detect genetically distinct subspecies or strains. Variant strains usually arise as a result of physical separation and evolution of the genome. If one homogeneous sample of cells is split and sent to two different locations, over time, changes (mutations) may occur that will distinguish the two populations as unique entities. The importance of this issue can be appreciated when considering tuberculosis (TB). Since the late 1980s, there has been a resurgence of this disease accompanied by the appearance of several new strains that are resistant to the standard antibiotic treatments (known as MDR-TB or multi-drug resistant TB). The use of genetic identification for rapid determination of which strain is present has been essential to protect health care workers and provide appropriate therapy for affected individuals.

The tools used for genetic studies include standard molecular technologies. Total sequencing of an organism's genome is one approach, but this method is time consuming and expensive. Southern blot analysis was used originally, but, in most laboratories, this has now been supplanted by newer technologies such as PCR (polymerase chain reaction). Solution-phase hybridization using DNA probes has proven effective for many organisms. In this procedure, probes labeled with a

WORDS TO KNOW

ASSAY: A determination of an amount of a particular compound in a sample (e.g., to make chemical tests to determine the relative amount of a particular substance in a sample). A method used to quantify a biological compound.

CHEMILUMINESCENT SIGNAL: A chemiluminescent signal is the production of light that results from a chemical reaction. A variety of tests to detect infectious organisms or target components of the organisms rely on the binding of a chemical-containing probe to the target and the subsequent development of light following the addition of a reactive compound.

DNA FINGERPRINTING: DNA fingerprinting is the term applied to a range of techniques that are used to show similarities and dissimilarities between the DNA present in different individuals (or organisms).

DNA PROBES: Substances (agents) that bind directly to a predefined specific sequence of nucleic acids in DNA.

GENOME: All of the genetic information for a cell or organism. The complete sequence of genes within a cell or virus.

HYBRIDIZATION: A process of combining two or more different molecules or organisms to create a new molecule or organism (oftentimes called a hybrid organism).

PCR (POLYMERASE CHAIN REACTION): The Polymerase Chain Reaction, or PCR, refers to a widely used technique in molecular biology involving the amplification of specific sequences of genomic DNA.

QUANTITATED: An act of determining the quantity of something, such as the number or concentration of bacteria in an infectious disease.

REVERSE TRANSCRIPTASE: An enzyme that makes it possible for a retrovirus to produce DNA (deoxyribonucleic acid) from RNA (ribonucleic acid).

SOUTHERN BLOT ANALYSIS: Southern blot refers to an electrophoresis technique where pieces of deoxyribonucleic acid (DNA) that have resulted from enzyme digestion are separated from one another on the basis of size, followed by the transfer of the DNA fragments to a flexible membrane. The membrane can then be exposed to various probes to identify target regions of the genetic material.

reporter molecule are combined with cells in solution and upon hybridization with target cells, a chemiluminescent signal that can be quantitated by a luminometer is emitted. A variation of this scheme is to capture the target cells by hybridization to a probe followed by a second hybridization that results in precipitation of the cells for quantitation. These assays are rapid, relatively inexpensive and highly sensitive. However, they require the presence of a relatively large number of organisms to be effective. Amplification technologies such as PCR, LCR (ligase change reaction), and, for viruses with a RNA genome, RT-PCR (reverse transcriptase PCR) allow detection of very low concentrations of organisms from cultures or patient specimens such as blood or body tissues. Primers are designed to selectively amplify genomic sequences unique to each species, and, by screening unknowns for the presence or absence these regions, the unknown is identified. To speed the process up, multiplex PCR can be used to discriminate between several different species in a single amplification reaction. Going one step further, microarray technology will allow comparisons among much larger numbers of microor-

ganisms and may be more successful at identifying specimens that contain more than one species.

■ Impacts and Issues

Microorganism identification technologies were important during the investigation of the anthrax outbreak in the United States in the fall of 2001. Because an anthrax infection can mimic cold or flu symptoms, the earliest victims did not realize they were harboring a deadly bacterium. After confirmation that anthrax was the causative agent in the first death, genetic technologies were utilized to confirm the presence of anthrax in other locations and for other potential victims. Results were available more rapidly than would have been possible using standard microbiological methodology and appropriate treatment regimens could be established immediately. Furthermore, unaffected individuals were quickly informed of their status, alleviating unnecessary anxiety.

The attention then turned to identification of the source of the anthrax used in the attacks. The evidence indicated that this event was not a random, natural phenomenon, and that an individual or individuals had most likely dispersed the cells as an act of bioterrorism. In response to this threat, government agencies collected samples from all sites for analysis. A key element in the search was the genetic identification of the cells found in patients and mail from Florida, New York, and Washington, D.C. The PCR studies suggested that the samples were derived from the same strain of anthrax, known as the "Ames strain". Although this strain has been distributed to many different research laboratories around the world, careful analysis revealed minor changes in the genome that allowed investigators to narrow the search to about fifteen United States laboratories. Unfortunately, despite further extensive genetic studies of these fifteen strains and comparison to the lethal anthrax genome, a final confirmation of the source of the anthrax used in the bioterrorism attacks still eludes investigators. This is due to the overall similarity between the strains and the lack of unique characters in the strain used in the attacks that could provide a definitive identification.

BIBLIOGRAPHY

Books

Dale, Jeremy W., and Simon F. Park. *Molecular Genetics.* New York: John Wiley & Sons, 2004.

James, Jenny Lynd. *Microbial Hazard Indentification in Fresh Fruits and Vegetables.* New York: Wiley-Interscience, 2006.

Persing, David H., et al, eds. *Molecular Microbiology: Diagnostic Principles and Practice.* Seattle: Corixa Corp, 2003.

Periodicals

Jernigan, D.B., et al. "Investigation of Bioterrorism-Related Anthrax, United States, 2001: Epidemiologic Findings." *Emerging Infectious Diseases.* 8 (2002): 1019–1028.

Peplies, Jorg, Frank Oliver Glockner, and Rudolf Amann. "Optimization Strategies for DNA Microarray-Based Detection of Bacteria with 16S rRNA-Targeting Oligonucleotide Probes." *Applied and Environmental Microbiology.* 69 (2003): 1397–1407.

Read, Timothy R., et al. "Comparative Genome Sequencing for Discovery of Novel Polymorphisms in *Bacillus anthracis.*" *Science.* 296 (2002): 2028–2033.

Constance Stein

IN CONTEXT: TERRORISM AND BIOLOGICAL WARFARE

The capability for detecting and identifying microorganisms quickly and accurately is required to protect both troops on the battlefields and civilians confronted with terrorist attacks using biological agents. Because the systems currently available for sensing biological molecules rely on technologies that require several steps to identify biological weapons, the procedures are both labor and time intensive. The Defense Advanced Research Projects Agency (DARPA) initiated the Biosensor Technologies program in 2002 to develop fast, sensitive, automatic technologies for the detection and identification of biological warfare agents. The program focuses on a variety of technologies including surface receptor properties, nucleic acid sequences, identification of molecules found in the breath and mass spectrometry.

Genital Herpes

■ Introduction

Genital herpes is a common sexually transmitted disease that affects over 45 million people in the United States alone. Genital herpes is caused most often by infection with the Herpes Simplex 2 virus (HSV-2), but occasionally, the Herpes Simplex 1 (HSV-1) virus is also responsible. Often, people infected with these Herpes viruses have no symptoms, but when symptoms of genital herpes do appear, they usually involve blisters in the area of the genitals or rectum. The blisters are normally fluid-filled at first, and then break to form tender, itchy ulcers that can take up to a month to heal. Although infection with HSV-1 or HSV-2 can last a lifetime in the body, future outbreaks of genital herpes blisters usually decline in frequency and severity. Genital herpes is spread among sexual partners when the virus is released from a blister (or occasionally from intact skin) during sexual contact.

Editors note: Further information about genital herpes can be found in the articles about the specific causative agents, Herpes Simplex 2 Virus and Herpes Simplex 1 Virus.

SEE ALSO *Herpes Simplex 1 Virus; Herpes Simplex 2 Virus.*

Germ Theory of Disease

■ Introduction

The germ theory of disease states that microorganisms—organisms that, with only one known exception, are too small to be seen without the aid of a microscope—are the cause of many diseases. The microorganisms include bacteria, viruses, fungi, algae, and protozoa. The germ theory of disease also states that the microbes that cause a disease are capable of being recovered and will cause the same disease when introduced into another creature. This theory has withstood scientific scrutiny for centuries. Indeed, it is known with certainty that many diseases are caused by microorganisms. Two examples are anthrax, which is caused by the bacterium *Bacillus anthracis*, and bacterial meningitis, which is caused by *Neisseria meningitidis*.

While now an accepted part of infectious disease microbiology and the foundation of a variety of disciplines, such as hygiene and epidemiology (the study of the origin and spread of infections), the exact reasons why some microbes cause disease remain poorly understood and are still being investigated.

■ History and Scientific Foundations

Millenia ago, when microorganisms were unknown, some diseases were thought to be a consequence of divine punishment for a person's bad behavior. Illnesses that affected groups of people were sometimes attributed to the foul smelling gases from a nearby swamp or the vapors from sewage lagoon. While it is true that some microbes can become airborne and can cause disease when inhaled (anthrax is one example), this was not recognized for a long time. Other purported causes of disease included vapors created by the rotation of Earth or disturbances within Earth, which was thought to be hollow.

A publication dating back to 36 BC proposed that some illness was the result of the inhalation of tiny creatures present in the air. However, this farsighted view was the exception for centuries. With the development of the microscope in the seventeenth century by Robert Hooke (1635–1703) and Anton van Leeuwenhoek (1632–1723), it became possible to examine specimens, such as water, and to visually detect living organisms.

At that time, the prevailing view was that life and disease arose spontaneously from non-living material.

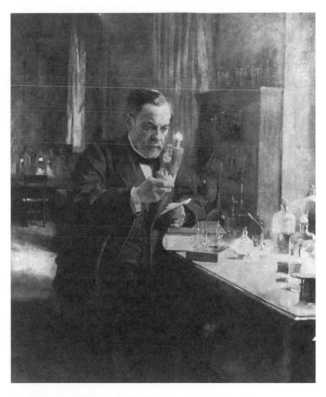

Louis Pasteur (1822–1895), the French chemist and microbiologist, developed vaccines for rabies and anthrax, among others. In addition, Pasteur is known for his work with sterilization and the pasteurization process. *Library of Congress.*

WORDS TO KNOW

ASEPSIS: Without germs, more specifically without microorganisms.

CARBOLIC ACID: An acidic compound that, when diluted with water, is used as an antiseptic and disinfectant.

COWPOX: Cowpox refers to a disease that is caused by the cowpox or catpox virus. The virus is a member of the orthopoxvirus family. Other viruses in this family include the smallpox and vaccinia viruses. Cowpox is a rare disease, and is mostly noteworthy as the basis of the formulation, over 200 years ago, of an injection by Edward Jenner that proved successful in curing smallpox.

EPIDEMIOLOGY: Epidemiology is the study of various factors that influence the occurrence, distribution, prevention, and control of disease, injury, and other health-related events in a defined human population. By the application of various analytical techniques including mathematical analysis of the data, the probable cause of an infectious outbreak can be pinpointed.

INFECTION CONTROL: Infection control refers to policies and procedures used to minimize the risk of spreading infections, especially in hospitals and health care facilities.

MICROORGANISM: Microorganisms are minute organisms. With the single yet-known exception of a bacterium that is large enough to be seen unaided, individual microorganisms are microscopic in size. To be seen, they must be magnified by an optical or electron microscope. The most common types of microorganisms are viruses, bacteria, blue-green bacteria, some algae, some fungi, yeasts, and protozoans.

PUERPERAL FEVER: Puerperal fever is a bacterial infection present in the blood (septicemia) that follows childbirth. The Latin word *puer*, meaning boy or child, is the root of this term. Puerperal fever was much more common before the advent of modern aseptic practices, but infections still occur. Louis Pasteur showed that puerperal fever is most often caused by *Streptococcus* bacteria, which is now treated with antibiotics.

SPONTANEOUS GENERATION: Also known as abiogenesis; the incorrect discarded assumption that living things can be generated from nonliving things.

VACCINATION: Vaccination is the inoculation, or use of vaccines, to prevent specific diseases within humans and animals by producing immunity to such diseases. The introduction of weakened or dead viruses or microorganisms into the body to create immunity by the production of specific antibodies.

Then, in 1668, the Italian scientist Francisco Redi (1627–1697) showed that maggots did not appear if decaying meat was kept in a sealed container, but that the maggots appeared if the meat was placed in the open air. This implied that the maggots were present in the air that contacted the meat, rather than spontaneously appearing on the meat.

Early in the eighteenth century, it was observed that people could be protected from developing smallpox by exposing them to pus from the lesions of other people with the illness. While we now recognize this as the basis of vaccination, at the time the idea—that something in the illness could protect others from the malady—was revolutionary. The English physician Edward Jenner (1749–1823) is recognized as the founder of the practice of vaccination. Jenner noticed that dairy workers who had been exposed to cowpox, a milder disease similar to smallpox, seldom contracted smallpox. He showed that injecting people with fluid from the cowpox blisters (which was subsequently shown to contain the cowpox virus, which is related to the smallpox virus) conferred protection against smallpox.

In 1848, Hungarian physician Ignaz Semmelweis (1818–1865) discovered that a disease called puerperal fever could be spread from corpses to living patients by attendants who did not wash their hands between the autopsy room and the hospital ward. Handwashing greatly reduced the number of these infections. In 1854, English physician John Snow (1813–1858) demonstrated that an ongoing cholera epidemic in London was caused by water coming from a particular pump. When the water flow from the pump was shut off, the outbreak ended.

However, even with the accumulating weight of evidence that some agent was responsible for various diseases, many physicians continued to maintain that these agents did not exist because they could not be seen with the unaided eye. If they did not exist, then they could not be the cause of disease. It remained for Agostino Bassi (1773–1856), Louis Pasteur (1822–1895), and Robert Koch (1843–1910) to perform the research necessary to finally convince the scientific community that germs did, indeed, cause disease.

In 1835, Bassi proposed the germ theory for the first time, when he hypothesized that a lethal disease of silkworms was due to a microscopic living organism. The agent was subsequently shown to be a fungus that was named *Beauveria bassiana*. Then, in a series of experiments in the middle of the nineteenth century, Pasteur convincingly demonstrated that the spoilage of wine, beer, and foods were caused by something in the air and not by the air itself.

In 1875, concrete evidence for the germ theory was provided by Robert Koch, who showed that *Bacillus anthracis* was the cause of anthrax in cattle and sheep.

Koch's step by step approach to his experiments laid the foundation for a series of conditions that must be met to demonstrate that a particular microorganism is the cause of a particular disease. The following conditions came to be known as Koch's postulates.

Koch's postulates drove the nail into the coffin of the theory of spontaneous generation. Once scientists accepted that the germ theory of disease was valid and began to search for more examples of microbial-caused diseases, the floodgates opened. By the end of the nineteenth century, it had been established that microbes were responsible for cholera, typhoid fever, diphtheria, pneumonia, tetanus, meningitis, and gonorrhea, as a few examples.

Also in the nineteenth century, English physician Joseph Lister (1827–1912) demonstrated that the development of infections in patients following surgery could be drastically reduced if a spray of carbolic acid was applied over the wound during surgery and surgical dressing put on the wound was soaked in the chemical. Since carbolic acid was known to kill microbes present in sewage, Lister helped convince people that microorganisms were important in post-operative infections.

■ Applications and Research

The germ theory is applied to infection control in hospitals, the treatment of food and water, and efforts to control the spread of infection in natural settings. Examples of the latter are the various vaccination and disease prevention programs that are spearheaded by agencies such as the World Health Organization (WHO) and the U.S. Centers for Disease Control and Prevention (CDC). Even in the present day, research continues to identify the microbes responsible for diseases, to rapidly and accurately detect their presence, and to devise strategies that will minimize or completely prevent the particular diseases.

■ Impacts and Issues

The germ theory is profoundly important in understanding and preventing a variety of diseases. Knowledge that

---

GERMAN PHYSICIAN ROBERT KOCH (1843–1910)

Robert Koch is considered to be one of the founders of the field of bacteriology. He pioneered principles and techniques in studying bacteria and discovered the specific agents that cause tuberculosis, cholera, and anthrax. For this he is also regarded as a pioneer of public health, aiding legislation and changing prevailing attitudes about hygiene to prevent the spread of various infectious diseases. For his work on tuberculosis, he was awarded the Nobel Prize in 1905.

Koch's postulates

- The particular microorganism must be present in every case of the disease.
- That microorganism must be able to be isolated from a person or other creature host with the particular disease and must be capable of being grown in a pure form free from other organisms. (This condition has since been modified, since not all organisms can be grown in the laboratory. However, with molecular techniques of organism identification that are based on the detection of certain unique sequences of genetic material, the microbe does not always need to be grown to fulfill this condition.)
- The microorganism that is recovered from the pure culture is capable of causing the disease when introduced into a previously healthy test creature.
- The microorganism can be recovered from the infected creature and can be shown to be the same as the originally recovered or detected microbe.

---

microorganisms can cause disease spawned efforts to prevent the microbes from coming into contact with people, food, water, and other materials. The practices of disinfection, sterilization, personal hygiene, and proper food preparation have their basis in germ theory.

Knowledge that many diseases are caused by microorganisms, and that the microbes can be spread from person-to-person and from an inanimate surface to a person spurred the development of techniques to minimize or prevent microbial spread. One example is asepsis—the treatment of living and non-living surfaces to kill or prevent the growth of associated microorganisms. Aseptic technique is one of the cornerstones of research microbiology and is crucially important in medicine. Up until the middle of the nineteenth century, the absence of aseptic techniques during operations made surgery a risky procedure. However, after the adoption of techniques to minimize microbial contamination of wounds and the airborne spread of microorganisms, the mortality rate following surgery plummeted. The infection control practices that are routine in hospitals today are a result of the germ theory.

Similarly, knowledge that some disease-causing bacteria, viruses, and protozoa—particularly those that normally reside in their intestinal tract—can be spread via the contamination of water by feces prompted the implementation of techniques of water treatment. Techniques of drinking water treatment that include filtration, chlorination, or exposure of the water to ozone or ultraviolet light are designed to kill potentially harmful microbes in the water.

The techniques of modern day molecular biology have an important place in germ theory. Detection and identification of microorganisms based on the presence of target sequences of genetic material is making infection control more rapid and efficient. Furthermore, the use of antibodies and other compounds to block the adherence of microbes to living and non-living surfaces is useful in minimizing the spread of infections.

The discipline of epidemiology is rooted in the germ theory. Epidemiology is essentially the germ theory in reverse. Rather than tracing the path from the source of a microbe to the disease, an epidemiologist begins with a disease and then, by various means, determines the source and geographical dissemination of that particular disease. For example, a 2006 outbreak of disease that occurred in several Midwestern states in the United States was traced to a crop of organic spinach contaminated with the bacterium *Escherichia coli* O157:H7. Epidemiology is also important in designing strategies to combat an ongoing disease outbreak and in minimizing the chances of future illnesses.

Strategies to minimize the spread of disease-causing microorganisms are often wise. However, concern with the potential for microbial safety in the home and workplace has fostered a sense of urgency that is out of proportion to the risk posed by the microbes. Supermarket shelves are lined with antibacterial products designed to keep a home almost free of microbes. While this may seem sensible, it has, in fact, spawned the development of increased resistance of some microbes to the chemicals being used to control or kill them. In addition, evidence is accumulating that the human immune system requires exposure to microorganisms to keep the system primed and capable of a rapid and efficient response. The strategy of disinfecting a house may be contributing to an increase in allergic diseases, since the immune system may over-react when confronted by a foreign substance, such as a microorganism.

SEE ALSO *Bloodborne Pathogens; Disinfection; Koch's Postulates.*

BIBLIOGRAPHY

Books

Ewald, Paul. *Plague Time: The New Germ Theory of Disease.* New York: Anchor, 2002.

Tierno, Philip M. *The Secret Life of Germs: What They Are, Why We Need Them, and How We Can Protect Ourselves Against Them.* New York: Atria, 2004.

Waller, John. *The Discovery of the Germ: Twenty Years That Transformed the Way We Think About Disease.* New York: Columbia University Press, 2003.

Brian Hoyle

Giardiasis

■ Introduction

Giardiasis (pronounced GEE-are-DYE-uh-sis) is intestinal infection with the protozoan parasite *Giardia lamblia* (also called *Giardia intestinalis* or *Giardia* (gee-ARE-dee-uh). Protozoa are single-celled animals with more complex features and behavior than bacteria, which are also single-celled organisms. Giardiasis is a waterborne disease found almost everywhere in the world. Its symptoms include diarrhea, gas, stomach cramps, fatigue, weight loss, and nausea. Giardiasis is transmitted by ingestion of cysts—extremely small, dormant, seedlike objects—that have been shed in the feces of an infected person or animal. Several drugs can be used to treat giardiasis, but healthy individuals can usually overcome the disease without treatment. The symptoms of untreated giardiasis usually last from two to six weeks.

■ Disease History, Characteristics, and Transmission

History

Giardiasis has probably been endemic since before modern humans evolved. *Giardia* were first described by the Dutch scientist Antony van Leeuwenhoek (1632–1723), who significantly improved the microscope and was the first person to observe single-celled organisms. He found *Giardia* living in his own feces. The organism was originally named *Cercomonas intestinalis* by the Czech physician Wilhelm Lambl (1814–1895) in 1859. It was renamed *Giardia lamblia* in 1915 to honor both Lambl and the French physician Alfred Giard (1846–1908), another early researcher of *Giardia*. Today, the term *Giardia intestinalis* is usually preferred by scientists.

In the twentieth century, five species of *Giardia* were identified. *Giardia intestinalis*, the species that afflicts humans, can be hosted by mammals, reptiles, and possibly birds.

Characteristics

Giardia is a protozoan flagellate, that is, a one-celled animal that propels itself using tiny, rapidly-waving hairs called flagella. It exists in two forms, the trophozoite and the cyst. A *Giardia* cyst is a microscopic, oval object about 1 to 12 µ (millionths of a meter) long and 7 to 10 µm wide. A *Giardia* infection occurs when a sufficiently large number of these cysts are ingested by an animal or human.

In the duodenum, the part of the small intestine just below the stomach, each cyst hatches and divides into

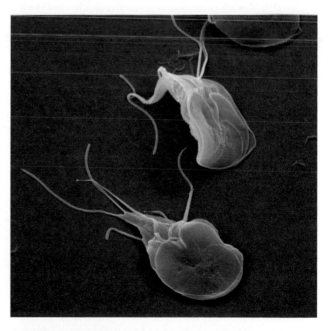

A color enhanced scanning electron micrograph (SEM) shows *Giardia lamblia*. This single-celled organism is a parasite that infects the small intestine in humans. *Oliver Meckes/Nicole Ottawa/ Photo Researchers, Inc.*

two trophic individuals or trophozoites. A *Giardia* trophozoite is shaped somewhat like a limpet with a short, pointed tail. It attaches its flat surface to the cells of the intestinal wall and feeds on them. In a few days, the trophozoites detach from the intestinal wall and divide into two identical individuals. Some are carried downstream through the digestive tract to the large intestine, where feces are formed. The harsh chemical conditions in the large intestine signal the trophozoites to become cysts. Cysts can survive for months in surface waters such as lakes and streams.

Giardia infection usually lasts two to six weeks. In some cases, however, the infection can become chronic or ongoing. Exactly how *Giardia* cause the symptoms of giardiasis is not known. Between 60% and 80% of people infected with *Giardia* have no symptoms.

Transmission

During bouts of diarrhea caused by giardiasis, both trophozoites and cysts exit the body in the feces. The trophozoites die outside the body, but the cysts may be ingested by another animal and continue the life cycle. There can be from 1,000,000 to 100,000,000 cysts per gram in stool samples that test positive for *Giardia*, but many stool samples of infected persons do not contain detectable levels of *Giardia* at all.

Cysts are almost always transmitted by the fecal-oral route—that is, by the ingestion of fecal material, generally in very small or dilute amount, through the mouth. This may occur through feces-hand-oral contact (common among children or those caring for children) or in drinking water. The drinking water route is common worldwide, but less so in developed countries. A 2001 New Zealand study found that persons who were changing diapers were four times more likely to test positive for *Giardia* than others. *Giardia* cysts may also be foodborne, that is, transmitted through contact between food and infected workers or family members.

Whether pets and animals are significant in spreading *Giardia* is debated. *Giardia* is common in pets, wild mammals, and farm animals, but there is little evidence that these are important sources of human infection, despite the association in the United States of *Giardia* with drinking open waters containing fecal matter from beavers. (The disease is sometimes called "beaver fever" in the United States.)

Scope and Distribution

Giardia is present in most surface waters of the world, at rates varying from 0.1 to over 1,000 cysts per 26 gallons (100 liters) of water. About 12% of the groundwater sources in the United States are contaminated either with *Giardia* or *Cryptosporidium*, another protozoan parasite.

Globally, about 200 million people, about 3% of the world's population, are infected with *Giardia* at any one time. Giardiasis is particularly common in children in poor countries. In industrialized countries, giardiasis is most common among children one to four years old, in adults caring for small children, and in those who have traveled recently to the developing world. It can also be contracted by people who drink untreated lake or stream water while visiting wilderness areas. However, drinking such water does not usually result in infection. The body can usually fend off infection if it has ingested only a small to moderate number of cysts.

Treatment and Prevention

The primary public-health approach to preventing giardiasis is to keep *Giardia* cysts out of drinking water supplies. This is accomplished by keeping water sources used for drinking water from *Giardia* contamination by sewage or livestock waste, and by treating drinking water before distributing it. Because *Giardia* and other protozoan cysts are resistant to chemicals such as chlorine at the levels ordinarily used to treat water, the primary means of treating water is filtering. Portable, hand-operated filters can be used by persons in wilderness areas to filter out not only *Giardia* cysts, but other parasites and bacteria. The U.S. Centers for Disease Control (CDC) recommends not drinking recreational water, untreated surface water, or untreated ice or drinking water while traveling in developing countries.

For healthy individuals, treatment for giardiasis is usually not necessary, as the body is capable of freeing itself from the infection. Where treatment is needed or desired, a number of drugs are available, including albendazole, furazolidone, metronidazole, nitazoxanide, and quinacrine.

Impacts and Issues

Infection with *Giardia intestinalis* is the most commonly reported protozoan parasite infection worldwide. In developing countries, about 20% of patients with diarrhea are positive for *Giardia* (the range is 5% to 43%). In developed regions such as the United States and Europe, about 3% of diarrhea patients have *Giardia*. Because untreated diarrhea can cause severe dehydration (loss of water and electrolytes from the body), it can be life endangering in persons with little access to medical care and with compromised immune systems, especially small children. Diarrhea causes 4% of all deaths worldwide. In 1998, for example, diarrhea killed some 2.2 million people, most of them children under the age of five. It is not known how many of these deaths are due to *Giardia* infection. Chronic *Giardia* infection may also cause failure to thrive in children due to impaired uptake of fats and vitamins A and B$_{12}$.

SEE ALSO *Cryptosporidiosis; Parasitic Diseases; Waterborne Disease.*

BIBLIOGRAPHY

Books

Erlandsen, Stanley, and Ernest Meyer. *Giardia and Giardiasis, Biology Pathogenesis, and Epidemiology.* New York: Springer, 2001.

Parker, James N., and Philip M. Parker. *The Official Patient's Sourcebook on Giardiasis.* San Diego, CA: Icon Health Publications, 2002.

Periodicals

Casemore, David P. "Foodborne Illness: Foodborne Protozoal Infection." *Lancet.* 336 (1990): 1427–1433.

Hawralek, Jason. "Giardiasis: Pathophysiology and Management." *Alternative Medicine Review.* 8.2 (2003): 129–143.

Hoque, M. Ekramul, et al. "Nappy Handling and Risk of Giardiasis." *Lancet.* 357 (2001): 1017.

Meng, Tze-Chiang, et al. "Inhibition of *Giardia lamblia* Excystation by Antibodies against Cyst Walls and by Wheat Germ Agglutinin." *Infection and Immunity.* 64 (1996): 2151–2157.

Reiner, David S., et al. "Identification and Localization of Cyst-Specific Antigens of *Giardia lamblia.*" *Infection and Immunity.* 57 (1989): 963–968.

Vogel, Gretchen. "Searching for Living Relics of the Cell's Early Days." *Science.* 277 (1997): 1604.

Web Sites

Centers for Disease Control (U.S. Government). "Parasitic Disease Information: Giardiasis." September 14, 2004 <http://www.cdc.gov/ncidod/dpd/parasites/giardiasis/> (accessed February 1, 2007).

IN CONTEXT: REAL-WORLD RISKS

The Centers for Disease Control and Prevention, National Center for Infectious Diseases, Division of Parasitic Diseases states that, "Anyone can get giardiasis. Persons more likely to become infected include:

- Children who attend day care centers, including diaper-aged children
- Child care workers
- Parents of infected children
- International travelers
- People who swallow water from contaminated sources
- Backpackers, hikers, and campers who drink unfiltered, untreated water
- Swimmers who swallow water while swimming in lakes, rivers, ponds, and streams
- People who drink from shallow wells."

"Contaminated water includes water that has not been boiled, filtered, or disinfected with chemicals. Several community-wide outbreaks of giardiasis have been linked to drinking municipal water or recreational water contaminated with Giardia."

SOURCE: *Centers for Disease Control and Prevention (CDC)*

GIDEON

■ Introduction

The Global Infectious Diseases and Epidemiology Online Network (GIDEON) is a web-based software system designed for use in geographic medicine, a branch of medicine that deals with international public health issues including infectious and tropical disease. GIDEON is located at <www.gideononline.com>, and helps physicians to diagnose any recognized infectious disease occurring in the world.

The first module of GIDEON generates a ranked list of potential diagnoses based on signs, symptoms, laboratory tests, country of acquisition, incubation period, exposure (foods, animals, insects) and other relevant details. This list is not intended to replace the expertise of health care workers, but rather, present a comprehensive group of diseases which can focus further analysis of the case, suggest additional diagnostic tests, and offer in-depth analysis of each individual disease. At this point, the user can "ask" GIDEON why additional diseases are not listed, display information on the country-specific status of each disease listed, or access links to specific therapy and diagnostic options.

Additional options allow for generation of a list of diseases compatible with bioterrorism, and simulation of disease scenarios not associated with a specific patient. For example, the user might access a list of all infectious diseases associated with diarrhea or diseases associated with diarrhea in the United States, and then limit the listing to agents of diarrhea associated with water, or diarrhea which might develop in the United States within 24 hours of ingesting water.

The second GIDEON module presents the epidemiology of individual diseases, including descriptive text (infective agent, route of infection, incubation period, diagnostic tests, therapy, vaccines), a global and historical overview of the disease, and its status in every country and region. Country notes include specific regions of activity within each country, local foods, insects, etc. involved in transmission, reported incidence and rates (cases per 100,000 population per year) and a chronology of regional outbreaks. The vaccination standards for every relevant disease in every country are also listed. As of February 2007, the epidemiology module contains three million words of text and 30,000 references in 16,000 text notes. Reference numbers are electronically linked to available abstracts and titles in the medical literature. Over 22,000 graphs and 342 maps are automatically generated to follow the status of all diseases, both worldwide and in each specific country. Five thousand images include life-cycle charts, photomicrographs, x-rays, skin lesions, and the like. More than 5,700 outbreaks and 11,000 surveys are listed; for example, all outbreaks of measles reported in scientific literature, prevalence studies of hookworm, AIDS and liver fluke in African countries; and studies for food contamination in all European countries.

The third module follows the pharmacology and usage of all anti-infective drugs and vaccines. Drugs of choice, contraindications, doses for special patient groups, and interaction with other drugs, are presented in great detail. An index of all drug trade names (over 10,000) reflects the international nature of the program. The user may access a list of drugs for a specific indication, such as AIDS or tuberculosis; or antibiotics associated with a specified form or toxicity or drug interaction.

The vaccines module presents similar information regarding all vaccines, including lesser-known preparations used to prevent diseases such as Kyasanur Forest disease and Argentine hemorrhagic fever. Dosage schedules, boosters, side effects, and trade names are accessed through interactive menus.

The fourth module is designed to identify, compare, and characterize all species of bacteria, mycobacteria (tuberculosislike organisms) and yeasts. Technical material used in evaluating susceptibility standards of bacteria to anti-infective agents is also available.

All text, maps, images, and graphs are designed for transfer to PowerPoint®, word processors, or e-mail for preparation of publications, syllabi, student handouts, and other formats. A built-in network option allows for installation on any computer network. The network manager can add custom notes in their own language to the program regarding any disease, drug, or pathogen (disease-causing agent) relevant to his own institution. A text box allows the user to append custom notes in their own font and language to the GIDEON text, including, for example, contact information, submission of specimens, pricing, or ongoing outbreaks.

■ Impacts and Issues

As of 2007, 342 generic infectious diseases are distributed haphazardly through 230 countries and regions, and are challenged by 350 drugs and vaccines. An average of two new infectious diseases are described in humans every three years. 2,500 pathogenic bacteria, viruses, parasites and fungi have been reported, and a new species is discovered almost every week. Books and journals are inadequate for disseminating information immediately when dealing with ongoing outbreaks, epidemics, and breakthroughs in diagnosis and treatment.

As GIDEON is a web-based program, the server could easily be adopted to follow all diseases analyzed by users. This form of "syndromic surveillance" is an example of bioinformatics (using computers as tools to manage data and solve problems in the biological sciences) that can be useful to health departments or other agencies worldwide for rapid identification of disease outbreaks or unusual disease patterns in the community.

SEE ALSO *Globalization and Infectious Disease; Notifiable Diseases; ProMED; Public Health and Infectious Disease; Travel and Infectious Disease.*

BIBLIOGRAPHY

Periodicals

Felitti, Vincent J. "GIDEON: Global Infectious Diseases and Epidemiology Online Network." *JAMA.* 293 (2005): 1674–1675.

Web Sites

GIDEON. "GIDEON Content-Outbreaks." <http://www.gideononline.com/content/outbreaks.htm> (accessed May 1, 2007).

Stephen A. Berger

WORDS TO KNOW

BIOINFORMATICS: Bioinformatics, or computational biology, refers to the development of new database methods to store genomic information (information related to genes and the genetic sequence), computational software programs, and methods to extract, process, and evaluate this information. Bioinformatics also refers to the refinement of existing techniques to acquire the genomic data. Finding genes and determining their function, predicting the structure of proteins and sequence of ribonucleic acid (RNA) from the available sequence of deoxyribonucleic acid (DNA), and determining the evolutionary relationship of proteins and DNA sequences are aspects of bioinformatics.

GEOGRAPHIC MEDICINE: Geographic medicine, also called geomedicine, is the study of how human health is affected by climate and environment.

INCUBATION PERIOD: Incubation period refers to the time between exposure to disease causing virus or bacteria and the appearance of symptoms of the infection. Depending on the microorganism, the incubation time can range from a few hours (an example is food poisoning due to *Salmonella*) to a decade or more (an example is acquired immunodeficiency syndrome, or AIDS).

INCIDENCE: The number of new cases of a disease or injury that occur in a population during a specified period of time.

OUTBREAK: The appearance of new cases of a disease in numbers greater than the established incidence rate, or the appearance of even one case of an emergent or rare disease in an area.

PATHOGEN: A disease causing agent, such as a bacteria, virus, fungus, etc.

IN CONTEXT: GIDEON

The *Journal of the American Medical Association* (JAMA) calls GIDEON ".an intellectual tour de force for helping physicians quickly and successfully respond to the diagnostic and therapeutic problems of seeing patients with infectious illnesses that either are intrinsically complex or may have originated in unfamiliar, foreign settings/"

SOURCE: *Vincent J. Felitti, MD, Reviewer for JAMA, 2005*

Glanders (Melioidosis)

■ Introduction

Glanders and melioidosis (also called pseudoglanders) are related infectious diseases caused by bacterial species in the *Burkholderia* genus. Both diseases produce similar symptoms and are diagnosed, treated, and prevented similarly. However, glanders and melioidosis differ with respect to where they originate and how they spread.

Glanders primarily infects horses, but can also infect donkeys, mules, cats, dogs, sheep, and goats. Such infected animals pass the infection on to humans either directly or indirectly. Melioidosis is found in contaminated water and soil. It spreads to humans and animals (the same ones as with glanders) by contact with such contaminated sources.

Glanders is caused by the bacterium *Burkholderia mallei*. The bacterium is found only in infected host animals and is not found in plants, soil, or water. Melioidosis is caused by the bacterium *Burkholderia pseudomallei*. Most animals that contract melioidosis do so by ingestion of contaminated food, soil, or water. Humans become infected with both glanders and melioidosis through openings in the skin, mucosal surfaces, and by inhalation.

■ Disease History, Characteristics, and Transmission

Glanders is transmitted by direct contact with infected animals, and the bacteria enter the human body through breaks in the skin or through the mucosal surfaces of the eyes and nose. Melioidosis is transmitted by direct contact with contaminated soil and surface waters, and the bacteria are thought in enter the body through breaks in the skin, inhalation of contaminated soil, and ingestion of contaminated water. Person-to-person transmission of both glanders and melioidosis also have been documented. Symptoms depend on the amount of bacteria in the human system. A few bacteria inside the body rarely cause any symptoms, however, more symptoms appear when more organisms are present.

In glanders infection, symptoms appear in about one to five days, while melioidosis symptoms may not develop for years. When symptoms occur, their characteristics depend on the mode of transmission (skin or mucosal surfaces) into the body and the form of the infection (acute or chronic).

An acute localized infection with glanders results in swollen lymph glands, fever, sweats, muscle pains, and

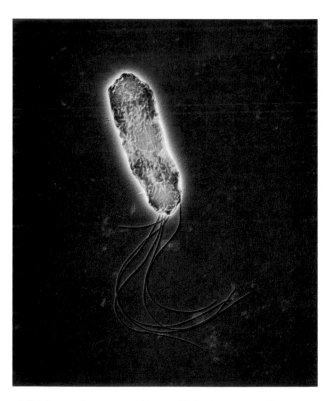

Melioidosis, a disease caused by *Burkholderia pseudomallei*, is considered to be a potential agent of biological warfare and biological terrorism. *Eye of Science/Photo Researchers, Inc.*

coughing. Other symptoms include eye tearing, light sensitivity, and diarrhea. Entrance into the body through the eyes, nose, and respiratory tract causes excessive and sometimes infectious mucus. The infection may also enter the bloodstream. This more serious bacterial infection in the bloodstream is called septicemia. Septicemia caused by *B. mallei* will usually cause death within seven to ten days.

An acute localized infection with melioidosis causes respiratory problems, headache, diarrhea, fever, pus-filled skin lesions, muscle soreness, and confusion. Usually the infection is resolved in a short period of time. However, people with unrelated serious illnesses such as renal failure, diabetes, and HIV (human immunodeficiency virus) infection can go into septic shock, resulting in multiple organ collapse and death.

Acute pulmonary infections in both glanders and melioidosis can cause symptoms ranging from mild bronchitis to severe pneumonia. Symptoms include fever, headache, anorexia, pulmonary abscesses, and muscle soreness.

Chronic infections of both diseases cause multiple abscesses within the arm and leg muscles or in the spleen or liver. For glanders, nasal and subcutaneous nodules (small lumps) form, followed with ulceration. Death can follow within a few months. Symptoms of chronic melioidosis are often similar to tuberculosis. Lung or spleen abscesses often cause abdominal pain and fever, while brain abscesses often cause neurological problems. Melioidosis infection also may travel into the bones, brain, lungs, and joints. It usually causes death when it infects the bloodstream, but is non-fatal in other areas. However, the severity of the infection and the timeliness of treatment is critical in the prognosis.

Scope and Distribution

Both diseases are rare in the United States. According to the Division of Bacterial and Mycotic Diseases (DBMD), of the U.S. Centers for Disease Control and Prevention (CDC), glanders has not appeared in the United States since 1945, and there are between zero to five cases of melioidosis annually, most often in travelers and immigrants.

Glanders is frequently found in Africa, Asia, Central and South America, and the Middle East. The disease has been controlled in North America, Australia, and most of Europe. Melioidosis is commonly found in parts of Southeast Asia (especially Thailand, Singapore, Malaysia, Myanmar, and Vietnam) and northern Australia. It is also occasionally found in Brunei, China, Hong Kong, India, Laos, Taiwan, and several countries in Africa, Central and South America, the Middle East, and the South Pacific.

WORDS TO KNOW

ABSCESS: An abscess is a pus-filled sore, usually caused by a bacterial infection. It results from the body's defensive reaction to foreign material. Abscesses are often found in the soft tissue under the skin, such as the armpit or the groin. However, they may develop in any organ, and they are commonly found in the breast and gums. Abscesses are far more serious and call for more specific treatment if they are located in deep organs such as the lung, liver, or brain.

ACUTE: An acute infection is one of rapid onset and of short duration, which either resolves or becomes chronic.

MORTALITY: Mortality is the condition of being susceptible to death. The term "mortality" comes from the Latin word *mors*, which means "death." Mortality can also refer to the rate of deaths caused by an illness or injury, i.e., "Rabies has a high mortality."

NODULE: A nodule is a small, roundish lump on the surface of the skin or of an internal organ.

Treatment and Prevention

Diagnosis of glanders and melioidosis is made with cultures of blood, sputum, or urine. A pus culture from an abscess also is used with melioidosis. Detecting and measuring the number of bacterial antibodies is another means to diagnosis.

Treatment for acute glanders is limited. According to the DBMD, the antibiotic sulfadiazine has been found to be effective. Other antibiotics used include amoxicillin-clavulanic, azlocillin, aztreonam, ceftazidime, ceftriaxone, doxycycline, imipenem, penicillin, and ticarcillin-vulanic acid. Statistics for glanders are difficult to obtain, but medical professionals contend that a large percentage of people infected still die when antibiotics are not given. The best way to prevent glanders is to eliminate the infection in animals.

Treatment of acute melioidosis includes intravenous cephalosporin antibiotics, often ceftazidime. According to the CDC, other antibiotics used include amoxicillin-clavulanate, meropenem, and imipenem. Antibiotics are given for 10–14 days. After the initial course of antibiotics is completed, the antibiotic pair co-trimoxazole and doxycycline is prescribed for 12–20 weeks to prevent another occurrence.

Before the use of antibiotics, acute melioidosis had a death rate of about 90%. Today, antibiotics have reduced the percentage to about 10% for simple cases that are early treated. However, untreated and severe cases still have a mortality rate of about 80%. Repeat occurrences of melioidosis happen about 10–20% of the time. In countries where melioidosis is prevalent, contact with soil, mud, flood waters, and surface waters should be avoided to prevent infection.

Medical researchers are still trying to develop a vaccine for both glanders and melioidosis.

■ Impacts and Issues

According to the DBMD, both glanders and melioidosis are considered potential biological weapons in warfare and terrorism due to the high incidence of death in infected humans. In the past, both have been studied intensively by the United States, the U.S.S.R. (now Russia), and other countries for use as military weapons. In addition, only a small number of the organisms need to be used to develop an effective biological warfare weapon. In wartime, enemy soldiers, civilians, and animals have been deliberately infected with them.

Glanders and melioidosis are also classified by the CDC in the Category B disease/agent grouping, the second highest grouping assigned to dangerous biological organisms.

Glanders is a major concern for the safety and health of people who regularly work around experimental or domestic animals. Therefore, people with high risk of glanders infection include those who are in close and frequent contact with infected animals such as animal caretakers, laboratory personnel, and veterinarians.

Melioidosis may remain dormant for many years before producing symptoms. Thus, it can be contracted without any visible signs of infection. As a result, travel to countries where melioidosis frequently occurs is considered risky. People with a higher than normal incidence of melioidosis infection include those engaging in frequent sexual activity with multiple partners and intravenous drug users.

SEE ALSO *Bacterial Disease; Emerging Infectious Diseases; Tropical Infectious Diseases; World Health Organization (WHO).*

BIBLIOGRAPHY

Books

Bannister, Barbara A. *Infection: Microbiology and Management.* Malden, MA: Blackwell Publishing, 2006.

Periodicals

Cheng, Allen C., and Bart J. Currie. "Melioidosis: Epidemiology, Pathophysiology, and Management." *Clinical Microbiology Reviews* 18 (April 2005): 383–416. Also available online at: <http://cmr.asm.org/cgi/content/full/18/2/383>.

Raja, N.S., M.Z. Ahmed, and N.N. Singh. "Melioidosis: An Emerging Infectious Disease." *Journal of Postgraduate Medicine* 51 (2005): 140–145. Also available online at: <http://www.jpgmonline.com/article.asp?issn=0022-3859;year=2005;volume=51;issue=2;spage=140;epage=145;aulast=Raja>.

Web Sites

Centers for Disease Control and Prevention. "Glanders." October 11, 2005. <http://www.cdc.gov/ncidod/dbmd/diseaseinfo/glanders_g.htm> (accessed April 26, 2007).

Centers for Disease Control and Prevention. "Melioidosis." October 12, 2005. <http://www.cdc.gov/ncidod/dbmd/diseaseinfo/melioidosis_g.htm> (accessed April 26, 2007).

Virginia Bioinformatics Institute, Virginia Tech. "*Burkholderia mallei.*" May 15, 2004. <http://pathport.vbi.vt.edu/pathinfo/pathogens/Burkholderia_mallei.html> (accessed April 26, 2007).

Globalization and Infectious Disease

■ Introduction

The rise of globalization has contributed significantly to the spread of infectious disease. As the AIDS epidemic has illustrated, a disease that emerges or re-emerges anywhere in the world can now move rapidly around the globe. With the increased ease of air travel and the growth of international trade, infectious diseases have more opportunities to spread than in previous eras. Dangerous microbes (pathogens) can arrive in people, in insects, in exotic animals, or in shipments of fruits, meats, or vegetables.

With globalization, diseases no longer have borders. Nations and international health organizations must now work together to prevent and control the spread of infectious diseases.

■ Disease History, Characteristics, and Transmission

Trade and travel can transmit infectious diseases. More than 760 million people travel internationally each year, according to the World Tourism Organization. It takes less than 36 hours to travel to almost any destination on the globe—far shorter than the usual incubation periods for most infectious diseases. A person can become infected in Sierra Leone, travel through Europe, and die in the United States within the space of a few days, as the American traveler Joseph Ghoson demonstrated in 2004.

Lassa fever, a zoonotic or animal-borne disease, can also be spread through person-to-person contact. Transmission occurs when a person comes into contact with blood, tissue, secretions, or excretions of an infected individual. In epidemics of Lassa fever, as many as 50% of infected individuals may die. When Lassa fever was confirmed as Joseph Ghoson's cause of death, the Centers for Disease Control (CDC) rushed to compile a list of 188 people known to have had contact with him while he was infectious. They included five family members; 139 health-care workers at the hospital where he died; 16 employees of commercial laboratories in Virginia and California, where Ghoson's blood samples were tested; and 19 people on the London, England, to Newark, New Jersey, flight that he took home. If infected, these individuals could spread Lassa fever.

The CDC could not locate every person who had contact with Ghoson in part because of reporting problems. The CDC does not have electronic access to airline records and or flight manifests without special arrangement. Accordingly, investigators from the CDC's Global Migration and Quarantine unit had to fly to Newark and sift through paper documents to identify Ghoson's fellow travelers. There was no way to identify other people who may have come into contact with Ghoson on his trek back from Africa.

■ Scope and Distribution

The exact scope of infectious diseases spread through globalization is unknown. Many cases probably go unreported each year because surveillance is passive. Physicians must recognize a disease, inquire about the patient's travel history, obtain proper diagnostic samples, and report the case. A physician who does not expect to see an illness that is rare or unknown in his country could misidentify the disease.

Additionally, inspections of cargo are declining even as imports, legal and illegal, increase. Monkeypox is a zoonotic, or animal-borne, disease that first appeared in the United States when contaminated African rodents that had been imported into the country were housed next to prairie dogs. The virus passed from the prairie dogs to humans in 2003 after the animals were sold as pets. Tens of thousands of exotic animals are smuggled into the United States each year as part of a global black market. Meanwhile, the globalization of food production has created a boom in food import and export

WORDS TO KNOW

EMERGING INFECTIOUS DISEASE: New infectious diseases such as SARS and West Nile virus, as well as previously known diseases such as malaria, tuberculosis, and bacterial pneumonias that are appearing in forms that are resistant to drug treatments, are termed emerging infectious diseases.

PATHOGEN: A disease causing agent, such as a bacteria, virus, fungus, etc.

VECTOR: Any agent, living or otherwise, that carries and transmits parasites and diseases. Also, an organism or chemical used to transport a gene into a new host cell.

ZOONOSES: Zoonoses are diseases of microbiological origin that can be transmitted from animals to people. The causes of the diseases can be bacteria, viruses, parasites, and fungi.

without an accompanying rise in inspectors. However, an infected insect or small animal in a corner of a large crate might elude even the most eagle-eyed official.

■ Treatment and Prevention

The CDC has revised its infectious disease priorities in response to globalization. International outbreak assistance is now a top priority. CDC plans to strengthen its diagnostic facilities and enhance its capacity for epidemiological investigations overseas. The CDC expects to offer follow-up assistance after infectious disease outbreaks as part of an effort to control new pathogens. It has also increased research on diseases that are uncommon in the United States. The CDC launched the International Emerging Infections Program, targeting disease sources in developing countries and working with international health organizations to prevent the spread of disease through travel, migration, and trade. It is also coordinating disease control and eradication efforts to stop the spread of malaria and tuberculosis.

The CDC is also attempting to strengthen preventive procedures at home. Prompted in part by the SARS epidemic of 2003 and the Ghoson incident, the CDC has asked Congress to toughen laws on disease reporting, increase the number of inspectors and quarantine stations, and require common carriers such as airlines and ships to maintain list of passengers for longer periods of time.

The CDC is also promoting the expansion of regional disease surveillance networks into a global network that could provide early warning of infectious diseases. With this strategy, the CDC works closely as a technical consultant with the World Health Organization (WHO). Like the CDC, WHO is charged with addressing health threats in the changing global landscape and it has focused on creating new strategies to coordinate response efforts.

■ Impacts and Issues

Coordination is the major issue that faces government agencies as they attempt to protect the public health. The CDC's Geographic Medicine and Health Promotion Branch has warned that there is inadequate national surveillance for zoonotic diseases. Human diseases are handled by the CDC, while animal diseases are addressed by the Department of Agriculture. Monkeypox is just one example of a zoonotic disease that has infected humans. Avian influenza, also known as H5N1, or bird flu, is a zoonotic disease that has the potential to cause enormous disruptions around the world. In 2005, World Bank economists forecast that a H5N1 pandemic could cost the global economy about 2% of the annual gross domestic product.

Vaccines offer a promising means of stopping infectious disease. Under the long-established WHO system, countries send influenza specimens to the agency, which then makes these samples available to the global community for public health purposes, including vaccine development. However, some developing countries have been reluctant to share viral samples for vaccine research because they want to ensure that their citizens have access to vaccines at affordable prices. Indonesia, the nation struck hardest by H5N1, announced in 2007 that it would not send human bird flu virus samples to WHO unless the agency could guarantee the specimens would not be used commercially. Indonesia and WHO subsequently came to an agreement that Indonesia would continue to send samples while WHO will stockpile vaccines in the event of an epidemic. A long-term WHO goal is that developing countries obtain enough technology and scientific training to produce vaccines.

Globalization also has positive effects for combating disease. Pharmaceutical companies have reached agreements with several nations and international health organizations to provide drugs and vaccines for some epidemic diseases at reduced cost. Increasing international attention on neglected diseases has garnered support for research and development of drugs and vaccines to fight illnesses rare in industrialized nations, are but endemic in under-developed nations. International agencies are better able to communicate vaccine and drug needs. Finally, an increasing amount of companies are producing vaccines and manufacturing therapeutic drugs in growing number of nations—India is poised to become one of the world's major suppliers of pharmaceuticals in the next several decades.

Increase in worldwide trade has posed unique challenges for disease prevention. In 1986, CDC investigators began an investigation of rising numbers of certain Asian mosquitoes in the United States. The invasive species served as vectors (transmitters) of disease, causing illnesses such as West Nile and dengue (DEN-gay) fever. Both illnesses were extremely rare in the United States, typically occurring only in people who traveled abroad. The CDC researchers discovered that ports of entry in California, Florida, New York, and Texas all had sizable populations of daytime biting mosquitoes native to Asia. Cargo ships were identified as the means of transport—especially those ships carrying large box containers or old tires.

To combat invasive species and vectors of disease, there are now more stringent laws governing inspection, decontamination, and quarantine of imported cargo. However, several invasive species have managed to establish sizable populations across the United States. The *Aedes albopictus* mosquito, associated with dengue virus found in varying numbers from Hawaii throughout the southeastern United States. Researchers tracked a sharp increase in the presence of day-biting mosquitoes to shipments of bamboo plants to California plant nurseries. Immediate control measures such as insecticide application and quarantine and decontamination of other shipments prevented the mosquitoes from establishing large local populations. Health officials warned nursery workers to use insect repellant and wear covering clothing to minimize the risk of bites. No cases of illness were linked to the event. Preventative measures have worked to combat similar cases of invasive mosquito species in 2004 and 2006.

■ Primary Source Connection

Airline travel can provide a vehicle for spreading infectious diseases. In June 2007, the first federal isolation order in the United States in over forty years was issued to traveler Andrew Speaker from Atlanta, Georgia, when he returned to the United States after boarding planes in Georgia, Italy, and France while he was infected with a highly resistant strain of tuberculosis. Although no active tuberculosis infections among Speaker's fellow travelers have been found, another case of air travel in 2003 by an infected person did result in spreading the newly-emerging disease known as SARS. In the following *New York Times* article, journalist Kieth Bradshear relates how SARS spread from one infected man to fellow passengers on a flight from Hong Kong to Beijing in 2003. Bradshear has been the Hong Kong Bureau Chief for the *New York Times* since 2001.

HONG KONG, April 10—Health officials announced here tonight that a man infected with a new respiratory disease had flown from Hong Kong to Munich, Barcelona, Frankfurt, London, Munich again, Frankfurt again and then back to Hong Kong before entering a hospital.

The Hong Kong Department of Health appealed for passengers and air crews from all seven flights to consult medical professionals. A health department spokeswoman said it was not yet known whether the man, who is 48, had infected anyone else on the flights with the disease—severe acute respiratory syndrome, or SARS.

All the flights were on Lufthansa. The airline said in a statement tonight that it had disinfected all the planes and was contacting the air crews and passengers. It said the chances of anyone's having become infected during the flights were "very remote."

Airlines have been saying that the filters aboard modern planes do a good job of removing viruses from the air. But according to the health department here, at least 13 people have fallen ill with SARS so far after they shared a flight from Hong Kong to Beijing last month with an elderly man who had been infected with the disease while visiting his brother in a hospital here.

Tonight's appeal for the Lufthansa crews and passengers to come forward follows nearly a dozen such calls by health officials and by airlines operating flights in and out of Hong Kong. Travelers have continued to board planes while feeling ill despite strenuous warnings from the World Health Organization and national health agencies that they not do so.

In the case that was announced tonight, the man flew on Lufthansa Flight 731 on March 30 from Hong Kong to Munich, and traveled the next day on Flight 4316 to Barcelona, according to an itinerary that was released here by the health department. He developed symptoms while in Barcelona.

The man then traveled on Flight 4303 to Frankfurt on April 2 and on to London the same day on Flight 4520. He went to Munich the next day on Flight 4671, then headed for Frankfurt on April 4 on Flight 265. He connected with Flight 738 the same day back to Hong Kong, arriving on April 5.

The man checked into a hospital here on April 8 and was confirmed today to have SARS.

Doctors do not yet know how infectious, if at all, people are in the early stages of SARS. Increasingly, doctors suspect that some people may be able to transmit the disease before the symptoms become evident. But Hong Kong's health secretary, Dr. Yeoh Eng-kiong, warned tonight that doctors here had become infected from people who had not yet shown the full symptoms identified by the World Health Organization.

Dr. Yeoh suggested that even someone with just diarrhea could be infectious.

The sick man's nationality was a mystery tonight. The health department's statement did not specify it, while the airline's statement described the man as "Chinese." A Lufthansa official said the company had been told by the health department only that the man was Chinese. The department spokeswoman, in turn, said that the man seemed to be of Chinese descent but that the agency had been unable to determine his nationality.

"He travels a lot," the spokeswoman said. "We don't know his passport."

Hong Kong, which is a special administrative region of China, still issues separate passports from mainland China, a legacy of its days as a British crown colony. Officials here sometimes refer to people as Chinese if they are from Taiwan, which Beijing regards as a renegade province, or if they are people of any nationality who happen to be of Chinese descent.

The infected man's travels could not come at a worse time for Hong Kong, as countries have begun limiting the entry of people traveling from here or imposing quarantines on them.

Malaysia stopped issuing visas today to practically all holders of passports from Hong Kong and mainland China. Cathay Pacific Airways, Hong Kong's main airline, said tonight that it had suspended all flights to Kuala Lumpur, the Malaysian capital, because there were few passengers.

Regina Ip, Hong Kong's security secretary, met with Malaysia's consul general here to protest the decision. "There is no reason why the mobility of Hong Kong residents who do not have any close contact with infected persons should be restricted," she said afterward.

Singapore also imposed a 10-day quarantine on all foreign workers earning less than $24,000 a year who have recently been in a SARS-affected country or territory. Employers must pay costs of the quarantine. Singapore has been trying for years to lure high-income employees in financial services and other lucrative industries, while making it harder for lower-income workers to go there and do jobs that less-educated Singaporeans might otherwise do.

Hong Kong's economy depends heavily on its role as Asia's transportation hub, the place from which businesses can control and coordinate factories and other businesses spread across the continent. Hong Kong has the world's busiest container port for sea freight, the world's busiest airport for international cargo shipments

and what was, until recently, Asia's busiest airport in terms of international air passenger departures.

But the availability of flights here is withering as many governments have warned citizens not to visit and many businesses have ordered their employees not to travel here.

Cathay Pacific has canceled a quarter of its daily flights here. Dragonair, an affiliated carrier that dominates the skies between Hong Kong and cities in mainland China, has stopped operating almost half its flights. Continental Airlines canceled its daily nonstop flight from Hong Kong to New York this week for lack of passengers.

The airport authority here said that a third of all flights originally scheduled to operate today had been canceled for various reasons.

Health officials have said that the virus causing SARS can probably survive no more than several hours outside the body, so that air and sea cargo shipments from Hong Kong, as well as mail, do not pose a risk to recipients.

Keith Bradhsear

BRADSHER, KEITH. "CARRIER OF SARS MADE SEVEN FLIGHTS BEFORE TREATMENT." *NEW YORK TIMES* (APRIL 10, 2003).

SEE ALSO *Developing Nations and Drug Delivery; Emerging Infectious Diseases; Re-emerging Infectious Diseases; World Trade and Infectious Disease.*

BIBLIOGRAPHY

Books

Centers for Disease Control and Prevention. *Protecting the Nation's Health in an Era of Globalization.* Atlanta: Office of Health Communication, National Center for Infectious Disease, Centers for Disease Control and Prevention, 2002.

Wamala, Sarah P., and Ichiro Kawachi. *Globalization and Health.* New York: Oxford University Press, 2006.

Web Sites

Centers for Disease Control and Prevention. "Lassa Fever." December 3, 2004 <http://www.cdc.gov/ncidod/dvrd/spb/mnpages/dispages/lassaf.htm> (accessed May 17, 2007).

Caryn E.Neumann

Gonorrhea

■ Introduction

Gonorrhea is one of the most common sexually transmitted diseases. It is caused by the bacterium *Neisseria gonorrhoeae* which infects parts of the reproductive tract such as the cervix, uterus, and Fallopian tubes in women and the urethra in both men and women.

    N. gonorrhoeae, sometimes known as gonococcus, is one of two pathogenic species in the *Neisseria* genus. The other, *N. meningitides*, is a leading cause of acute bacterial meningitis, an inflammation of the membranes covering the brain and spinal cord. Gonorrhea is curable and treatment is important as the disease can cause serious complications that may lead to both female and male infertility. Treatment must extend to the sexual partners of those who are diagnosed with the disease in order to help control its spread. Strains of gonorrhea that are resistant to antibiotics appear to be increasing in importance; for this reason, researchers need to develop new antibiotics that can carry on fighting the disease.

■ Disease History, Characteristics, and Transmission

The word gonorrhea comes from the Greek words *gono* for seed and *rhoea*, meaning flow. The disease was first described in AD 170 by the Greek physician and philosopher Galen (c.129–216). It was thought that the characteristic discharge of gonorrhea in men consisted of semen. The causative agent, *N. gonorrhoeae*, was discovered in 1879 by Albert Neisser (1855–1916) who gave the bacterium its name. This was just one of many important advances during late nineteenth and early twentieth centuries in the understanding of the causes of venereal diseases (now know as sexually transmitted diseases, or STDs). *N. gonorrhoeae* is a coccus, a round-shaped bacterium that is Gram negative (a term referring to the way it is stained for microscopic examination). The *N. gonorrhoeae* bacteria tend to associate in pairs, a feature that aids identification.

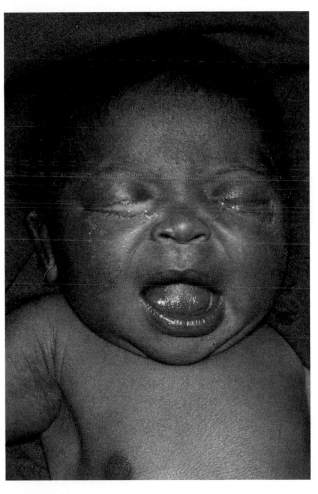

An infants's eyes ooze pus due to an infection caused by *Neisseria gonorrhoeae* bacterium. This congenital (present at birth) infection was passed from mother to baby during childbirth. *Dr. M.A. Ansary/ Photo Researchers, Inc.*

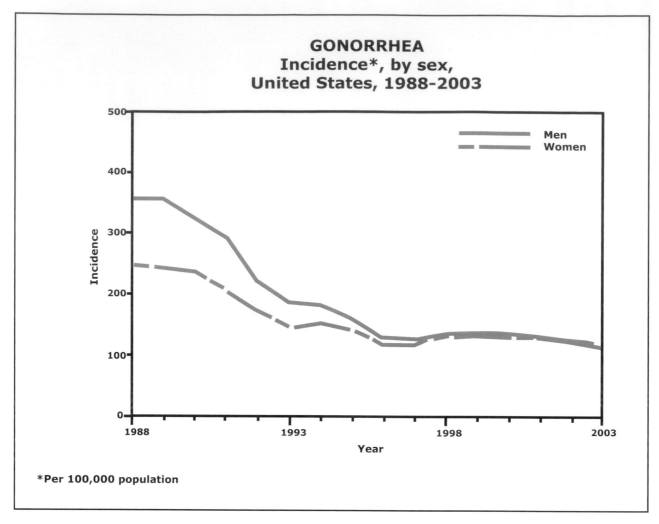

Graph showing the overall decrease in gonorrhea infections between 1988 and 2003 in both males and females in the United States. *Data courtesy of Centers for Disease Control.*

Infection with *N. gonorrhoeae* causes urethritis (inflammation of the lining of the urethra) among men and cervicitis (inflammation of the cervix) in women. The time of onset of symptoms following infection varies from one day to 30 days. In men, the first symptom of gonorrhea is usually painful urination, followed by a thick purulent (pus-containing) discharge from the ure-thra. The presence of pus makes the discharge yellow, white, or green, and it may be flecked with blood. In some cases, there is swelling in the testicles. However, many men have no symptoms. In women, painful uri-nation is also the first symptom of gonorrhea—this may be followed by a vaginal discharge and possible bleeding. Sometimes the symptoms in women are so minor that they are mistaken for a vaginal or urinary infection. Most women with gonorrhea have no symptoms at all.

Untreated, gonorrhea tends to resolve after several weeks. However, during this time complications may set

in and the person remains infectious. In men, the epidi-dymis (the coiled tube leading sperm from the testicles) may become inflamed, which can lead to infertility. Gon-orrhea in women can lead to salpingitis, which is inflam-mation of the Fallopian tubes. It is also a leading cause of pelvic inflammatory disease (PID), which affects around one million women a year in the United States. Symp-toms of PID can include severe abdominal pain and fever, and the condition may lead to the development of pus-filled abscesses, long-lasting pelvic pain, and infertility. PID can also scar the Fallopian tubes, increasing the risk of ectopic pregnancy. (An ectopic pregnancy occurs when a fertilized egg starts to develop inside a Fallopian tube instead of within the uterus; it requires immediate medical attention.) In around one percent of cases, gon-orrhea spreads throughout the body and causes severe arthritis—inflammation of the joints—and skin lesions. Neonatal gonorrhea contracted during childbirth causes very severe conjunctivitis, an inflammation of the conjunctiva (the mucus membrane that lines the inner surface of the eyelid) covering the cornea, and may lead to blindness.

Gonorrhea is spread through contact with the anus, mouth, penis, or vagina—typically from various forms of unprotected sexual intercourse. Ejaculation is not necessary for infection to occur. The chance of a man contracting gonorrhea from an infected woman is 20%. The corresponding risk for a woman is 50%. A few 'core transmitters' spread the disease through having unprotected sex with many different partners. Those without symptoms are more likely to spread the disease than those who do have symptoms. As the infection affects the cervix in women, an infected woman can transmit the disease to the fetus during childbirth.

■ Scope and Distribution

After chlamydia, gonorrhea is the most common sexually-transmitted disease in the United States. In 2004, the Centers for Disease Control and Prevention (CDC) recorded 330,132 new cases and the true figure is probably nearer to 700,000 because of under-reporting. Worldwide, there are around 62 million new cases of gonorrhea every year. Teenagers, young adults, and African-Americans appear to be most at risk of gonorrhea. It is also more common within lower socio-economic groups.

■ Treatment and Prevention

Penicillin was the first treatment for gonorrhea. Many other antibiotics, including ceftriaxone and ciprofloxacin, are used, but they can only treat the primary infection, not the complications. It is important that any sexual partners of the infected person are traced and treated to stop spreading the infection. Nearly half of those infected with *N. gonorrhoeae* are infected with *C. trachomatis* as well. Antibiotic resistance can be a problem, as strains of *N. gonorrhoeae* resistant to penicillin and the fluoroquinolone antibiotics have emerged in recent years. Pregnant women should be tested for gonorrhea and treated to prevent the infection passing to their babies. Newborn's are routinely treated with silver nitrate drops or other drugs to prevent conjunctivitis and reduce the risk of blindness.

Sexual abstinence or a monogamous sexual relationship with an uninfected partner are the most effective means of preventing the spread of gonorrhea. Condoms, used correctly and consistently, can also help prevent infection. Vaccines and microbiocides against *N. gonorrhoeae* are under development.

WORDS TO KNOW

GRAM-NEGATIVE BACTERIA: All types of bacteria identified and classified as a group that does not retain crystal-violet dye during Gram's method of staining.

PURULENT: Any part of the body that contains or releases pus is said to be purulent. Pus is a fluid produced by inflamed, infected tissues and is made up of white blood cells, fragments of dead cells, and a liquid containing various proteins.

SEXUALLY TRANSMITTED DISEASE (STD): Sexually transmitted diseases (STDs) vary in their susceptibility to treatment, their signs and symptoms, and the consequences if they are left untreated. Some are caused by bacteria. These usually can be treated and cured. Others are caused by viruses and can typically be treated but not cured. More than 15 million new cases of STD are diagnosed annually in the United States.

IN CONTEXT: A TOP SECRET WEAPON AGAINST GONORRHEA

The Unites States Army made immediate use of penicillin in World War II (1941–1945). In hospitals near the front, the new therapeutic agent saved thousands of soldiers from post-battle-field wound infections, and also proved an effective agent in treating many cases of syphilis and gonorrhea among the troops. Penicillin was initially considered a war asset and war secret in the United States and Britain but by the end of 1945, commercial manufacturing plants were capable of producing enough penicillin so that physicians also could prescribe it to their civilian patients.

■ Impacts and Issues

Gonorrhea is a serious public health problem because it can inflict long-term damage upon the female—and, to a lesser extent—male reproductive systems without an individual being aware that he or she is infected. There may be no symptoms associated with either the primary infection or the complications. According to the CDC, after a two-decade decline in the number of cases of gonorrhea in the United States, reported cases began

IN CONTEXT: TRENDS AND STATISTICS

Researchers are increasingly concerned about antimicrobial resistance shown by *N. gonorrhoeae*. The problem presents an important global public health challenge in the struggle to control gonorrhea.

Gonococcal strains have been demonstrated that are resistant to fluoroquinolones, penicillins, spectinomycin, and tetracyclines. Moreover, strains that resist treatment doses of the antibiotics ciprofloxacin and ofloxacin that exceed the CDC recommended treatment doses have been discovered. According to World Health Organization (WHO) data and reports such resistant strains may be encountered in more than 40% of cases treated in some Asian countries.

SOURCE: *Centers for Disease Control and Prevention, Division of Sexually Transmitted Disease (STD)*

rising again in the 1990s. The CDC estimates that about five percent of people in the United States ages 18–35 are unknowingly infected with gonorrhea. Meanwhile, the antibiotic drugs used to control *N. gonorrhoeae* could be losing their effectiveness, as resistance spreads from Southeast Asia through Hawaii to the west coast of the United States.

Gonorrhea and HIV infection are closely related; those with both conditions are more likely to transmit HIV. People with gonorrhea who are HIV negative are also more likely to be infected with HIV than someone without gonorrhea. Without a vaccine against *N. gonorrhoeae*, prevention efforts focused on safer sex practices, regular STD testing, and routine gynecological examination remain essential to controlling the spread of gonorrhea.

SEE ALSO *Antibiotic Resistance; Bacterial Disease; Sexually Transmitted Diseases.*

BIBLIOGRAPHY

Books

Wilson, Walter R., and Merle A. Sande. *Current Diagnosis & Treatment in Infectious Diseases.* New York: McGraw Hill, 2001.

Web Sites

Centers for Disease Control and Prevention (CDC). "Gonorrhea." April 2006 <http://www.cdc.gov/std/Gonorrhea/STDFact-gonorrhea.htm> (accessed April 9, 2007).

National Institute of Allergy and Infectious Diseases. "Gonorrhea." August 2006 <http://www.niaid.nih.gov/factsheets/stdgon.htm> (accessed February 23, 2007).

Susan Aldridge

H5N1

■ Introduction

The H5N1 virus is classified as an influenza A virus. This type of virus is normally found in avian species (birds) and is both highly contagious and highly lethal to bird populations ranging from wild migrating birds to chickens on commercial poultry farms.

The influenza in humans resulting from H5N1 infection is highly lethal. High death rates are not uncommon, including cases where infection resulted in death in more than 75% of persons infected during an outbreak.

As of May 2007, H5N1 was not easily transmissible to humans. Most of the cases of human infection with H5N1 involved infections resulting from close contact with infected bird populations. Situations, for example, where people lived in proximity to infected birds (mostly poultry), handled infected birds, or had contact with H5N1-contaminated surfaces. Globally, epidemiologists (scientists who study the origin of disease) had documented only a few cases of human-to-human transmission of H5N1 and all of the documented cases involved close contact (e.g., a family member caring for an infected relative, etc).

■ History and Scientific Foundations

Genetic testing of the H5N1 flu virus shows it to be a highly mutable virus. H5N1 has been documented to infected pigs and pigs serve as a host for flu viruses that historically mutate easily into a form that can infect humans. Accordingly, the World Health Organization (WHO) has made the study and containment of H5N1 and other avian flu viruses originating in Asia its top priority. WHO officials fear a potentially devastating global pandemic if H5N1 is able to mutate into a form easier to transmit to humans or a form easier for humans to transmit to other humans.

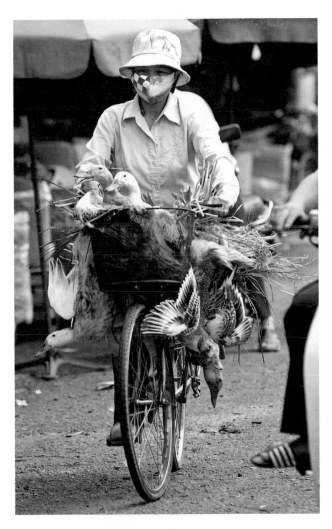

A Vietnamese woman transports ducks from a poultry market in Hanoi, Vietnam, in August 2004. The World Health Organization reported that tests in Vietnam have shown the presence of the H5N1 strain in one of three people who have died of bird flu. *AP Images.*

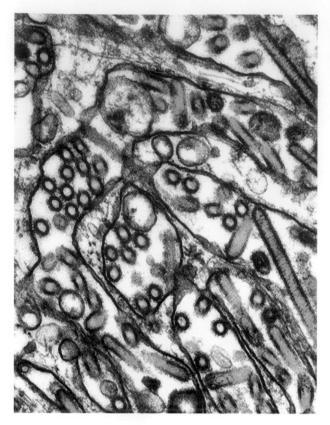

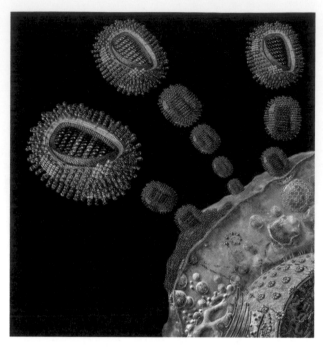

A colored transmission electron micrograph (TEM) shows influenza A virus particles (green). This is the H5N1 strain. The red cells are MDCK (Madin-Darby canine kidney) culture cells, which are used in vaccine and virus research.   *CDC/Photo Researchers, Inc.*

In this computer rendering, two subtypes of influenza virus are combining to form a new strain. The influenza belongs to the orthomyxovirus class of RNA (ribonucleic acid) viruses. Viruses use the machinery of a host cell (bottom right) to replicate their genomes. If a cell is infected with two influenza strains (purple genome and orange genome) simultaneously, the viral RNA may be mixed and repackaged to form a new strain (purple and orange genome). This could happen between a bird flu and a human strain of the virus. The resulting strain may be transmissible from human to human and spread rapidly though the population.   *Russell Kightley/Photo Researchers, Inc.*

Mechanism of action

The avian flu viruses attack human cells by first attaching themselves to the outer cell membrane with pointed probe-like hemagglutin (HA) molecules that are capable of binding to specific sites on the cell membrane.

Hemagglutinin (designated as HA) and neuraminidase (designated as NA) are glycoproteins (proteins that contain a short chain of sugar as part of its structure). Hemagglutinin and neuraminidase protrude from the outer surface of the influenza virus and neuraminidase is a constituent of the enveloping membrane that surrounds the viral contents. A typical influenza virus particle contains hundreds of molecules of hemagglutinin and neuraminidase studded across the viral surface.

Because the binding must be specific—that is, the HA molecule must be of a certain structure and configuration to bind to the membrane receptor sites—the vast majority of viruses that infect birds are not capable of binding to human cell membranes. Small and subtle changes, driven by the process of mutation, in either the protein structure or in protein configuration (the protein's shape in three dimensional space) can, however, permit binding to human cell membranes. This

allows the virus to infect the human cell, and make the jump from birds to humans.

■ Applications and Research

Researchers and health officials find optimism for containing the current outbreaks of flu in the data obtained from comparative analysis of flu strains that show the structure of the H5N1 HA molecules from the strain responsible for the recent outbreaks in China and Vietnam is actually quite different from the structure of the HA molecules associate with the 1918 flu pandemic.

However, scientists remain vigilant—and public health officials remain concerned—because the changes required to make the jump to humans also occurred in the viruses responsible for during global outbreaks of influenza in 1957 and 1968.

■ Impacts and Issues

Biologically, however, there is little that can be done to stop the virus from spreading and mutating, except to reduce its host environment. Governments of the affected countries (especially Thailand, Viet Nam, Laos, Cambodia, Republic of Korea, Indonesia, and in more than a dozen provinces, municipalities and autonomous regions on the Chinese mainland) have often ordered the wholesale slaughter of sick, potentially infected, and exposed birds as a response to Avian flu outbreaks (the disease H5N1 causes in avian populations).

Millions of chickens, for example, have been culled in order to attempt to inhibit the spread to other flocks as governments imposed prompt and sometimes severe quarantine restrictions. In other countries chickens have been given vaccines (some with questionable effectiveness) against the disease in an attempt to minimize the potentially overwhelming negative economic impacts of H5N1 on commercial bird species.

The specific H5N1 virus linked to human deaths is especially dangerous because it is resistant to both amantadine and rimantadine, two commonly used antiviral drugs used to treat influenza. Other antiviral medications, oseltamivir (Tamiflu) and zanamavir, have shown effectiveness but the full extent (or limits of effectiveness) were, as of May 2007, still subject to additional testing. Although research programs (and clinical trials) existed in several countries, as of May 2007, no vaccine against H5N1 was yet formally approved for use in humans.

SEE ALSO *Avian Influenza; Developing Nations and Drug Delivery; Emerging Infectious Diseases; Influenza; Influenza, Tracking Seasonal Influences and Virus Mutation; Influenza Pandemic of 1918; Notifiable Diseases; Pandemic Preparedness; Vaccines and Vaccine Development.*

BIBLIOGRAPHY

Periodicals

Gorman C. "The Avian Flu: How Scared Should We Be?" *Time.* (October 17, 2005): 30.

Web Sites

Centers for Disease Control and Prevention (CDC). "CDCSite Index A-Z." <http://www.cdc.gov/flu/avian/> (accessed May 21, 2007).

World Health Organization. "WHO Statistical Information System (WHOSIS)." <http://www3.who.int/whosis/menu.cfm> (accessed May 21, 2007).

World Health Organization. "WHO Weekly Epidemiologic Record (WER)." <http://www.who.int/wer/en> (accessed May 21, 2007).

Paul Davies

WORDS TO KNOW

ANTIVIRAL DRUGS: Antiviral drugs are compounds that are used to prevent or treat viral infections, via the disruption of an infectious mechanism used by the virus, or to treat the symptoms of an infection.

CELL MEMBRANE: The cell is bound by an outer membrane that, as described by a membrane model termed the fluid mosaic model, is comprised of a phospholipid lipid bilayer with proteins—molecules that also act as receptor sites—interspersed within the phospholipid bilayer. Varieties of channels exist within the membrane. In eukaryotes (cells with a true nucleus) there are a number of internal cellular membranes that can partition regions within the cells' interior. Some of these membranes ultimately become continuous with the nuclear membrane. Bacteria and viruses do not have inner membranes.

EPIDEMIOLOGIST: Epidemiologists study the various factors that influence the occurrence, distribution, prevention, and control of disease, injury, and other health-related events in a defined human population. By the application of various analytical techniques including mathematical analysis of the data, the probable cause of an infectious outbreak can be pinpointed.

HEMAGGLUTININ: Designated (HA) a glycoprotein, a protein that contains a short chain of sugar as part of its structure.

MUTABLE VIRUS: A mutable virus is one whose DNA changes rapidly so that drugs and vaccines against it may not be effective.

NEURAMINIDASE: Designated (NA) a glycoprotein, a protein that contains a short chain of sugar as part of its structure.

Haemophilus Influenzae

■ Introduction

Haemophilus influenzae is a bacterium that can cause upper respiratory disease mainly in young children. *H. influenzae* type b, or Hib for short, is a particular cause for meningitis.

H. influenzae are Gram negative—this means that their cell wall consists of two membranes that are on either side of a thin, but strong layer called the peptidoglycan. The bacteria can be shaped like ovals or can adopt different shapes, and so are described as being pleomorphic. When grown on a solid nutrient, clumps of bacteria tend to form in the vicinity of another bacterium called *Staphylococcus* when the latter are present. This behavior can be important in identifying *H. influenzae*.

While vaccination against Hib has reduced the occurrence of infections in developed countries, *H. influenzae* remains responsible for many lower respiratory infections in children in other regions of the world.

■ Disease History, Characteristics, and Transmission

H. influenzae was first described Richard Johannes Pfeiffer (1858–1945) in 1892 during an influenza epidemic. The name for the bacterium reflects an early misunderstanding that it was the cause of the flu. In 1933, scientists demonstrated that influenza was instead caused by a virus. *H. influenzae*, however, was subsequently shown to be the cause of several other diseases.

Some types (strains) of *H. influenzae* are surrounded by a sugary coat called a capsule, while other strains do not have a capsule. The strains with a capsule tend to be more of a health concern, since the capsule helps protect a bacterium from attack by a host's immune system. Nonetheless, some strains without a capsule are also pathogenic (disease-causing) and can

cause bronchitis, ear infections, and epiglottitis, an inflammation in the esophagus. Complications of epiglottis can produce a blockage of the airway that can be fatal in children under the age of five.

H. influenzae is normally found in the throat and nose of many people. The bacteria residing there are

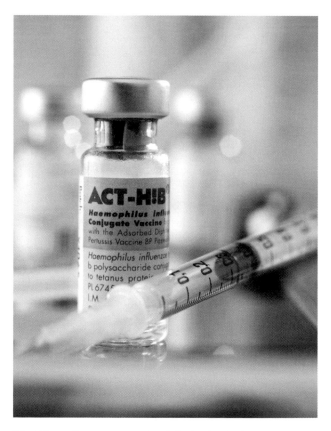

The Hib vaccine protects against infection by the bacterium *Haemophilus influenzae* type B, which can cause a range of serious illnesses in children, including meningitis and pneumonia. The vaccine is given in several doses during the first year of a baby's life. *Tek Image/Photo Researchers, Inc.*

usually harmless. But, if the bacteria spreads to other areas of the body or if a person's immune system is compromised, the bacteria can cause infection. Thus, *H. influenzae* represents an opportunistic pathogen.

Only humans are known to be susceptible to *H. influenzae* infections. This has complicated research on the mechanisms of infection and vaccine development, since animal models of the disease cannot be established.

H. influenzae can be spread from person to person in the droplets that are expelled when someone coughs or sneezes. The bacterium most often affects children, where strains that possess a capsule can cause a lung infection (pneumonia). More seriously, the bacteria can infect the blood and spread. Joints can be affected, producing arthritis. A heart infection called pericarditis can occur. *H. influenzae* infections may also attack the lining of nerves such as those in the brain. The resulting inflammation is a form of bacterial meningitis, a potentially life-threatening complication. Stiffness in the neck accompanied by flulike symptoms can be an early indication of bacterial meningitis.

Hib infections were previously a much more common and dangerous threat. The availability of infant-and childhood-based vaccines against Hib, and their widespread use beginning in the late 1990s, included in the series of vaccinations that many children receive during their first decade of life, has reduced the prevalence of Hib meningitis dramatically. In the United States, the incidence of Hib infections in children less than five years old has dropped from 40–100 children per 100,000 in the 1990s, to less than two of every 100,000 children in 2006.

■ Scope and Distribution

H. influenzae is worldwide in distribution. Most affected are children who are in close contact with one another. There is no indication that girls, boys, or members any particular race group are more susceptible to infection.

H. influenzae pneumonia and meningitis are greater problems in developing countries. Agencies including the United States Centers for Disease Control and Prevention (CDC) and the World Health Organization (WHO) assist countries in determining the prevalence and geographical distribution of infections, which helps in infection control programs.

■ Treatment and Prevention

H. influenzae can be treated by a number of different antibiotics, although there have been reports of antibiotic resistance.

Hib pneumonia and meningitis are preventable. Vaccination in a series of inoculations, which can begin

WORDS TO KNOW

DROPLETS: A drop of water or other fluid that is less than 5 microns (a millionth of a meter) in diameter.

GRAM NEGATIVE BACTERIA: Gram-negative bacteria are bacteria whose cell wall is comprised of an inner and outer membrane that are separated from one another by a region called the periplasm. The periplasm also contains a thin but rigid layer called the peptidoglycan.

STRAIN: A subclass or a specific genetic variation of an organism.

HATTIE ELIZABETH ALEXANDER (1901–1968)

Hattie Elizabeth Alexander was a pediatrician and microbiologist who made fundamental contributions in the early studies of the genetic basis of bacterial antibiotic resistance, specifically the resistance displayed by *Hemophilus influenzae*, the cause of influenzal meningitis (swelling of the nerves in the spinal cord and brain). Her pioneering studies paved the way for advances in treatment saved countless lives.

Alexander pioneered studies of the antibiotic resistance and susceptibility of *Hemophilus influenzae*. In 1939, she successfully utilized an anti-pneumonia serum that had been developed at Rockefeller University to cure infants of influenzal meningitis. Until then, infection with *Hemophilus influenzae* type b almost always resulted in death. Her antiserum reduced the death rate by almost 80%. Further research led to the use of sulfa drugs and other antibiotics in the treatment of the meningitis.

In addition to her research, Alexander devoted much time to teaching and clinical duties. She was elected the first woman president of the American Pediatric Society in 1965.

as early as six months of age, protects children. The discovery and widespread use of the three Hib vaccines have been invaluable in reducing the cases of childhood pneumonia and meningitis. Prior to the use of the vaccine, Hib was the most common cause of bacterial meningitis in countries such as Canada, where it caused more cases than all other forms of bacterial meningitis combined. The illness ravaged the young; almost 70% of cases involved children less than 18 months of age. Up to 30% of those affected had permanent brain damage.

IN CONTEXT: DISEASE IN DEVELOPING NATIONS

The World Health Organization (WHO) estimates that the "*Haemophilus influenzae* type b, or Hib, is a bacterium estimated to be responsible for some three million serious illnesses and an estimated 386,000 deaths per year, chiefly through meningitis and pneumonia. Almost all victims are children under the age of five, with those between four and 18 months of age especially vulnerable."

"In developing countries, where the vast majority of Hib deaths occur, pneumonia accounts for a larger number of deaths than meningitis. However, Hib meningitis is also a serious problem in such countries with mortality rates several times higher than seen in developed countries; it leaves 15 to 35% of survivors with permanent disabilities such as mental retardation or deafness."

SOURCE: *World Health Organization (WHO)*

Following the introduction of vaccine formulations for children (1987) and infants (1990), the number of cases of Hib meningitis decreased by over 80% in Canada and the United States within five years.

■ Impacts and Issues

Despite the overwhelming success of Hib vaccines in combating meningitis, *H. influenzae* continues to be a problem in developing countries. The World Health Organization (WHO) estimates that Hib causes three million serious illnesses and almost 400,000 deaths each year, mainly due to pneumonia. Meninigitis also is a health and economic threat is these countries; 15–35% of survivors are left with brain damage and hearing loss, which impairs their ability to function in family care and to work.

The vaccination rate for the approximately 90 countries who have Hib vaccination programs is over 90%. However, in developing countries, only about 42% of people are vaccinated, and in under-developed regions such as Sub-Saharan Africa the vaccination rate is less than 10%.

The major reason for the gulf between the developed and developing world in the prevention of *H. influenzae* disease is the cost of the vaccines. International assistance through agencies that includes CDC and WHO are aimed at increasing the availability and use of these vaccines in less-developed regions. For example, WHO is actively involved in implementing the GAVI Hib Intitiative, which will help countries most effectively vaccinate children. Agencies including WHO and UNICEF have developed the Global Immunization Vision and Strategy (GIVS), which seeks make vaccination against diseases including Hib more efficient.

SEE ALSO *Bacterial Disease; Childhood Infectious Diseases, Immunization Impacts; Developing Nations and Drug Delivery; Meningitis, Bacterial.*

BIBLIOGRAPHY

Books

Bloom, Barry R., and Paul-Henri Lambert. *The Vaccine Book*. Oxford: Academic Press, 2002.

Ferreiros, C. *Emerging Strategies in the Fight against Meningitis*. Oxford: Garland Science, 2002.

Web Sites

Centers for Disease Control and Prevention. "*Haemophilus influenzae/e* Serotype b (Hib) Disease." <http://www.cdc.gov/ncidod/dbmd/diseaseinfo/haeminfluserob_t.htm> (accessed April 10, 2007).

Brian Hoyle

Hand, Foot, and Mouth Disease

■ Introduction

Hand, foot, and mouth disease (HFMD) is a mild, self-limiting disease caused by the enterovirus family of viruses. HFMD usually affects infants and children under the age of ten. It is endemic around the world, with periodic outbreaks. Symptoms include fever, nausea, ulcers in the mouth, and sores on the hands and feet. Infected individuals generally recover within two weeks; complications are rare. The disease is considered contagious and spreads through contact with fluids from infected persons.

Although there is no treatment for the disease and there are no formal preventative measures, the majority of persons with HFMD recover without any complica-tions. However, more severe strains of enteroviruses have emerged, causing potentially fatal diseases, high-lighting the need to monitor HFMD.

HFMD is not to be confused with foot-and-mouth disease, which is an unrelated disease that only affects cattle, sheep, and swine.

■ Disease History, Characteristics, and Transmission

Hand, foot, and mouth disease was first diagnosed dur-ing an outbreak in Canada in 1957, but the name was not assigned until 1960 when Birmingham, England,

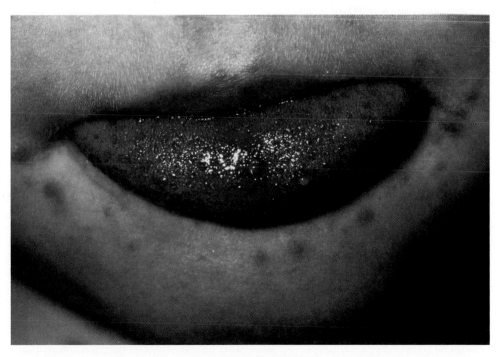

Skin lesions are shown on the tongue and around the mouth of a five-year-old boy who has contracted hand, foot, and mouth disease (HFM), common in children. *Dr P. Marazzi/Photo Researchers, Inc.*

WORDS TO KNOW

ENTEROVIRUS: Enteroviruses are a group of viruses that contain ribonucleic acid as their genetic material. They are members of the picornavirus family. The various types of enteroviruses that infect humans are referred to as serotypes, in recognition of their different antigenic patterns. The different immune response is important, as infection with one type of enterovirus does not necessarily confer protection to infection by a different type of enterovirus. There are 64 different enterovirus serotypes. The serotypes include polio viruses, coxsackie A and B viruses, echoviruses and a large number of what are referred to as non-polio enteroviruses.

COHORT: A cohort is a group of people (or any species) sharing a common characteristic. Cohorts are identified and grouped in cohort studies to determine the frequency of diseases or the kinds of disease outcomes over time.

suffered a similar outbreak. Individual cases of HFMD occur worldwide with a peak occurrence in late summer and early fall.

The disease, most common in children, results from infection by a group of enteroviruses, namely coxsackievirus A16. More severe forms of infection have appeared due to human enterovirus-71, causing epidemics with associated fatalities from HFMD-associated meningitis or encephalitis in countries such as Japan, Taiwan, Singapore, Malaysia, and Indonesia.

The onset of disease symptoms is usually three to seven days, after which children will suffer from a mild fever, loss of appetite, nausea, abdominal cramping, and a sore throat. After one to two days, the fever will heighten. In addition, painful sores will develop on the tongue, gums, and cheeks; these begin as small dots but quickly blister and ulcerate. At this point, patients will usually also display a rash affecting the palms of hands, soles of feet, and often the buttocks.

HFMD is considered moderately to highly contagious during the first week of infection and can be transmitted through contact with nose and throat discharge, blister fluids, and stools of those affected. There is no evidence of transmission from mother to infant during pregnancy, but mothers infected just prior to delivery may pass the virus on to the newborn baby. The risk of severe infection among babies is highest during the first two weeks of life.

■ Scope and Distribution

The people most commonly infected with HFMD are infants and children below the age of ten, although some cases may occur in adults. Children are the most susceptible to the disease due to their lack of previous exposure to the antigens and therefore lack of inbuilt immune defense.

The development of outbreaks and epidemics of this infection is rapid among cohorted children attending childcare facilities and schools, due to the high degree of physical contact and child interaction aiding transmission. The ratio of boys affected to girls is 1:1 and there does not appear to be a higher susceptibility to infection among certain races or ethnic groups.

Both individual cases and outbreaks of HFMD occur worldwide with no regions demonstrating a higher predisposition to the disease caused by infection with the coxsackievirus. However, HFMD presents two very different disease states depending upon the specific enterovirus causing infection and demonstrates a varied distribution.

The more severe illness, which is caused by the human enterovirus-71, presented in the first outbreak in Singapore in 1970, then occurred in Malaysia in 1997, in Taiwan in 1998, and again in Singapore in 2000. As an example of the scope of this disease, 1.5 million people were reportedly affected during the outbreak in Taiwan, including 78 child fatalities. In nearly all of the above-mentioned outbreaks, fatalities occurred as a result of infection leading to viral meningitis or encephalitis. The mortality rates and chances of complication were higher in later epidemics than those previous, which raised much concern amongst health care facilities in these countries.

Despite the fatalities occurring during outbreaks associated with this disease, HFMD caused by coxsackievirus infection is generally still considered to be a mild disease with global distribution.

■ Treatment and Prevention

HFMD is caused by a viral infection and there is no specific treatment for the infection. The infection is self-limiting, so patients will usually recover once the virus has run its course, usually within ten days. The most common complication of HFMD is dehydration due to the pain experienced when swallowing. As such it is important for patients to maintain adequate fluid intake during the course of the illness. Medication may also be administered to manage symptoms, such as non-steroidal anti-inflammatory medication for pain and fever.

There is no vaccination or formal prevention available for HFMD, but transmission may be minimized by hygiene practices such as cleaning contaminated surfaces and preventing the sharing of utensils. It is also important to limit exposure of those infected, so infected children should avoid group environments until sores have healed and the fever subsided.

In cases of disease with a strong potential for outbreak, prevention must be maintained at both the individual and societal levels. Health ministries in Singapore have been made aware of the possible severity of enterovirus infection and have made laws requiring childcare centers and general practitioners to report any suspected outbreaks of HFMD. This creates a heightened awareness among the community of the possibility of infection and increases the chances of preventing an epidemic.

■ Impacts and Issues

One important feature of HFMD is the speed and ease with which it can be transmitted. In addition to the weeklong incubation period during which infected persons display no symptoms, the virus may remain present in the saliva for up to ten days and in the stool for months. This combination means that children may be contagious for months, even if symptoms have been displayed only for a short time, making implementation of successful prevention strategies difficult.

Once a person has had HFMD, they will no longer be susceptible to infection from that particular strain of enterovirus. However, the person will remain susceptible to infection from other enteroviruses, which means that previous infection does not infer complete immunity. Studies into outbreaks of HFMD involving human enterovirus-71 have suggested that previous infection by other enteroviruses, including coxsackievirus A16, may cause increased sensitivity to the disease, as well as increased severity.

Although generally HFMD enterovirus infection is mild and self-limiting, there has been an emergence of more critical forms of disease. The high numbers of fatalities among later outbreaks suggests that certain strains of infection are gaining virulence, while populations remain defenseless against them. Discrepancies exist among symptoms and presentation of persons with HFMD in epidemics involving fatalities. Some patients display the usual symptoms of HFMD before experiencing further complications, while others display no signs at all. The onset of complicating viral meningitis, encephalitis, or endocarditis following enterovirus infection is rapid, which further limits the treatment opportunities for persons affected with these strains of enterovirus.

IN CONTEXT: EFFECTIVE RULES AND REGULATIONS.

With regard to public health concerns Centers for Disease Control and Prevention (CDC) states that CDC has "no specific recommendations regarding the exclusion of children with HFMD from child care programs, schools, or other group settings. Children are often excluded from group settings during the first few days of the illness, which may reduce the spread of infection, but will not completely interrupt it. Exclusion of ill persons may not prevent additional cases since the virus may be excreted for weeks after the symptoms have disappeared. Also, some persons excreting the virus, including most adults, may have no symptoms. Some benefit may be gained, however, by excluding children who have blisters in their mouths and drool or who have weeping lesions on their hands."

SOURCE: *Centers for Disease Control and Prevention (CDC)*

SEE ALSO *Childhood Infectious Diseases, Immunization Impacts; Contact Precautions; Emerging Infectious Diseases; Handwashing; Microbial Evolution; Notifiable Diseases; Polio (Poliomyelitis); Viral Disease.*

BIBLIOGRAPHY

Books

Mandell, G.L., J.E. Bennett, and R. Dolin. *Principles and Practice of Infectious Diseases*, Vol. 2. Philadelphia, PA: Elsevier, 2005.

Mims, C., et al. *Medical Microbiology*. St. Louis, MO: Mosby, 2004.

Periodicals

Chan, K.P., K.T. Goh, and C.Y. Chong. "Epidemic Hand, Foot and Mouth Disease caused by Human Enterovirus 71, Singapore." *Emerging Infectious Diseases*. 9, 1 (2003): 78–85.

McMinn, P.C. "An Overview of the Evolution of Enterovirus 71 and its Clinical and Public Health Significance." *FEMS Microbiology Reviews*. 26, 1 (2002): 91–107.

Web Sites

Centers for Disease Control (CDC). "Hand, Foot, & Mouth Disease." Sep. 5, 2006 <http://www.cdc.gov/ncidod/dvrd/revb/enterovirus/hfhf.htm> (accessed Feb. 23, 2007).

Handwashing

■ Introduction

Handwashing (or hand hygiene) is the single most important method of preventing the spread of infection—in the hospital, at home, and in the community. Experts agree that regular and proper handwashing using soap and water is the simplest and most effective way to promote personal hygiene and reduce infections at school and in most workplaces. In the hospital, however, studies have shown that using alcohol-based hand sanitizers are effective in reducing the numbers of transient pathogens (infectious microorganisms) residing on the hands, and, as they are quicker to use, they are used more often by busy hospital personnel.

Handwashing minimizes the spread of pathogens between people, or between other living things and people. Fomites, or inanimate objects and surfaces, such as contaminated computer keyboards, desk tops, stair rails, and cutlery often provide surfaces that harbor microorganisms that are easily transferred to membranes of the mouth, nose, and eyes via the hands.

■ History and Scientific Foundations

As early as the mid-nineteenth century, doctors and nurses began to assert that handwashing could reduce illness. Florence Nightingale (1820–1910), an English pioneer of the nursing profession, wrote about her perceived relationship between unsanitary conditions and

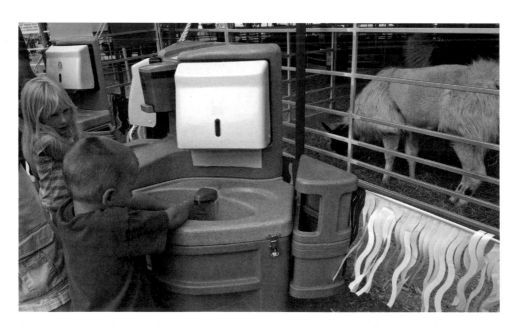

Children wash their hands as they leave a petting zoo. To reduce illness and disease transmission, the sponsors use hand-washing stations along with signs telling children to wash up after touching the animals. *AP Images.*

disease based on her nursing experiences during the Crimean War in 1855. At about the same time, the Viennese physician Ignaz Philipp Semmelweis (1818–1865) noted the connection between mortalities (deaths) in hospital patients and contact with physicians who often moved from patient to patient without washing their hands. After Semmelweis introduced handwashing with a solution containing chloride, the incidence of mortality due to puerperal fever (infection after childbirth) diminished from 18% to less than 3%.

Today, handwashing protocols are a cornerstone of the infection control program in any healthcare facility. Standard precautions, the most basic concept of infection control (which assumes that all body fluids are potential sources of infection), state that handwashing should occur both before and after routine contact with body fluids, even though latex gloves are worn. For surgery or other involved procedures, handwashing is accomplished with a non-irritating antimicrobial preparation that has fast, long-lasting, broad-spectrum activity against pathogens.

■ Applications and Research

In 2005, the American Society for Microbiology (ASM) and The Soap and Detergent Association (SDA) released the results of a study showing that people do not wash their hands as often as they report doing so. The study first conducted a telephone survey about hand hygiene habits, and then observed people in public restrooms at six public attractions in four major cities: Atlanta (Turner Field), Chicago (Museum of Science and Industry, Shedd Aquarium), New York City (Grand Central Station, Penn Station), and San Francisco (Ferry Terminal Farmers Market). Results showed that 91% of American adults say they always wash their hands after using public restrooms, but only 83% actually did so. Women washed their hands more than men after using public restrooms (90% versus 75%).

In the telephone survey, women were reportedly also slightly better than men at washing their hands after coughing or sneezing, although at only 39% and 24% respectively, hand hygiene after a cough or sneeze was reportedly low. The viruses that cause colds and influenza are spread more often by contaminated hands that come in contact with mucous membranes in the eyes, mouth, and nose than are spread through the air during sneezing, according to the Secretary of the ASM.

To maximize effectiveness, careful attention must be paid to proper handwashing technique. The act of handwashing is best accomplished by vigorous rubbing together of the hands and fingers. This is because the removal of microorganisms is accomplished not only by the presence of the soap or antiseptic, but also by the friction of the opposing skin surfaces rubbing together. Warm water, soap, and friction loosen dirt and grime.

The soap does not need to specifically labeled as "antibacterial," but liquid soap lasts longer without hosting bacterial growth than bar soap. Far more important than the type of soap is the effort put into washing. Friction is key and it is important to work the soap into lather on both sides of the hands, wrists, between the fingers, and on the fingertips. Careful attention should also be given to areas around nail beds that may harbor bacteria in broken cuticles. It is important to wash for about 15 seconds (contact time is often critical in effectively killing germs) before rinsing well without touching the faucet or sides of the washbasin, and drying with an air dryer or disposable towel (preferred) or clean cloth towel. Equally important is to avoid recontamination by turning the water faucet off with the paper towel or cloth. Children can be taught to count, repeat a simple rhyme, or to softly sing a "washing song" to make sure they invest the needed time in washing.

■ Impacts and Issues

Although it is difficult to estimate the financial impact of proper hygienic practices, conservative estimates by the U.S. Centers for Disease Control place the savings due to successful handwashing in clinical settings at over one billion dollars per year. As more than 20 million school days are lost due to the common cold alone, the savings of proper handwashing in schools and in the workplace could exceed this figure by a significant factor.

The American Society for Microbiology began focusing on increasing public awareness about the importance of handwashing in regular campaigns since 1996. The ASM also belongs to the Clean Hands Coalition, along with the Centers for Disease Control and Prevention (CDC) and other partners, which sponsors yearly handwashing awareness programs throughout the United States, usually in September near the start of the school year.

Especially during influenza season, both the CDC and World Health Organization (WHO) recommend the "elbow bump" greeting as a replacement for the handshake. Cold and influenza viruses that remain on the hands after a sneeze (and before handwashing) are often passed on through a handshake, then the recipient infects himself when touching his eyes or mouth with the contaminated hand. As it is difficult to contaminate the elbow with a sneeze, bumping elbows transfers fewer pathogens. WHO and CDC scientists responding to outbreaks of infectious disease where infrastructure is lacking commonly use the elbow bump greeting. In the event of an influenza pandemic, the U.S. government recommends the elbow bump greeting as a measure of social distancing in addition to regular handwashing to prevent the spread of infection.

■ Primary Source Connection

Handwashing is a primary means of stopping the spread of germs and preventing routine infectious diseases such as influenza and common colds. Shaking hands, a common greeting in several nations, can transmit germs from person to person. While handwashing is recommended as part of a routine of basic hygiene, it is not always possible. The article below discusses the use of hand sanitizer gels on the political campaign trail. Political candidates in the United States often meet and exchange greetings with thousands of people every day. Some politicians use gel hand sanitizers to ward off infection. Others assert that the practice is not particularly beneficial—at least to their image.

The article's author, Mark Leibovich, is a writer and political correspondent for the *New York Times*.

In Clean Politics, Flesh Is Pressed, Then Sanitized

WASHINGTON, Oct. 27—Campaigns are filthy. Not only in terms of last-minute smears and dirty tricks. But also as in germs, parasites and all the bacterial unpleasantness that is spread around through so much glad-handing and flesh-pressing.

"You can't always get to a sink to wash your hands," said Anne Ryun, wife of Representative Jim Ryun, Republican of Kansas.

Hands would be the untidy appendages that transmit infectious disease.

Like so many other people involved in politics these days, Mrs. Ryun has become obsessive about using hand sanitizer and ensuring that others do, too. She squirted Purell, the antiseptic goop of choice on the stump and self-proclaimed killer of "99.99 percent of most common germs that may cause illness," on people lined up to meet Vice President Dick Cheney this month at a fund-raiser in Topeka.

When Mr. Cheney was done meeting and greeting, he, too, rubbed his hands vigorously with the stuff, dispensed in dollops by an aide when the vice president was out of public view.

That has become routine in this peak season of handshaking, practiced by everyone from the most powerful leaders to the lowliest hopefuls. Politics is personal at all levels, and germs do not discriminate. Like chicken dinners and lobbyists, they afflict Democrats and Republicans alike. It would be difficult to find an entourage that does not have at least one aide packing Purell.

Some people find that unseemly in itself.

"It's condescending to the voters," said Gov. Bill Richardson of New Mexico, a Democrat.

A fervent nonuser of hand sanitizer, Mr. Richardson holds the Guinness Book of World Records mark for shaking the most hands over an eight-hour period (13,392, at the New Mexico State Fair in 2002).

Indeed, what message does it send when politicians, the putative leaders in a government by the people, for the people, feel compelled to wipe off the residues of said people immediately after meeting them?

"The great part about politics is that you're touching humanity," Mr. Richardson said. "You're going to collect bacteria just by existing."

Still, politics can be an especially dirty place to exist.

"Every time you're with big groups of people, you're going to be exposed to rhinoviruses, adenoviruses and the viruses that cause gastroenteritis," said Senator Tom Coburn, an Oklahoma Republican and physician.

Mr. Coburn said he washed his hands whenever possible but did not use any antigerm lotions. Being a doctor, he said, he has been exposed to more bugs and, thus, enjoys greater immunity than most other people.

For what it is worth, Howard Dean, also a doctor and the chairman of the Democratic National Committee, said he did not bother with the stuff, either.

"If you've had children, you're immune to everything," said Mr. Dean, a father of two.

As with most things, this places Mr. Dean at loggerheads with President Bush.

"Good stuff, keeps you from getting colds," Mr. Bush raved about hand sanitizer to Senator Barack Obama, Democrat of Illinois, at a White House encounter early last year.

Mr. Obama, who recounts the episode in his new book, says that after rubbing a blob of it on his own hands, the president offered him some, which he accepted ("not wanting to appear unhygienic.")

Mr. Obama has since started carrying Purell in his traveling bag, a spokesman said.

It is not clear when politicians became so awash in the gel. In one semifamous cleanliness lapse in the 1992 presidential campaign, Bill Clinton, who had just shaken dozens of hands at a tavern in Boston, was handed a pie but no fork on his way to the car. The ravenous Mr. Clinton promptly devoured it using his unwashed hand. He eventually became a serious user of hand wipes and lotions at the urging of his doctor, an aide said.

Senator John McCain, Republican of Arizona, said he learned about hand sanitizer from observing Senator Bob Dole's abundant use of it in his 1996 presidential run. Mr. McCain remains vigilant today.

"I use it all the time," he said through a representative. "I carry it with me in my briefcase."

Purell, which is made by GOJO Industries of Akron, Ohio, came on the market as a consumer product in 1997 and became popular in campaign vans, holding rooms and traveling bags in the 2000 campaign. Donald Trump, the billionaire germophobe who contemplated running for president, even distributed little bottles of it to reporters.

"One of the curses of American society is the simple act of shaking hands," Mr. Trump wrote in his book *Comeback*. "I happen to be a clean-hands freak."

Al Gore is, too. He turned his running mate, Senator Joseph I. Lieberman, onto sanitizer in 2000, and Mr. Lieberman became an evangelist.

"He said it was one thing he learned from Gore," said an aide to Senator Harry Reid of Nevada, Rebecca Kirszner, who became a popular dispenser of Purell on a senatorial trip to New Orleans after Hurricane Katrina.

Mr. Richardson said that if he ran for president, as he is considering, he had no intention of conforming to the norms of his antiseptic peers.

"I just won't use the sanitizer," he said. "I've been offered it, but I've turned it down."

This positions Mr. Richardson as the early hygienic maverick of 2008.

"I'm not afraid to get my hands dirty," he said.

Mark Leibovich

LEIBOVICH, MARK. "IN CLEAN POLITICS, FLESH IS PRESSED, THEN SANITIZED." *NEW YORK TIMES.* OCTOBER 28, 2006. <HTTP://WWW.NYTIMES.COM/2006/10/28/US/POLITICS/28DIRTY.HTML?_R=1&TH&EMC=TH&OREF=SLOGIN> (ACCESSED JUNE 12, 2007).

SEE ALSO *Antimicrobial Soaps; Infection Control and Asepsis.*

BIBLIOGRAPHY

Periodicals

Goldmann, Donald. "System Failure versus Personal Accountability—The Case for Clean Hands" *NEJM* (July 13, 2006): 355: 121–123.

Web Sites

American Society for Microbiology. "Don't Get Caught Dirty Handed." <http://www.washup.org/> (accessed June 10, 2007).

American Society for Microbiology. "Gross...You Didn't Wash Your Hands?" <http://www.microbeworld.org/know/wash.aspx> (accessed June 10, 2007).

Centers for Disease Control and Prevention (CDC). "An Ounce of Prevention Keeps the Germs Away." <http://www.cdc.gov/ncidod/op/gt;. (accessed June 10, 2007).

National Food Service Management Institute. "Wash Your Hands." <http://www.nfsmi.org/Information/handsindex.html>. (accessed June 10, 2007).

Brenda Wilmoth Lerner

Hantavirus

■ Introduction

During the 1950s, more than 6,000 United Nations military personnel serving in Korea were stricken by a mysterious illness characterized by high fever, kidney failure, and spontaneous bleeding. Few realize that this disease continues to claim victims in the region, with 418 cases reported in 2006 alone. Eventually a group of viruses was identified as the cause of this "Korean hemorrhagic fever" and [the group] was named Hantaan virus, after the Hantaan River, which flows through Gangwon and Gyeonggi Provinces.

Subsequently, similar illnesses of varying severity in Asia and Europe were found to be caused by a number of distinct viruses, and the group came to be known as the Hantaviruses. In 1993, a new illness was reported in the southwestern United States. Unlike the Korean disease, prominent features included rapidly progressive lung infection with high mortality (death rates). Despite the unique nature of the disease, a viral agent was discovered which had all of the common biological features of the older Hantavirus group. The new illness was therefore referred to as Hantavirus pulmonary syndrome (HPS). 396 cases were reported by 32 American states as of July 6, 2005, including 142 fatal cases. As in the Asian variety, a large number of additional Hantavirus species have since been identified in the United States, as well as Central and South America.

■ Disease History, Characteristics, and Transmission

Regardless of differences in clinical presentation and geographic occurrence, all of the Hantaviruses are found in rodents. Man acquires the disease through inhalation of dried rodent excreta, or occasionally through ingestion of milk and other foods that had been contaminated by these animals. In fact, the ability of the virus to survive in dust and the contagious nature of infected material have suggested Hantaviruses as potential agents of biorerrorism.

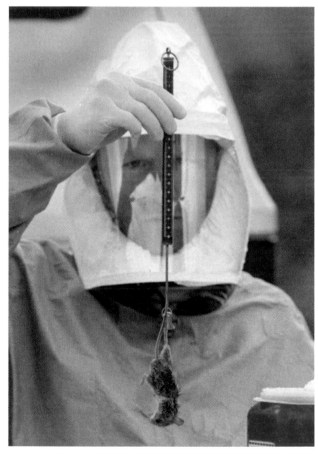

A researcher from the University of New Mexico weighs a mouse caught in an trap during a study of the Hantavirus in 1996. *AP Images.*

362

■ Scope and Distribution

The following is a summary of the clinical features, distribution, and epidemiology (patterns, characteristics, and causes) of Hantaviruses that infect humans. Specific viruses (strains, or types) are arranged alphabetically.

Old World Hantaviruses

Clinical features Infection by the European and Asian Hantaviruses is characterized by sudden onset, with intense headache, backache, fever, and chills. Hemorrhage is manifested during the febrile phase as a flushing of the face or injection of the conjunctiva (membranes lining the eye) and mucous membranes. A petechial rash (tiny, red dots) may appear on the palate and axillary (underarm) skin folds. Extreme albuminuria (protein in the urine), typically appearing on the fourth day, is characteristic of severe hemorrhagic fever renal syndrome (HFRS).

As the febrile (with fever) stage ends, hypotension (low blood pressure) may develop and last for hours to days, accompanied by nausea and vomiting. One-third of deaths occur during this phase, related to vascular leakage (bleeding) and shock. Approximately 50% of deaths occur during the subsequent oliguric phase (when the kidneys produce very little urine). Patients who survive and progress to the diuretic phase show improved renal function, but may still die of shock or pulmonary (lung) complications. The final (convalescent) phase can last weeks to months.

Case-fatality rates (rates calculated to show the severity of disease; the number of deaths divided by number of cases expressed as a percentage) range from less than 0.1% for hemorrhagic fever renal syndrome (HFRS) caused by Puumala [PUU] virus to approximately 5% to 10% for HFRS caused by Hantaan (HTN) virus.

Epidemiology Dobrava/Belgrade virus causes severe hemorrhagic fever with renal (kidney) syndrome. The reservoirs (organisms that maintain the infective agent), *Apodemus flavicolis* (the yellow-necked mouse) and *Apodemus agrarius*, are found from England and Wales, through northwest Spain, France, southern Scandinavia, European Russia to the Urals, southern Italy, the Balkans, Syria, Lebanon, and Israel.

Hantaan virus causes epidemic hemorrhagic fever (Korean hemorrhagic fever and hemorrhagic fever with renal syndrome). The reservoir, the striped field mouse (*Apodemus agrarius*), is found in Central Europe south to Thrace, the Caucasus and Tien Shan Mountains, the Amur River to East Xijiang and East Hunnan, West Sichuan, Fujian, and Taiwan.

Puumala virus causes nephropathia epidemica (a usually less severe form of hemorrhagic fever). The reservoir, the bank vole (*Clethrionomys glariolus*) is found in the West Palearctic from France and Scandinavia to

Lake Baikal, south to northern Spain, northern Italy, the Balkans, western Turkey, northern Kazakhstan, the Altai and Sayan Mountains, Great Britain, and southwestern Ireland. The house mouse (*Mus musculus*) is implicated in Serbia, and *Clethrionomys rutilis* in western Russia. The muskrat (*Ondatra zibethicus*) has been implicated as a disease reservoir in Germany. Note that Puumala virus may remain infective in the environment for as long as 12 to 15 days.

Saaremaa virus has been associated with human disease in Estonia, and is closely related to Dobrava virus.

Seoul virus causes less severe hemorrhagic fever with renal syndrome. The reservoir rat (*Rattus norvegicus*) is found worldwide. Wounds inflicted by other rats appear to be a major source for transmission among rats.

Thailand virus has been identified in humans and bandicoot rats (*Bandicota indica, B. savilei*) in Thailand.

Note: There are no proven cases of Hantaan or Seoul virus infections either from Europe or from western Russia (west of the Urals)—as of 2000, all claimed cases have turned out to be caused by Dobrava virus. Dobrava virus has been confirmed in the former Yugoslavia, Albania, Greece, Germany, Estonia and Russia. This is in contrast to the Balkan region, where Dobrova virus seems to be carried mainly by *Apodemus flavicollis*. In Estonia and Russia, the virus has only been found in *Apodemus agrarius*.

Hantavirus pulmonary syndrome

Clinical features The typical illness is characterized by fever, chills, headache, and occasionally gastrointestinal symptoms. Five days after onset, patients develop dyspnea (difficult breathing), with rapid progression to pulmonary edema/ARDS (adult respiratory distress syndrome) within as little as 24 hours. Recently, cases of prodromic infection (having symptoms of oncoming disease) without severe pulmonary disease have been reported.

Epidemiology Andes virus is transmitted by the long-tailed pygmy rice rat (*Oligoryzomys longicaudatus*), found in the north central to southern Andes, approximately 50 degrees S latitude, in Chile, and Argentina (and possibly Uruguay).

Bermejo virus (reservoir *Oligoryzomys species*) has been associated with human infections in Bolivia.

Bayou virus is transmitted by the rice rat (*Oryzomys palustris*) in Louisiana and eastern Texas.

Black Creek Canal virus is transmitted by the cotton rat (*Sigmodon hispidus*), found in the eastern and southern United States from southern Nebraska to central Virginia, south to Southeastern Arizona and peninsular Florida; and from central to eastern Mexico through Central America and central Panama to northern Colombia and northern Venezuela.

Cano Delgadito virus (clinical significance unknown) is found in rodents in central Venezuela.

Central plata virus is associated with human infections in Uruguay, and is transmitted by the yellow pygmy rice rat (*Oligoryzomys flavescens*).

Choclo virus (reservoir *Oligoryzomys fulvescens*) is implicated in human infections in Panama. Calabazo virus (clinical significance unknown) has been identified in *Zygodontomys brevicauda* in Panama.

Convict Creek virus (similar, possibly identical to Sin Nombre virus) has been identified in California, and was implicated in a fatal case in Ontario, Canada.

Juquitiba virus, Araraquare virus and Castelos dos Sonhos virus have been implicated in human infections in Brazil; HU39694 (yet unnamed) in Argentina—reservoirs unknown.

Laguna negra virus has caused human disease in Argentina, Chile and Paraguay, and is transmitted by the vesper mouse (*Calomys laucha*). This rodent is found in northern Argentina and Uruguay, southeastern Bolivia, Chile, western Paraguay, and west-central Brazil.

Maporal virus (clinical significance unknown) has been identified in the fulvous pygmy rice rat (*Oligoryzomys fulvescens*) in western Venezuela.

Monongahela virus (similar, possibly identical to Sin Nombre virus) is found in the eastern United States and Canada, and carried by the white-footed mouse (*Peromyscus leucopus*) and possibly *P. maniculatus nubiterrae*.

New York-1 virus is transmitted by the white-footed mouse (*Peromyscus leucopus*), found in the Central and Eastern United States to Southern Ontario, Southern Alberta, Quebec and Nova Scotia; and Northern Durango and along the Caribbean coast of Mexico to the Isthmus of Tehuantepec and Yucatan Peninsula.

Oran virus (reservoir *Ol. Longicaudatus*), Lechiguanas virus (*reservoir Or. Flavescens*) and Andes virus (reservoir *Ol. Longicaudatus*) are found in Argentina.

Rio Mamore virus (reservoir *Neacomys spinosus*) has been associated with human infections in Peru.

Sin Nombre virus is transmitted by the deer mouse (*Peromyscus maniculatus*) in the southwestern United States. The reservoir is found from the Alaska panhandle across Northern Mexico, Canada, most of the continental United States, to southernmost Baja California and north central Oaxaca, Mexico. The mouse itself shows evidence of pneumonia. The virus has also been found in *Pe. boylii*, *Pe. truei*, *Reithrodontomys* spp., *Mus musculus* and *Tamias* spp.

■ Treatment and Prevention

Although the viruses in this group can be cultivated using standard techniques, viral culture is limited to a small number of institutions which meet strict standards of bio-safety. Diagnosis can also be established through testing for serum antibodies in specialized laboratories. Treatment is directed at support of renal, pulmonary and other systems affected by the viruses. The value of specific antiviral agents is not proven, but some authorities have suggested Ribavirin in the treatment of the Old Word Hantaviruses. A vaccine (Hantavax) has also been developed for the Old World variety.

■ Impacts and Issues

The Hantavirus pulmonary syndrome (HPS) was first identified as such in May 1993, in the so-called "Four Corners" region of the United States, where the states of New Mexico, Utah, Arizona, and Colorado meet. Initially, it was unclear what was able to quickly kill healthy adults in this region. Virologists from the U.S. Center of Disease Control (CDC) used techniques that allow an analysis of a virus at the molecular level, to link the pulmonary illness to a previously unknown type of hantavirus, which was later named *Sin Nombre* (Spanish for without name).

In addition to molecular and clinical studies, scientists are studying HPS through the study of rodent populations (which often requires the trapping and collection of various mice species), weather patterns, and climate change,

Research in the southwestern United States has linked the years having higher levels of precipitation with a larger population of rodents, as the moisture leads to a greater supply of food for rodents, as well as higher vegetation growth, which provides ample habitat and protection for the rodents. Associated with the weather phenomenon El Niño in 1991 and 1993, rainfall levels increased in the southwestern United States. The population density of deer mice in New Mexico then increased from one deer mouse per hectare (2.47 acres) to twenty to thirty per hectare during that time period. It is thought that this large population of mice led to the first identified outbreak of HPS in May 1993.

Although rare, HPS has since been found throughout the United States. As of May 2007, rodent control remains the primary defense against the hantavirus.

SEE ALSO *Emerging Infectious Diseases; Hemorrhagic Fevers.*

BIBLIOGRAPHY

Books

Harper, David R., and Andrea S. Meyer. *Of Mice, Men, and Microbes: Hantavirus.* Burlington, MA: Academic Press, 1999.

Leuenroth, Stephanie J. *Hantavirus Pulmonary Syndrome (Deadly Diseases and Epidemics).* New York: Chelsea House, 2006.

Periodicals

Kreeger, Karen Young "Stalking the Deadly Hantavirus: A Study in Teamwork." *The Scientist.* 8 (July 1994): 1–4.

Web sites

Centers for Disease Control and Prevention. "All About Hantaviruses." <http://www.cdc.gov/ncidod/diseases/hanta/hps/index.htmgt; (accessed May 10, 2007).

Stephen A. Berger

Helicobacter pylori

◼ Introduction

Helicobacter pylori are bacteria that live in the lining of the stomach and sometimes cause stomach inflammation and ulcers. The discovery of *H. pylori* changed scientists' thinking about the nature of stomach ulcers, and led to the broader study of bacteria and other pathogens (infectious agents) as possible contributors to other well-known diseases, including heart disease and some types of cancer.

◼ History and Scientific Foundations

In 1975, J. Robin Warren of Australia discovered the presence of helical (spiral-shaped) bacteria in the antrum, the section of the stomach that empties into the duodenum (the top part of the upper intestine) through the pyloric valve. At that time, Warren observed that the bacteria were present in 50% persons who had stomach biopsies, and that infected persons invariably showed signs of stomach inflammation. Later, he named the bacterium *Helicobacter pylori* after working with fellow Australian Barry J. Marshall to cultivate the species from biopsied patients.

The two scientists hypothesized that an *H. pylori* infection played a part in stomach disorders, including gastritis and peptic ulcers. Many of their peers in the medical community considered this hypothesis to be preposterous, since the theory that ulcers were caused by lifestyle and psychological stress was widely accepted by both the scientific community and the general public. Robin observed that no one else noticed the bacterium in affected patients before, and that for some time after its discovery, his research team was virtually alone in investigating *H. pylori*.

Perhaps the greatest barrier to acceptance of such a simple explanation as a bacterial infection was the simplicity of the potential cure, a course of antibiotics and

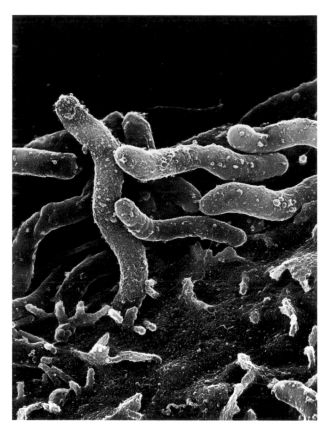

A colored scanning electron micrograph (SEM) shows *Helicobacter pylori bacteria* (red) on the surface of a human stomach. *SPL/Photo Researchers, Inc.*

acid secretion inhibitors for a serious chronic and often disabling condition. The idea of stress and lifestyle as the cause of stomach ulcers was so pervasive and impervious to new evidence that Marshall undertook drastic action, putting himself at risk to demonstrate the role of *H. pylori* in disease. He allowed colleagues to obtain a sample of his stomach tissue in a biopsy to show that he was free of infection, then infected himself with the bacterium and subsequently, contracted gastritis. This act of personal commitment and courage had a decisive impact on the medical profession, which began to accept his work, although the *H. pylori* hypothesis as a major cause of peptic ulcers did not gain worldwide acceptance until 1991.

■ Applications and Research

Subsequent studies have shown that about half of all humans have chronic *H. pylori* infection, and clinical experience confirms that this infection and the consequent destruction of the stomach lining and predisposition for stomach cancer can be halted by antibiotic treatment. Thus, Warren and Marshall brought about a paradigm shift, or a fundamental change in thinking regarding the relative importance of infectious agents as opposed to psychosocial factors in the cause and origin of gastric disease. This paradigm shift in turn led to a marked improvement in the health and quality of life for the large population stomach ulcer sufferers around the world, and led to research about the possible role of infectious agents in other diseases. For example, scientists are currently studying the potential role of infectious agents in inflammation of the walls of blood vessels that could relate to heart disease and strokes.

Thus, chronic gastritis is a disorder influenced by bacterial and the genetic predispositions of the human host. A 2007 study in which gastric biopsies were evaluated showed that the presence of *H. pylori* is strongly associated with both acute and chronic inflammation. The presence of neutrophils (the most common white blood cell involved in immune system function and which attacks infected tissue with inflammatory biochemicals, called cytokines) on biopsy is predictive of the presence of *H. pylori* as well as the extent of inflamed tissue. Long-term inflammation leads to atrophy (wasting, or decreasing size) of the stomach lining. This persistent inflammation appears to be due either to a weakness in the immune system in which the predisposed individual is unable to eliminate the bacterium, or a physiological weakness in the structure of the stomach lining that fosters the growth of *H. pylori* colonies (populations).

■ Impacts and Issues

As a persistent colonizer of the human stomach, *Helicobacter pylori* is now known to be involved in the development of gastric cancer as well as extra-intestinal diseases. Public awareness of its contribution in the development of gastric cancer is less than 15 years old. Current antibiotic therapies against *H. pylori* have been limited by antibiotic resistance and recurrence of infection, probably due to the predisposing factors in susceptible individuals

WORDS TO KNOW

ATROPHY: Decreasing in size or wasting away of a body part or tissue.

CHRONIC INFECTION: Chronic infections persist for prolonged periods of time—months an even years—in the host. This lengthy persistence is due to a number of factors including masking of the bacteria from the immune system, invasion of host cells, and the establishment of an infection that is resistance to antibacterial agents.

COLONIZATION: Colonization is the process of occupation and increase in number of microorganisms at a specific site.

PATHOGEN: A disease causing agent, such as a bacteria, virus, fungus, etc.

discussed above. Consequently, promising vaccine development programs have been mounted as an effective preventive measure. So far, however, developmental vaccines have failed the transition from animal models to human trials. *H. pylori* is implicated not only in gastric cancer, but also childhood lymphomas. The latter type of cancer probably could arise from the proliferation of lymphocytes in the stomach lining in the inflammatory response to chronic infection mentioned earlier. Such proliferation could raise the probability of a lymphocyte replication error that results in cancer.

Paradoxically, scientists have found an inverse association between *Helicobacter pylori* infection and esophageal cancer. This inverse relationship has been attributed to reduced stomach acidity that can damage the esophagus because of the atrophy of the gastric lining.

Epidemiologists might wonder about genetic or environmental factors that differentiate the 50% of the population chronically infected with the bacterium from the 50% that show no infection. Chronic infection with *Helicobacter pylori* illustrates the damage that can occur when the genetic variability of individuals results favorable conditions for a pathogen (disease-causing organism) that is harmless to a large proportion of the human population. The inability of the immune system and even antibiotic treatment to conclusively end the infection in these individuals can result in severe tissue damage and possibly, cancer. Perhaps the larger lesson to be taken from *H. pylori* infection is that humans and microbes are in a constant struggle to adapt to one another, and some of the resulting infections resemble a chronic and desultory war that eventually wears down the host. The work of Marshall and Warren is all the more important for having provided the basis for relieving a significant amount of the misery caused by this stubborn microbial foe. Marshall and Warren were awarded the Nobel Prize for the discovery of the role of *Helicobacter pylori* infection in the development of stomach ulcers in 2005.

SEE ALSO *Cancer and Infectious Disease; Exposed: Scientists Who Risked Disease for Discovery.*

BIBLIOGRAPHY

Web Sites

Helicobacter Foundation. "*H. pylori.*" <http://www. helico.com/h_general.html> (accessed May 30, 2007).
Nobelprize.org. "The Nobel Prize in Physiology or Medicine 2005." Press Release, October 3, 2005. <http://nobelprize.org/nobel_prizes/medicine/ laureatgt; (accessed June 7, 2007).

Kenneth T. LaPensee

Helminth Disease

■ Introduction

Helminth diseases are caused by parasitic worms known as helminths. These worms are categorized into three main categories: roundworms, tapeworms, and flukes. There are around 300 identified helminths that infect humans. Transmission of helminths typically involves direct contact with the parasite, or ingestion of the parasite via contaminated food or water. In some cases, the parasites can pass through human skin from infected water or soil.

Symptoms range depending on the type of helminth causing the disease. There may be general symptoms, or more specific symptoms as certain regions of the body are affected. Furthermore, while full recovery is possible from some infections, death or debilitating disabilities occurs with other infections. Treatment, when possible, usually involves administration of anti-inflammatory drugs alone or in combination with anti-helminth drugs that kill the existing parasites in various stages of their development.

Helminths cause human disease worldwide, although climate conditions limit many species of helminths to tropical or semi-tropical areas. However, with changes in climate, certain infections are becoming widespread. Developing or poverty-stricken countries are heavily affected with helminth diseases, a problem compounded by lack of education, funding, and additional problems in these countries such as HIV infection, lagging infrastructure, political instability, and war.

■ Disease History, Characteristics, and Transmission

Helminths are parasitic worms, that is, they infect a host and survive by feeding off the host's nutrients, a process that usually harms the host. The adverse effects of the helminth lead to the development of disease within the host. There are roughly 300 recognized helminths that infect humans. Helminths are thought to have been present in humans as far back as ancient Egyptian times, and gradually, specific disease-causing species were identified over the centuries. The study of helminths increased in the twentieth century, which caused the number of recognized helminths to increase from 28 to over 300.

Helminths are separated into three main categories based on morphology (structure) and mode of transmission. These categories are roundworms or nematodes, tapeworms or cestodes, and flukes or trematodes.

Most roundworms hatch and live in the intestines. The eggs of roundworms enter the body of the host and travel towards the intestines, where they hatch. Depending on their subtype, they remain in the intestine or migrate to other regions of the body. Transmission of roundworms occurs when contaminated material enters the body. This could be via ingestion of contaminated food or water, entry of eggs via the anal or genital tracts, or ingestion of, or contact with, contaminated soil. Symptoms of roundworm infection vary depending on the type of worm. Some cause general symptoms such as abdominal pain, diarrhea, fatigue, itching, and fever, while others can be more specific and cause damage to certain regions of the body.

Tapeworms generally live in the intestines. Their eggs are normally ingested when meat containing the parasites is undercooked or raw. While symptoms may not occur, some patients will experience abdominal pain, fatigue, and diarrhea.

Flukes are a group of helminths that live in various regions of the body including the spleen, liver, lungs, and intestines. The lifecycle of these worms involves freshwater snails as intermediate hosts. Following the release of larval forms of the worm from the snail into fresh water, the larval worms can enter humans via contact with the skin. Most cases of fluke infection do not cause initial symptoms, and the parasites pass out of the body. However, reinfection can occur. If it occurs continuously over time, this can cause damage to body

HELMINTH: A representative of various phyla of worm-like animals.

HYGIENE: Hygiene refers to the health practices that minimize the spread of infectious microorganisms between people or between other living things and people. Inanimate objects and surfaces such as contaminated cutlery or a cutting board may be a secondary part of this process.

MORPHOLOGY: The study of form and structure of animals and plants. The outward physical form possessed by an organism.

SANITATION: Sanitation is the use of hygienic recycling and disposal measures that prevent disease and promote health through sewage disposal, solid waste disposal, waste material recycling, and food processing and preparation.

organs. In symptomatic cases, infection usually results in a rash, itching, muscle aches, coughing, chills, and fever. Severe infections involve flukes entering the liver, lung, or brain and spinal cord.

■ Scope and Distribution

Helminth diseases occur worldwide. However, different types of infections are present in different regions. One factor that influences where an infection can occur is climate. Some helminths survive only in tropical climates, while others require temperate conditions.

Soil-transmitted helminths and schistosomes, a type of trematode, are the cause of most of the world's helminth disease burden. Regions that are poverty-stricken, in the midst of conflict, or have low sanitation standards have a high prevalence of infection. Poverty-stricken countries in the developing world, located in Africa, China, East Asia, and the Americas, account for most of the world's helminth infections.

However, some infections of helminths are common in developed countries. For example, infection by the pinworm, a nematode that causes itching, is common in temperate areas such as Western Europe and North America. Large infection rates are recorded for these regions. Cambridge University reports infection in 30% to 80% of Caucasian children in the United States, Canada, and Europe. Despite its large prevalence in the temperate zone, this infection is rare in the tropics.

■ Treatment and Prevention

As there are a large variety of helminths that cause disease in humans, there is no specific treatment. However, most infections can be treated via the use of vermifuges, which are anti-worm drugs that effectively kill parasitic worms. In addition, while some helminth infections can be cured within a short period of time, others may take months or years to heal, and in some cases, patients are left with debilitating disabilities due to organ and limb damage.

There are several ways to prevent infection from helminths. First, avoiding contact with the parasites ensures infection does not occur. Contact can be prevented by frequent washing of hands, maintaining a clean bathroom and kitchen, and avoiding contact with infected animals. Furthermore, thorough cooking of food, particularly pork and beef that may potentially carry parasites, prevents ingestion of parasites. Chlorinating, filtering, or boiling drinking water prevents parasites being ingested while drinking. To avoid parasite uptake while bathing or swimming in infected water, a problem particularly for fluke parasites, water can be boiled prior to bathing, or avoided completely.

Another way to prevent infection is to lower the prevalence of helminths within a community. This is achieved through regular deworming, or administration of anti-worm treatments to infected people. This can effectively reduce the long-term effects of the parasites on infected persons, as well as reduce the prevalence of the parasite within a community.

In order to effectively implement prevention methods in communities affected by helminth infestations, communities can be educated about hygiene, sanitation, and proper food preparation. Together with helminth treatments, these methods help to reduce the prevalence and effects of helminths on communities.

■ Impacts and Issues

Parasitic infections are a worldwide issue as millions of people become infected by helminths every year. Although knowledge about helminths is increasing, the prevalence of infections is also increasing rather than declining. There are a number of reasons for this occurrence.

The Human Immunodeficiency Virus (HIV) and AIDS causes decreased immunity in infected people, and makes them more susceptible to infection by emerging parasites that are taking advantage of weakened immune systems. Furthermore, existing helminth infections also take advantage of people with low immunity and have increased as a result. This problem compounds when countries with a high prevalence of HIV infection also have a high prevalence of helminth infection.

Helminth invasion into new areas has also become a major contributor to global increases in infection. This is initiated by changes in the climate that make previously helminth-free regions suitable for helminths to survive and reproduce. In addition, war and its resulting social upheaval results in lower standards of sanitation and nutrition that has lead to re-emergence of helminth infections in some populations. Helminth resistance to anti-worm drugs has also caused issues in controlling and treating infections.

The World Health Organization (WHO) estimates that nearly one billion people worldwide do not have access to clean drinking water. Water polluted by sewage, refuse, and agricultural byproducts (such as manure) spreads some helminths. Several international organizations help communities build wells, water purification stations, and sewage collection systems.

Several world leaders serve as advocates for international, cooperative anti-helminth efforts, including former United States President Jimmy Carter (1924–), Amadou Toumani Touré (1948–) of Mali, and Yakubu Gowon (1934–) former Nigerian head of state. The Carter Center's International Task Force for Disease Eradication, with support from the Bill & Melinda Gates Foundation, sponsors anti-helminth programs with the aim of eradicating dracunculiasis (Guinea worm disease) and lymphatic filariasis across the globe, eradicating onchocerciasis (river blindness) in the Americas, and controlling schistosomiasis.

SEE ALSO *AIDS (Acquired Immunodeficiency Syndrome); Bilharzia (Schistosomiasis); Climate Change and Infectious Disease; Dracunculiasis; Emerging Infectious Diseases; Handwashing; HIV; Hookworm (Ancylostoma) Infection; Liver Fluke Infections; Lung Fluke (Paragonimus) Infection; Opportunistic Infection; Pinworm (Enterobius vermicularis) Infection; River Blindness (Onchocerciasis); Roundworm (Ascariasis) infection; Sanitation; Tapeworm Infections; War and Infectious Disease; Water-borne Disease.*

IN CONTEXT: DISEASE IN DEVELOPING NATIONS

Helminth diseases are most likely to strike children, especially in the developing world, causing malnutrition and illness. Malnutrition during childhood has life-long effects on an estimated 182 million children worldwide, from increased rates of illness and stagnated development, to disability and premature death. Thus, the World Health Organization (WHO), in partnership with UNICEF, focuses its anti-helminth efforts on children and schools. In areas where helminths thrive in local water or soil, efforts to curb helminth diseases include food safety, hygiene, and sanitation education, as well at the widespread administration of anti-helminth drugs. Such comprehensive public health measures have reduced incidence of helminth diseases in limited parts of Indonesia by as much as 50%.

BIBLIOGRAPHY

Books

Crompton, D.W.T., A. Montresor, and M.C. Nesheim. *Controlling Disease Due to Helminth Infections.* Geneva: World Health Organization, 2004.

Mims, C., H. Dockrell, R. Goering, I. Roitt, D. Wakelin, and M. Zuckerman. *Medical Microbiology.* St. Louis, MO: Mosby, 2004.

Periodicals

Cox, F.E.G. "History of Human Parasitology." *Clinical Microbiology Reviews.* vol. 15, no. 4 (2002): 595–612.

Web Sites

Cambridge University. "Helminth Infections of Man." Oct. 5, 1998 <http://www.path.cam.ac.uk/~schisto/General_Parasitology/Hm.helminths.html> (accessed Feb. 23, 2007).

Hemorrhagic Fevers

■ Introduction

Hemorrhagic diseases are caused by infection with certain viruses and, rarely, bacteria. Hemorrhage is severe and uncontrolled bleeding. As implied by their name, a central feature of hemorrhagic fevers is this uncontrolled bleeding, which is caused by the destruction of cells inside the body as the virus makes new copies of itself.

Hemorrhagic fevers are terrifying to those affected, to those attempting to care for the sick, and to those who read about or watch images of an outbreak. Hemorrhagic infections cause symptoms that appear and progress swiftly. Because outbreaks of hemorrhagic fevers appear and sweep through a population very rapidly before disappearing, very little is known of the details of the various viral infections.

■ Disease History, Characteristics, and Transmission

Hemorrhagic diseases are mainly caused by viruses. They are also known collectively as viral hemorrhagic fevers. Bacterial hemorrhagic infections are rare, but one example of such a disease is scrub typhus.

Viral hemorrhagic fevers are caused by viruses in four groups—arenaviruses, filoviruses, bunyaviruses, and the flaviviruses. Arenaviruses are a family of RNA viruses (their genetic material is not composed of DNA, only RNA) that are associated with human diseases transmitted by rodents. They cause a number of hemorrhagic fevers, including Lassa fever (caused by the Lassa virus), Argentine hemorrhagic fever (caused by the Junin virus), Bolivian hemorrhagic fever (caused by the Machupo virus), Venezuelan hemorrhagic fever (caused by the Guananto virus), and Brazilian hemorrhagic fever (caused by Sabia).

The first arenavirus was isolated in 1933 during an investigation into an outbreak of St. Louis encephalitis. The virus was found not to be the cause of the outbreak,

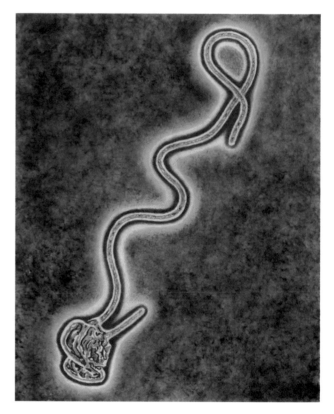

This colored transmission electron micrograph (TEM) shows a single Ebola virus, the cause of Ebola hemorrhagic fever (Ebola HF). Although the virus appears similar to the Marburg virus that causes green monkey disease, different antibodies are used for treatment. Both viruses cause fever, skin rash, and hemorrhaging. *CAMR/A. Barry Dowsett/Photo Researchers, Inc.*

but the severity of its health threat was revealed. The limited studies that have been done in the intervening decades (studies are limited because of the great danger in working with the viruses) have shown that arenaviruses are typically transmitted to humans via animals such as rodents. These viruses are characterized as zoonotic, which

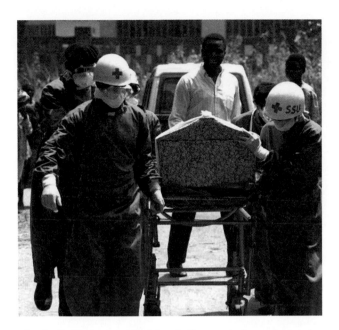

The deadly Ebola virus killed four Italian nuns who worked at the Kikwit hospital in Zaire (now the Democratic Republic of Congo) in 1995. *AP Images.*

means that they reside in another host (a wild or domesticated animal) but are capable of causing disease when transmitted to humans.

Bunyaviruses are a family of RNA viruses that are associated with rodent- or insect-borne diseases in humans. Viruses in this family are known to cause Crimean-Congo hemorrhagic fever, Rift Valley fever, and Hantavirus pulmonary syndrome. Congo-Crimean fever, a disease known for many years in eastern Europe and central Asia, is caused by a virus that is transmitted to humans and a variety of domestic and wild animals by ticks. Humans can become infected when they come into close contact with infected cattle, and slaughterhouses have been involved in disease outbreaks. Rift Valley fever is generally found in areas of eastern and southern Africa where cattle and sheep are raised. The virus responsible for the disease primarily affects livestock, but humans can also contract the disease when they are bitten by mosquitoes infected with the virus or when they come into contract with the blood or body parts of infected animals. Hantavirus disease is transmitted to humans mainly through the inhalation of aerosolized virus particles from dried mouse feces. Investigation of a disease outbreak that occurred in the United States in 1993 determined that a virus called the Sin Nombre virus (a type of hantavirus) was a cause. Another virus called that Hantaan virus causes Hantavirus pulmonary syndrome. This virus was isolated during an investigation of a disease outbreak that occurred in the 1950s near the Hantan River in Korea.

Filoviruses cause severe hemorrhagic diseases in humans and other primates, including Ebola hemorrhagic fever and Marburg hemorrhagic fever. Flaviviruses cause a wide range of human diseases, including tick-borne encephalitis, yellow fever, Dengue hemorrhagic fever, Kyasanur Forest disease, and Omsk hemorrhagic fever. Depending on the virus, the disease may be transmitted to humans via rodents, ticks, and mosquitoes. In some cases, such as Ebola, the host is still not known. Bats are a suspected natural reservoir of the virus that causes Ebola, but the virus has yet to be isolated from these animals.

The various viral hemorrhagic viruses differ in structure. For example, arenaviruses are spherical, while filoviruses, such as the Marburg virus, can be U-shaped, O-shaped, or even shaped like the number 6. Although these hemorrhagic viruses differ, they do share some common features. For example, they all contain ribonucleic acid (RNA) as their genetic material. In addition, humans are not their normal host. While the viruses are able to live without severely affecting natural hosts, such as cattle, the infection caused in humans is severe. This is the primary reason that human outbreaks of hemorrhagic fever disappear so rapidly. The high death rate makes it impossible for the virus to persist in a human population for very long once an outbreak has been recognized and treatment measures, such as isolation of those who are infected, is initiated.

Most hemorrhagic viruses share another feature in common. Once a human is infected he or she can then transfer the virus to other people (person-to-person transmission), often via contaminated body fluids. Caregivers can become infected in this way. This transmission can occur in a hospital or clinic, and such hospital-acquired infections are called nosocomial infections.

While the various viral hemorrhagic fevers have their own distinct symptoms, they do share some symptoms and a pattern of symptoms over time. The diseases typically begin a sudden fever, a general feeling of fatigue, myalgia, dizziness, pain and stiffness in the neck and back, diarrhea, and severe headache (which can be so bad that a person becomes nauseated and vomits, and becomes very sensitive to light). Some people do recover, and recovery can be as rapid as the onset of the disease. However, others deteriorate further, and begin to hemorrhage from the mouth, eyes, and ears. This bleeding is only the external manifestation of the massive bleeding that is occurring inside the body, as various organs become infected. In the final stages of a hemorrhagic fever, organs fail and the nervous system breaks down, leading to coma, seizures, and death.

■ Scope and Distribution

The filoviruses that cause Marburg hemorrhagic fever and Ebola are found in various regions of the Africa continent. Three of the four known species of Ebola are named for the regions in which they were first discovered—Ivory Coast, Sudan, and Zaire.

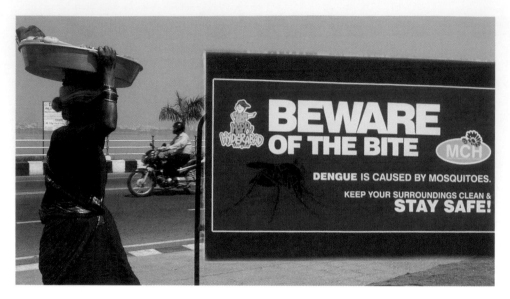

An Indian woman carries vegetables on her head as she passes by a sign warning people about the risk of contracting dengue fever. The sign is part of an awareness campaign launched by the Municipal Corporation of Hyderabad in India's southern state of Andhra Pradesh in 2006. *Noah Seelam/AFP/Getty Images.*

WORDS TO KNOW

BIOSAFETY LEVEL FOUR LABORATORY: A specially equipped, secured laboratory where scientists study the most dangerous known microbes. These labs are designed to contain infectious agents and disease-causing microbes, prevent their dissemination, and protect researchers from exposure.

HEMORRHAGE: Very severe, massive bleeding which is difficult to control.

MYALGIA: Muscular aches and pain.

ZOONOSES: Zoonoses are diseases of microbiological origin that can be transmitted from animals to people. The causes of the diseases can be bacteria, viruses, parasites, and fungi.

The occurrence of viral hemorrhagic fevers in areas as widely separated as Korea, Arizona, and Africa highlight the global distribution of the virus that cause hemorrhagic fevers. A particular virus may be more localized; for example, the viruses that cause Ebola appear to be localized to a few regions in Africa. However, because so little is still known about viral hemorrhagic fevers, it is possible that the true distribution of the various viruses is not yet known.

■ Treatment and Prevention

Hemorrhagic diseases are difficult to treat because outbreaks occur quickly, often in remote regions of the world. The speed and ferocity of the infection often means that patients are near death by the time they are seen by a health care provider. Vaccines are available only for yellow fever and Argentine hemorrhagic fever. For the remaining hemorrhagic fevers, the best prevention is to avoid contact with animals that are known to be hosts of the particular virus. However, in many cases, a population has little knowledge of the infections and their exposure risks, making prevention virtually impossible. One exception is hantavirus pulmonary syndrome in the United States. This disease has been well publicized and many people are aware that it is spread by rodents. When insects are involved in the transmission of a virus, spraying programs that kill insect populations, especially during their breeding season, can be helpful.

When combating an outbreak, isolating infected patients from other patients can help reduce the spread of the disease. In addition, all protective clothing and soiled material used in patient treatment should be stored in a secure container until it can be destroyed (usually by incineration).

■ Impacts and Issues

While relatively little is known about viral hemorrhagic fevers, they may have a serious impact on life in the areas of the world where they occur. For example, it is estimated that 100,000–300,000 Lassa fever infections occur annually in regions of West Africa where that virus is most prevalent, and about 5,000 of those infected die of the disease. But, since the rodent species that carries the virus is found much more widely, the actual range of Lassa fever may be much greater. In regions where the virus is found, about 15% of people admitted to hospital have Lassa fever; many more people never make it to a hospital, so the actual impact of the disease is difficult to determine.

As of 2007, much less is known about hemorrhagic fevers than remains to be discovered. One reason for this lack of knowledge is that the infections are very difficult to study during an outbreak. Health care providers faced with an outbreak struggle to mount a quick and efficient response that can save lives. Sometimes, cultural norms and taboos in remote regions hinder efforts to contain outbreaks and study their cause. For instance, during the 2005 Ebola outbreak in the Cuvette Ouest region of the Republic of Congo, medical workers from United Nations aid agencies arrived at the scene wearing white protective biohazard suits and were met with skepticism and hostility, as the color white is associated with evil in the remote village where the outbreak first occurred.

Viral hemorrhagic fevers can only be studied in a few specialized laboratories known as biosafety level four (BSL-4) laboratories. These laboratories are designed with safety and containment features that make it safe for researchers to work with the viruses and that prevent escape of the viruses outside of the lab. In BSL-4 laboratories, hemorrhagic fevers are studied in a high-containment environment, where incoming and outgoing airflow is controlled and where researchers wear protective clothing that includes one-piece positive pressure suits with separate ventilation systems. Protocols for studying the viruses that cause hemorrhagic fevers include restricted access to the laboratory, working under Class III biological safety cabinets, and decontamination following work with the virus. Currently, there are about 30 BSL-4 laboratories in the world, 10 of which are in the United States.

SEE ALSO *Ebola; Marburg Hemorrhagic Fever.*

IN CONTEXT: SCIENTIFIC QUESTIONS

Ebola virus and Marburg virus are the two known members of the filovirus family that cause hemorrhagic fevers. Ebola viruses were first isolated from humans during concurrent outbreaks of VHF in northern Zaire and southern Sudan in 1976. An earlier outbreak of VHF caused by Marburg virus occurred in Marburg, Germany, in 1967 when laboratory workers were exposed to infected tissue from monkeys imported from Uganda. Two subtypes of Ebola virus—Ebola-Sudan and Ebola-Zaire—previously have been associated with disease in humans. In 1994, a single case of infection from a newly described Ebola virus occurred in a person in Cote d'Ivoire. In 1989, an outbreak among monkeys imported into the United States from the Philippines was caused by another Ebola virus but was not associated with human disease.

Initial clinical manifestations of Ebola hemorrhagic fever include fever, headache, chills, myalgia (muscle aches throughout the body), and malaise; subsequent manifestations include severe abdominal pain, vomiting, and diarrhea. In reported outbreaks, fifty percent to ninety percent of cases have been fatal.

The natural reservoirs for these viruses are not known. Although nonhuman primates were involved in the 1967 Marburg outbreak, the 1989 U.S. outbreak, and the 1994 Côte d'Ivoire case, their role as virus reservoirs is unknown. Transmission of the virus to secondary cases occurs through close personal contact with infectious blood or other body fluids or tissue. In previous outbreaks, secondary cases occurred among persons who provided medical care for patients; secondary cases also occurred among patients exposed to reused needles. Although aerosol spread has not been documented among humans, this mode of transmission has been demonstrated among nonhuman primates. Based on this information, the high fatality rate, and lack of specific treatment or a vaccine, work with this virus in the laboratory setting requires biosafety level four containment.

BIBLIOGRAPHY

Books

Drexler, Madeline. *Secret Agents: The Menace of Emerging Infections.* New York: Penguin, 2003.

Powell, Michael, and Oliver Fischer. *101 Diseases You Don't Want to Get.* New York: Thunder's Mouth Press, 2005.

Zimmerman, Barry E., and David J. Zimmerman. *Killer Germs.* New York: McGraw-Hill, 2002.

Brian Hoyle

Hepatitis A

Introduction

Hepatitis is an inflammation of the liver that can be caused by exposure to chemicals including alcohol, or by any one of six hepatitis viruses. Hepatitis A infection is caused by the Hepatitis A virus (HAV), and was formerly known as infectious hepatitis. HAV was discovered in the early 1970s in the stool of a patient incubating the disease. Hepatitis A is an acute disease, with symptoms including nausea, malaise, diarrhea and enlarged liver. Some infected people, particularly children, have no symptoms. Unlike other forms of hepatitis, it does not progress to chronic disease, which damages the liver.

Hepatitis A has been on the decline in developed countries since the 1970s, although epidemics still occur, especially under conditions of overcrowding and poor hygiene. It is still a risk to travelers, as HAV can be spread through seafood, fruit, and vegetables that have been in contact with contaminated water. Those at risk can be protected through vaccination against HAV.

Disease History, Characteristics, and Transmission

Hepatitis A is a single-stranded RNA virus (that is, its genetic material is made of RNA, not DNA), unrelated to the other hepatitis viruses. During its average incubation time of 28 days, it first infects the intestines and then passes through the blood into the liver. The onset of symptoms including nausea, loss of appetite, diarrhea and fever, is acute. The person with hepatitis A may have an enlarged liver with pain and tenderness in the upper

	Hepatitis A				
Number of Acute Clinical Cases Reported	**2005**	**2004**	**2003**	**2002**	**2001**
	4,488	5,683	7,653	8,795	10,616
Estimated Number of Acute Clinical Cases	19,000	24,000	33,000	38,000	45,000
Estimated Number of New Infections — Current	42,000	56,000	61,000	73,000	93,000
Historical			**mean**	**min**	**max**
1990-1999			301,000	181,000	373,000
1980-1989			254,000	221,000	380,000
Number of Persons with Chronic Infection	no chronic infection				
Estimated Annual Number of Chronic Liver Disease Deaths	no chronic infection				
Percent Ever Infected	31.3%				

Table showing the number of hepatitis A cases from 2001 to 2005. *Data courtesy of Centers for Disease Control.*

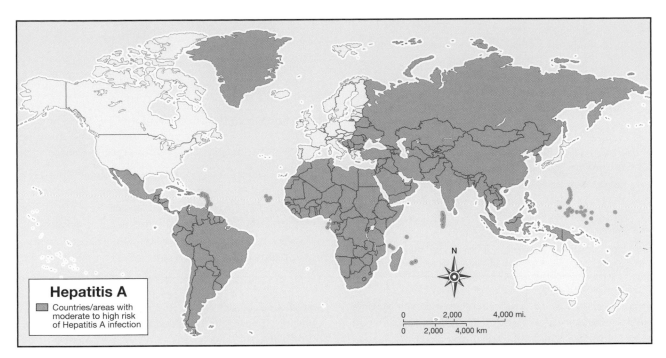

Hepatitis A

■ Countries/areas with moderate to high risk of Hepatitis A infection

0   2,000   4,000 mi.
0   2,000   4,000 km

Map showing outbreaks of hepatitis A in 2003.   © *Copyright World Health Organization (WHO). Reproduced by permission.*

right abdomen. Many go on to develop jaundice, a yellowing of the skin and eyes resulting from liver inflammation. The urine may be dark and stools a pale clay color.

The vast majority of cases of hepatitis A clear up within a week or so, although 15% are prolonged and relapsing over a period of months. The disease does not, however, become chronic like hepatitis B and hepatitis C. Only 0.3% of the cases reported to the Centers for Disease Control and Prevention (CDC) prove fatal, although the mortality rate rises to nearly two percent in those over 50 years of age. Hepatitis A is transmitted through the fecal-oral route, commonly through eating seafood, raw fruit, or vegetables that have come into contact with water contaminated with infected sewage.

■ Scope and Distribution

Adults are more likely than children to develop symptoms of hepatitis A. Household and sexual partners of those with hepatitis A are at elevated risk of contracting the disease, as are men who have sex with men, and both injecting and non-injecting drug users. Epidemic of hepatitis A are fairly common in institutions such as prisons and nursing homes, and among those of low socioeconomic status living in overcrowded conditions.

According to CDC data, there were 4,488 cases of acute hepatitis A in the USA in 2005. Computer modeling of this data suggests the true number of new infec-

tions that year was about 42,000 (many of which would have been asymptomatic). This represents the lowest figure since 2001, which is a reflection of the decline in hepatitis A in developed countries, although epidemics may still occur where hygiene is poor. Hepatitis A most often represents a risk to those traveling into less developed countries where the disease is common.

■ Treatment and Prevention

There is no definitive treatment for hepatitis A, and often the disease resolves with adequate nutrition and rest. Those at risk of infection can be given either immune serum globulin, prepared from pooled plasma, or a vaccine against hepatitis A (or both). There are two hepatitis A vaccines, both made of inactivated virus. One protects against hepatitis A only, while the other is a combined hepatitis A and hepatitis B vaccine.

■ Impacts and Issues

People travel more widely today than ever before which means they may be exposed to diseases they otherwise would not be. For travelers, Hepatitis A is the most common preventable infection. The extent of the risk depends upon the length of stay, the living conditions in the place visited, and the level of hepatitis A in the country visited. In general, the risk of contracting

WORDS TO KNOW

FECAL-ORAL ROUTE: The transmission of minute particles of fecal material from one organism (human or animal) to the mouth of another organism.

IMMUNE GLOBULIN: Globulins are a type of protein found in blood. The immunoglobulins (also called immune globulins) are Y-shaped globulins that act as antibodies, attaching themselves to invasive cells or materials in the body so that they can be identified and attacked by the immune system. There are five immune globulins, designated IgM, IgG, IgA, IgD, and IgE.

INACTIVATED VIRUS: Inactivated virus is incapable of causing disease but still stimulates the immune system to respond by forming antibodies.

JAUNDICE: Jaundice is a condition in which a person's skin and the whites of the eyes are discolored a shade of yellow due to an increased level of bile pigments in the blood resulting from liver disease. Jaundice is sometimes called icterus, from a Greek word for the condition.

hepatitis A is low in North America (except Mexico), New Zealand, Australia and developed European countries. However, epidemics still occur even on standard tourist itineraries. Before traveling, it is advisable to check out the latest information on proposed destinations through public health departments and the Centers for Disease Control and Prevention.

In destinations where high standards of hygiene and sanitation may be lacking, it is recommended to stick to bottled water and avoid ice, seafood, raw fruit and vegetables, and foods sold by street venders. Personal hygiene is also essential—thorough handwashing after the bathroom and before eating or preparing food will help avoid transmission of HAV.

Despite food safety measures, outbreaks of Hepatitis A sometimes occur wherever food is prepared and served. In February 2007, an employee at a well-known catering company in Los Angeles, California was diagnosed with Hepatitis A, sparking an investigation into

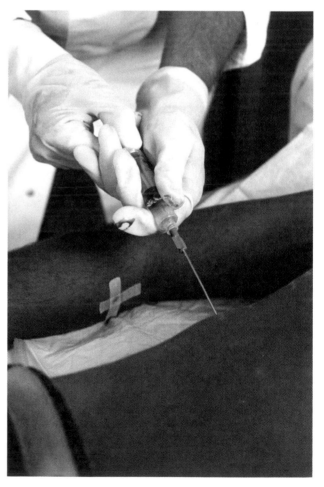

A doctor removes a sample of liver tissue to test for hepatitis or cirrhosis (scarring of the liver). *Phanie/Photo Researchers, Inc.*

IN CONTEXT: PERSONAL RESPONSIBILITY AND PREVENTION

The National Center for HIV/AIDs, Viral Hepatitis, STD and TB prevention recommends that with regard to prevention of Viral Hepatitis A:

- Hepatitis A vaccine is the best protection.
- Short-term protection against hepatitis A is available from immune globulin. It can be given before and within 2 weeks after coming in contact with HAV.
- Always wash your hands with soap and water after using the bathroom, changing a diaper, and before preparing and eating food.

SOURCE: *Centers for Disease Control and Prevention (CDC)*

events the company had catered during the concurrent Hollywood entertainment industry awards season. Several celebrities and movie industry executives were contacted by health authorities, recommending immune globulin injections to prevent Hepatitis A infection after they were possibly exposed to the disease by food served during the festivities.

SEE ALSO *Food-borne Disease and Food Safety; Hepatitis B; Hepatitis C; Travel and Infectious Disease.*

BIBLIOGRAPHY

Books

Achord, James L. *Understanding Hepatitis.* Oxford, MS: University of Mississippi Press, 2002.

Web Sites

Centers for Disease Control and Prevention (CDC). "Hepatitis A Fact Sheet." October 4, 2006 <http://www.cdc.gov/hepatitis> (accessed March 2, 2007).

Hepatitis B

■ Introduction

Hepatitis B (HBV) is one of six viruses which cause hepatitis, an inflammation of the liver. Formerly known as post-transfusion or serum hepatitis, HBV is transmitted through infected blood and other body fluids, rather than by food or casual contact. Infection can cause acute disease, with symptoms including nausea, malaise, diarrhea, joint pain, and abdominal pain. In some cases, HBV infection progresses to chronic disease, damaging the liver and causing cirrhosis and liver cancer, which may be fatal. In countries where HBV infection is com-

mon, liver cancer rates are relatively high. Since the advent of screening of blood for HBV in developed countries, rates of infection have gone down, although people are still at risk through injecting drug use and sexual contact. An effective vaccine helps to protect babies from mother-to-child transmission and to stop those who work with blood from being infected with HBV through accidental exposure.

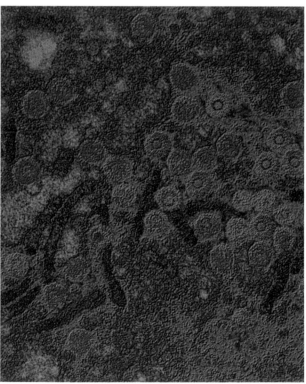

A virologist holds a sample tray with sections that contain live hepatitis B viruses.   *Will & Deni McIntyre/Photo Researchers, Inc.*

Micrograph of the hepatitis B virus shows orange spheres with red cores, known as Dane particles, which are the complete virus. The brown rods, parts of the disassembled virus, are inactive.   *Eye of Science/Photo Researchers, Inc.*

Number of Acute Clinical Cases Reported	Hepatitis B				
	2005	**2004**	**2003**	**2002**	**2001**
	5,494	6,212	7,526	8,064	7,844
Estimated Number of Acute Clinical Cases	15,000	17,000	21,000	23,000	22,000
Estimated Number of New Infections Current	51,000	60,000	73,000	79,000	78,000
Historical			**mean**	**min**	**max**
1990-1999			140,000	79,000	232,000
1980-1989			259,000	208,000	287,000
Number of Persons with Chronic Infection	1.25 million persons				
Estimated Annual Number of Chronic Liver Disease Deaths	3,000-5,000				
Percent Ever Infected	4.9%				

Table depicting the number of hepatitis B cases from 2001 to 2005. *Data courtesy of Centers for Disease Control.*

■ Disease History, Characteristics, and Transmission

HBV is unrelated to any known human virus, although similar liver viruses are found in other animal species. It exists as spherical particles with double stranded DNA as the genetic material. Around 70% of those infected with HBV will develop symptoms around 12 weeks after exposure. These symptoms include nausea, diarrhea, joint pain, abdominal discomfort, fatigue, and loss of appetite. Jaundice—a yellowing of the skin and whites of the eyes—may develop, along with dark urine and clay colored stools. The symptoms may continue for several months. In around 10 percent of cases, the HBV infection causes chronic viral hepatitis. Around 15–25 percent of those who develop chronic HBV will die of the disease, through cirrhosis (scarring) of the liver or liver cancer.

Transmission of HBV occurs through infected blood and other body fluids. Sex contact with an infected person, or injecting drug use with sharing of needles and other items, is strongly associated with HBV transmission. The virus is highly infectious; experiments have shown that it can be spread through a mere 0.0001 ml of blood. But for most people the HBV infection clears up within a few weeks. However, those with chronic disease remain infectious, even if they do not have symptoms. HBV infection can also pass from mother to child through contact with infected blood during childbirth.

WORDS TO KNOW

CIRRHOSIS: Cirrhosis is a chronic, degenerative, irreversible liver disease in which normal liver cells are damaged and are then replaced by scar tissue. Cirrhosis changes the structure of the liver and the blood vessels that nourish it. The disease reduces the liver's ability to manufacture proteins and process hormones, nutrients, medications, and poisons.

INTRAVENOUS: It the vein. For example, the insertion of a hypodermic needle into a vein to instill a fluid, withdraw or transfuse blood, or start an intravenous feeding.

JAUNDICE: Jaundice is a condition in which a person's skin and the whites of the eyes are discolored a shade of yellow due to an increased level of bile pigments in the blood resulting from liver disease. Jaundice is sometimes called icterus, from a Greek word for the condition.

■ Scope and Distribution

The Centers for Disease Control and Prevention (CDC) recorded 5,494 cases of acute HBV infection in the United States in 2005. Using this data, the CDC

IN CONTEXT: SOCIAL AND PERSONAL RESPONSIBILITY

The National Center for HIV, STD, and TB Prevention, Divisions of HIV/AIDS Prevention at Centers for Disease Control and Prevention (CDC) states that the following are the best practices to reduce the risk of contracting Hepatitis B:

- "Hepatitis B vaccine is the best protection.
- If you are having sex, but not with one steady partner, use latex condoms correctly and every time you have sex. The efficacy of latex condoms in preventing infection with HBV is unknown, but their proper use may reduce transmission.
- If you are pregnant, you should get a blood test for hepatitis B; Infants born to HBV-infected mothers should be given HBIG (hepatitis B immune globulin) and vaccine within 12 hours after birth.
- Do not shoot drugs; if you shoot drugs, stop and get into a treatment program; if you can't stop, never share drugs, needles, syringes, water, or 'works,' and get vaccinated against hepatitis A and B.
- Do not share personal care items that might have blood on them (razors, toothbrushes).
- Consider the risks if you are thinking about getting a tattoo or body piercing. You might get infected if the tools have someone else's blood on them or if the artist or piercer does not follow good health practices.
- If you have or had hepatitis B, do not donate blood, organs, or tissue.
- If you are a health care or public safety worker, get vaccinated against hepatitis B, and always follow routine barrier precautions and safely handle needles and other sharps."

predicted that there were around 51,000 total new HBV infections that year. The incidence of infection is on the decline in the United States, but there are 1.25 million people already carrying the infection. Each year, between 3,000 and 5,000 people in the United States die of complications of chronic HBV infection such as liver cirrhosis and liver cancer.

Infants are most at risk of developing chronic HBV infection even though they are unlikely to have symptoms of acute disease. Others at high risk include sex and household partners of those with chronic HBV, men who have sex with men (especially if they have more than one sexual partner), intravenous drug users, and people whose work brings them into contact with blood, such as healthcare workers.

Around 10% of those with the human immunodeficiency virus (HIV) are also chronic carriers of HBV. The risk of HBV infection has also been shown to be higher

among those whose parents were born in Southeast Asia, Africa, the Amazon basin, the Pacific Islands, and the Middle East. Rates of HBV in part of Africa and Asia are high and liver cancer accounts for 20–30 percent of all cancer cases in these areas.

■ Treatment and Prevention

There is no specific treatment for acute HBV infection once acquired. Adequate nutrition and rest are most often recommended to ease symptoms. Chronic infection can be treated with interferon, an immune system protein, and antiviral drugs such as lamivudine.

The hepatitis B vaccine is manufactured through genetic engineering, a process that involves inserting the HBV gene into yeast cells. It was introduced in 1982 and is highly effective against infection. The vaccine is now recommended for all newborns. Adults with an increased risk of exposure to HBV through work, travel, sexual practices, or drug use are also encouraged to get vaccinated.

■ Impacts and Issues

HBV is a bloodborne infection. Those who are, or have been, infected should not donate blood, organs, or tissue. People should not share razors or toothbrushes, which may carry invisible traces of blood. People who inject drugs should never reuse or share needles. Needle exchange programs in some countries have demonstrated limited success in reducing incidence of HBV among intravenous drug users.

Nearly one million people die each year from cirrhosis or liver cancer caused by HBV. Deaths from HBV-related illnesses disproportionately affect the developing world. HBV is endemic in some regions. In China, as much as 10 percent of the population is HBV infected. In certain parts of Eastern and Southeast Asia, 7–10 percent of all pregnant women are infected; 70–90 percent of the children born to these women become infected during childbirth. Though HBV is vaccine-preventable, the vaccine remains significantly more costly than other childhood vaccines.

Though most HBV infections are acquired during infancy or childhood, HBV has life-long effects. The social and economic effects of populations with high rates of HBV infections are substantial. Care of patients with chronic HBV is costly. HBV is one of the few viruses that can lead to cancer, although the way in which it does so is not well understood. HBV-related liver cancer and cirrhosis increase demand for liver transplants in an environment already strained by a lack of suitable donor organs. If the HBV vaccine could be made more readily available in those countries where infection is common, it could reduce the number of cases of liver cancer among the population.

SEE ALSO *Blood Supply and Infectious Disease; Bloodborne Pathogens; Hepatitis C.*

BIBLIOGRAPHY

Books

Koff, R.S., and G.Y. Wu. *Chronic Viral Hepatitis.* Totowa: Humana Press, 2002.

Wilson, Walter R., and Merle A. Sande. *Current Diagnosis & Treatment in Infectious Diseases.* New York: McGraw Hill, 2001

Web Sites

Centers for Disease Control and Prevention (CDC). "Hepatitis B Fact Sheet." November 7, 2006 <http://www.cdc.gov/hepatitis> (accessed April 25, 2007).

Hepatitis C

■ Introduction

The Hepatitis C virus (HCV) is one of six viruses that cause hepatitis, an inflammation of the liver. Formerly known as non-A non-B hepatitis (HCV was not discovered until 1989), Hepatitis C accounts for the majority of cases acquired through infected blood transfusions that cannot be attributed to Hepatitis B virus (HBV). Unlike Hepatitis A and Hepatitis B, Hepatitis C rarely causes an acute infection, but many cases progress to chronic hepatitis, which can cause liver damage and eventually lead to liver cancer. Hepatitis C is a major indication for liver transplantation.

Antiviral treatment is available for hepatitis C, but there is, as yet, no vaccine to protect against the disease. For many people around the world, especially in the Far East, hepatitis C is a silent killer as even those with chronic infection may have no symptoms until liver disease is well advanced.

■ Disease History, Characteristics, and Transmission

HCV is an RNA virus (that is, its genetic material consists of RNA rather than DNA) and is a flavivirus, related

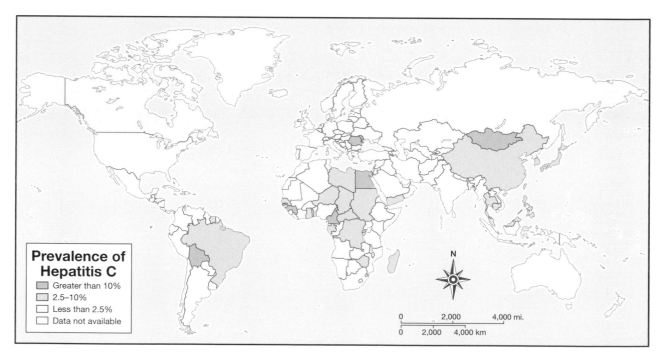

Prevalence of Hepatitis C
- Greater than 10%
- 2.5–10%
- Less than 2.5%
- Data not available

Map showing the prevalence of hepatitis C infection throughout the world in 2003. © Copyright World Health Organization (WHO). Reproduced by permission.

Hepatitis C					
	2005	**2004**	**2003**	**2002**	**2001**
Number of Acute Clinical Cases Reported	no data		no data	no data	
Estimated Number of Acute Clinical Cases	3200	4200	4500	4800	3900
Estimated Number of New Infections — Current	20,000	26,000	28,000	29,000	24,000
Historical			**mean**	**min**	**max**
1990-1999			67,000	36,000	179,000
1980-1989			232,000	180,000	291,000
Number of Persons with Chronic Infection	3.2 million persons				
Estimated Annual Number of Chronic Liver Disease Deaths	8,000-10,000				
Percent Ever Infected	1.6%				

Table illuminating the number of hepatitis C cases from 2001 to 2005. *Data courtesy of Centers for Disease Control.*

to the viruses causing yellow fever and dengue. It exists in six different genotypes which have varying distributions around the world and which respond differently to treatment. The incubation period for HCV is 6 to 12 weeks and most acute infections do not cause any symptoms. In 55 to 85% of cases, HCV becomes chronic over a period of several years, during which time the liver becomes progressively inflamed and damaged. Around 70% of those who are chronically infected with HCV will develop significant liver disease, including cirrhosis (scarring) and/or liver cancer.

HCV is a bloodborne pathogen, that is, a disease-causing organism transmitted through infected blood and body fluids that may contain blood. With the screening and treatment of blood and blood products, transmission of HCV by blood transfusion or receipt of blood clotting factors is now rare in Western countries. This leaves injection drug use as the main route of HCV infection in North America and Europe. To a lesser extent, Hepatitis C is transmitted through body fluids during sexual contact. Occupational exposure, through needlestick injuries by healthcare workers, may also transmit HCV. Hepatitis C can also pass from an infected mother to her baby during childbirth, although the risk is relatively low. Hepatitis C is not spread through coughing, sneezing, kissing, or casual contact between people.

Scope and Distribution

The Centers for Disease Control and Prevention (CDC) estimates that there were 20,000 new HCV infections in 2005, which is a decrease over previous years. Around 3.2 million people in the United States have chronic hepatitis C and about 1.6% of the population have probably been infected at some stage during their lifetime. Injecting drug users are at high risk of HCV and thousands of people with hemophilia (a blood disorder requiring the administration of blood clotting factors) became infected through receipt of blood products before 1987. Sex with an infected person or with multiple partners carries an intermediate risk of infection.

Treatment and Prevention

Treatment for hepatitis C consists of injections of interferon, an immune system protein, which may be combined with the oral antiviral drug ribavirin over a period of months. Response to treatment depends upon the genotype of HCV with which the patient is infected. Those with genotype 1 are less likely to respond to antiviral treatment than those with genotype 2 or 3 and will require a longer course of treatment. There are side effects, such as flulike symptoms, anemia, and depression associated with hepatitis C treatment; not all patients are able to tolerate it.

To reduce the risk of spreading HCV, people who inject drugs should not share needles or other drug-related items. Toothbrushes, razors, and other personal items that could contain invisible traces of blood should not be shared. A person with hepatitis C cannot donate blood, organs, or tissue. Condoms may provide some protection to those having sex with an infected person. Occupational exposures for healthcare workers can be avoided by following the appropriate guidance on cleaning up blood spills, using needles with protective shields, and other infection control procedures. As there is no

WORDS TO KNOW

BLOODBORNE PATHOGEN: Disease-causing agents carried or transported in the blood. Bloodborne infections are those in which the infectious agent is transmitted from one person to another via contaminated blood.

INCUBATION PERIOD: Incubation period refers to the time between exposure to disease causing virus or bacteria and the appearance of symptoms of the infection. Depending on the microorganism, the incubation time can range from a few hours (an example is food poisoning due to *Salmonella*) to a decade or more (an example is acquired immunodeficiency syndrome, or AIDS).

STRAIN: A subclass or a specific genetic variation of an organism.

vaccine against HCV, these practical precautions against infection offer the most efficient protection strategies.

■ Impacts and Issues

Hepatitis C is a silent killer because many people do not realize they are infected and can pass the virus on to others. Moreover, the infection causes progressive damage to the liver, but may not produce any symptoms for many years. HCV is the most common cause of unexplained liver disease around the world and responsible for many deaths from liver cancer. The CDC recommends that those at risk of infection be tested for HCV in order to help identify infections early and maximize the chances for successful treatment.

Many persons with tattoos and body piercings may also be at higher risk of harboring the Hepatitis C virus than previously thought. Research at the University of Texas Southwestern Medical Center has shown that commercially acquired tattoos among persons in one study group accounted for more than twice as many hepatitis C infections as injection-drug use. Data from the CDC does not support this conclusion, as only a small percentage of hepatitis C cases reported to the CDC involve people with a documented history of receiving tattoos. CDC officials have found, however, that outbreaks of hepatitis C can be traced back to tattoo and piercing establishments, and that often oversight of sterilization techniques at such establishments are lacking and not adequately monitored by health authorities. Currently, the CDC is conducting a large-scale study that could provide definitive scientific evidence of any links that exist between tattooing and body piercing and the incidence of hepatitis C.

The World Health Organization estimates that worldwide, for every one person infected with the virus that causes AIDS, four people are infected with HCV. Within the next two decades, many of these persons now displaying relatively few symptoms will progress to the

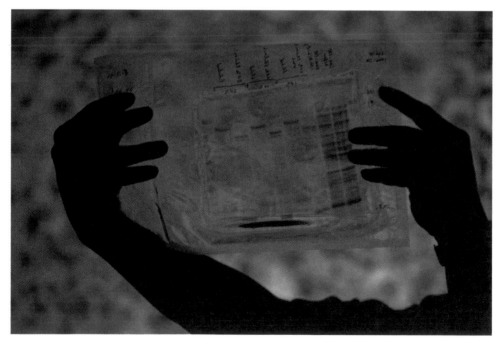

A research scientist studies a DNA map of the hepatitis C virus. *Richard T. Nowitz/Photo Researchers, Inc.*

end stages of the disease. The number of cases of cirrhosis, hepatocellular carcinoma (liver cancer), and liver failure are expected to dramatically increase, placing a major burden on healthcare resources. The need for donor livers for transplantation is expected to increase more than 500% during this time.

In 2006, scientists reproduced the Hepatitis C virus in mice cells, and identified a gene called protein kinase R (PKR) that blocks the virus from replicating within the cell. This could provide clues as to why interferon, which stimulates PKR to keep the HCV in check, works better against some genotypes (strains) of Hepatitis C virus than others. This research is in its initial stages, but by understanding how the virus responds to interferon treatment, scientists hope to design more effective long-term treatments for HCV. In the meantime, the blooming hepatitis C epidemic has sparked some of the largest and most varied efforts at promoting alternative and holistic treatments for HCV. No complimentary or alternative treatment has yet been proven both safe and effective for Hepatitis C infection. The National Center for Complementary and Alternative Medicine, however, is sponsoring a second (phase II) clinical trial to determine possible benefits of silymarin compounds in milk thistle for liver disease associated with hepatitis C.

SEE ALSO *Blood Supply and Infectious Disease; Bloodborne Pathogens; Hepatitis B.*

BIBLIOGRAPHY

Books

Askari, Fred. *Hepatitis C: The Silent Epidemic.* Cambridge, MA: Da Capo, 2005.

Koff, R.S and Wu, G.Y. *Chronic Viral Hepatitis.* Totowa: Humana Press, 2002.

IN CONTEXT: PERSONAL RESPONSIBILITY AND PREVENTION

The National Center for HIV/AIDs, Viral Hepatitis, STD and TB prevention states that the following persons may be at risk for hepatitis C and should contact their medical care provider for a blood test:

- If you were notified that you received blood from a donor who later tested positive for Hepatitis C.
- If you have ever injected illegal drugs, even if you experimented a few times many years ago.
- If you received a blood transfusion or solid organ transplant before July, 1992.
- If you were a recipient of clotting factor(s) made before 1987.
- If you have ever been on long-term kidney dialysis.
- If you have evidence of liver disease (e.g., persistently abnormal ALT levels).

SOURCE: *Centers for Disease Control and Prevention (CDC)*

Web Sites

Centers for Disease Control and Prevention (CDC). "Hepatitis C Fact Sheet." May 24, 2005 <http://www.cdc.gov/hepatitis> (accessed February 25, 2007).

Susan Aldridge

Hepatitis D

■ Introduction

The Hepatitis D virus (HDV) is one of six viruses that cause hepatitis, an inflammation of the liver. It is unusual in that it is found only with Hepatitis B virus (HBV) infection. HDV is transmitted in a similar way to HBV, that is, through infected blood and other body fluids, rather than by food or casual contact. HDV infection can cause acute disease, with symptoms similar to that of HBV, including nausea, malaise, diarrhea, joint pain and abdominal pain. People with HBV and HDV tend to be at higher risk of serious liver damage and death than those with HBV alone. However, HDV is uncommon in the United States, and most cases occur in injecting drug users.

■ Disease History, Characteristics, and Transmission

HDV is a single-stranded RNA virus which exists as one of seven genotypes (genetic identities). There are two types of HDV infection. Hepatitis D may occur as a co-infection, that is, simultaneously with HBV, or it may be seen as a superinfection in someone who already has chronic HBV infection. The symptoms of acute HDV infection are difficult to distinguish from those of hepatitis A and hepatitis B, and include jaundice, a yellowing of the skin and whites of the eyes, fatigue, abdominal pain, loss of appetite, nausea, vomiting, joint pain, and dark urine. A condition called fulminant hepatitis, which is a sudden, severe form of the disease with rapid onset, is more likely to develop from acute HDV infection than with Hepatitis A or Hepatitis B. Around 2–20% of those with co-infection will develop acute liver failure, which is often fatal. Superinfection causes a worsening in the severity and progression of Hepatitis B; those affected are likely to develop chronic cirrhosis of the liver or liver cancer.

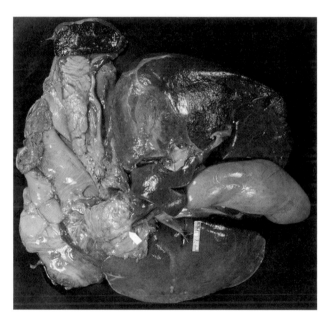

A human liver shows the effects of hepatitis.   *Martin M. Rotker/Photo Researchers, Inc.*

Transmission of HDV is similar to that of HBV, that is, through infected blood and other body fluids. Sexual contact with an infected person, or injecting drugs with shared needles is strongly associated with HDV transmission. Rarely, HDV infection can pass from mother to child through contact with infected blood during childbirth.

■ Scope and Distribution

There are little surveillance data for hepatitis D, but the disease is less prominent in the United States (where there is no routine surveillance data), Northern Europe, and Japan. It is found mainly in Southern Europe, Africa, and South America. Estimates put the number of people infected with Hepatitis D at about 15 million people worldwide. Those at risk include injecting drug users, those on hemodialysis (filtering the blood by machine), sexual contacts of people with the infection, men who have sex with men, and those who may be exposed to HDV through their occupation.

■ Treatment and Prevention

There is no treatment for hepatitis D other than rest and adequate nutrition. Chronic infection can be treated with interferon, although response is less effective than if the person is infected only with Hepatitis B. Higher doses of interferon may be necessary with co-infection. Liver failure can be treated with liver transplant. Transmission of HDV is prevented in the same way as HBV, preventing contact with infected blood.

Blood is not screened specifically for HBV and HDV in all countries, so this is a possible route of infection, particularly when traveling abroad, for someone who already has hepatitis B. If someone is protected against HBV, then they are automatically protected from HDV as well. Therefore, the HBV vaccine is an effective method of preventing HDV transmission. Researchers are working on a vaccine specific for HDV.

■ Impacts and Issues

Hepatitis D is an unusual virus in that it cannot infect people on its own. It requires the presence of hepatitis B. Anyone who is at risk of hepatitis B infection may also be at risk of hepatitis D if they live an area where the virus is common. Being infected with both viruses leads to a poorer prognosis than being infected with hepatitis B alone.

In those parts of the world where hepatitis D is common, more widespread access to hepatitis B vaccine and screening and treatment of the blood supply could considerably cut the death toll from liver disease. Recent research suggests a decrease in HDV among drug users and prostitutes in Taipei, China. However, the virus has a new potential reservoir among the populations of male and immigrant prostitutes moving into the area. Increased surveillance of the health of these groups could help stop the spread of HDV in the area.

> ## WORDS TO KNOW
>
> **BLOODBORNE PATHOGEN:** Disease-causing agents carried or transported in the blood. Bloodborne infections are those in which the infectious agent is transmitted from one person to another via contaminated blood.
>
> **FULMINANT:** A fulminant infection is an infection that appears suddenly and whose symptoms are immediately severe.
>
> **RNA VIRUS:** An RNA virus is one whose genetic material consists of either single or double-stranded ribonucleic acid (RNA) rather than deoxyribonucleic acid (DNA).
>
> **SUPERINFECTION:** When a new infection occurs in a patient who already has some other infection, it is called a superinfection. For example, a bacterial infection appearing in a person who already had viral pneumonia would be a superinfection.

SEE ALSO *Blood Supply and Infectious Disease; Bloodborne Pathogens; Hepatitis B.*

BIBLIOGRAPHY

Books

Achord, James L. *Understanding Hepatitis.* Oxford, MS: University of Mississippi, 2002.

Web Sites

Centers for Disease Control and Prevention (CDC). "Hepatitis D Fact Sheet." <http://www.cdc.gov/hepatitis> (accessed March 5, 2007).

Stanford University. "Hepatitis D virus." <http://www.stanford.edu/group/virus/delta/2004hammon/Deltavirus.htm> (accessed March 5, 2007).

Hepatitis E

■ Introduction

Hepatitis is an inflammation of the liver that can be caused by exposure to chemicals, including alcohol, or by any one of six hepatitis viruses. Hepatitis E infection is caused by the Hepatitis E virus (HEV), and was shown to be a separate form of hepatitis in 1980. Hepatitis E infection is always acute, like hepatitis A virus (HAV) infection. It causes symptoms such as nausea, malaise, diarrhea, and enlarged liver. Occasionally HEV infection can be severe, especially among pregnant women. It is rare in the United States, but common in Asia and Africa, where epidemics may occur, Like HAV, HEV is spread through contaminated water and food. It is, therefore, a risk to travelers to areas where sanitation standards are poor. There is no commercially available vaccine against HEV; therefore prevention relies upon maintaining personal hygiene and avoiding potential sources of exposure.

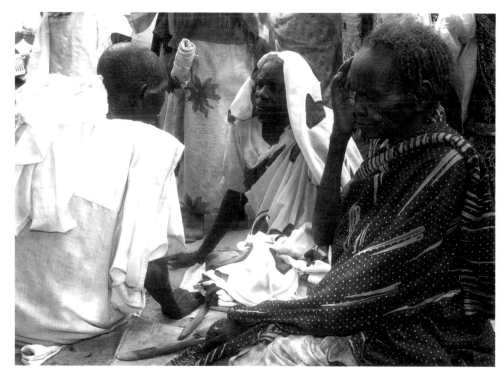

A group of displaced persons in the Darfur region of the Sudan wait for a medical visit in 2004. The UN health organization said that although the health situation in Darfur was stable at that time, an increasing number of cases of hepatitis E were spreading due to the consumption of contaminated water. Thousands of displaced people live in such camps.   *AP Images.*

■ Disease History, Characteristics, and Transmission

The hepatitis E virus is a single-stranded RNA virus, with no outer envelope, but distinguished by the appearance of spikelike structures on its surface. The incubation time of HEV is three to eight weeks. Infection may give rise to no symptoms or just very mild illness. Symptoms of HEV can infection include jaundice, a yellowing of the skin and whites of the eyes, nausea, vomiting, diarrhea, fatigue, fever, dark urine, and pale stools. In 0.5 to 4% of cases, HEV infection is fulminant, that is, severe and rapid in onset. Fulminant hepatitis E is fatal to mother and child in about 20% of cases if it occurs during late pregnancy. It is difficult to distinguish HEV from HAV infection and other forms of acute viral hepatitis. It does not progress to chronic disease, unlike hepatitis B and hepatitis C.

Hepatitis E is transmitted by the fecal-oral route, via contaminated water and foods such as shellfish and raw fruits and vegetables. Unlike Hepatitis B and Hepatitis C, Hepatitis E is not transmitted sexually or through blood.

■ Scope and Distribution

Testing for antibodies against HEV has suggested that strains of the virus occur around the world. However, HEV infection is more of a problem in developing countries and epidemics occur in Central and Southeast Asia, North and West Africa, and Mexico. The risk is highest where access to clean water is restricted and where sanitation is poor. Travelers to such area are at risk of HEV infection, as they are to infection with HAV. Symptomatic infection with HEV is most common in the 15–40 age group. Children get infected also, but are more likely to be asymptomatic.

■ Treatment and Prevention

Hepatitis E infection is usually self-limiting and there is no specific treatment for it, other than rest and adequate nutrition. A vaccine against HEV is under development. In the absence of a widely available vaccine, prevention of HEV infection, depends upon maintaining a good standard of personal hygiene, including handwashing after using the bathroom and before eating or preparing food.

■ Impacts and Issues

Hepatitis E is rare in the United States, but those who live or travel to developing countries may be at risk of exposure. While the disease is generally not serious, it occasionally develops in a potentially fatal form called fulminant hepatitis that can be especially dangerous in pregnant women. Therefore, travelers to areas where HEV is endemic are advised to take precautions. In destinations where high standards of hygiene and sanitation may be lacking, it is best to drink bottled water and avoid ice, seafood, and raw fruit and vegetables. For those who live in developing countries, improvement of the infrastructure with respect to access to clean drinking water and adequate sanitation is the most effective method of preventing outbreaks with viruses like HEV. If research on a vaccine against HEV is successful, then it may prove worthwhile to carry out mass vaccination among populations at risk. Meanwhile, outbreaks of Hepatitis E can be limited by adequate surveillance measures.

SEE ALSO *Hepatitis A; Hepatitis B; Travel and Infectious Disease.*

BIBLIOGRAPHY

Periodicals

Seppa, N. "Hepatitis E Vaccine Passes Critical Test." *Science News* 171 (March 3, 2007): 9, 131.

Web Sites

Centers for Disease Control and Prevention (CDC). "Hepatitis E Fact Sheet." Nov 1, 2005 <http://www.cdc.gov/hepatitis> (accessed March 5, 2007).
World Health Organization. "Hepatitis E." <http://www.who.int/mediacentre/factsheets/fs280/en/print.html> (accessed March 7, 2007).

WORDS TO KNOW

FECAL-ORAL ROUTE: The transmission of minute particles of fecal material from one organism (human or animal) to the mouth of another organism.

FULMINANT: A fulminant infection is an infection that appears suddenly and whose symptoms are immediately severe.

JAUNDICE: Jaundice is a condition in which a person's skin and the whites of the eyes are discolored a shade of yellow due to an increased level of bile pigments in the blood resulting from liver disease. Jaundice is sometimes called icterus, from a Greek word for the condition.

STRAIN: A subclass or a specific genetic variation of an organism.

Herpes Simplex 1 Virus

■ Introduction

The Herpes Simplex 1 virus (HSV-1) causes painful sores, known as cold sores, on the skin or in the eyes. Less frequently, HSV-1 can cause genital ulcers. HSV-1 is closely related to HSV-2, which is the virus generally associated with similar lesions in the genital area (known sometimes just as "herpes"). Both HSVs belong to the Herpes family of viruses, all of which exist as viral particles of diameter around 200 nm (nanometers), consisting of a protein exterior enclosing a molecule of double-stranded DNA. Other significant Herpes viruses include the Varicella-Zoster virus, which causes chicken pox, Epstein-Barr virus, and Cytomegalovirus (CMV). The Herpes virus invades cells, such as neurons, and may lie dormant for many years, causing no obvious symptoms. However, a herpes infection can be activated at any time and may often recur during life. Symptoms tend to occur only when the Herpes virus is active. Although the virus itself cannot be eliminated, symptoms of active infection, like cold sores, can be treated with antiviral drugs.

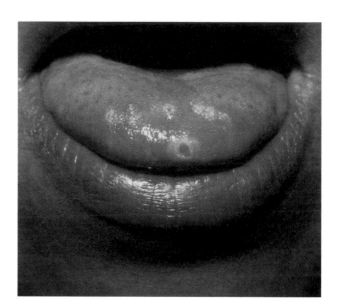

A cold sore on the tongue caused by the Herpes Simplex type I virus. © *Dr. Milton Reisch/Corbis.*

■ Disease History, Characteristics, and Transmission

HSV-1 often causes no symptoms when it first enters the body, creating a latent infection within nerve cells. However, in around one-quarter to one-third of those infected, it will eventually become active. Triggers for activation of HSV-1 include stress, sunlight exposure, fever, broken skin, and menstruation. When HSV-1 activation occurs, new virus particles are formed and may move from neurons to the mucous membranes of the body, such as the mouth, skin, and eyes.

HSV-1 reactivation is not always accompanied by symptoms. However, the virus particles may continue to replicate within surface cells, which then begin to swell, releasing fluid. This forms a blister—usually referred to as a fever blister or cold sore. Each blister contains millions of new virus particles and is highly infectious. A single blister or a cluster of them may occur, and they often recur around the same location on the upper or lower lip, nose, chin, cheeks, or inside of the mouth. The formation of a cold sore is often preceded by burning, tingling, itching, or pain in the area where the blister is going to form. The time between the warning signs and the appearance of the cold sore is typically a few hours to a day or so. Once the blister has formed, it breaks and produces a yellow crust. This falls off within a few days, leaving behind pinkish skin that heals without forming a scar. The whole process normally takes 8-10 days.

The fingers, generally around the fingernails (where the virus may enter through torn cuticles), are a common site of HSV-1 infection, which results in a painful condition known as herpetic whitlow. This area is especially vulnerable because it contains many nerve endings through which HSV-1 can be transmitted. Also, HSV-1 is the cause of *Herpes gladiatorum*—sometimes called "wrestler's herpes"—a herpes infection on the face, neck, chest, or arms that is spread via skin contact.

HSV-1 may also cause fever and swollen glands in children and tonsillitis, pharyngitis (throat infection), and even encephalitis (infection of the brain) among adults. Although HSV-1 encephalitis is rare, it still accounts for about 10 percent of cases of this infection in the United States.

HSV-1 is transmitted by person-to-person contact, via the mucous membranes—that is, through kissing and sexual intercourse. Contact with infected secretions from items such as cups, glasses, towels, and food is also a significant mode of transmission. In a person with an intact immune system, symptoms of reactivation may not be apparent, but they still make new copies of the HSV-1 virus. This phenomenon is known as viral shedding and leads to people without symptoms spreading HSV-1 unknowingly through the usual modes of transmission. HSV-1 can also be transmitted from mother to baby during childbirth, resulting in general infection of the newborn and possibly encephalitis.

■ Scope and Distribution

Herpes infections are found all around the world, but prevalence is influenced by age and socioeconomic status. In less developed countries, about one-third of children are infected by five years of age and this goes up to 70–80 percent by early adolescence. In developed countries, around 20 percent of children are infected by the age of five and 40–60 percent by early adulthood. People with weakened immunity, such as transplant recipients and HIV/AIDS patients, are more susceptible to serious HSV-1 infections. Those with eczema—whose skin is frequently broken or damaged—are often affected with widespread HSV-1 infection, a condition known as eczema herpeticum, which requires prompt treatment with antiviral drugs. Healthcare workers, such as anesthesiologists and dentists, are at risk of herpetic whitlow if their fingers come into contact with patients who have cold sores or through viral shedding from patients who are infected but do not have symptoms.

■ Treatment and Prevention

There is no cure for HSV-1 infection. Once the virus is present in cells, it is there for life, even though it may not cause any symptoms. However, there are a number of antiviral drugs that can treat the symptoms of cold sores. The main ones are acyclovir, valacyclovir, and famciclovir; the former can be used as a cream, a tablet, or an intravenous injection, but the other two are only available in tablet form. These drugs are most effective in

treating a first episode of cold sores. An outbreak of cold sores can be prevented by using lip balm—to avoid broken skin—and minimizing stress and sun exposure. People who have cold sores should not kiss others and should keep any items such as cups, washcloths, and towels separate.

The TORCH test, which is sometimes called the TORCH panel, belongs to a category of blood tests called infectious-disease antibody titer tests. This type of blood test measures the presence of antibodies (protein molecules produced by the human immune system in response to a specific disease agent) and their level of concentration in the blood. The name of the test comes from the initial letters of the five disease categories. The TORCH test measures the levels of an infant's antibodies against five groups of chronic infections: Toxoplasmosis, Other infections, Rubella, CMV, and HSV. The

IN CONTEXT: REAL-WORLD RISKS

The Herpes 1 virus is also the cause of a condition known as *Herpes gladiatorum* (a skin infection common in wrestlers, rugby players, and other athletes playing sports with extensive skin contact between competitors). First described in the 1960s, the Centers for Disease Control and Prevention (CDC) states that, "In a national survey of 1477 trainers of athletes approximately 3% of high school wrestlers were reported to have developed HSV skin infections during the 1984-85 season. Lesions occur most often on the head and neck. Primary infection may cause constitutional symptoms with fever, malaise, weight loss, and regional lymphadenopathy (a swelling of the lymph nodes). Ocular (eye) involvement includes keratitis (a swelling or inflamation of the transparent covering at the front of the eye that protects the iris and pupil), conjunctivitis (a swelling or inflammation of the conjunctiva often termed 'pinkeye'), and blepharitis (a swelling or inflammation of the eyelids). Transmission occurs primarily through skin-to-skin contact."

The CDC further states that, "Control methods should include education of athletes and trainers regarding *herpes gladiatorum*, routine skin examinations before wrestling contact, and exclusion of wrestlers with suspicious skin lesions."

SOURCE: *Morbidity and Mortality Weekly Report (February 9, 1990),* Centers for Disease Control and Prevention.

category of other infections usually includes syphilis, hepatitis B, Coxsackie virus, Epstein-Barr virus, Varicella-Zoster virus, and Human Parvovirus.

▪ Impacts and Issues

HSV-1 is a common infection that usually lies dormant in the body within the nervous system. It causes health problems mainly in immunocompromised people, although the infection may be triggered in anyone carrying the virus through stress or sunlight exposure. People without symptoms may easily pass on the infection to those who are more vulnerable, so anyone who has ever had an outbreak of cold sores should consider themselves infected with HIV-1 and should take extra care with hygiene. Although antiviral drugs can treat the symptoms of cold sores, lessening their duration, they do not cure the infection itself.

HSV-1 infection is occasionally life-threatening. Untreated, HSV-1 encephalitis has a mortality rate of 70 percent and requires intravenous acyclovir to bring the infection under control. Neonatal (newborn) HSV-1 infection, although rare, can have a mortality rate of 60 percent, since the infant immune system is incapable of fighting it. Babies who survive often have severe neurological problems. Although for many people HSV-1 infection is of little consequence, for those who are already vulnerable, it may be extremely serious.

SEE ALSO *Chickenpox (Varicella); CMV (Cytomegalovirus) Infection; Herpes Simplex 2 Virus; Shingles (Herpes Zoster) Infection.*

BIBLIOGRAPHY

Books

Gates, Robert H. *Infectious Disease Secrets.* 2nd ed. Philadelphia: Hanley and Beltus, 2003.

Gillespie S., and K. Bamford. *Medical Microbiology and Infection at a Glance.* Malden, U.K.: Blackwell, 2000.

Wilson, Walter R., and Merle A. Sande. *Current Diagnosis & Treatment in Infectious Diseases.* New York: McGraw Hill, 2001.

Web Sites

SkinCareGuide Network. "Herpes Guide—From Cold Sores to Genital Herpes." November 1, 2006. <http://www.herpesguide.ca> (accessed February 3, 2007).

Susan Aldridge

Herpes Simplex 2 Virus

■ Introduction

Genital herpes (often known just as herpes) is an infection by the Herpes Simplex virus (HSV) which leads to the formation of painful sores in the genital area. Most cases of genital herpes are caused by HSV-2, but the closely related HSV-1, which normally causes cold sores, is occasionally involved. Both HSVs belong to the herpes family of viruses, all of which exist as viral particles of a diameter around 200 nm (nanometers). Other significant herpes viruses include the Varicella-Zoster virus, which causes chicken pox, Epstein-Barr virus, and Cyto-megalovirus (CMV). The herpes virus invades cells and may lie dormant for many years, causing no obvious symptoms. However, a herpes infection can be activated at any time and often recur throughout life. Symptoms typically are present only when the herpes virus is active. Although the virus itself cannot be eliminated, symptoms of active infection, like genital sores, can be treated with antiviral drugs.

■ Disease History, Characteristics, and Transmission

HSV-2 frequently causes no symptoms when it enters the body, creating a latent infection within nerve cells. However, HSV-2 infection can be activated—or re-activated—by triggers such as stress, sunlight exposure, fever, broken skin, and menstruation. New virus particles then move towards the genital area where they start to multiply in surface cells, causing them to swell and release fluid. This leads to the formation of groups of small, painful blisters, which may eventually rupture to give an ulcer or sore. Men develop genital sores on the tip or shaft of the penis and in the rectal area. Women develop the sores in the vulva, perineum, cervix, vagina, and rectal area. The symptoms are often more severe among women. The first episode of genital herpes may be accompanied, in around 10% of cases, by symptoms such as fever, malaise, aches and pains,

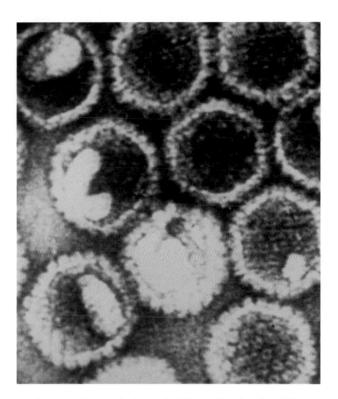

An electron micrograph shows the Herpes Simplex virus. The virus can cause genital lesions and is generally transmitted through sexual contact. © Lester V. Bergman/Corbis.

and a swollen groin. Meningitis, an illness involving inflammation of the membranes covering the brain and spinal cord, is an occasional complication of genital herpes. The symptoms typically lessen or disappear within four to five days. Sores usually heal within two weeks. Women infected with HSV-2 may transmit herpes to their babies during childbirth. Neonatal herpes (herpes infections in newborns) varies in its severity, but has an overall mortality rate as high as 60% and can cause long-term neurological complications. As many as 1% of childbirthing women in

WORDS TO KNOW

ASYMPTOMATIC: A state in which an individual does not exhibit or experience symptoms of a disease.

DORMANT: Inactive, but still alive. A resting non-active state.

LATENT INFECTION: An infection already established in the body but not yet causing symptoms, or having ceased to cause symptoms after an active period, is a latent infection.

LESIONS: The tissue disruption or the loss of function caused by a particular disease process.

PRODROMAL SYMPTOMS: Prodromal symptoms are the earliest symptoms of a disease.

the United States shed HSV-2 during delivery, and 6% of the babies thus exposed develop neonatal herpes. HSV-1 is much less likely to lead to neonatal herpes.

In 80% of cases, genital herpes recurs. However, symptoms are most often less severe during recurrence. Prodromal symptoms (early signs that herald an illness), such as a tingling sensation in the genital area, often precede a recurrence of genital herpes.

HSV-2 infection is transmitted through sexual contact with an infected person and is one of the most common of the sexually transmitted diseases. An infected, asymptomatic person (a person who has no symptoms) can still infect sexual partners. The time between sexual contact and the appearance of symptoms, if any, is about five days.

■ Scope and Distribution

HSV-2 infection is found around the world and is the most common cause of genital ulcers. However, detection of HSV-2 antibody, a sign of infection, is unusual before puberty. Around one third of sexually active adults in the Western world have HSV-2 antibody. It has been isolated from the cervix or urethra of between 5–12% of adults attending sexual health clinics. Mostly these patients are asymptomatic or have tiny, unnoticed genital lesions.

In the United States, it is estimated that there are around half a million new cases of HSV-2 per year. Women are more at risk of contracting HSV-2 infection than men. Risk increases for both men and women who have multiple sexual partners. A heterosexual woman

with one partner has a 10% chance of contracting the infection. A heterosexual man in the same situation has a negligible risk. Homosexual men run a higher risk of developing HSV-2.

HSV-2 infection also makes transmission of the human immunodeficiency virus (HIV) more likely.

■ Treatment and Prevention

There is no cure or vaccine for HSV-2 infection. There are a number of antiviral drugs that can be used to treat outbreaks of genital herpes, such as acyclovir, valacylcovir, and famciclovir. Those who know they are infected, because of past outbreaks, can help protect their sexual partners by using condoms. People with active genital sores should not have sexual contact with others even if using a condom, since sores and lesions can appear outside of the area covered by the condom.

The Division of Sexually Transmitted Disease (STD) at Centers for Disease Control and Prevention (CDC) recommends that "all pregnant women should be asked whether they have a history of genital herpes. At the onset of labor, all women should be questioned carefully about symptoms of genital herpes, including prodromal symptoms, and all women should be examined carefully for herpetic lesions."

■ Impacts and Issues

HSV-2 usually lies dormant within the body, with people being unaware that they can infect others through sexual contact. As herpes infections can be life threatening in the newborn and in those with impaired immunity, the risk of infection is a serious concern. HSV-2 infection has also been found to promote HIV transmission. The link between genital ulcers and HIV has been known for over 20 years, but more sensitive methods of detecting HSV-2 infection has allowed detailed investigation of the connection. Genital ulceration, even if it is not visible, attracts the CD4 cells that HIV infects. More recent research, from India, has shown that HIV infection is twice as likely among people with newly acquired HSV-2 infection, as compared to those with long-standing infections. Activation of HSV-2 infection in those who also have HIV may also make them even more likely to transmit HIV to an uninfected partner. These findings suggest a new approach to reducing HIV infection. Treatment with acyclovir, a relatively cheap drug, could help prevent reactivation of HSV-2 thereby potentially reducing the risk of HIV transmission.

According to the Centers for Disease Control (CDC) from the 1970s to the early 1990s, the prevalence of

IN CONTEXT: REAL-WORLD RISKS

Centers for Disease Control and Prevention, Sexually Transmitted Diseases Treatment Guidelines 2006 states that the following recommendations apply to counseling of persons with HSV infection:

- Persons who have genital herpes should be educated concerning the natural history of the disease, with emphasis on the potential for recurrent episodes, asymptomatic viral shedding, and the attendant risks of sexual transmission.
- Persons experiencing a first episode of genital herpes should be advised that suppressive therapy is available and is effective in preventing symptomatic recurrent episodes and that episodic therapy sometimes is useful in shortening the duration of recurrent episodes.
- All persons with genital HSV infection should be encouraged to inform their current sex partners that they have genital herpes and to inform future partners before initiating a sexual relationship.
- Sexual transmission of HSV can occur during asymptomatic periods. Asymptomatic viral shedding is more frequent in genital HSV-2 infection than genital HSV-1 infection and is most frequent during the first 12 months after acquiring HSV-2.
- All persons with genital herpes should remain abstinent from sexual activity with uninfected partners when lesions or prodromal symptoms are present.
- The risk of HSV-2 sexual transmission can be decreased by the daily use of valacyclovir by the infected person.

- Recent studies indicate that latex condoms, when used consistently and correctly, might reduce the risk for genital herpes transmission.
- Sex partners of infected persons should be advised that they might be infected even if they have no symptoms. Type-specific serologic testing of asymptomatic partners of persons with genital herpes is recommended to determine whether risk for HSV acquisition exists.
- The risk for neonatal HSV infection should be explained to all persons, including men. Pregnant women and women of childbearing age who have genital herpes should inform their providers who care for them during pregnancy and those who will care for their newborn infant. Pregnant women who are not infected with HSV-2 should be advised to avoid intercourse during the third trimester with men who have genital herpes. Similarly, pregnant women who are not infected with HSV-1 should be counseled to avoid genital exposure to HSV-1 during the third trimester (e.g., oral sex with a partner with oral herpes and vaginal intercourse with a partner with genital HSV-1 infection).
- Asymptomatic persons diagnosed with HSV-2 infection by type-specific serologic testing should receive the same counseling messages as persons with symptomatic infection. In addition, such persons should be taught about the clinical manifestations of genital herpes.

SOURCE: *Centers for Disease Control and Prevention, Sexually Transmitted Diseases Treatment Guidelines 2006*

---

herpes cases in the United States increased by 30%. The most dramatic rise in new cases occurred among teens and young adults. Since the late 1990s, the incidence of herpes infections in young people has stabilized. Many credit aggressive education campaigns about safer sex practices for this change. Medical testing and care, honest discussion between sexual partners about health issues, and the habitual and proper use of condoms can help reduce—but not eliminate—the risk of transmitting HSV-2.

SEE ALSO *Chickenpox (Varicella); Herpes Simplex 1 Virus; Shingles (Herpes Zoster) Infection.*

BIBLIOGRAPHY

Books

Gates, Robert H. *Infectious Disease Secrets.* 2nd ed. Philadelphia: Hanley and Beltus, 2003.

Gillespie, S., and K. Bamford *Medical Microbiology and Infection at a Glance.* Malden: Blackwell, 2000.

Wilson, Walter R., and Merle A. Sande *Current Diagnosis & Treatment in Infectious Diseases.* New York: McGraw Hill, 2001.

IN CONTEXT: REAL-WORLD FACTS

Centers for Disease Control and Prevention, Sexually Transmitted Diseases Treatment Guidelines 2006 state that "genital herpes is a chronic, life-long viral infection. Two types of HSV have been identified, HSV-1 and HSV-2. The majority of cases of recurrent genital herpes are caused by HSV-2, although HSV-1 might become more common as a cause of first episode genital herpes. At least 50 million persons in the United States have genital HSV infection. The majority of persons infected with HSV-2 have not been diagnosed with genital herpes. Many such persons have mild or unrecognized infections but shed virus intermittently in the genital tract."

"The majority of genital herpes infections are transmitted by persons unaware that they have the infection or who are asymptomatic (without observable symptoms) when transmission occurs."

SOURCE: *Centers for Disease Control and Prevention, Sexually Transmitted Diseases Treatment Guidelines 2006*

Periodicals

Wald, A., and L. Corey. "How Does Herpes Simplex Virus Type 2 Influence Human Immunodeficiency Virus Infection and Pathogenesis?" *The Journal of Infectious Diseases.* 187 (2003): 1519–1512.

Web Sites

SkinCareGuide Network. "Herpes Guide—from Cold Sores to Genital Herpes." February 21, 2007 <http://www.herpesguide.ca> (accessed February 22, 2007).

Susan Aldridge

Histoplasmosis

Introduction

Histoplasmosis is a disease caused by a mycotic (fungal) infection of *Histoplasma capsulatum* fungal spores. The infection develops when fungal spores are inhaled, and the resulting disease affects the lungs. The fungus is found globally and is endemic (occurs normally) in some areas of America. The key factor about these spores is their resilience in the environment and their ability to become airborne when the ground is disturbed. Those at risk of disease are people exposed to contaminated soils, caves, and bat and bird housings. The disease is not transmissible between humans.

In the majority of cases, infection will not result in disease, but in severe cases, persons with histoplasmosis may present with chronic tuberculosis-like symptoms. People with existing immune system problems are at an increased risk of the disease spreading to other organs of the body, which can be potentially fatal if untreated. Treatment commonly includes anti-fungal medication.

Disease History, Characteristics, and Transmission

Histoplasmosis was first reported in the United States in 1926. It occurs worldwide and is endemic in some parts of the United States. It primarily affects the lungs, but in some cases spreads to other organs in the body. Histoplasmosis is also known as Darling's disease, Ohio River Valley Fever, Mississippi River Valley disease, and Appalachian Mountain disease.

Approximately 95% of people infected with this disease remain asymptomatic (without symptoms) or have symptoms that heal spontaneously; in most cases these people will develop partial immunity against re-infection. If symptoms do occur, they will usually develop within 3–18 days. Acute symptomatic pulmonary histoplasmosis has a short duration, with possible symptoms including fever, chills, chest pain, and a non-productive cough.

Chronic pulmonary histoplasmosis presents with longer-lasting symptoms that are similar to tuberculosis: chest pain, loss of breath, coughing, sweating, and fever. Disseminated histoplasmosis is the most serious form of the disease; it is only common among immunosuppressed people and can be fatal if left untreated. In these cases, the disease spreads from the lungs to other organs, and symptoms include neck stiffness, skin lesions, and mouth sores.

Histoplasmosis is contracted by inhalation of the *Histoplasma* fungal spores, which thrive in damp, organically rich soil, and some animal droppings, such as those of birds and bats. Once these microscopic spores enter the lungs, they imbed in the small air sacs and trigger an immune reaction that, in serious cases, leads to inflammation, scarring, and calcium deposits on the lungs. The extent of histoplasmosis infection is dependent both on the number of spores inhaled and the immunity of the host.

Scope and Distribution

Histoplasmosis is primarily located in the temperate regions of the world and is endemic in areas of America, including the south-eastern, mid-Atlantic, and central states of Arkansas, Kentucky, Missouri, Tennessee, West Virginia, Ohio, and Texas, as well as Central and South America. Most cases of the disease are sporadic, but point source outbreaks have been previously described.

The fungal spores are commonly found in fertile soils, caves, poultry houses, bird roosts, and areas harboring bats. The spores frequently become airborne when disturbed; are extremely resilient; and remain viable in the environment for long periods of time. In fact, plants fertilized with droppings may contain spores and produce infectious smoke when burned. This gives the spores the ability to transfer large distances from the initial source and still retain viability in causing disease.

WORDS TO KNOW

MYCOTIC: Mycotic means having to do with or caused by a fungus. Any medical condition caused by a fungus is a mycotic condition, also called a mycosis.

IMMUNOSUPPRESSION: A reduction of the ability of the immune system to recognize and respond to the presence of foreign material.

SPORE: A dormant form assumed by some bacteria, such as anthrax, that enable the bacterium to survive high temperatures, dryness, and lack of nourishment for long periods of time. Under proper conditions, the spore may revert to the actively multiplying form of the bacteria.

Due to the high prevalence of histoplasmosis fungi, infection is common, and 80% of people living in fungal rich areas of the United States could exhibit a positive skin test for the presence of histoplasmosis fungi. However, development of disease is rare and is only considered a risk to people with weakened immune systems, such as very young children, elderly people, organ transplant and chemotherapy patients, and persons with autoimmune disease. The ages of people affected range from children to adults, and there is no increased incidence among either sex, although chronic lung infections are more common in men than women.

Although quite infrequent, outbreaks of histoplasmosis have been previously described and generally result from a single event causing the disruption of a large area housing the fungus, such as construction, clearing, cleaning, and cave exploration. One such outbreak occurred in 2001 in Indiana and infected 523 school students. The cause of the outbreak was rototilling of a courtyard containing the fungus.

■ Treatment and Prevention

Histoplasmosis may present symptoms similar to other diseases, and as such, diagnosis is achieved through blood tests or laboratory culture. Generally, histoplasmosis fungal infections do not lead to the development of disease, and, even in mild cases, the disease usually resolves without treatment. When required in severe disease states, the most common treatment for histoplasmosis is anti-fungal medication. In most cases, previous infection will result in partial protection against reinfection.

Awareness is a key factor in ensuring successful disease prevention, so before beginning a job or activity with a potential risk of exposure to the histoplasmosis fungi, it is important to investigate all of the potential risk factors involved. When working in areas carrying a high risk of making contact with the fungal spores, it is also important to wear appropriate protective clothing, such as disposable coveralls, to prevent transfer of the spores from the worksite and a dust mask that covers both the nose and the mouth to filters out all particles larger than 2 microns in size.

Due to the natural widespread occurrence of *Histoplasma capsulatum*, it would be virtually impossible to decontaminate all infected sites. Prevention is commonly achieved by minimizing the disruption of soils in affected areas in addition to limiting the exposure of persons to dust in contaminated environments. In areas where soil disruption is unavoidable, spraying infected areas thoroughly with water mist prior to beginning excavation reduces the number of aerosols produced.

■ Impacts and Issues

Cases of chronic disease caused by histoplasmosis are on the rise, and are attributed mainly to the increasing number of persons living with HIV and weakened immune systems due to chemotherapy, organ transplant, or autoimmune disease. It has also been seen that immunosuppression later in life may also result in reactivation of quiescent infection born from earlier exposure. As the number of people living with immune disorders increases, scientists expect there will be a proportional increase in the prevalence of chronic histoplasmosis. For this reason, scientists consider histoplasmosis to be an emerging infectious disease.

Land use might also play a part in the resurgence of histoplasmosis. Development of lands traditionally used for farming in the nitrogen-rich belt of the central and Southern United States could also be a factor in the increased number of reported cases.

Scientists have learned that histoplasmosis infection can also lead to ocular histoplasmosis syndrome (OHS). OHS is a condition that damages blood vessels in the eyes and leads to impaired vision. It is thought that the fungal spores travel from the lungs to the eye and lodge in the blood vessels leading to the retina. This causes no initial damage to eyesight, although it does leave recognizable histo spots on the blood vessels. Vision loss can occur years after the initial infection. Detecting the histo spots can indicate future vision loss, and laser eye surgery can reduce the likelihood of vision loss by 50%. The National Eye Institute recommends that individuals that live in areas where histoplasmosis is endemic have their eyes checked regularly, and for medical practitioners to consider the presence of histo spots as an indication that vision loss may occur.

Awareness of this disease acts to minimize unnecessary exposure to contaminated areas and promote the use of protective equipment when required. The National Institute for Occupational Safety and Health, along with the Center for Disease Control and Prevention (CDC), engages in promotions geared to educate employers and workers about the risks and prevention strategies for histoplasmosis.

SEE ALSO *AIDS (Acquired Immunodeficiency Syndrome); Emerging Infectious Diseases; HIV; Land Utilization and Disease; Opportunistic Infection; Tuberculosis.*

BIBLIOGRAPHY

Books

Mandell, G.L., J.E. Bennett, and R. Dolin. *Principles and Practice of Infectious Diseases*, Vol. 2. Philadelphia, PA: Elsevier, 2005.

Periodicals

Chamany, S., et al. "A Large Histoplasmosis Outbreak Among High School Students in Indiana, 2001." *Pediatric Infectious Disease Journal*. Vol. 23, no. 10 (2004): 909–914.

Web Sites

Directors of Health Promotion and Education. "Histoplasmosis." 2005 <http://www.dhpe.org/ infect/histo.html> (accessed February 23, 2007).

National Eye Institute. "Histoplasmosis." December 2006 <http://www.nei.nih.gov/health/histoplasmosis/ index.asp> (accessed February 23, 2007).

IN CONTEXT: REAL-WORLD RISKS

The Division of Bacterial and Mycotic Diseases, Centers for Disease Control and Prevention (CDC) list the following as "risk groups" for histoplasmosis:

- Persons in areas with endemic disease with exposures to accumulations of bird or bat droppings (e.g., construction or agricultural workers, spelunkers).
- High risk groups are immunocompromised persons (e.g., persons with cancer, transplant recipients, persons with HIV infection).

No national surveillance exists.

SOURCE: *Coordinating Center for Infectious Diseases/Division of Bacterial and Mycotic Diseases, Centers for Disease Control and Prevention.*

HIV

■ Introduction

The Human Immunodeficiency Virus (HIV) is the microorganism responsible for acquired immunodeficiency syndrome, or AIDS. HIV attacks the immune system, and eventually leaves the body vulnerable to potentially fatal opportunistic infections. An estimated 36 million people worldwide are infected with HIV.

■ History and Scientific Foundations

HIV is a type of "retrovirus" with a genetic code that is comprised of RNA rather than DNA. As it has no DNA, which is necessary to create RNA viral genome (genetic material) copies, it uses the DNA of infected host cells to create a new RNA genome for replicates (copies) of the virus. A retrovirus replicates by using a DNA intermediary, i.e., an infected cell's DNA. Retroviruses rely on the enzyme reverse transcriptase in order to perform the reverse transcription of its genetic code from its RNA into DNA, which can then be inserted into the host cell's genome using another enzyme. The virus then replicates as part of the cell's DNA. One of the major classes of HIV drugs targets reverse transcriptase, inhibiting the virus' ability to create the DNA segment for insertion into the infected cell's DNA.

One of the most important features of HIV replication is its ability to generate large numbers of new genetic combinations through a process known as recombination. This, together with a high rate of genetic mutations of individual genes, enables HIV to rapidly create new drug-resistant strains. After HIV was identified as the cause of AIDS, researchers suspected that genetic recombination could also play a key role in the evolution of the virus. Very recently, studies of HIV infections worldwide have produced an estimate for the occurrence of HIV genetic recombination and have revealed that recombination frequencies appear to be

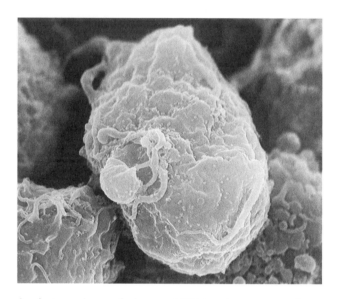

An electron micrograph shows an HIV virus that was grown in cultured lymphocytes.   © *CDC/PHIL/Corbis.*

much higher than expected. Recombination is currently regarded as a central aspect of the HIV infectious cycle.

HIV has a globular structure with a spiked envelope. The spikes on HIV virus carry the mystery of how the virus is attracted to CD4+ cells (a type of white blood cell) that play an important role in the immune system. The spikes on the HIV virus control the process by which the virus fuses with the targeted CD4+ cells. Despite intensive efforts by scientists, the spikes have been slow to reveal their structural and functional secrets. Recent advances are providing the first glimpses of the overall three-dimensional structure of the spiked envelope. Increasing knowledge of the viral envelope's component atomic structures offers new insights into the structural elements within the spike and could lead to entirely new avenues for the treatment of AIDS. The new treatments would target the ability of HIV to fuse with target cells, while current therapies interrupt viral replication.

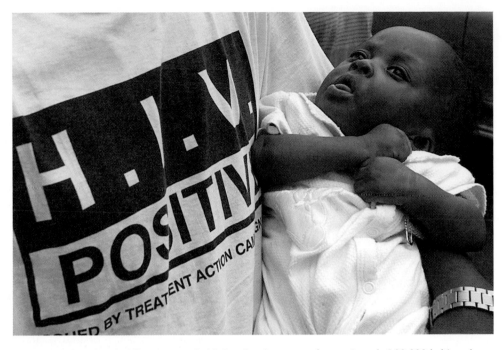

An HIV-positive South African woman holds her daughter, one of approximately 100,000 babies who are born HIV-positive annually in South Africa. Activists often wear similar t-shirts in support of those who are HIV-positive. They claim that the government's anti-viral program for pregnant women is not effective enough. © *Reuters/Corbis.*

The immune system has a so-called innate component (innate immunity) comprised of white blood cells called phagocytes, which migrate to affected areas and engulf disease-causing organisms (pathogens). Special cells of innate immunity called dendritic cells are particularly important for regulating immune response. When dendritic cells encounter foreign material, they have unique receptors that allow them to distinguish harmless and pathogenic (disease-causing) organisms. These cells carry fragments of pathogen to the lymph nodes, where they could stimulate a response by the adaptive immune system (called adaptive immunity), depending on the ability of the foreign material to cause disease.

If dendritic cells decide that the material is pathogenic (part of a virus or bacteria), they activate CD4+ helper T cells. (CD4+ refers to a surface protein on this type of T cell.) Helper T cells can then stimulate another group of white blood cells called B cells to produce antibodies that bind to the specific antigen and immobilize it, preventing it from causing infection. Antibodies are specific for only one antigen. Once activated, memory cells are produced that insure faster and stronger immune response when the body is re-exposed to the same pathogen.

Pathogens that escape antibody detection can enter and infect body tissue cells. The cell membrane of infected cells changes in a way that is recognized by T cells. Cytotoxic T cells kill infected cells, preventing them from producing more pathogen. Cytotoxic T cells must interact with Helper T cells to regulate the destruction of infected cells, in order to destroy cells that are infected by the specific microbe that has been presented to the helper cells by the dendritic cells.

HIV specifically attacks Helper T cells. Without an adequate number of Helper T cells, the immune system cannot signal B cells to produce antibodies to kill infected cells. When HIV has critically depleted the Helper T cell population, the body can no longer launch an adaptive immune response and becomes susceptible to many opportunistic infections, thus resulting in the immunodeficiency that characterizes AIDS. Research shows that the CD4+ membrane proteins are targets for HIV infection. Thus, memory helper T cells are quickly infected and destroyed in the mucus membranes of tissues. Only recently, researchers have recognized that the memory cell destruction occurs in the first several days after HIV infection, suggesting that therapies should begin as soon as the infection is detected.

Mysteries remain about how HIV causes disease, particularly the reason why there is uncontrolled viral replication in the majority of infected patients. In the past several years, investigation into HIV disease has focused on T regulatory (Treg) cells, a subset of CD4+ T-cells whose main function is to maintain a certain amount of tolerance in order to avoid autoimmunity (in which the immune system attacks the body's own tissues). Preliminary data point to two main roles for Treg cells in HIV: a detrimental effect in which

WORDS TO KNOW

AUTOIMMUNITY: Autoimmune diseases are conditions in which the immune system attacks the body's own cells, causing tissue destruction. Autoimmune diseases are classified as either general, in which the autoimmune reaction takes place simultaneously in a number of tissues, or organ specific, in which the autoimmune reaction targets a single organ. Autoimmunity is accepted as the cause of a wide range of disorders, and is suspected to be responsible for many more. Among the most common diseases attributed to autoimmune disorders are rheumatoid arthritis, systemic lupus erythematosis (lupus), multiple sclerosis, myasthenia gravis, pernicious anemia, and scleroderma.

CD4+ T CELLS: CD4 cells are a type of T cell found in the immune system, which are characterized by the presence of a CD4 antigen protein on their surface. These are the cells most often destroyed as a result of HIV infection.

CYTOTOXIC: A cytotoxic agent is one that kills cells. Cytotoxic drugs kill cancer cells but may also have application in killing bacteria

OPPORTUNISTIC INFECTION: An opportunistic infection is so named because it occurs in people whose immune systems are diminished or are not functioning normally; such infections are opportunistic insofar as the infectious agents take advantage of their hosts' compromised immune systems and invade to cause disease.

PATHOGEN: A disease causing agent, such as a bacteria, virus, fungus, etc.

RECOMBINATION: Recombination is a process during which genetic material is shuffled during reproduction to form new combinations. This mixing is important from an evolutionary standpoint because it allows the expression of different traits between generations. The process involves a physical exchange of nucleotides between duplicate strands of deoxyribonucleic acid (DNA).

HIV-specific immune responses are muted and a beneficial effect that limits immune activation (thus limiting the helper T-cell targets of HIV). There is currently a lack of standardized assays to measure levels and function of Treg cells, which continues to hamper research into this promising area. Thus, it is possible that HIV takes advantage of a feature of the immune system that naturally limits immune response.

■ Impact and Issues

The level of specificity of the science required to provide breakthroughs in the battle against HIV is unprecedented. Most disease cures and treatments that have been discovered during the past 100 years have been based on only limited knowledge of a microbe's ability to causes disease. As with the fight against cancer, the effort to find a cure for AIDS is leading scientists into ever more minute aspects of the pathogen, all the way down to the atomic structure of viral envelope spikes and the molecular mechanisms of genetic replication.

HIV is an amazingly versatile and adaptive enemy, probably owing to millennia of evolution in non-human primates and now being offered a new and relatively open ecological niche within humanity. While HIV transmission is preventable, a variety of social and behavioral factors have led to what will ultimately become the worst epidemic in terms of lives lost in the history of the human species. Also, as with the struggle against cancer, contending with the perplexing mysteries of HIV will leave a mark not only on the history and future development of medicine, but on human behavior and social evolution for the foreseeable future.

SEE ALSO *AIDS (Acquired Immunodeficiency Syndrome); AIDS: Origin of the Modern Pandemic; Viral Disease.*

BIBLIOGRAPHY

Books

Palladino, Michael A., and David Wesner. *HIV and AIDS (Special Topics in Biology Series)*. San Francisco: Benjamin Cummings, 2005.

Periodicals

Sempere J.M., V. Soriano, and J.M. Benito. "T Regulatory Cells and HIV Infection." *AIDS Rev.* (January–March 2007): 9 (1): 54–60.

Web Sites

University of Arizona: The Biology Project. "Immunology and HIV. Immune System's Response to HIV." <http://www.biology.arizona.edu/immunology/tutorials/AIDS> (accessed June 8, 2007).

Kenneth T. LaPensee

Hookworm (*Ancylostoma*) Infection

■ Introduction

Ancylostoma (an-cy-LO-sto-ma) infection, also called hookworm infection, is an infection of one of two different roundworms: *Ancylostoma duodenale* or *Necator americanus*. Depending on maturity, the roundworms range from 0.3 to 0.5 inches (0.7 to 1.3 cm) in length.

Hookworms are parasitic roundworms, specifically infesting the intestines of their host. They have hooklike appendages, from which they take their name. Hookworms belong to the class Nematoda. Moderate infestation of hookworms in humans is considered by the World Health Organization (WHO) to be between 2,000 and 3,999 eggs per gram of feces. Heavy infestation is counted at 4,000 or more eggs per gram of feces.

Hookworm infection is most common with areas of rural poverty and low socioeconomic status, especially in southern China, the Indian subcontinent, and in parts of the Americas. The worldwide number of cases was first estimated in 1990 to be 740 million people. By 2005, the number of cases worldwide was about double that initial estimate.

■ Disease History, Characteristics, and Transmission

Hookworms deposit eggs on ground containing warm, moist, shaded soil. Such conditions allow eggs to develop into larvae. The larvae are barely visible; however, they are easily able to penetrate human skin. They frequently enter the body through the soles of the feet or when humans handle feces. Children often are infected because they frequently play in dirt and go barefoot. Humans cannot infect other humans.

Once inside the body, larvae travel through the bloodstream to the lungs and respiratory tract, and on to the trachea. They are swallowed into the digestive tract and stomach where they end up in the small intes-

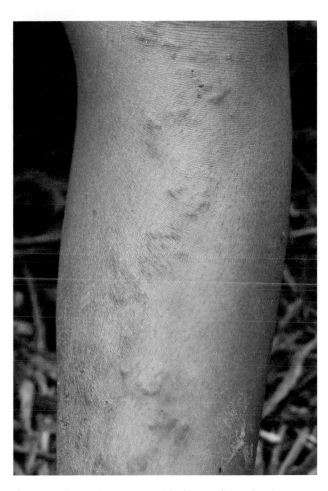

Cutaneous larva migrans, a parasitic skin condition showing subcutaneous (under the skin) burrowing tracks of hookworm (*Ancylostoma braziliense*) larva, are visible on the lower leg of a child in Peru. *Gregory G. Dimijian, M.D./Photo Researchers, Inc.*

tines. From skin to intestines, the trip takes, on average, about one week. At this point, larvae develop into adult worms about 0.5 inches (1.3 cm) in length. They attach

405

WORDS TO KNOW

HELMINTH: A representative of various phyla of worm-like animals.

MORBIDITY: The term "morbidity" comes from the Latin word "morbus," which means sick. In medicine it refers not just to the state of being ill, but also to the severity of the illness. A serious disease is said to have a high morbidity.

PARASITE: An organism that lives in or on a host organism and that gets its nourishment from that host. The parasite usually gains all the benefits of this relationship, while the host may suffer from various diseases and discomforts, or show no signs of the infection. The life cycle of a typical parasite usually includes several developmental stages and morphological changes as the parasite lives and moves through the environment and one or more hosts. Parasites that remain on a host's body surface to feed are called ectoparasites, while those that live inside a host's body are called endoparasites. Parasitism is a highly successful biological adaptation. There are more known parasitic species than nonparasitic ones, and parasites affect just about every form of life, including most all animals, plants, and even bacteria.

IN CONTEXT: DISEASE IN DEVELOPING NATIONS

The World Health Organization (WHO) states that hookworm infection "is a leading cause of anaemia and protein malnutrition. The largest numbers of cases occur in impoverished rural areas of sub-Saharan Africa, Latin America, South-East Asia and China."

SOURCE: *World Health Organization (WHO)*

---

themselves to the walls of the small intestine where they suck blood. The hookworm causes symptoms to its host when the worms drain blood and nourishment from the intestinal wall. One adult worm can produce thousands of eggs and live up to ten years. Eggs are expelled in feces. Under the proper conditions, the eggs hatch, molt, and develop into infective larvae after five to ten days.

Most of the time, there are no symptoms. However, symptoms can occur at any point within the worm's life cycle. Initial symptoms include itching and a rash at the larvae's entrance site to the host. Asthma- or pneumonia-like symptoms may occur when worms are in the lungs. Symptoms from intestinal infection include anemia, loss of appetite and weight loss, excessive intestinal gases, cramps and abdominal pain, and diarrhea. In chronic infections, symptoms may include malnutrition, breathing difficulties, dizziness, pale complexion, tiredness and weakness, swelling and bloating, impotence, enlargement of the heart, and irregular heartbeat.

In children, physical development and growth can be slowed or not fully attained because of loss of sufficient amounts of iron and protein. Infection can be especially problematic for newborn and infant children, pregnant women, and people who are malnourished. Death is uncommon but can occur, especially in newborn and infant children.

■ Scope and Distribution

Hookworm infection occurs mostly in tropical and subtropical regions of the world. *Ancylostoma duodenale* is found in China, India, Japan, and Mediterranean countries. *Ancylostoma americanus* is located in the tropical areas of Africa, Asia, and the Americas. According to the Division of Parasitic Diseases of the Centers for Disease Control and Prevention (CDC), approximately 1.3 to 1.6 billion people are infected worldwide, about one-fourth to one-fifth of the world's population.

■ Treatment and Prevention

Diagnosis is often accomplished by identifying hookworm eggs in a stool sample with the use of a microscope. A blood sample is also used because positive results show iron or protein deficiency.

Treatment consists of anthelmintic drugs (that is, drugs proven to effectively remove worms), along with iron supplements and a high protein diet. In particular, the drug mebendazole (MBZ) is used because it causes immobilization and eventual death of the worms by restricting the ingestion of nutrients. It is often branded under the names Antiox®, Ovex®, Pripsen®, and Vermox®. It cures the infection about 99% of the time when given twice a day for three days. Other drugs also given are albendazole (Albenza®) and pyrantel (Antiminth®), which are given once each day for three days. They should not be given to pregnant woman.

Hookworm infection is prevented by promoting safe sanitary practices. Feces should be disposed of properly and contaminated areas cleansed thoroughly. Wearing shoes, avoiding swimming in contaminated pools, and treating or boiling contaminated water before drinking also help prevent hookworm infection.

■ Impacts and Issues

Hookworm infection is the leading cause of iron deficiency anemia in developing countries. In developing countries where food is scarce, people with heavy hookworm infections are sometimes unable to eat enough calories to compensate for those lost due to intestinal iron and protein depletion brought on by hookworms. In the past, hookworm infection has been neglected due to its concentration among the world's poorest peoples. Generally, in the past, international coordination involving the infection has not been accomplished. Over the decades of the 1990s and 2000s, however, there has been increasing concern over the global incidence of hookworm infection. International efforts are increasing to control the occurrence of hookworm, flatworm, and related helminth (parasitic worm) infections. The World Health Organization estimates that over two billion people worldwide suffer from illnesses associated with helminths.

Children are especially susceptible to hookworm infection because of the amount of time they spend outdoors. WHO estimates that about 400 million school-aged children are annually infected. Once infected, the children often suffer morbidity that includes physical and mental problems such as anemia, attention deficits, learning disabilities, and school absenteeism. Children who are not properly treated are permanently affected.

WHO adopted in 2001 a resolution to target all countries where helminth infections occur most frequently. The project called Partners for Parasite Control (PPC) aims to regularly treat at least 75% of all school children at risk by the year 2010. PPC also supports local health facilities so that they have adequate supplies of anti-helminth drugs and perform regular treatment to high-risk groups.

SEE ALSO *Bilharzia (Schistosomiasis); Helminth Disease; Roundworm (Ascariasis) infection.*

IN CONTEXT: REAL-WORLD RISKS

The Centers for Disease Control and Prevention (CDC), Division of Parasitic Diseases states that hookworm infection cause any serious health problems and that "The most serious results of hookworm infection are the development of anemia and protein deficiency caused by blood loss. When children are continuously infected by many worms, the loss of iron and protein can retard growth and mental development, sometimes irreversibly. Hookworm infection can also cause tiredness, difficulty breathing, enlargement of the heart, and irregular heartbeat. Sometimes hookworm infection is fatal, especially among infants."

SOURCE: *The Centers for Disease Control and Prevention (CDC), Division of Parasitic Diseases*

BIBLIOGRAPHY

Books

Holland, Celia V., and Malcolm W. Kennedy, eds. *The Geohelminths: Ascaris, Trichuris, and Hookworm.* Boston, MA: Kluwer Academic Publishers, 2002.

Periodicals

Hotez, Peter J., et al. "Hookworm Infection." *New England Journal of Medicine.* 351, 8 (August 19, 2004): 799–807.

Web Sites

Division of Parasitic Diseases of the Centers for Disease Control and Prevention (CDC). "Hookworm Infection." <http://www.cdc.gov/ncidod/dpd/parasites/hookworm/factsht_hookworm.htm> (accessed March 14, 2007).

World Health Organization. "Partners for Parasite Control (PPC)." <http://www.who.int/wormcontrol/en/> (accessed March 14, 2007).

Host and Vector

■ Introduction

The terms host and vector refer to the route of transmission of some infectious diseases to humans and animals.

The host is the living being that the bacteria, virus, protozoan, or other disease-causing microorganism normally resides in. Some bird species, for example are normal hosts to arboviruses such as West Nile virus. Typically, the microorganism does little or no harm to the host, which is important if the disease-causing organism is to successfully persist in that host over time. Occasionally, the host population maintains the organism even though some members suffer from infection caused by it. Several species of birds in North America have experienced West Nile infection although they are considered the natural host.

A reservoir host, or simply a reservoir, refers to a living (human, animal, insect, or plant) or non-living (soil, water) entity where a disease-causing organism can normally live and multiply. A host in which a parasite resides to sexual maturity is called a primary host, and a host in which a parasite spends only part of its life cycle or does not reach sexual maturity is called an intermediate host. Certain species of snails, for example, are the intermediate host of the *Schistosoma* larvae that are responsible for causing the disease bilharzia in humans.

A vector is an organism that helps transmit infection from one host to another. For example, the mosquito serves as the vector to infect humans with the West Nile virus. The mosquito acquires the virus from birds when it takes a blood meal. If the same mosquito subsequently feeds on a human, the virus can be transferred, and the result can be West Nile disease in humans.

■ Disease History, Characteristics, and Transmission

The host-vector route of transmission is responsible for a number of diseases including several types of encephalitis

that sicken humans and horses (Western equine encephalitis, Eastern equine encephalitis, and St. Louis encephalitis). Malaria, which is caused by a number of protozoans of the genus *Plasmodium* (the most common and serious forms of malaria are caused by *P. falciparum* and *P. vivax*) is also a vector-borne disease. The vector for transmission of the malaria protozoa is also the mosquito. Typically, the host is another human whose blood harbors the protozoan. As with encephalitis, the mosquito acquires the microbe when it feeds on the infected host, and transfers the microbe to a susceptible human host when it seeks another blood meal.

Mosquitoes also function as the vectors in the transmission of arbovirus species that cause Yellow fever and Dengue fever in humans. Other examples of potential disease vectors include flies, mites, fleas, ticks, rats, skunks, and even dogs.

■ Scope and Distribution

The host-vector route of disease transmission occurs globally. Some diseases are confined to certain regions of the world. One example is malaria, which is associated with equatorial regions. Malaria's influence is huge; the World Health Organization estimates that 350 to 500 million cases of malaria and up to three million deaths occur each year. Other vector-borne diseases can be present even in colder climates. For example, West Nile disease is increasing in Canada.

■ Treatment and Prevention

The best way to eliminate host-vector diseases is to break the vector-mediated chain of transmission between the infected host and the susceptible person or animal that will become a new host. In the case of malaria, for example, spraying areas that are breeding grounds for mosquitoes can help curb their population, and so reduce the likelihood of disease transmission. In some malaria-prone areas of Africa, the use of dichloro-diphenyl-trichloroethane (DDT) is being advocated as a means of mosquito control. Despite the infamous history of DDT due to its overuse and resulting environmental harm, its controlled application may be a relatively safe means of host-vector control.

Another means of malaria host-vector control that is becoming more widely practiced is the use of mosquito netting to protect people while they sleep. This inexpensive and easy-to-use method prevents the mosquito from feeding on a sleeping person and interrupts the transmission path of the *Plasmodium* protozoan.

Similarly, protective clothing can minimize the chance that a vector will be able to get access to unexposed skin.

More exotic vector control approaches are being explored by scientists. An example is an ongoing program to breed and release male mosquitoes that cannot breed into malaria-prone regions. The intention is that, since malaria is transmitted only by female mosquitoes, the lack of availability of a male breeding partner will drive down the female population over time.

■ Impacts and Issues

Changing the behavior of vectors influences the transmission of a disease. Knowledge of a vector's habitat, life cycle, behavior, and migratory patterns, for example, is vital to efforts to curb the spread of disease. Vector-borne diseases with simple transmission cycles can be difficult to treat and prevent. This is because the vectors are living things that are often capable of moving from one location to another, sometimes over thousands of miles.

Threats from vector-borne diseases with complicated transmission cycles that involve one or more intermediate hosts are sometimes easier to eliminate. This is because breaking only one link in the disease transmission chain will result in fewer infections. Guinea worm disease, for example, infected 3 to 5 million people in Asia and Africa about 20 years ago. Through an international effort, ponds in endemic areas were treated with a simple insecticide that eliminated the intermediate host, a copepod or "water flea", but left the water potable (drinkable). By 2006, cases of Guinea worm infection numbered fewer than 12,000 in Africa, and the disease was eliminated from Asia.

A looming issue for host-vector diseases involves climate change. As vector-borne diseases such as malaria are associated with warmer climates, some researchers have warned that the increasing warming of the Earth's atmosphere could expand the habitat of mosquito species, and so increase the prevalence of mosquito-borne diseases such as malaria.

SEE ALSO *Arthropod-borne Disease; Bloodborne Pathogens; Climate Change and Infectious Disease; Dengue and*

WORDS TO KNOW

INTERMEDIATE HOST: An organism infected by a parasite while the parasite is in a developmental form, not sexually mature.

PRIMARY HOST: The primary host is an organism that provides food and shelter for a parasite while allowing it to become sexually mature, while a secondary host is one occupied by a parasite during the larval or asexual stages of its life cycle.

RESERVOIR: The animal or organism in which the virus or parasite normally resides.

VECTOR: Any agent, living or otherwise, that carries and transmits parasites and diseases. Also, an organism or chemical used to transport a gene into a new host cell.

IN CONTEXT: REDUCING COSTS AND RISKS OF VECTOR CONTROL

Integrated vector management (IVM) strategies are emerging as part of an effort to achieve effective disease-control at costs countries can afford and at the same time minimize potential negative impacts on biodiversity, ecosystems, and public health (e.g., reduce risks related to pesticides, bioaccumulation of toxic or potentially toxic chemicals).

The World Health Organization (WHO) Global Strategic Framework for Integrated Vector Management defines IVM as a strategy to "improve the efficacy, cost-effectiveness, ecological soundness and sustainability of disease vector control. IVM encourages a multi-disease control approach, integration with other disease control measures and the considered and systematic application of a range of interventions, often in combination and synergistically."

The IVM approach is also designed to reduce the development of vector resistance to vector control measures (e.g., increasing resistance to pesticides).

Cost effectiveness is an important aspect of IVM strategy. For example, officials in Sri Lanka initially indicate that "costs of periodic river flushing to eliminate mosquito breeding habitats compared favourably with the use of insecticide-impregnated bednets as a mosquito-control measure."

SOURCE: *World Health Organization*

Dengue Hemorrhagic Fever; Encephalitis; Malaria; Vector-borne Disease; Zoonoses.

BIBLIOGRAPHY

Books

Honigsbaum, Mark. *The Fever Trail: In Search of the Cure for Malaria.* New York: Picador, 2003.

Marquardt, William H. *Biology of Disease Vectors. 2nd ed.* New York: Academic Press, 2004.

Marqulies, Phillip. *West Nile Virus: Epidemics Deadly Diseases throughout History.* New York: Rosen Publishing Group, 2003.

Web Sites

Centers for Disease Control and Prevention. "Division of Vector-Borne Diseases" <http://www.cdc.gov/ncidod/dvbid/> (accessed April 2, 2007).

Brian Hoyle

Hot Tub Rash (*Pseudomonas aeruginosa* Dermatitis)

■ Introduction

Hot tub rash is a form of skin irritation that results from an infection caused by the bacterium *Pseudomonas aeruginosa*. This bacterium is commonly found in environments such as water and soil.

■ Disease History, Characteristics, and Transmission

Hot tub rash is a skin infection that is known as dermatitis. The infected skin becomes itchy, and a red rash develops 48 hours to several weeks after contact with contaminated water. The depressions in the skin that surround hair follicles can also become contaminated, which can lead to the development of pus-filled blisters, a condition known as folliculitis. Less commonly, hot tub rash can lead to other and more serious infections in the eye, breast, lung, and urinary tract.

The term hot tub rash reflects the prevalence of the infection in hot tubs, where warm water can provide ideal conditions for the growth of *P. aeruginosa*, but hot tub rash is not exclusive to hot tubs. The skin infection can also occur from swimming in a contaminated lake or pool, and *P. aeruginosa* skin infections have also been documented in waterslides and bathtubs, as well as following the use of diving suits that have not been properly washed between use, particularly when someone has a cut or scratch in the skin. Any opening on the skin surface increases the likelihood that *P. aeruginosa* can establish an infection. Skin that is covered by a bathing suit can develop a more severe infection, as the contaminated water is held in closer and has more prolonged contact with the skin.

Chemicals such as chlorine, which are added to keep the water free from microorganisms, lose their potency more quickly at the elevated water temperatures in hot tubs. Back-yard or commercial hot tubs are sometimes inadequately disinfected, which also creates opportunity for the growth of *P. aeruginosa*.

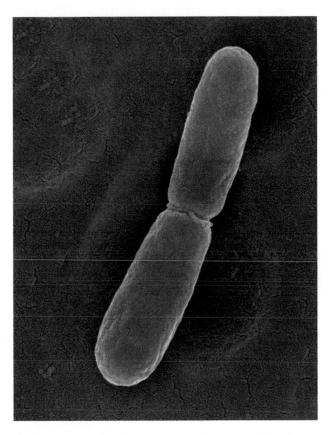

Pseudomonas aeruginosa is a rod bacteria that causes skin and urinary tract infections and septicemia. It produces a blue-green pigment, pyocyanin, which causes the bluish pus produced by the infections. © *Visuals Unlimited/Corbis.*

The construction of a hot tub can contribute to *P. aeruginosa* growth. Many hot tubs are made of wood. Even if the tub's inner surface looks smooth, the wood will contain many tiny cracks in which the bacteria can grow. When growing on surfaces, *P. aeruginosa* often produces a sugary coating called an exopolysaccharide. The resulting exopolysaccharide-enclosed population of bacteria (which is

WORDS TO KNOW

BIOFILM: Biofilms are populations of microorganisms that form following the adhesion of bacteria, algae, yeast, or fungi to a surface. These surface growths can be found in natural settings such as on rocks in streams, and in infections such as can occur on catheters. Microorganisms can colonize living and inert natural and synthetic surfaces.

IN CONTEXT: PERSONAL RESPONSIBILITY AND PREVENTION

To ensure safe and healty use, The Centers for Disease Control and Prevention (CDC) recommends that spa users observe the following rules to protect against recreational water illnesses:

- Refrain from entering a spa when you have diarrhea.
- Avoid swallowing spa water or even getting it into your mouth.
- Shower or bathe with soap before entering the spa.
- Observe limits, if posted, on the maximum allowable number of bathers.
- Exclude children less than 5 years of age from using spas.
- If pregnant, consult a physician before spa use, particularly in the first trimester.

SOURCE: *Centers for Disease Control and Prevention (CDC)*

called a biofilm) can become very resistant to chlorine and other disinfectants. Bacteria can slough off from the biofilm into the water; if someone is in the hot tub there can be an opportunity for the skin infection to develop. Even plastic hot tubs can have surface-adhering *P. aeruginosa* biofilms.

■ Scope and Distribution

As *P. aeruginosa* is widespread in the environment, hot tub rash is also common. In a hospital, the infection is more of a concern, especially for patients with malfunctioning immune systems. In these patients, *P. aeruginosa* often causes infection in the moist tissues of the lung.

There is no age, race, gender, or geographical influence on the occurrence of hot tub rash.

■ Treatment and Prevention

Hot tub rash tends to clear without treatment in several weeks. However, some people can benefit from the use of an antibiotic-containing ointment that is rubbed onto the affected areas of the skin. This treatment may be ineffective, however, as some strains of *P. aeruginosa* are resistant to a variety of antibiotics.

For people at higher risk of more serious infection (such as those with an inefficient immune system), treatment with the antibiotic ciprofloxacin can be useful.

Hot tub rash can be prevented by avoiding environments where *P. aeruginosa*-contaminated water might be found. Most commonly, this means avoiding the use of a domestic hot tub, or not using a crowded hot tub. If this is unrealistic, then regular disinfection of the tub water and cleaning of the inside surface of the tub should be considered essential maintenance.

■ Impacts and Issues

While hot tub rash is often an inconvenience rather than a health concern, the infection can be serious for someone whose immune system is less able to fight off infection. In such people *P. aeruginosa* becomes an opportunistic pathogen—an organism that does not normally cause disease but which is capable of causing disease under the appropriate circumstances.

In an public environments such as hospitals or spas, whirlpools and hot tubs need to be regularly maintained and the water tested for the presence of microorganisms. The Centers for Disease Control and Prevention (CDC) recommends maintaining the free-chlorine or bromine level of the hot tub or pool between 2–5 parts per million and maintaining the pH level of the water at 7.5–7.8. As well, the whirlpool or tub should be located in a well-ventilated room, as the agitation of the hot water could create aerosolized bacteria. If the bacteria become aerosolized, they can be inhaled, which can result in a lung infection. The possibility of a lung infection is especially serious for persons who have cystic fibrosis, since *P. aeruginosa* can establish a persistent infection that can progressively damage the lung tissue.

SEE ALSO *Swimmer's Ear and Swimmer's Itch (Cercarial Dermatitis).*

BIBLIOGRAPHY

Books

Tortora, Gerard J., Berell R. Funke, and Christine L. Case. *Microbiology: An Introduction.* New York: Benjamin Cummings, 2006.

Brunelle, Lynn, and Barbara Ravage. *Bacteria.* Milwaukee: Gareth Stevens Publishing, 2003.

Web Sites

Centers for Disease Control and Prevention. "Hot Tub Rash." <http://www.cdc.gov/healthyswimming/derm.htm> (accessed March 1, 2007).

Brian Hoyle

HPV (Human Papillomavirus) Infection

■ Introduction

The human papillomavirus (HPV) grows exclusively in the epithelial cells making up the surface of the skin, including the cervix, vagina, and anus. While HPV infection often causes no symptoms, it sometimes triggers benign tumors known as papillomas or warts on the hands and feet, or in the genital area. Most HPV infections clear up on their own, but they are also capable of causing cancers in the cervix and, more rarely, in the vagina, vulva, penis, and anus. The link between HPV and cancer is not well understood, but the virus could trigger abnormal growth and multiplication in the cells it infects. The genetic material (DNA) of HPV has been found in the majority of cervical cancers studied and the disease is a major killer of women in certain parts of the world. However, there is now a vaccine that can protect girls and young women against the main types of HPV causing both genital warts and cervical cancer.

■ Disease History, Characteristics, and Transmission

Over 100 types of HPV have been identified—about 60 of them cause skin warts, while another 40 or so cause

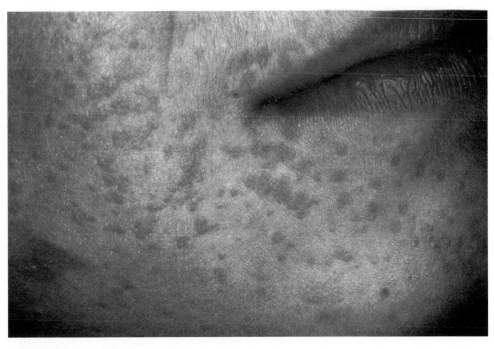

Warts are contagious, yet harmless, skin growths caused by the human papillomavirus (HPV). *CNRI/Photo Researchers, Inc.*

WORDS TO KNOW

DYSPLASIA: Abnormal changes in tissue or cell development.

MORTALITY: Mortality is the condition of being susceptible to death. The term "mortality" comes from the Latin word *mors*, which means "death." Mortality can also refer to the rate of deaths caused by an illness or injury, i.e., "Rabies has a high mortality."

PREVALENCE: The actual number of cases of disease (or injury) that exist in a population.

SEXUALLY TRANSMITTED DISEASE (STD): Sexually transmitted diseases (STDs) vary in their susceptibility to treatment, their signs and symptoms, and the consequences if they are left untreated. Some are caused by bacteria. These usually can be treated and cured. Others are caused by viruses and can typically be treated but not cured. More than 15 million new cases of STD are diagnosed annually in the United States.

genital warts. Most people with HPV infection will not have symptoms, although they can still transmit the infection to others. Skin warts are either flat (shallow) or plantar (deep), occurring mainly on the hands and feet in children and young adults. Sometimes papillomas grow in the mouth or on the larynx (voicebox). Anogenital warts can occur anywhere in the external genitalia, in the vagina, on the cervix, or around the anus. They consist of soft, moist, pink or flesh-colored swellings. In an otherwise healthy person, these warts are benign. Ninety percent of anogenital warts are caused by HPV type 6 or HPV type 11.

HPV can also cause cervical cancer, with HPV type 16 or HPV type 18 being involved in around 70% of cases. Microscopic evaluation of cells from the cervix taken in a Pap test (a routine screen for cervical cancer) can reveal a series of changes that may lead to cervical cancer. The first stage is known as dysplasia, an abnormality that often reverts to normal by the time a second test is taken. However, these changes may progress to a condition known as cervical intraepithelial dysplasia (CIN), which is generally regarded as being precancerous and likely to develop into cervical cancer within ten years, if left untreated. Most genital HPV infections do not develop into cervical cancer, however.

HPV infection is transmitted by skin contact and, in the case of genital warts, through sexual contact, usually involving intercourse. Rarely, a mother can transmit an HPV infection to her newborn baby, who may then develop warts in the throat or larynx.

■ Scope and Distribution

Infection with HPV is very common around the world. It is estimated that 50–75% of all those who have ever had sexual intercourse will have HPV infection at some time in their lives, although this will usually not cause symptoms. About 1% of sexually active men and women have genital warts. A recent study for the Centers for Disease Control and Prevention (CDC) revealed that the prevalence of HPV infection among women aged 14–59 in the United States is probably higher than previously estimated. Vaginal swabs were tested for the presence of HPV DNA and found to be positive in 27% of the group. In women aged 20–24, the rate of HPV infection was 44.8% and in the 14–24 age group, the rate was 33.8%. When the infections were analyzed by HPV type, 3.4% of the women were infected with type 6, 11, 16, and 18, which are responsible for the majority of genital warts and cervical cancer. If extrapolated to the whole U.S. population, this study suggests that the number of HPV infections among women aged 14–59 is 7.5 million, rather than the 4.5 million previously estimated.

Men also can get HPV and, for both sexes, the risk of infection goes up as the number of sexual partners increases. Having sex with someone who has had many sexual partners is also risky. In other words, the risk of HPV goes up with the number of possible exposures to the virus.

Globally, HPV infection exacts a significant toll in the form of cervical cancer. One in ten of all cancers in women, worldwide, are cervical cancer. It is the most commonly diagnosed cancer among women in southern Africa and Central America. The disease causes more than 273,000 deaths every year, accounting for 9% of cancer mortality in women.

■ Treatment and Prevention

Often, no treatment is needed for the symptoms of HPV infection, because both skin and genital warts tend to disappear over time. Ninety percent are gone within two years. If warts are large or painful, they can be destroyed by burning (electrocautery), freezing (cryotherapy), and chemical treatment. Laryngeal papillomas can be surgically removed.

Sexual abstinence is the only sure way of avoiding genital HPV infection. Limiting the number of sexual contacts and using condoms will provide some protection. Women who are sexually active should have regular Pap smears to check for the early signs of cervical cancer. In countries that have a national screening program, cervical cancer has become far less common than previously and cases tend to occur among women who have never had a Pap test. Finally, a vaccine against HPV types 6, 11, 16 and 18 has recently (2006) become available.

■ Impacts and Issues

Gardasil®, the HPV vaccine, was approved for use in the United States in June 2006, and is recommended for use in girls aged 11–12. The vaccine has been shown to be safe and effective in females aged 9–26. Research is ongoing into whether the vaccine works for older women and boys, and how long the protection lasts. The vaccine is made from the proteins that compose the outer coat of the HPV virus. Research has shown that it affords the highest level of protection against genital warts and cervical cancer among those who have not been exposed to HPV infection already— that is, those who have not become sexually active. Females who have been exposed may gain some protection, but the vaccine cannot cure any existing infection. It is important for those who have been vaccinated to still receive regular Pap tests, because the current vaccine does not protect against all the HPV types that can cause cervical cancer. If Pap screening and the HPV vaccine became available worldwide, it is possible that cervical cancer might be eradicated.

In early 2007, Texas Governor Rick Perry issued an executive order requiring HPV vaccination for all schoolgirls entering the sixth grade for the 2008–2009 school year. With this order, Texas became the first state to require vaccination against HPV. The governor's order was intended to bypass political objections in the state legislature and local some communities, including objections by parents' groups to giving young girls a vaccine that prevents a complication of a sexually transmitted disease before the girls become sexually active. Perry also ordered Texas health agencies to provide the vaccine free or at a reduced cost to girls without health insurance, as well as to those without health coverage for routine vaccinations. As of April 2007, the state legislature was considering a new bill that would remove the HPV vaccine from the list of required vaccinations for Texas school children, and the debate about mandatory HPV vaccination remains unresolved.

SEE ALSO *Cancer and Infectious Disease; Sexually Transmitted Diseases.*

IN CONTEXT: SOCIAL AND PERSONAL RESPONSIBILITY

The Division of Sexually Transmitted Disease (STD) Prevention of the Centers for Disease Control (CDC) states that "the surest way to eliminate risk for genital HPV infection is to refrain from any genital contact with another individual."

For individuals who take the risks of sexual activity the CDC states that "a long-term, mutually monogamous relationship with an uninfected partner is the strategy most likely to prevent future genital HPV infections. However, it is difficult to determine whether a partner who has been sexually active in the past is currently infected."

The CDC further recommends that "for those choosing to be sexually active and who are not in long-term mutually monogamous relationships, reducing the number of sexual partners and choosing a partner less likely to be infected may reduce the risk of genital HPV infection. Partners less likely to be infected include those who have had no or few prior sex partners."

With regard to condom use, the CDC states "HPV infection can occur in both male and female genital areas that are covered or protected by a latex condom, as well as in areas that are not covered. While the effect of condoms in preventing HPV infection is unknown, condom use has been associated with a lower rate of cervical cancer, an HPV-associated disease."

SOURCE: *Centers for Disease Control and Prevention, Division of Sexually Transmitted Disease (STD)*

IN CONTEXT: TRENDS AND STATISTICS

The Division of Sexually Transmitted Disease (STD) Prevention of the Centers for Disease Control (CDC) states that "every year, about 5.5 million people acquire a genital HPV infection. While there is no way to know for sure if HPV is increasing, there are no signs of a significant decline. With improved testing technology, researchers have been able to get a much clearer picture of the true extent of HPV in certain groups in recent years, and the infection is even more common than originally asserted."

SOURCE: *Centers for Disease Control and Prevention, Division of Sexually Transmitted Disease (STD)*

BIBLIOGRAPHY

Books

Wilson, Walter R., and Merle A. Sande. *Current Diagnosis & Treatment in Infectious Diseases.* New York: McGraw Hill, 2001.

Periodicals

Dunne, E.F., et al. "Prevalence of HPV Infection Among Females in the United States." *Journal of the American Medical Association* 297 (February 28, 2007): 813–819.

Web Sites

American Cancer Society. "Frequently Asked Questions About Human Papilloma Virus (HPV) Vaccines." <http://www.cancer.org/docroot/CRI/content/CRI_2_6x_FAQ_HPV_Vaccines.asp> (accessed February 25, 2007).

Cancer Research UK. "Cervical Cancer. International Statistics." <http://info.cancerresearchuk.org/cancerstats/types/cervix/international/> (accessed February 25, 2007).

Centers for Disease Control and Prevention. "Genital HPV Infection—CDC Fact Sheet." May 2004. <http://www.cdc.gov/std/hpv/STDFact-HPV.htm> (accessed February 25, 2007).

Susan Aldridge

Immigration and Infectious Disease

■ Introduction

Every day, an estimated two million people cross an international boundary. Many of these people are simply travelers who have planned short visits. Others are immigrants, either refugees or voluntary migrants. Some migrants never cross national borders but are displaced within their own nations. As of 2007, there are an estimated 25–45 million internally displaced persons (IDPs) worldwide. IDPs typically migrate or are forced to move because of war, ecological disaster, disease, or economic collapse. This increasing movement of people across the globe plays a significant role in the spread of disease.

Since antiquity, health hazards have moved across long distances through movement of people. Travel, trade, exploration, and war forged nations but also spread disease. Travel by horse or on foot was slow, serving as a limited barrier to the transport of infectious disease—those who fell ill often died or were no longer ill by the time they reached other population centers. Ships spread diseases faster as a disease could linger on ship for months, infecting whole crews. Also, the large cargo load of ships posed a unique disease risk. In the case of the Black Death (plague), rats aboard cargo ships likely hosted fleas responsible for spreading plague throughout Asia, the Middle East, and Europe. In the modern era, the spread of air travel and its reduced costs have greatly increased the number of travelers as well as heightened the risk of disease. Air travel permits infected persons and diseases to reach new populations—often in distant locations—within hours.

Immigration raises many of the same disease issues as voluntary travel. However, immigrants also have unique health needs. Some immigrant populations come from areas with parasites or other infectious diseases that are endemic to their homeland, but have been eliminated in the industrialized world. Immigrants may not have had access to routine healthcare in their home countries. Providing effective healthcare to immigrant groups requires training healthcare professionals to recognize the health needs of diverse immigrant groups.

■ Disease History, Characteristics, and Transmission

Cholera, dysentery, typhoid, tuberculosis, HIV/AIDS, and malaria are only a few of the infectious diseases that migration and immigration have helped to spread. Illnesses that have been largely eliminated from some areas, such as malaria or tuberculosis, can be reintroduced by migrants, and such cases of disease are labeled imported cases.

Cholera, dysentery, and typhoid are major killers that are spread by poor sanitation. Densely packed refugee camps with improper sanitation and poor hygienic conditions foster outbreaks of infectious disease. In 2007, one person died and 30 others were hospitalized after a cholera outbreak at a Congolese refugee camp in Uganda. The refugees were subsequently advised by Ugandan officials to observe precautionary measures like washing hands, avoiding raw foods, and using clean utensils. These measures, as well as construction of latrines, helped reduce some incidence of infectious disease. Such measures are not always possible at severely under-resourced, overcrowded, and hastily constructed camps. Food shortages and malnutrition in refugee and IDP camps also contribute to the spread of disease.

■ Scope and Distribution

It is difficult to measure the scope and distribution of infectious disease spread by immigrants because of reporting difficulties. Health care systems in some countries, including developing nations that have received large numbers of refugees from neighboring nations, are too inadequate to correctly identify diseases and complete the necessary procedures for effective reporting.

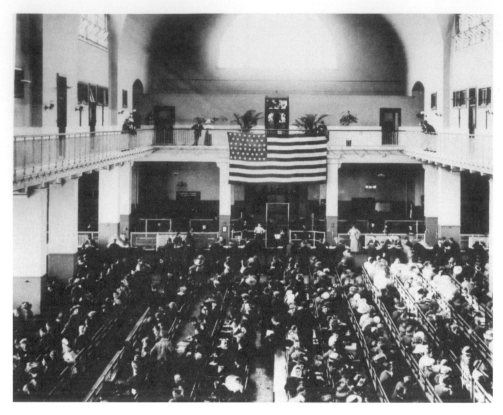

Hundreds of immigrants sit in the Great Hall of Ellis Island in New York City awaiting possible entry into the United States. Approximately 16 million hopeful immigrants arrived at Ellis Island between 1892 and 1924; 20 percent were refused entry due to poor health or their political backgrounds. *AP Images.*

However, the Centers for Disease Control (CDC) and the World Health Organization (WHO) have helped identify areas of concern.

Haiti has sent large numbers of economic and political refugees to the United States and to other Caribbean nations. In 2006, the Jamaican Health Ministry reported that there was a link between Haitian immigrants and a recent outbreak of malaria in Jamaica. DNA testing by the CDC tied an outbreak in Kingston to a single source consistent with the *Falciparum* malaria parasite found in Haiti. At least 302 Jamaicans were infected. The government conducted an island-wide surveillance of breeding sites for the *Anopheles* (malaria-spreading) mosquito and destroyed about 450 *Anopheles* breeding sites in 256 communities.

Tuberculosis, an infectious disease that in some forms is resistant to treatment, is spread through air droplets expelled when infected persons cough, sneeze, speak, or sing. It had largely been eliminated from some nations, notably the United States and the United Kingdom, until immigration brought it back. In 2001, 61.4% of all tuberculosis cases in the Netherlands occurred among foreign citizens. Tuberculosis transmission during air travel has been documented by WHO.

Varicella, the chickenpox virus, is yet another disease that can be spread by immigrants. In tropical coun-

tries, varicella does not generally infect in early childhood as it does in temperate zones. In the tropics, infections typically occur in the late teens and 20s, meaning immigrants from those countries don't have the same high level of immunity to chickenpox as do young adults who grew up in temperate countries.

■ Treatment and Prevention

The International Health Regulations (IHR), a WHO-designed legal instrument, aims to provide maximum security against the international spread of diseases with a minimum interference with world traffic. The first IHR, approved in 1969, only targeted cholera, yellow fever, and plague. The rise of globalization prompted a revised IHR, which took effect on June 15, 2007. Among its many measures, the IHR establishes a single code of procedures and practices for routine public health measures at international airports and ports and some ground crossings. The regulations focus on ensuring early detection, confirmation, investigation and rapid response for any emergencies of international concern.

However, some nations are having difficulty with the IHR. As the deadline for the enforcement of the IHR approached, Kenya's borders continued to be frontiers for the spread of communicable diseases. Meanwhile, an unprecedented resurgence of communicable diseases such as tuberculosis, malaria, avian influenza, and SARS is causing international concern. Kenya, as one example, reported outbreaks of polio and Rift Valley fever in 2006. Kenya is hosting refugees from Somalia, Sudan, Rwanda, and the Congo.

■ Impacts and Issues

Infectious diseases do not recognize borders. Accordingly, nations need to improve their medical surveillance to safeguard the health of their citizens. The IHR is one step in this direction. Screening and immunization programs would protect the health of immigrants and established residents. Canadian medical researchers have recommended that family doctors should ask young adult immigrants and refugees whether they have ever had chickenpox, test those who answer in the negative, and offer to vaccinate those who are susceptible to the disease.

Somalia until recently had an HIV prevalence rate of about one percent, which was lower than that of many African countries. After much cross-border movement of HIV-infected refugees from Ethiopia, the HIV infection rates in Somalia subsequently increased. By 2006, United Nations AIDS (UNAIDS) officials expressed fears that Somalia will experience a general AIDS epidemic within ten years. Condoms are generally unavailable in Somalia and there is a lack of adequate healthcare. Other African nations have experienced similar patterns of disease progression with HIV. Eleven African nations have HIV prevalence rates over 13%.

Political issues are also affecting international public health. Taiwan lacks full membership in WHO because of an historically strained relationship with mainland China. Taiwan has had more success than any other East Asian country in fighting H5N1, or avian influenza. Nevertheless, WHO has refused Taiwan's applications to attend avian flu-related international conferences, thus preventing Taiwan from effectively sharing its valuable experience in disease prevention. According to Taiwan's National Immigration Agency, an average of 1,200 people travel between Taiwan and China each day, and the number of Taiwanese traveling to the United States averages more than 1,600 per day.

In May 2007, a man with a strain of tuberculosis that is highly resistant to current drug therapies was the subject of the first federal order for isolation issued in the United States for over forty years after he re-entered the country from Canada. The man had traveled by air among several countries including France and Italy against the advice of his physicians who determined that he had tuberculosis. While abroad, medical personnel determined that his tuberculosis was the extremely resistant type (XDR-TB), and finally persuaded him to seek medical care, but only

after he had returned to the United States. The CDC then began intensive efforts to track possible contacts that were in close contact with the infected man, including his fellow aircraft passengers and flight attendants.

The United Nations estimated that there were nearly 200 million international migrants in 2006—approximately 3% of the total global population. The annual number of migrants worldwide is likely increase. While immigration has the potential to spread disease, it also has brought attention to many health issues. Industrialized nations with large immigrant populations, such as the United States, have renewed interest in combating neglected diseases (diseases rare or eliminated in developed nations) across the globe. For example, international cooperative projects have sought to reduce incidence of

WORDS TO KNOW

IMMIGRATION: The relocation of people to a different region or country for their native lands; also refers to the movement of organisms into an area in which they were previously absent.

IMPORTED CASE OF DISEASE: Imported cases of disease happen when an infected person who is not yet showing symptoms travels from his home country to another country and develops symptoms of his disease there.

INTERNATIONAL HEALTH REGULATIONS: International regulations introduced by the World Health Organization (WHO) that aim to control, monitor, prevent, protect against and respond to the spread of disease across national borders while avoiding unnecessary interference with international movement and trade.

ISOLATION: Isolation, within the health community, refers to the precautions that are taken in the hospital to prevent the spread of an infectious agent from an infected or colonized patient to susceptible persons. Isolation practices are designed to minimize the transmission of infection.

MIGRATION: In medicine, migration is the movement of a disease symptom from one part of the body to another, apparently without cause.

PREVALENCE: The actual number of cases of disease (or injury) that exist in a population.

STRAIN: A subclass or a specific genetic variation of an organism.

tuberculosis and endemic parasitic diseases in Central and South America, as well as encourage screening and treatment for immigrants from those regions.

■ Primary Source Connection

The letter below to the editor of the journal *Pediatrics* highlights the special vaccination needs of children immigrating to the United States. Since Laurie C. Miller, a Boston-based physician specializing in internationally adopted children, wrote this letter in 1999, more than 100,000 additional children have been adopted by adults living in the United States. Miller is an associate professor of pediatrics and director of the International Adoption Clinic at Tufts University School of Medicine. She is the author of *The Handbook of International Adoption Medicine: A Guide for Physicians, Parents, and Providers.*

Internationally Adopted Children—Immigration Status

To the Editor,—

The number of internationally adopted children arriving in the United States has increased dramatically (13,620 in 1997, compared with 9,945 in 1986). Many children have received vaccines in their birth countries; however, the efficacy [effectiveness] of the vaccines and the accuracy of the records are sometimes questionable. Hostetter, et al. have reported protective diphtheria and tetanus titers in only 38 percent of Chinese, Russian, or Eastern European children with written evidence of age-appropriate vaccines.

We have observed that polio titers also may not be protective. Four children in our clinic with written evidence of 3 to 6 polio vaccines were found to have incompletely protective titers. The children were from Lithuania (1), Russia (2), and China (1). They ranged in age from 12 months to 8 years. In 3 children, protective titers to Type

1 and Type 2 polio were found, but no titers to Type 3 polio were measured. In one child, protective titers to Type 1 were absent, but were present for Types 2 and 3. Although the *Red Book* recommends that "written documentation should be accepted as evidence of prior immunization," clinicians caring for internationally adopted children should be aware of the possibility of incomplete immunity to polio, and should either revaccinate or verify immunity to all 3 types of polio. Revaccination or verification of protective titers should be considered for all immunizations in this population.

LAURIE C. MILLER, MD

International Adoption Clinic

New England Medical Center

Boston, MA 02111

Laurie C. Miller

MILLER, LAURIE C. "INTERNATIONALLY ADOPTED CHILDREN–IMMIGRATION STATUS." LETTER TO THE EDITOR. *PEDIATRICS.* 103.5 (MAY 1999): P1078(1).

BIBLIOGRAPHY

Books

Clark, Robert P. *Global Life Systems: Population, Food, and Disease in the Process of Globalization.* Lanham, MD: Rowman and Littlefield, 2000.

Web Sites

World Health Organization. "International Health Regulations." 2006 <http://www.who.int/csr/ihr/en/> (accessed May 17, 2007).

World Health Organization. "Tuberculosis and Air Travel: Guidelines for Prevention and Control." 2006 <http://www.who.int/tb/publications/2006/who_htm_tb_2006_363.pdf> (accessed May 17, 2007).

Caryn E. Neumann

Immune Response to Infection

■ Introduction

The immune system is a series of cells, tissues, organs, and processes in the body that differentiates the self from foreign bodies, fights infections, and develops immunity against future attack. The function of the immune system is to identify pathogens (disease-causing organisms) of all types and to destroy them through immune processes. Bacteria, viruses, fungi, parasites, cancerous cells, and single-celled organisms such as amoebas can all attack the body and cause disease. The immune system must recognize and act on these pathogens without attacking its own healthy tissues, thereby causing illness. The immune system also works to keep dangerous pathogens out of the body. This is an important function of the skin and mucous membranes, which have high concentrations of immune system cells: resisting, trapping, and killing microorganisms, preventing them from causing disease.

■ Scientific Foundations

One of the most important jobs of the immune system is to differentiate the self from the non-self. Almost all the cells of the body have specific proteins on their surfaces that identify them as "self." This is referred to at the major histocompatibility complex (MHC) protein. Foreign bodies, like bacteria, viruses, or cells belonging to another organism lack the appropriate MHC protein and are thus identified as "non-self." The healthy immune system reacts to things identified as non-self and not to things identified as self.

Many organs in the body are regarded as part of the immune system because they produce, transport, coordinate, or help mature immune cells. The bone marrow is often considered first because it is the source of all blood and immune cells. The thymus is the developing ground for T-cells (a lymphocyte, or white blood cell that fights pathogens), where large numbers of unsuit-

able cells undergo apoptosis (programmed cell death) for each mature T-cell that is produced. One of the functions of the spleen is to store and release generalized immune cells to respond to infection. Other lymphoid organs, such as the tonsils, adenoids, and appendix, are

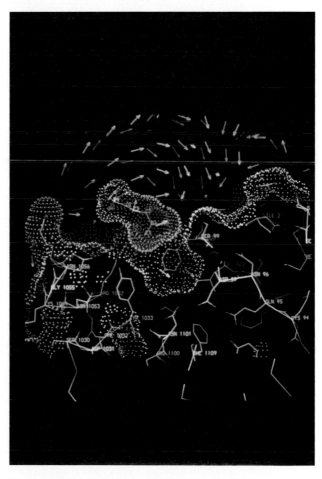

The first sightings of actual antibody-antigen docking are seen via X-ray crystallography. © *Ted Spiegel/Corbis.*

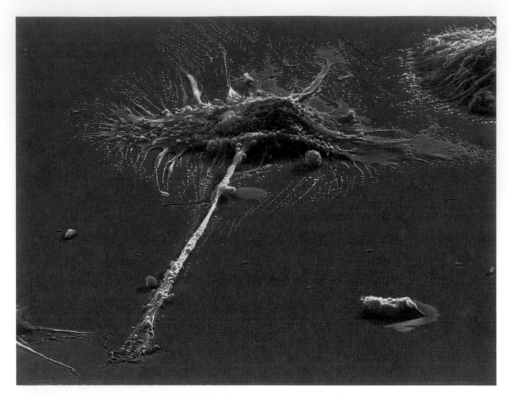

This colored scanning electron micrograph (SEM) shows a macrophage white blood cell (brown) attacking a group of *Borrelia* bacteria (blue, lower left). The macrophage extends a long pseudopod toward the bacteria prior to engulfing and destroying them. Several diseases are caused by various types of *Borrelia* bacteria, including Lyme disease and relapsing fever.   *Eye of Science/Photo Researchers, Inc.*

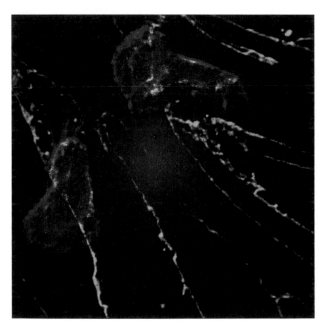

A confocal light micrograph shows white blood cells (red) moving through the intact walls of a blood vessel (green) in a process known as diapedesis. This is characteristic of the inflammatory response that occurs at the site of an injury. The cells leave the blood for the surrounding tissues so that they can destroy any invading organisms that may be present.   *David Becker/Photo Researchers, Inc.*

placed strategically in the respiratory and digestive tracts to intercept infectious agents before they enter further into the body.

The lymphatic system is a complex network of vessels and nodes that transport lymph, a fluid very similar to blood plasma. The lymph system connects the organs of the immune system with one another and with the rest of the body, carrying immune cells to their necessary locations. Lymph nodes are small compartments that provide space for immune cells to interact with antigens and begin their response. They also allow transfer of immune cells between the lymph system and the circulatory system. Unlike the blood, which is pumped around the body at high pressure by the heart, the lymph fluid is slow-moving and at low pressure, lacking a central pump. The lymph fluid is extracted from the body's tissues by osmosis, and then is transported around the body by the movement of muscles. Because of its slow-moving nature, lymph fluid can sometimes build up in the limbs, causing swelling and the possibility of infection. This is called lymphedema.

Anything that the immune system responds to, whether it is a microbe, protein, virus, or fragment of a pathogen, is called an antigen. The presence of antigens activates specific immune cells to destroy the pathogen and

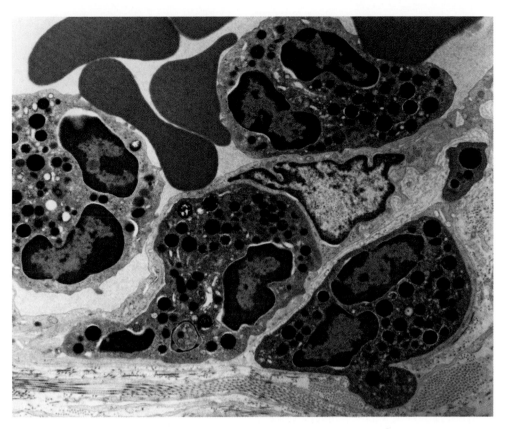

A neutrophil, a type of white blood cell, is shown as it moves from inside a capillary of an endothelial cell into the site of an infection in neighboring connective tissue. Neutrophils attack invaders and engulf them by phagocytosis. *© Visuals Unlimited/Corbis.*

teach the immune system to recognize it in the future. There are two major kinds of immune cells: those that react generally to all pathogens and those that are keyed to a specific disease-causing agent. Generalized immune cells include neutrophils, which consume pathogens and kill them with powerful chemical granules, and then send signals to other cells. Macrophages then arrive to consume the foreign bodies. Natural killer cells also use toxic granules to kill disease agents, responding to cells lacking the correct MHC proteins.

Lymphocytes, also known as white blood cells, are produced in the bone marrow and are present in the blood. From the bone marrow, certain lymphocytes known as T-cells travel to an organ known as the thymus to mature. Lymphocytes are also carried around the body by the lymphatic system. Two major types of lymphocytes react to specific pathogens. B-cells create antibodies, while T-cells destroy invaders and coordinate the overall immune response. Antibodies are special markers that lock onto antigens and alert the T-cells to destroy them. Cells use proteins called cytokines to communicate that they are injured and to organize immune cells.

After a pathogen has been detected and destroyed, a small number of antibodies and specialized T-cells remain to guard against future attack. When that same pathogen is encountered again, the number of specialized cells multiplies to mount an immune response.

■ Impacts and Issues

The generalized immune system cells provide innate immunity, the ability to identify a foreign body and destroy it without having been exposed to it previously. Once the immune system has encountered a pathogen, activated its immune cells, and developed antibodies, the body is said to have developed acquired (or adaptive) immunity. Vaccines provide resistance from diseases that the body has not encountered by causing the production of antibodies. Thus, vaccines induce a kind of acquired immunity. Nursing infants also obtain antibodies and immune system proteins from their mothers when they breast-feed. This is widely recognized as one of the benefits of nursing, since the immune system of infants is immature at birth.

One of the first bodily responses to infection or injury is inflammation, the familiar redness, swelling, heat, and pain associated with trauma. Inflammation is initiated locally by the blood vessels in the infected area.

WORDS TO KNOW

ACQUIRED (ADAPTIVE) IMMUNITY: Immunity is the ability to resist infection and is sub-divided into innate immunity, which an individual is born with, and acquired, or adaptive, immunity, which develops according to circumstances and is targeted to a specific pathogen. There are two types of acquired immunity, known as active and passive. Active immunity is either humoral, involving production of antibody molecules against a bacterium or virus, or cell-mediated, where T-cells are mobilized against infected cells. Infection and immunization can both induce acquired immunity. Passive immunity is induced by injection of the serum of a person who is already immune to a particular infection.

ANTIBODY: Antibodies, or Y-shaped immunoglobulins, are proteins found in the blood that help to fight against foreign substances called antigens. Antigens, which are usually proteins or polysaccharides, stimulate the immune system to produce antibodies. The antibodies inactivate the antigen and help to remove it from the body. While antigens can be the source of infections from pathogenic bacteria and viruses, organic molecules detrimental to the body from internal or environmental sources also act as antigens. Genetic engineering and the use of various mutational mechanisms allow the construction of a vast array of antibodies (each with a unique genetic sequence).

ANTIGEN: Antigens, which are usually proteins or polysaccharides, stimulate the immune system to produce antibodies. The antibodies inactivate the antigen and help to remove it from the body. While antigens can be the source of infections from pathogenic bacteria and viruses, organic molecules detrimental to the body from internal or environmental sources also act as antigens. Genetic engineering and the use of various mutational mechanisms allow the construction of a vast array of antibodies (each with a unique genetic sequence).

CYTOKINE: Cytokines are a family of small proteins that mediate an organism's response to injury or infection. Cytokines operate by transmitting signals between cells in an organism. Minute quantities of cytokines are secreted, each by a single cell type, and regulate functions in other cells by binding with specific receptors. Their interactions with the receptors produce secondary signals that inhibit or enhance the action of certain genes within the cell. Unlike endocrine hormones, which can act throughout the body, most cytokines act locally near the cells that produced them.

INNATE IMMUNITY: Innate immunity is the resistance against disease that an individual is born with, as distinct from acquired immunity that develops with exposure to infectious agents.

LYMPHOCYTE: A type of white blood cell; includes B and T lymphocytes. A type of white blood cell that functions as part of the lymphatic and immune systems by stimulating antibody formation to attack specific invading substances.

MAJOR HISTOCOMPATIBILITY COMPLEX (MHC): The proteins that protrude from the surface of a cell that identify the cell as "self." In humans, the proteins coded by the genes of the major histocompatibility complex (MHC) include human leukocyte antigens (HLA), as well as other proteins. HLA proteins are present on the surface of most of the body's cells and are important in helping the immune system distinguish "self" from "non-self" molecules, cells, and other objects.

NEUTROPHIL: An immune cell that releases a bacteria-killing chemical; neutrophils are prominent in the inflammatory response. A type of white blood cell that phagocytizes foreign microorganisms; also releases lysozyme.

PATHOGEN: A disease causing agent, such as a bacteria, virus, fungus, etc.

The activated vessels release fluids, which cause the swelling, as well as cytokines, which send signals to the immune system. This causes white blood cells of all types to rush to the area. The white blood cells begin acting on pathogens in their customary ways, identifying and consuming pathogens and creating antibodies. The cytotoxic (toxic to cells) chemicals present in neutrophils and other granulocytes are also responsible for reinforcing the inflammatory response. Inflammation can become harmful when it moves from a localized response to a systemic condition. Some heart problems, asthma, blood vessel disease, colitis (bowel disease), arthritis, fibromyalgia, and nephritis (kidney disease) are all associated with excessive or inappropriate inflammation.

Disorders of the immune system can cause serious disease. HIV is a well-known virus that attacks the helper T-cells, which activate and manage immune response. Once levels of helper T-cells fall to sufficiently low levels, the normal immune response breaks down and the victim becomes more susceptible to opportunistic infections. Many types of autoimmune diseases are the result of the immune system attacking the body. Crohn's disease, type I diabetes, rheumatoid arthritis, multiple sclerosis, myasthenia gravis, celiac disease, and Addison's disease are among the serious conditions associated with misdirected immune response. It should be noted that some developmental processes and the destruction of cancer require the immune system to act upon the self, and so not all autoimmune responses are harmful.

All organisms require defense from invasive pathogens. In humans and other vertebrates, the intricate and multi-layered protection provided by the organs, cells, proteins, and chemicals of the immune systems provides resistance to many kinds of attack. Even single-celled organisms use chemical substances to defend themselves. The proper function of the immune system is necessary for the health of the organism, avoiding both infection and autoimmune disease. Without the immune system, the body would be susceptible to endless attack, shortening lifespan or even making life impossible.

■ Primary Source Connection

Why an unequal society is an unhealthy society: poor relationships and low status don't just make people envious. They also interfere with the immune system and damage health.

Among those who see the mind as the work of natural selection, there is a sense that the time has come: we are beginning to understand what we really are.

From the construction boom in Darwinian theory, two major propositions have emerged, sustained by confidence that supporting data will increasingly be delivered in hard genetic currency. One is that human nature is evolved and universal; the other is that variations in personality and mental capabilities are substantially inherited. The first speaks of the species and the second about individuals. That leaves society—and here a third big idea is taking shape. In two words, inequality kills.

The phrase (which is that of Richard Wilkinson, one of the leading researchers in the field) sticks out from the current consensus like a sore thumb. For the most part, the major biological ideas concerning human nature and mental capabilities tend to confirm the way the world has turned out.

But what might be the biggest biological idea of all, in terms of its implications for human health and happiness, shows the world in a very different light. It finds that society has a profound influence over the length and quality of individuals' lives. The bodies of data are legion and the message from them is clear: unequal societies are unhealthy societies. They are unhealthy not just in the strict sense, but also in the wider one, that they are hostile, suspicious, antagonistic societies.

The most celebrated studies in this school of thought are those conducted among Whitehall civil servants by Michael Marmot, who presents his ideas in popular form in his recent book *Status Syndrome*. He and his colleagues found a steady gradient in rates of death between the lowest and the highest ranks of the civil service hierarchy. Top civil servants were less likely to die of heart disease than their immediate subordinates, and so on down the ladder; at the bottom, the lowest grades were four times more likely to die than the uppermost.

The main features of these findings were that the gradient was continuous, and that only about a third of the effect vanished when account was taken of the usual lifestyle suspects such as smoking and fatty food. This influence upon life and death affected everybody in the hierarchy, according to their position in it. Differences in wealth were an implausible cause in themselves, for most of the civil servants were comfortably off and even the lowest-paid were not poor. The fatal differences were those of status.

What goes for Whitehall seems to go for the world. In rich countries, death rates appear to be related to the differences between incomes, rather than to absolute income levels. The more unequally wealth is distributed, the higher homicide rates are likely to be. Although the findings about income inequality are controversial, the broad picture is consistent; and remains so when softer criteria than death are measured—for instance, trust or social cohesion. Inequality promotes hostility, frustrates trust and damages health.

It is hard to make sense of these findings outside a framework based on the idea of an evolved psychology. However, understanding humans as evolved social beings, made what we are by the selective pressures of life in groups of intelligent beings, it is easy to see that our minds and bodies depend upon our relations with our kind. These relations assume central importance for our health once economic development has minimised the dangers of infectious disease and relegated starvation to history.

Studies of baboons, social primates obliged by their nature to form hierarchies, tell the same story. A state of subordination is stressful; such stress may put the body into a mode that is vital in emergencies but corrosive as a permanent condition, interfering with the immune system and increasing the risk of heart disease. Conversely, human relationships formed on a broadly equal basis may support the immune system and promote health.

An American researcher, Sheldon Cohen, demonstrated this by dripping cold viruses into volunteers' noses, and then asking them about the range and frequency of their social relationships. The more connections they had—with acquaintances, colleagues, neighbours and fellow club members as well as with nearest and dearest—the less likely they were to develop colds.

The relationship between the length of life and its everyday quality is the relationship between its biological and social dimensions, which demands an evolutionary explanation; and the findings seem to demand egalitarian measures. Such Darwinian readings of the data on health and equality do not confound claims that humans are innately unequal. They do, however, lead to different views of how to make the best of people.

So do the prior ethical commitments that evolutionary thinkers bring to their projects. In his book *The Blank Slate*, having stated that all human characteristics are substantially impervious to parental influence, the psychologist Steven Pinker denounces the past century's art and related theories of art. Folk wisdom and popular taste are right, he affirms; "elite art" is perverse and wrong. The argument, built upon the idea that we all share an evolved human nature, is a standard-issue right-leaning castigation of the liberal elite.

Pinker takes his moral bearings from literary reference points, such as *Nineteen Eighty-Four*, that affirm the individual and condemn attempts to impose equality upon humankind's natural inequality. Modern Darwinism of this kind holds that evolutionary processes act on individual organisms rather than upon groups of organisms.

It makes no particularly strong predictions about variations among individual minds. That part of the picture comes from the behaviour geneticists, who compare identical twins with fraternal twins (or study their prize specimens, identical twins who have been reared apart) and conclude that a large proportion of the variation between individuals' personality traits, temperaments and intelligence is due to inherited differences.

Such findings readily lend themselves to a view of the world which attaches great importance to allowing individuals to fulfil their potential, while regarding social programmes to reduce inequalities as vain at best. Equality of opportunity is a fundamental principle; equality of outcome is a pernicious fantasy.

The result is an upbeat fatalism: upbeat about the prospects for scientific understanding of human psychology, fatalistic about the prospects that society might be improved by such understanding, and upbeat, also, in the confidence that society needs no radical alteration. Many of those who dislike such visions collude in them by acquiescing in the assumption that the effects of environments can be altered, but those of genes cannot.

The big idea that provides much of the driving force for evolutionary psychology, the project to describe a universal human nature, is that the sexes have different reproductive interests. The sex which invests the most in reproduction will be the one which takes more care in choosing its mates. Among humans, this implies that women will tend to be more discriminating than males in their choice of partners. It also implies that men and women will have different emotional propensities—as Stephen Jay Gould put it, conceding the central principle of evolutionary psychology in the very act of deploring the neoDarwinian school. It does not imply that every woman will be more circumspect in choice of partners than every man, or that every man will be readier to take risks than every woman, any more than the tendency for men to be taller than women means that all men are taller than all women. Through the widespread failure to recognise that evolved behaviours and ways of thinking are tendencies, evolutionary psychology has determinism thrust upon it.

In the application of evolutionary perspectives to health and equality, however, the prospect of a better society—or at least of better communities or workplaces—is unmistakable. This way of understanding human nature has the qualities that have marked great Darwinian ideas since *The Origin of Species*: it is profound in its implications, potentially transformative, and it challenges existing wisdom. On the one hand, it calls into question the idea that equality of opportunity should be pursued without regard for equality of outcome. On the other, it goes beyond the assumption that the task of "progressive" politics is to ensure that the least well-off have enough, and instead emphasises that how much is enough depends on how much others have.

The application of natural selection to social justice replaces vestigial sentiments about the abstract virtue of co-ops and community spirit with hard data about life and death, implying that we would all (or almost all) be healthier and happier if we were prepared to share more of what we have. Above all, it speaks to the world we live in, where want is marginal but trust is precarious. In Richard Wilkinson's words, it is "the science of social justice."

Like other big evolutionary ideas, however, it may be honoured more by denial than by engagement.

Marek Kohn

KOHN, MAREK. "WHY AN UNEQUAL SOCIETY IS AN UNHEALTHY SOCIETY: POOR RELATIONSHIPS AND LOW STATUS DON'T JUST MAKE PEOPLE ENVIOUS. THEY ALSO INTERFERE WITH THE IMMUNE SYSTEM AND DAMAGE HEALTH." *NEW STATESMAN* (1996) 133.4698 (JULY 26, 2004): P30(2).

SEE ALSO *Bacterial Disease; HIV; Vaccines and Vaccine Development; Viral Disease; Water-borne Disease.*

BIBLIOGRAPHY

Web Sites

Bugl, Paul. "Immune System." *University of Hartford.* <http://uhaweb.hartford.edu/BUGL/immune.htm> (accessed June 13, 2007).

Carter, J. Stein. "Immune System." *University of Cincinnati.* <http://biology.clc.uc.edu/Courses/bio105/immune.htm> (accessed June 13, 2007).

National Center for Biotechnology Information. "Diseases of the Immune System." <http://www.ncbi.nlm.nih.gov/disease/Immune.html> (accessed June 13, 2007).

National Institute of Allergy and Infectious Disease. "Understanding the Immune System." <http://health.nih.gov/viewPublication.asp?disease_id=63&publication_id=2841&pdf=yesgt; (accessed June 13, 2007).

Kenneth T. LaPensee

Impetigo

■ Introduction

Impetigo is a skin disorder characterized by crusting lesions and commonly occurs among children at an early school age. Infection is due to either *Staphylococcus* or *Streptococcus* bacteria and occurs at sites of skin trauma such as bites, scratches, or cuts.

Symptoms present as a tiny cluster of fluid-filled blisters that weep after bursting and form a crust. Fluids at these sites, as well as the nasal fluids of persons who harbor the causative agent in their nose, carry infection and allow for easy transmission between people. Washing sores with antibacterial soap and covering them can prevent transmission of the bacteria.

Treatment with antibiotics is usually very effective, and sores generally heal slowly without scarring. Prevention is achieved through good hygiene practices such as handwashing and treatment of other skin sores to prevent establishment of infection. Impetigo and its causative pathogens (disease-causing organisms) are found throughout the world.

■ Disease History, Characteristics, and Transmission

Impetigo is a skin disorder that results from bacterial infection, commonly by *Staphylococcus aureus* but also by

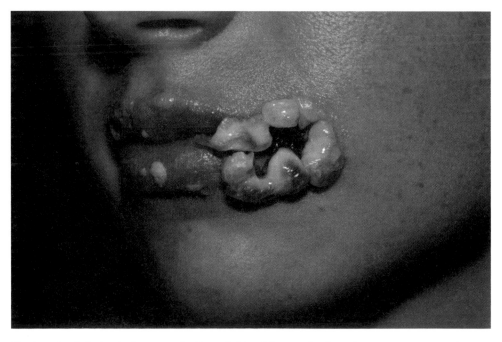

The impetigo infection is shown on the lips and side of the mouth of a patient. *Dr. M.A. Ansary/Photo Researchers, Inc.*

Streptococcus bacteria. Infection usually occurs when the protective barrier of the skin is irritated or breached due to cuts, scratches, insect bites, or eczema.

The disease is one of the most common among children and is characterized by crusting skin lesions usually located around the nose, mouth, hands, and forearms. Symptoms begin as small pimplelike sores surrounded by reddened skin, which quickly develop into fluid-filled blisters. Once the blisters rupture, that patch of skin will continue to weep and a yellowish crust will develop over four to six days. The lesions may vary slightly depending on the causative agent, but generally symptoms have the same presentation and will appear around two to three days after infection.

Impetigo is extremely contagious and transmission occurs through contact with the infected site, nasal fluid, or fomites (items such as clothing and bedding that contain infected material on their surface). Scratching may also spread the lesions.

■ Scope and Distribution

Those most commonly affected by impetigo are toddlers and school children between the ages of two and six years old, with peak incidence usually occurring in the hot and humid weather of the summer months. The disease tends to occur in small outbreaks, although epidemics are rare.

Impetigo often follows a recent upper respiratory tract infection caused by streptococcus bacteria, and people who suffer from cold sores may also have a higher chance of developing the disease.

There is often no apparent source of infection for impetigo. This is due largely to the fact that *Staphylococcus aureus* is part of the human body's normal flora, which means that it is one of many bacteria that readily colonize areas of the human body without causing infection. *Staphylococcus* bacteria are commonly found on the skin's surface, nose, and mouth and cause infection when they enter open wounds at these sites.

■ Treatment and Prevention

The focus of treatment for impetigo is to cure the infection and to relieve symptoms. If the infection is limited to a small area, a topical antibiotic ointment will generally be sufficient. If this is not effective, oral antibiotics may be required. Healing will begin within a few days of treatment and sores generally clear within ten days without severe scarring.

Prevention of impetigo may be achieved by maintaining good hygiene practices such as regular handwashing, bathing, and tending to skin injuries such as cuts, scrapes, bites, and rashes. To prevent passing along infection, infected sites should be covered and items such as linen and cutlery should not be shared

WORDS TO KNOW

COLONIZATION: Colonization is the process of occupation and increase in number of microorganisms at a specific site.

FOMITE: A fomite is an object or a surface to which an infectious microorganism such as bacteria or viruses can adhere and be transmitted. Transmission is often by touch.

PATHOGEN: A disease causing agent, such as a bacteria, virus, fungus, etc.

IN CONTEXT: REAL-WORLD RISKS

Impetigo refers to a very localized bacterial infection of the skin. It tends to afflict primarily children, but can occur in people of any age. Impetigo caused by the bacteria *Staphylococcus aureus* (or staph) affects children of all ages, while impetigo caused by the bacteria called group A streptococci (*Streptoccus pyogenes* or strep) are most common in children ages two to five years.

■ Impacts and Issues

Impetigo, although often widespread, generally poses little threat to communities and treatment is readily available in developed countries. The ease of transmission between people infected is heightened among groups of young children where limiting contact can prove difficult. In situations of outbreak among school groups, it is important that parents and teachers work together to ensure the infected children are appropriately and effectively treated while those not infected are successfully protected.

Evidence suggests that geography and climate will influence the primary infective organism causing impetigo. In developing nations and warmer climates, *Streptococcus* bacteria is the most common. In rare cases, impetigo caused by *Streptococcus* bacteria can progress deeper than the skin. One such complication arising from infection by *Streptococcus* may lead to damage of the kidneys, heart, or other organs. This makes early detection and treatment important in these developing regions.

SEE ALSO *Bacterial Disease; Childhood Infectious Diseases; Immunization Impacts; Handwashing;*

IN CONTEXT: EFFECTIVE RULES AND REGULATIONS

The Centers for Disease Control and Prevention (CDC), Coordinating Center for Infectious Diseases, Division of Bacterial and Mycotic Diseases states that The spread of all types of GAS infection (Group A Streptococcal Disease (strep throat, necrotizing fasciitis, impetigo) can be reduced by good handwashing, especially after coughing and sneezing and before preparing foods or eating. Persons with sore throats should be seen by a doctor who can perform tests to find out whether the illness is strep throat. If the test result shows strep throat, the person should stay home from work, school, or day care until 24 hours after taking an antibiotic. All wounds should be kept clean and watched for possible signs of infection such as redness, swelling, drainage, and pain at the wound site. A person with signs of an infected wound, especially if fever occurs, should seek medical care. It is not necessary for all persons exposed to someone with an invasive group A strep infection (i.e. necrotizing fasciitis or strep toxic shock syndrome) to receive antibiotic therapy to prevent infection. However, in certain circumstances, antibiotic therapy may be appropriate. That decision should be made after consulting with your doctor.

SOURCE: *Centers for Disease Control and Prevention (CDC), Coordinating Center for Infectious Diseases, Division of Bacterial and Mycotic Diseases*

Microorganisms; Staphylococcus aureus Infections; Strep Throat.

BIBLIOGRAPHY

Books

Mandell, G.L., J.E. Bennett, and R. Dolin. *Principles and Practice of Infectious Diseases, vol. 2.* Philadelphia, PA: Elsevier, 2005.

Mims, C., H. Dockrell, R. Goering, I. Roitt, D. Wakelin, and M. Zuckerman. *Medical Microbiology.* St. Louis, MO: Mosby, 2004.

Web Sites

Health Protection Agency. "Impetigo: Factsheet for Schools." <http://www.hpa.org.uk/infections/topics_az/wfhfactsheets/WFHImpetigo.htm> (accessed March 6, 2007).

Medline Plus. "Impetigo." Feb. 26, 2007 <http://www.nlm.nih.gov/medlineplus/ency/article/000860.htm> (accessed March 6, 2007).

Infection Control and Asepsis

Introduction

Steps that are taken to reduce or prevent infection in health care settings are known as infection control. Almost two million people in the United States acquire a nosocomial (hospital or health-care-related) infection each year, adding more than five billion dollars to health care costs annually. Most hospitals have dedicated infection control practitioners on staff, whose job it is to oversee the infection control procedures as specified by the United States Centers for Disease Control and Prevention (CDC) and the Association for Professionals in Infection Control and Epidemiology (APIC). Infection control professionals (ICPs) are usually nurses, physicians, medical technologists, or epidemiologists, and their main focus is to investigate and gather data about existing infections in order to take the appropriate actions to contain them and prevent future infections.

History and Scientific Foundations

Before infection control and asepsis were recognized, surgery was often a death sentence for the patient. Up until the mid-nineteenth century, the death rate following surgeries was over 50%. Instead of being a life-saving measure, surgery was a desperate last resort when all other treatments had failed. British surgeon and scientist Joseph Lister (1827–1912) changed the role of surgery by demonstrating the value of infection control. When he applied a spray of disinfectant over a patient's wound during surgery, Lister showed that post-operative infections could be markedly reduced. Later, this was shown to be due to the killing of bacteria that were present in the air of the operating room or on the clothing or gloves of the health care providers. By killing the bacteria before or immediately after they contacted the wound, infection was minimized. In the decades after Lister's method became popular, post-

operative patient deaths dropped to less than 1%. This was the beginning of the modern concept of aseptic technique.

Asepsis is defined as the absence or removal of disease-causing (pathogenic) microorganisms. Compounds that are used to achieve asepsis are termed antiseptics. Asepsis is designed to leave a surface sterile, free from microorganisms, and is used in surgery and for procedures where surfaces of medical equipment such as instruments or wound dressings will come in contact with sterile areas of the body. Sanitization is sufficient for other surfaces in the healthcare setting (and at home or in the community) to prevent infections. Sanitization does not leave surfaces sterile, but reduces the amount of disease-causing microorganisms to an insignificant level.

The cornerstone of infection control involves breaking the cycle of infection and interrupting the transmission of disease-causing organisms. The concept of standard precautions is the infection control foundation for healthcare workers, and is used universally in the developed world. Standard precautions assumes that any patient's body fluid, tissue, or secretion could be potentially infectious until determined otherwise, and along with hand-washing, barrier protection such as latex (or a latex-alternative) gloves, disposable gowns, and masks should be used as appropriate to avoid exposure to them. Likewise, barrier protections are used to prevent patients from being exposed to body fluids or surface disease-causing organisms that might be present on or in the healthcare worker.

Additional infection control measures are based upon isolating or grouping together (cohorting) persons with infectious diseases according to how the disease is spread. Isolation means setting apart a person with a known infection. Additional sets of precautions are used for persons with documented infections and include airborne precautions, droplet precautions, and contact precautions. When airborne precautions are implemented, as with a person who has an active tuberculosis infection, negative-pressure airflow rooms assure that the extremely small tuberculosis bacteria will not enter other patient

WORDS TO KNOW

ASEPSIS: Without germs, more specifically without microorganisms.

BIOFILM: Biofilms are populations of microorganisms that form following the adhesion of bacteria, algae, yeast, or fungi to a surface. These surface growths can be found in natural settings such as on rocks in streams, and in infections such as can occur on catheters. Microorganisms can colonize living and inert natural and synthetic surfaces.

COHORTING: Cohorting is the practice grouping persons with like infections or symptoms together in order to reduce transmission to others.

INFECTION CONTROL PROFESSIONAL (ICP): Infection control professionals are a group of nurses, doctors, laboratory workers, microbiologists, public health officials, and others who have specialized training in the prevention and control of infectious disease. Infection control professionals develop methods to control infection and instruct others in their use. These methods include proper hand washing, correct wearing of protective masks, eye-guards, gloves, and other specialized clothing, vaccination, monitoring for infection, and investigating ways to

treat and prevent infection. Courses and certifications are available for those wishing to become infection control professionals.

ISOLATION: Isolation, within the health community, refers to the precautions that are taken in the hospital to prevent the spread of an infectious agent from an infected or colonized patient to susceptible persons. Isolation practices are designed to minimize the transmission of infection.

NOSOCOMIAL INFECTION: A nosocomial infection is an infection that is acquired in a hospital. More precisely, the Centers for Disease Control in Atlanta, Georgia, defines a nosocomial infection as a localized infection or one that is widely spread throughout the body that results from an adverse reaction to an infectious microorganism or toxin that was not present at the time of admission to the hospital.

STANDARD PRECAUTIONS: Standard precautions are the safety measures taken to prevent the transmission of disease-causing bacteria. These include proper hand washing, wearing gloves, goggles, and other protective clothing, proper handling of needles, and sterilization of equipment.

rooms, and specialized masks are used by both hospital staff and the patient to prevent the spread of tuberculosis. Droplet precautions are used for persons with known or suspected diseases that can be spread through larger infectious particles that are released by coughing or sneezing, such as polio or measles. Gown, masks, and gloves are usually worn by healthcare personnel and visitors when they are in the room of a patient with droplet precautions. Contact precautions are used with persons who have infections that can be transmitted by direct or indirect skin-to-skin contact, such as wounds infected with resistant bacteria. Regardless of the type of specialized precautions implemented in persons with infections, standard precautions are always additionally in effect.

Other key elements to infection control in the healthcare setting include disposing infectious waste (such as gloves and wound dressings) in separate containers that receive special handling and are labeled "biohazard", disposing of needles, scalpels, and other sharp medical equipment in thick, biohazard labeled containers, limiting patient or visitor exposures, and specialized housekeeping and laundry methods.

Asepsis has long been a valuable means of infection control. One of the first laboratory procedures a microbiology student learns is to wipe down the working surface with an alcohol solution before and after doing any work involving bacteria. This simple step kills most bacteria that are adhering to the work surface. This is because the alcohol dissolves the membrane(s) of bacteria. Bacterial membranes are composed mainly of phospholipids—molecules that have a water-loving (hydrophilic) ends and a central portion that is water-hating (hydrophobic). This allows phospholipids to spontaneously associate with the hydrophilic portions oriented to the outside of the membrane and the hydrophobic regions buried inside; this products a barrier that is vital for the structure and the survival of the bacteria. Alcohol, which is also hydrophobic, can induce hydrophobic portions of the phospholipids to associate with it instead of remaining as an intact membrane. As a result, the bacterial membrane dissolves, killing the microbe. The simple act of wiping down a work surface prevents the spread of potentially harmful bacteria.

■ Applications and Research

Many infections are contagious and so are capable of being spread from person to person and from another host to a person. People may even contaminate themselves and contract an infection. An example of the latter is the fecal-oral route, where hands soiled by feces during a bowel movement and which have not been properly cleaned come in contact with in the mouth or other parts of the body. A common example is the infections that occur in day care facilities. Infants can handle their soiled diaper and subsequently put a hand in their mouth or another persons's mouth. Another example is at the other end of the age spectrum. Elderly people who may be incontinent and whose attentiveness to their sanitary habits may have deteriorated can unknowingly transfer feces to the urinary tract through inadequate hygiene after a bowel movement. This route of transfer can also allow the fecal bacteria to enter the bloodstream. The subsequent blood infection (sepsis) can spread through the body quickly, lethally overwhelming the ability of the immune system to fight the infection.

A simple and time-tested way to minimize person to person transmission of microbes is handwashing. Proper handwashing is the most effective way to prevent the spread of infection. In the home, the use of household soap and vigorous scrubbing of the hands for 30–60 seconds has been shown to eliminate most microorganisms of concern from the hands. This is especially important for those who are involved in food preparation, since fecally-acquired bacteria and virus can contaminate food during handling. In a related step, the cleaning of cutting boards and utensils such as knives helps prevent transfer of microbes. As an example, on of the main reasons for the millions of foodborne contamination with the bacterium *Campylobacter jejuni* that occurs each year in the United States is not washing cutting boards used to process raw poultry before the board is used for another food. The bacteria sticking to the board are transferred to the other food which, if not cooked or undercooked, can cause illness when eaten.

In the hospital setting, handwashing is done according to CDC guidelines. These specify that healthcare providers wash their hands before and after seeing each patient and, if gloves have also been worn, as the final step when the gloves have been removed and put in the proper disposal container. Many hospitals are equipped with an alcohol-based washstand at the foot of each patient bed or in the room. Handwashing using alcohol takes only seconds—the time savings can be important in a healthcare providers busy schedule.

Various infection control procedures are in place in most hospitals to lessen the spread of infection. This is important for several reasons. Firstly, bacteria that are resistant to most antibiotics are becoming more prevalent. An example is methicillin-resistant *Staphylococcus*

aureus (MRSA); the prevalence of MRSA in hospitals has gone from sporadic and rare in the early 1980s to over 90% of all clinical *S. aureus* isolates in hospitals in the United States and United Kingdom in 2006. In fact, in the UK, MRSA infections now make up over half of all hospital infections. The fact that only a few antibiotics remain effective against MRSA is frightening, and makes control of the bacterium's presence and spread in a hospital critical for patient health and survival.

A second reason for infection control is the emergence of new infectious viral and bacterial diseases that are easily spread from person to person. An example is the viral disease called severe acute respiratory syndrome, or SARS. Another example of a disease that is poised to become a global problem is avian influenza (bird flu). As of 2007, the virus that causes avian influenza, which has been capable of transmission from birds to humans and which has been of limited concern, is adapting to be capable of person to person transmission. The World Health Organization and CDC are monitoring avian influenza cases closely.

Infection control measures are also important because diseases that used to be rampant but which were controlled decades ago are now re-emerging to become a significant health threat. One example is the form of tuberculosis caused by the bacterium *Mycobacterium tuberculosis*.

Research laboratories and hospitals often have a variety of CDC- and APIC-mandated infection control procedures in place. Depending on the organism being studied or encountered, most countries have a series of mandated safety controls, with more dangerous microbes requiring more stringent safety and infection control measures. One example is the use of filters in the ventilation system that trap bacteria and even particles as small as viruses. The filters prevent the movement of the microbes from the room to other parts of the building or outside. Some work surfaces can be inside of an enclosed structure called a fume hood, which is separate from the rest of the lab. The fume hood can be open to the rest of the room; just having a semi-enclosed space cuts down on air movement. Fume hoods can also be completely enclosed, with the work begin done by means of plastic gloves that the person slips their hands into. Equipment and other items can be introduced into the chamber of the fume hood by a two-way door that does not allow air inside the fume hood to move to the outside. Even the work surface itself is designed for infection control. A century ago, the work surfaces in labs were made of wood; while pretty, the surfaces had cracks and crevasses that were ideal breeding grounds for infectious bacteria. Modern lab surfaces are made of chemically-resilient plastic that is very smooth, watertight, and free of gaps. The same principle can be used in the operating theater, where the floor is a single, crack-free unit that is made of material that can be easily cleaned.

Another infection control procedure in a hospital is the use of protective hand wear and clothing. This helps protect the health care provider from contamination from a patient, and, because the protective gear is discarded when moving from patient to patient, minimizes the chance that the health care provider will become a vehicle of transfer of an infection. The use of protective gear depends on the risk posed by a patient. For example, the CDC guidelines indicate that if there is a reasonable chance that someone could be exposed to the splashing or spraying of blood (such as can occur in an Ebola infection, where copious bleeding can occur), a protective gown and perhaps a face mask should be worn. The gown may need to be made of a water-resistant material.

Highly infectious patients will tend to be isolated from other patients in a hospital, and wards containing people who are particularly susceptible to infection (such as transplant recipients, whose immune system is usually deliberately suppressed to reduce the chance of rejection of the transplanted organ) may be in an area of the hospital that has less daily traffic. Contact precautions specify that such patients should be housed in a private room or with similarly-affected people.

Infection control actions can also be taken in the community; an example is malaria. The disease is transmitted by mosquitoes, so steps to control mosquito populations, especially during the insect's breeding season, can help lessen the infection. Spraying prime breeding grounds with insecticide is a common strategy. As well, more high-tech science approaches are being used. For example, a program in malaria-prone regions of Africa that releases genetically altered and infertile male mosquitoes has shown promise. The males are unable to successfully mate with female mosquitoes, which reduce the numbers of the next generation. As malaria is transmitted only be female mosquitoes, reduced numbers of new females means there is less opportunity for the spread of malaria. Another simple and effective infection control mechanism for insect-borne diseases is the use of mosquito netting over a bed during sleep. Organizations including WHO and World Vision conduct campaigns that solicit money for the purchase of mosquito netting and the delivery of the netting to rural villages in malaria-prone regions of Africa. This simple step saves many lives by preventing the mosquito-borne transmission of the infection.

The use of antimicrobial or antiviral agents can help overcome an infection and, in the case of vaccines, can prevent someone from contracting an infection. An example of the power of a vaccine is polio. Prior to the 1950s, polio was a dreaded childhood viral illness that paralyzed many children. After the introduction and refinement of two polio vaccines, polio has become a rare event. The Polio Eradication Initiative launched by the World Health Organization (WHO) in 1988 has reduced the global number of polio cases by over 99%. In 2006, four countries had polio epidemics, as compared to 125 countries in 1988.

The WHO campaign also highlights the importance of maintaining an infection control program. During 2006, the interruption of the campaign in Nigeria due to a military conflict caused a renewed polio outbreak. Infection control cannot be done once and then forgotten; vigilance must be continual.

Even with vigilance, infection control can be difficult. An example is the use of antibiotics. In the decades of 1940s–1960s following the introduction of penicillin and the discovery or synthesis of new antibiotics, these agents were hugely successful at dealing with bacterial infections. But, as with the polio campaign, initial success does not guarantee long-term success. Bacteria haven proven to be capable of adaptation to many of the antibiotics that have been introduced. This resistance can appear within only a few years, and can spread. Strains of enterococci and *Staphylococcus aureus* that are resistant to virtually all known antibiotics currently in use pose a challenge in patient care.

Antibiotic resistance can spread through a bacterial population quickly because the genetic information that specifies the protein involved in the resistance is often located on a piece of genetic material that is not part of the main chromosome, but which is more mobile. This means that the information is more capable of being transferred from one bacterium to another bacterium that it comes into contact with.

The hospital is a prime breeding ground for antibiotic resistance. The heavy use of antibiotics and disinfectants in a hospital imposes a selection pressure on bacteria. Those bacteria that can adapt to be resistant stand a better chance of surviving and thriving.

■ Impacts and Issues

Infection control and asepsis will always be fundamentally important measures in hospitals. One reason is evident from the prevalence of hospital-acquired (nosocomial) infections. In the United States, nosocomial infections kill 90,000 patients each year according to CDC, which in 2005 issued new recommendations aimed at lessening the toll from these infections.

Infection control and asepsis are also becoming more important in the prevention of infections, as infectious diseases become more resistant and as new diseases emerge. People are more at risk for infections, especially since the populations of many developed countries are aging. In general, the elderly are increasingly vulnerable to infections as their immune systems and overall resilience declines. As the population of a country like the United States ages, the costs of health care will grow. In 2007, the costs of delivering health care in the United States and elsewhere are skyrocketing, as the many infection control measures and the development of new effective weapons against microbial diseases is expensive. As health care becomes increasingly more expensive to deliver, the ability to supply the needed care becomes more difficult. Governments in countries such as the United States, Canada, and England are recognizing that the current systems of health care are likely not sustainable. Reducing the need for health care by improved infection control is also recognized as an economical, vital strategy to ensure good health for future generations.

Traditionally, infection control strategies for bacterial disease have been geared towards the types of bacteria studied in the laboratory. Scientists now know, however, that these bacteria that live and grow while floating in the lab growth medium are not at all like the populations found in the real world. Infections are often caused by bacteria that grow by adhering to surfaces. These so-called biofilms are more resistant to drugs that would easily kill their floating counterparts. This means that infection control strategies need to change to more realistically deal with the real world of biofilm-caused bacterial infections.

■ Primary Source Connection

Institutions such as schools, hospitals, and nurseries are especially prone to infectious disease that spread through casual contact or the fecal-oral route. A 2006 outbreak of *E. coli* in nurseries in Scotland highlighted the importance of institutional hygiene and infectious disease control practices in preventing disease.

Nurseries Told to Clean Up Their Act

FILTHY CONDITIONS have been uncovered at scores of Scotland's nurseries, the Sunday Mail can reveal today.

The alarming hygiene failures at the nurseries can be exposed as suspected cases of potentially fatal E Coli linked to a nursery in Fife hit 25.

Inspectors have ordered 84 nurseries to clean up their act after discovering:

Vermin in a nursery classroom.

Toddlers asked to do their own cleaning with chemicals.

Dishes being washed in a toilet.

Tots being asked to share facecloths.

The Care Commission assessed 2380 nurseries and playgroups.

Of those, 84 were ordered to change their practices on infection control.

Inspectors found signs of vermin in a cabin used as Auchtertyre Primary School's nursery in the Highlands.

Bosses of the school in Kyle of Lochalsh were told to destroy the cabin.

They had been warned about the health hazard last year but took no action.

The warning was repeated in findings published in February, yet the building is still standing.

A spokesman for Highland Council said: "It is planned for demolition.

"Vermin control measures have been and are in place at the school but because of the rural nature of the site, mice can sometimes be an issue."

At Dundee's Wonderland nursery, staff gave kids chemicals to clean up.

The inspectors reported: "The nursery must review its practice of permitting children to use a chemical cleaning agent to clean the tables.

"Staff should also ensure that cleaning materials remain in the original container."

At the time of the inspection, the youngsters were eating sandwiches without plates.

The inspectors added: "They should provide plates for the children at meal times to improve hygiene.

Owner Graham MacDonald said: "For years, we had been allowing the children to use anti-bacterial sprays to clean up.

"We thought it was a good way to teach them about hygiene but have stopped it.

"The children do get given plates to eat from but on the day of the inspection, they were having sandwiches."

Staff at Beauly Playgroup in Invernessshire were told to make changes after inspectors discovered the only sink to wash dishes was in the toilet. Yesterday, the owners were unavailable for comment.

Coringa Day Care in Dundee was told to produce an infection-control procedure immediately and were slammed for using communal bedding and face-cloths. In April, the centre was reopened as Sweeties Day Care.

The new owner, Jane McDonald, is eager to distance herself from the report.

She said: "I am getting antibacterial mats for the children. I will only use bedding for the cots and it will be washed every day."

Also in April, organisers of the Kiwi Pre-school Playgroup in East Kilbride, Lanarkshire, were told to clean up dirty toilets.

The inspectors' report said: "The toilet area was uninviting. It was dark and dirty and had not been well maintained."

A spokesman for South Lanarkshire Council said: "Kiwi Pre-School Playgroup will take forward the points raised and improvements to the toilet area will be in their plan of action."

Toilets also featured in the inspectors' remarks about Langholm Primary School Nursery Class in 2005. Toys were found stored there.

The experts said: "The nursery is required to make proper provision for the health and welfare of the children and to ensure appropriate attention to infection control by making alterations to flush mechanisms, washbasin taps and hot water supply and making appropriate arrangements for the storage of play resources."

A spokesman for Dumfries and Galloway Council said an alternative area had been found to store the toys.

Croft Park Nursery in Airdrie, Lanarkshire, was criticized because food was not being served at the correct temperature.

Janette Rose, of the Early Years Service which runs the nursery, said they had amended their food preparation practice.

A commission spokesman said: "All care staff must adopt the highest standards with regard to hygiene and infection control to minimise the risk to children."

Himaya Quasem and Heather Greenaway

QUASEM, HIMAYA, AND HEATHER GREENAWAY. "NURSERIES TOLD TO CLEAN UP THEIR ACT; EXCLUSIVE THE E COLI CRISIS." *SUNDAY MAIL*, MAY 14, 2006. P.5.

SEE ALSO *Airborne Precautions; Contact Precautions; Handwashing; Standard Precautions; Water-borne Disease.*

BIBLIOGRAPHY

Books

Bankston, John. *Joseph Lister and the Story of Antiseptics.* Hockessin, DE: Mitchell Lane Publishers, 2004.

Lawrence, Jean, and Dee May. *Infection Control in the Community.* New York: Churchill Livingstone, 2003.

Websites

Yale-New Haven Hospital. "YNHH Infection Control; Introduction." <http://www.med.yale.edu/ynhh/infection/precautions/intro.html> (accessed June 13, 2007).

Brian Hoyle

Influenza

■ Introduction

Influenza is a viral disease that has plagued humans since the time of learning to walk upright. The medical writings of antiquity contain evidence that implicates influenza in causing epidemics of death and disease. A form of the influenza virus exists in nearly all animals, including domesticated birds and pigs, and these animal viruses bear a close genetic relationship to human influenza viruses.

A typical attack of influenza starts with high fever, chills, muscle aches, a dry cough, and feeling distinctly ill. Soon a sore throat with nasal congestion and a runny nose develops. The cough worsens and misery results. In healthy adults and children, a case of influenza lasts about a week and recovery is complete. Many think the illness is nothing more than a particularly severe "cold." However, influenza can be unpredictable, and can kill healthy adults and children.

■ Disease History, Characteristics, and Transmission

Most often, influenza primarily attacks the nose, throat, and lungs, but any part of the body can be infected. Sometimes influenza will cause abdominal pain, nausea,

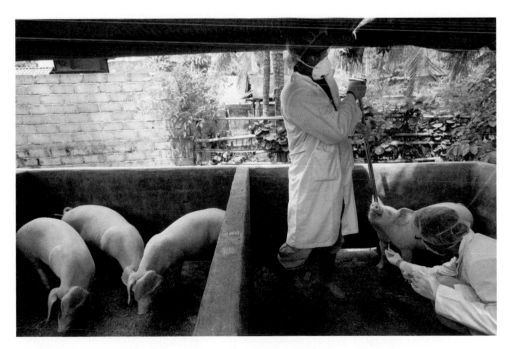

In Bali, Indonesia, scientists swab a pig's nostril to obtain a sample for their study of the evolution of influenza viruses in late 2006. Earlier that year, two cases of H5N1 (bird flu) were found in pigs, which are susceptible to many of the viruses that infect humans. *Dimas Ardian/Getty Images.*

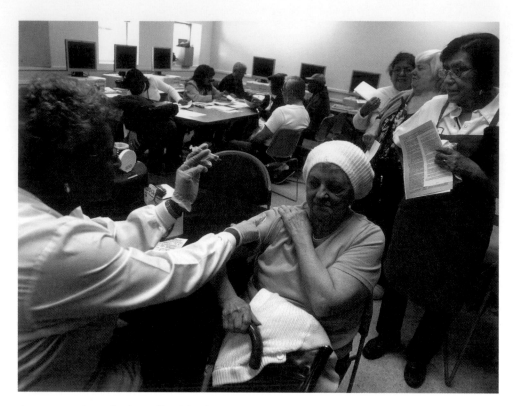

A woman receives a flu shot, offered free by the city of Chicago in October 2006. In a switch from recent years, vaccine makers produced an ample supply, and health officials administered more than 100 million doses nationwide by the end of the year. *Tim Boyle/Getty Images.*

and diarrhea. Rarely, the muscles will be infected and can be severely damaged. Infants may develop a severe form of viral pneumonia with the heart and lungs struggling to sustain life. Influenza can infect the brain as well, resulting in seizures and coma. Influenza is predictably unpredictable in how severe the disease may be in any one person.

Other diseases can take advantage of the weakened state of the body after a case of influenza and cause a secondary infection. Bacteria such as group A streptococcus, *Staph aureus*, and strep pneumonia are particularly efficient at causing a lethal pneumonia after influenza damages the lungs. About 10% of children will develop a secondary infection while recovering from influenza, and ear infections frequently afflict infants and young children just as they are trying to recover from influenza. The secondary infections often cause another visit to the doctor when parents discover their child, who seemed to be recovering, is ill again.

Influenza is highly contagious and primarily spreads person to person in virus-laden droplets produced by sneezing or coughing. Alternatively, the droplets land on a surface and contaminate the hands that, if not washed, carry the virus to the mouth or nose. School-aged children are the main culprits in spreading influenza. Usually 10–40% of school-aged children will get

influenza in any one season. They swap virus at school and bring it home to infect family members. Children are contagious before they even appear or feel ill, and the virus is present in nasal mucous and cough droplets for over a week after apparent recovery from influenza.

The microbiology of the influenza virus is quite complex. Influenza viruses consist of three different major types known as A, B, and C. Of the three types, only A and B cause significant disease in humans. Both A and B types cause the seasonal epidemics around the world, but at any one time there may be hundreds of different variations of each type circulating the globe. This multitude of subtly different varieties presents a challenge to the human immune system.

Both influenza A and B virus change their structure often enough such that the immune system can never develop long-lasting immunity. Influenza B virus changes much more slowly than influenza A and usually causes milder illness compared to influenza A. However, influenza B can cause severe disease in the elderly, those with impaired immunity, or those with chronic lung or heart disease.

Influenza A generally causes more severe disease and is the most unpredictable. The yearly season epidemics of the "flu" are primarily the result of influenza A. The virus has two specific proteins on its surface, which are important for infecting humans. These proteins, known as antigens, bear the names hemagglutinin (HA) and neuraminidase (NA). The HA and NA proteins vary in their chemical structure from year to year. This process, termed antigenic drift, results in virus particle proteins with subtle variations in structure. Fifteen different HA subtypes are known to exist while there are nine NA subtypes. These slightly different proteins get different number designations, and the various influenza strains are named by the specific HA and NA proteins on the virus. The H3N1 virus contains HA protein 3 and NA protein 1.

Influenza A employs an additional means of evading the immune system. When two different viral strains infect someone at the same time, the two viral variants will swap component genes and create yet another slightly different form of influenza. The new virus will contain some proteins of one variety of influenza A and some proteins of the other variety. This sloppy way of making new virus particles extends to swapping genetic material with animal or bird influenza viruses. This process, termed antigenic shift, will sometimes create an influenza virus for which humans have no immunity at all. A novel virus produced this way has the potential to spread worldwide, resulting in a pandemic.

Three influenza pandemics have occurred in the twentieth century. The influenza pandemic in 1918 killed at least twenty million people, and some experts think there were fifty million deaths within a period of 24 weeks. Nearly as many United States soldiers died of influenza in 1918 as died in battle in all of World War I. In the United States, the 1957 pandemic resulted in 70,000 deaths while in 1968 about 30,000 died. During influenza pandemics, a larger proportion of healthy adults die than during the yearly "flu season" outbreaks.

■ Treatment and Prevention

Medicine has developed weapons with which to combat influenza, specifically the adamantanes and the neuraminidase inhibitor drugs. The adamantanes treat only influenza A while the neuraminidase inhibitors will treat both influenza A and B. Both of these classes of medicines interfere with the ability of the influenza virus to make more virus particles. They either stop production of the viral genetic material or prevent the viral particles from escaping from infected cells to infect other cells. In order to help relieve symptoms or shorten the course of influenza, one must take these drugs early in the course of influenza. Once the illness is established and new influenza virus particles have replicated, the medications are largely ineffective. Many of the symptoms of influenza are due to the damage the virus does to the body during the making of new virus particles so stopping the virus early provides the greatest relief in symptoms.

Until effective medications became available to treat influenza, determining who has influenza rather than one

---

WORDS TO KNOW

ANTIGEN: Antigens, which are usually proteins or polysaccharides, stimulate the immune system to produce antibodies. The antibodies inactivate the antigen and help to remove it from the body. While antigens can be the source of infections from pathogenic bacteria and viruses, organic molecules detrimental to the body from internal or environmental sources also act as antigens. Genetic engineering and the use of various mutational mechanisms allow the construction of a vast array of antibodies (each with a unique genetic sequence).

ANTIGENIC SHIFT: Antigenic shift describes an abrupt and major genetic change (e.g. in genes coding for surface proteins of a virus).

DROPLET TRANSMISSION: Droplet transmission is the spread of microorganisms from one space to another (including from person to person) via droplets that are larger than 5 microns in diameter. Droplets are typically expelled into the air by coughing and sneezing.

PANDEMIC: Pandemic, which means all the people, describes an epidemic that occurs in more than one country or population simultaneously.

STRAIN: A subclass or a specific genetic variation of an organism.

---

of a similar multitude of viral respiratory illnesses was of little use. Treatment involved decreasing the fever, resting, and drinking plenty of fluids. This treatment is appropriate for most viral illnesses, but now with medications available, there is a difference whether the illness is a "cold" or the "flu" and testing for influenza is often done.

Several rapid tests are available to detect the influenza virus. These tests, often run in a doctor's office, use a sample of mucus taken from the nose or from the back of the throat. The tests are rapid usually taking only five minutes and will detect influenza virus accurately about 75-85% of the time if properly done.

Contrary to popular belief, antibiotics are not effective treatment for influenza. Antibiotics are useful in the treatment of bacterial infections and have no benefit during viral illnesses. Antibiotics may be helpful if secondary bacterial infections develop during the course of influenza.

Drugs provide a treatment option unavailable in past decades, but they do not provide the best option for control of influenza. Many will not realize their illness is influenza until it is too late for medications to be effective. Additionally they have usually already spread influenza to family members and co-workers.

Influenza vaccination provides the most effective treatment by preventing the disease, but the influenza virus poses a challenge for vaccine development. Since the virus changes slightly year to year and changes dramatically at unpredictable intervals, vaccines also need altering from year to year. Each year, public health officials make an educated guess as to what will be the prevalent strains circulating in the next season, and vaccine preparation commences targeting those strains.

Influenza vaccines provide excellent protection when administered at least two weeks before exposure to the influenza virus, and vaccination is needed each year. The vaccine itself does not cause influenza, but depending on the exact form of vaccine administered, side effects may include soreness at the injection site, muscle aches, runny nose, or sore throat. Young children often need two doses of vaccine for full protection. In the United States, the current vaccine recommendations include everyone older than 65 years, those between six months and five years, and everyone with chronic health problems involving the lungs or heart.

■ Scope and Distribution

Every year about 35,000 deaths occur in the United States due to influenza. Most of these deaths are those older than 65 years, but more children die of influenza or its complications each year than all the deaths due to whooping cough and measles combined. The World Health Organization credits influenza with causing between 250,000 and 500,000 deaths yearly throughout the world. For example, in 2002, an influenza outbreak started in Madagascar. Over a period of three months, 27,000 people developed influenza, and despite rapid medical intervention, 800 deaths occurred.

■ Impacts and Issues

Unless a family member or close friend dies of influenza, many people do not really give much thought to the impact influenza has on their health and pocketbook. Influenza ranks far behind heart disease and cancer as a worldwide cause of death, yet its economic impact is considerable. Public health experts have estimated a cost of $60-$4,000 for every case of influenza in a healthy adult in the United States. These costs include direct medical expenses, lost wages, and lost productivity at work. For parents, the cost often includes lost work while caring for the sick child, and afterwards, lost work from the case of influenza caught from the child.

A pandemic raises great concern for public health officials worldwide. Influenza pandemics occur several times a century but are unpredictable as to the exact

timing. Each of the past three influenza pandemics (in 1918, 1957, and 1968) resulted from human influenza virus sharing genetic material with a bird influenza virus. Human immune systems had never encountered the new virus, and everyone was susceptible to the new form of influenza. As a result, the new virus swept through countries throughout the globe.

The pandemic of 1918 deserves further explanation as medical history warns that a similar event at some point in the future is highly likely. In the 1918 pandemic, about one third of the world's population suffered a severe case of influenza, and nearly 3% of those infected with the virus died. An unusually high percentage of the young and healthy died during this pandemic. All current strains of influenza A virus are descended from the 1918 virus, but the current strains have weakened considerably. Now less than 0.1% of people die when infected by today's forms of influenza.

Given that the medical system has advanced since 1918, what would be the impact of a new, more lethal influenza virus today? The answer is that the impact could be devastating. Public health experts predict an estimated 90,000–200,000 deaths, over 700,000 hospital admissions, and about forty million visits to doctors in the United States alone. The estimated economic impact exceeds $160 billion, not including the disruptions due to illness in the police, transportation workers, and the health workers themselves.

Over the past several years, a particularly vicious strain (type) of avian (bird) flu, known as H5N1 influenza, has caused many cases of disease and death in humans. Presently, transmission of this virus from human to human does not readily occur. Close contact with infected birds is required to catch this form of influenza. If this bird virus ever acquires the ability to infect humans from one person to another, a new pandemic could occur. The Center for Disease Control and the World Health organization recognize this possibility, and planning for the potential pandemic continues.

■ Primary Source Connection

Scientists at the Centers for Disease Control and Prevention play a key role in accessing influenza viruses and formulating vaccines for them. In order to prepare for a future pandemic influenza, CDC scientists studied the characteristics of the 1918 pandemic flu virus. The CDC press release below, released in February 2007, relates that by manipulating the 1918 virus, CDC scientists have found a way to render it less capable of spreading among animals that were in close contact with each other. This type of research could prove beneficial in reducing the ability of future influenza viruses to spread rapidly across heavily populated regions and cause a pandemic.

Small Changes in 1918 Pandemic Virus Knocks Out Transmission: Research Provides Clues for Assessing Pandemic Potential of New Influenza Viruses

Press Release

Embargoed Until 2 p.m. EST: February 1, 2007

Contact:

CDC Media Relations

(404) 639-3286

Experts at the Centers for Disease Control and Prevention have shown that a molecular change in the 1918 pandemic influenza virus stops its transmission in ferrets that were in close proximity, shedding light on the properties that allowed the 1918 pandemic virus to spread so quickly and potentially providing important clues that could help scientists assess emerging influenza viruses, such as H5N1.

The study, which is published in the Feb. 5 issue of *Science*, showed that a modest change of two amino acids in the main protein found on the surface of the 1918 virus did not change the virus's ability to cause disease, but stopped respiratory droplet transmission of the virus between ferrets placed in close proximity. The experiments were conducted with ferrets because their reaction to influenza viruses closely mimics how the disease affects humans.

"With this vital research, we are learning more about what may have contributed to the spread and deadliness of the 1918 pandemic," said CDC Director Dr. Julie Gerberding. "By better understanding how this virus spreads, we can be better positioned to slow down or stop the spread of the pandemic virus and hence be better prepared for the next pandemic."

To spread and cause illness, the influenza virus must first bind to host cells found in humans and animals. The *Science* study suggests that the hemagglutinin (HA), a type of protein found on the surface of influenza viruses, plays an important role in the 1918 virus's ability to transmit from one host to another efficiently. This research suggests that, for an influenza virus to spread efficiently, the virus's HA must prefer attaching to cells that are found predominately in the human upper airway instead of cells found predominately in the gastrointestinal tracts of birds. Other changes may be necessary as well. Current H5N1 viruses prefer attaching to avian cells, suggesting the virus would need to make genetic changes before it could pass easily between humans.

"Work on the 1918 virus is providing clues that are helping us evaluate other influenza viruses with pandemic potential, such as H5N1, that may emerge," said Dr. Terrence Tumpey, lead author of the paper and a CDC senior microbiologist. "Though we still don't know what changes might be necessary for H5N1 to transmit easily among people, it's likely that changes in more than one virus protein would be required for the H5N1 virus to be transmitted among humans."

Influenza pandemics occur when a new strain emerges to which people have little or no immunity. Most experts argue another pandemic will occur, but it is impossible to predict which strain will emerge as the next pandemic strain, when it will occur or how severe it will be.

The 1918 pandemic caused an estimated 675,000 deaths in the United States and up to 50 million worldwide, in the worst pandemic of the past century.

The research was done in collaboration with Mount Sinai School of Medicine and the Southeast Poultry Research Laboratory. All laboratory work with 1918 virus was conducted at CDC in a high containment Biosafety Level 3 laboratory with enhancements, using stringent biosecurity precautions to protect both laboratory workers and the public from exposure to the virus. Currently available antiviral drugs have been shown to be effective against the 1918 influenza virus and similar viruses.

Centers for Disease Control and Prevention (CDC)

CENTERS FOR DISEASE CONTROL AND PREVENTION (CDC). "SMALL CHANGES IN 1918 PANDEMIC VIRUS KNOCKS OUT TRANSMISSION." PRESS RELEASE. FEBRUARY 1, 2007. <HTTP:// WWW.CDC.GOV/OD/OC/MEDIA/PRESSREL/2007/ R070201.HTM> (ACCESSED JUNE 4, 2007).

SEE ALSO *Droplet Precautions; H5N1 Virus; Influenza Pandemic of 1918; Influenza Pandemic of 1957; Influenza, Tracking Seasonal Influences and Virus Mutation; Pandemic Preparedness; Vaccines and Vaccine Development; Viral Disease.*

BIBLIOGRAPHY

Books

Barry, John M. *The Great Influenza: The Story of the Deadliest Pandemic in History.* New York: Penguin Books, 2004.

Goldsmith, Connie. *Influenza: The Next Pandemic?* Brookfield, CT: Twenty-first Century Books, 2006.

Web Sites

Centers for Disease Control and Prevention. "Influenza (Flu)." <http://www.cdc.gov/flu> (accessed June 4, 2007).

World Health Organization. "Influenza." <http:// www.who.int/topics/influenza/en> (accessed June 4, 2007).

Lloyd Scott Clements

Influenza Pandemic of 1918

■ Introduction

Influenza ("flu" for short) is an infection of the lungs and bronchial tubes by an influenza virus. Common symptoms of flu include cough, muscle aches, vomiting, loss of appetite, and fever. Flu can also cause death, usually from respiratory failure and in people with weakened immune systems. The 1918 influenza pandemic, a global wave of flu infection in 1918–1919, was one of the most deadly infectious-disease events in human history. A figure of 20–50 million deaths has traditionally been attributed to the pan-

demic, but in 2002, the *Bulletin of the History of Medicine* estimated that the toll was more likely between 50 and 100 million. The pandemic killed about 675,000 people in the United States, some 18 million in India (about 5% of the population at that time), and similar percentages elsewhere. The virus eventually evolved into less harmful forms. The lethal 1918 influenza virus was re-created by U.S. government scientists in 2005 for medical research purposes. There have been a number of flu outbreaks since 1918, but none have been anywhere near as deadly as that which occurred in 1918.

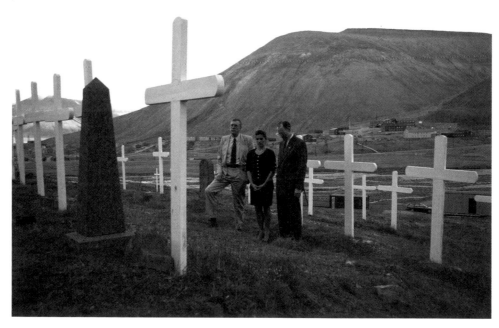

In 1998 scientists pay homage to victims of the 1918 influenza pandemic before exhuming their bodies, which were buried on an island off the coast of Norway. By collecting naturally preserved samples buried in the permafrost, scientists determined the composition, genetic structure, and nature of the 1918 virus. © *K.Moe/Svalnard Posten/Corbis Sygma.*

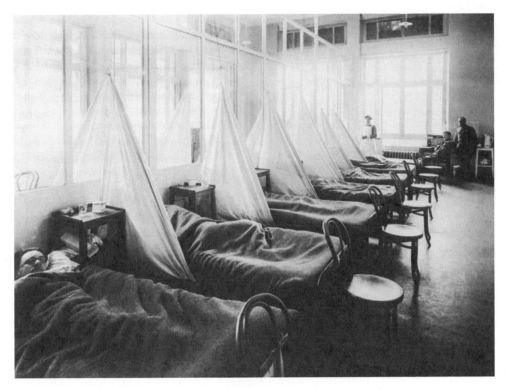

Influenza patients rest in a U.S. Army camp hospital in Aix-les-Baines, France, in 1918. Soldiers returning home from World War I helped fuel the spread of the influenza into one of the largest and deadliest pandemics in human history. *© Corbis.*

■ Disease History, Characteristics, and Transmission

Disease History

The exact origin of the virus strain that caused the 1918 flu pandemic is still a mystery. Although the flu was called the Spanish Flu at the time, it may have originated not in Spain but, like most new flu varieties, in Asia. Another hypothesis, based upon epidemiological evidence, places the origin in the United States.

Normally, in the United States, about 5% to 20% of the population gets a symptomatic flu infection each year. One hundred thousand to 200,000 people are hospitalized with flu complications annually, and up to 36,000 people, mostly elderly, die. Similar figures apply to most countries of the world in proportion to population. In the 1918 pandemic, however, 25–40% of the world population contracted flu and 2.5–5% of those persons died. In the United States, about 2.5% of persons with the flu died, resulting in about 675,000 deaths—about 10 times as many Americans as died in World War I (1914–1918). Two hundred thousand people died in the United States in October 1918 alone. Previous influenza outbreaks had death rates of about 0.1% in the United States, only one twenty-fifth as high as the 2.5% rate of 1918–1919.

The 1918 flu appeared 28 years after the pandemic of 1890, sweeping the world suddenly in September 1918. The flu was called Spanish Flu in the United States because it was especially deadly in Spain early in its history, killing as many as 8 million people. The 1918 flu was unique in that it was deadlier for young people than for the elderly: 99% of its victims were under age 65. Victims sometimes died within a few hours of infection. It should be noted that the great majority of those infected did not die. It struck rich, poor, and middle-class alike, with similar death rates for all groups.

By late November 1918, the death rate from the flu was tapering off in the United States. By early 1919, the pandemic was over, both in the United States and most of the rest of the world.

Disease Characteristics

Influenza is an infection of the lungs and other parts of the respiratory tract (breathing organs) that is caused by a virus. Viruses are tiny clusters of molecules that are smaller than a cell. Each individual virus, called a virion or virus particle, consists of a sheath or covering called a capsid, which is made of proteins (proteins are a type of complex molecule basic to life). The capsid carries a core of RNA (sometimes DNA). A virus cannot live on its own, but reproduces by attaching to a true cell such as a

WORDS TO KNOW

CAPSID: The protein shell surrounding a virus particle.

CREPITANT: A crackling sound that accompanies breathing, a common symptom of pneumonia, or other diseases of the lungs.

PANDEMIC: Pandemic, which means all the people, describes an epidemic that occurs in more than one country or population simultaneously.

RALES: French term for a rattling sound in the throat or chest.

REASSORTMENT: A condition resulting when two or more different types of viruses exchange genetic material to form a new, genetically different virus.

bacterium or human body cell and injecting its RNA or DNA into that cell. The cell is tricked into using the viral RNA or DNA to manufacture new virus particles, which can then infect other cells.

A global influenza pandemic occurs when a form of flu virus evolves that can be easily transmitted between human beings. There were three global flu pandemics in the twentieth century (1918–1919, 1957–1958, and 1967–1968). There had been none in the twenty-first century as of early 2007.

There are three basic types of flu virus, termed influenza A, B, and C. Influenza A viruses are the most common. They are also called avian viruses because "avian" means having to do with birds and these viruses are hosted by birds as well as by humans and some other mammals. The 1918 flu virus was an influenza A virus.

Each influenza A capsid consists of eleven different proteins. Two of these proteins tend to vary widely among flu strains. These are hemagglutinin (HA) and neuraminidase (NA). Strains of influenza A virus are named for which kinds of HA and NA protein they contain. For example, there are H1N1 flu viruses, H3N2 flu viruses, and dozens of others. The strain that caused the 1918 flu was an H1N1 virus. Not all H1N1 viruses are identical, as there are other proteins in the virus that can differ, and the H1 (HA number 1) protein itself can take on slightly different forms.

These differences are a matter of life and death. In the body, the immune system fights viral infections by destroying virus particles and the cells that have been infected by them. It decides what cells or particles to destroy by detecting molecules that belong to the virus. These molecules are called antigens. The HA protein of an influenza A virus is an especially important antigen. When the body's immune system knows to attack a particular form of HA, it can effectively fight the virus bearing that form of HA. If a form of HA is unknown to the immune system, however, the virus is free to spread through the body while the immune system is learning how to identify it. If a person survives that variety of flu, they are permanently immune to it afterward because their immune system remembers it.

From about 1919–2005, the 1918 H1N1 flu strain was considered extinct. However, samples of the virus's RNA were recovered in the 1990s from an Inuit Eskimo woman who had died of the flu in 1918 in Alaska and whose body had been frozen in permafrost since that time, as well as from preserved laboratory samples of lung tissue of four U.S. soldiers who died of flu in 1918. The full RNA sequence of the virus, which was reconstructed by scientists studying these samples and published in the journal *Science* in 2005, showed that the 1918 virus was probably transmitted directly from birds—which are a large natural reservoir of influenza A viruses—to human beings, unlike later pandemic influenzas, which are thought to have originated via reassortment. Reassortment can occur when two different (but related) viruses infect a single cell. Their RNA fragments, mixing inside the cell, can be reassembled into a new virus, a reassortant that contains RNA from both. The pandemic flu strains of 1957 and 1968 were probably reassortant viruses that mixed human flu viruses with avian flu viruses, but the 1918 flu was apparently a purely avian flu virus.

Re-creation of the 1918 flu virus has yielded some understanding of why this particular influenza A virus was so deadly. First, the virus replicates rapidly in the body's tissues. How it does so is not entirely understood, but it was known as of early 2007 that the particular form of HA protein possessed by the 1918 virus was necessary to this rapid spreading. The HA protein is used by a flu virus to stick to host cells, and the form of HA protein possessed by the 1918 virus may be more efficient at doing this job. Also, the 1918 virus spreads more widely in the body than most flu viruses. Most flu viruses use a molecule called trypsin to activate HA molecules and attach to cells. The trypsin must usually come from the cell being attacked. Lung cells are rich in trypsin, which is why flu viruses thrive in lung tissue. In contrast, the NA protein of the 1918 virus can activate the virus's own HA attachment molecule without help from cellular trypsin. The 1918 virus, therefore, was equipped to rapidly attack a wider variety of cells.

A second factor in the deadliness of the 1918 virus is that it triggers an excessive immune response from the body. Excess amounts of the chemicals called interferons, cytokines, and chemokines are produced by the tissues attacked by the virus, and these substances themselves damage the tissues—an event called by immunologists a "cytokine storm." Cells of the immune system also attack the tissues in response to these chemicals. In effect, the 1918 virus not only attacks the body but also tricks the body into attacking itself. This explains why the 1918 virus was most fatal to young adults—the population that has, on average, the strongest immune system.

Disease Transmission

Flu virus is spread mostly through contact with droplets emitted during coughing and sneezing. It is also spread through direct skin contact. The contagious period, during which a person infected with the disease can spread virus particles to an uninfected person, is about one day before symptoms appear to five days after symptoms appear. Typically, about half of all flu infections are asymptomatic (the person does not feel sick). Whether this was true of the 1918 flu is not known, because the viral nature of the disease was not understood until 1933, so asymptomatic cases could not be discovered.

The 1918 flu may have been more easily transmitted than later strains of flu because of the extreme number of virus particles probably produced in lung tissue of people that contracted it. Experiments in 2005 showed that 50 times more virus particles were released from human lung tissue growing in laboratory culture than were released when the tissue was infected by a modern H1N1 flu strain called the Texas virus. Mouse lungs infected with the 1918 virus contained 39,000 times more virus particles after 4 days than mouse lungs infected with the modern virus. However, a 2004 study published in *Nature* concluded from historical information that the transmissibility of the 1918 flu was "not large relative to many other infectious diseases."

Transportation systems such as ships and planes contribute to the global spread of viruses. The worldwide travel activity of troops during World War I (1914–1918) probably helped the 1918 flu pandemic to occur by spreading the virus quickly between countries and continents. Today, commercial jet travel is the usual means of global flu transport.

■ Scope and Distribution

H1N1 flu virus varieties are widespread today in humans and pigs. However, a number of genetic differences distinguish the present-day strains of H1N1 from the deadly 1918 strain. Today, the precise strain of H1N1 that caused the 1918 flu pandemic exists only in a few laboratories.

■ Treatment and Prevention

In 1918 the viral natural of influenza was not understood. No antiviral drugs had yet been discovered, and even antibiotics were not available. Antibiotics are drugs that kill bacteria; they are not useful directly against viral

A LEGACY OF DEATH

The influenza pandemic of 1918 killed more people—mostly otherwise healthy young adults—than any other disease of similar duration in world history. Exact numbers of those struck by influenza are unknown. In 1919, a U.S. Public Health Service survey of eleven cities and towns discovered that about 280 out of 1,000 persons had influenza during the pandemic, yielding an estimated national infection rate of over 25 million afflicted Americans in 1918–1919.

infections because they do not destroy virus particles, but they can help patients survive bacterial infections that may occur when the body is weakened by the primary, viral infection.

Influenza vaccines are now considered the best way to prevent flu. Each year, a new dominant type of influenza reliably appears in Asia. Medical researchers identify the strain and produce a vaccine that is distributed in parts of the world that have not yet experienced the new virus strain. A vaccine is a preparation that contains antigens—chemicals that alert the body's immune system to fight back against a specific invader. After being trained on specific antigens by a vaccine, the body can attack a disease agent carrying those antigens as soon as it appears. In the case of a flu vaccine, the HA protein, which is harmless by itself, is often used as the antigen. Virus particles that have been damaged so that they cannot cause an infection are also used in vaccines.

International surveillance of new influenza viruses is coordinated by the World Health Organization (WHO) Influenza Surveillance Network, set up in 1952. Scores of medical institutions in 83 countries collect flu specimens and send them to four centers (one each in Australia, Japan, the United Kingdom, and the United States) for analysis. WHO scientists study these samples each year to design vaccines for the northern and southern hemispheres, then send these vaccine designs to manufacturers for mass production. The Influenza Surveillance network works well for the industrialized countries of the world, but according to the U.S. National Academy of Science, the network is not as effective in Africa and Asia. This leaves more people vulnerable to flu pandemic in those places.

Today, vaccines are not the only tool for fighting a flu pandemic. Several antiviral drugs are available that would probably be effective against the 1918 virus or a similar virus. These drugs are designed to interfere with the functioning of one or more of the proteins a virus uses to reproduce. For instance, relenza and tamiflu are

RECONSTRUCTING PAST PANDEMICS, PREPARING FOR THE FUTURE?

In 2005, scientists announced that they had sequenced the genetic structure of the virus responsible for the 1918 influenza pandemic. By analyzing tissue samples recovered from a 1918 flu victim found frozen in the Alaskan tundra, along with preserved lung tissue samples from affected World War I soldiers, scientists were able to determine that the virus is a variety of avian (bird) influenza, known as the H1N1 strain. In 2005, the World Health Organization warned that the H5N1 avian influenza strain (commonly known as the "bird flu"), which recently emerged in Asia, may lead to the next global influenza pandemic. Evidence suggests that the H5N1 flu is genetically similar to the virus that caused the 1918 pandemic.

IN CONTEXT: TRENDS AND STATISTICS

Deaths from the 1918 flu in the United States reduced the statistical average life span of an American by 10 years. In the age range of 15 to 34 years, the death rate in 1918 due to pneumonia and influenza was 20 times higher than the normal rate. The large number of deaths in many of the young generation had an economic effect for decades to come. South America, Asia, and the South Pacific were also devastated by the infection.

In the United States the influenza outbreak greatly affected daily life. Gatherings of people, such as at funerals, parades, or even sales at commercial establishments were either banned or were of very short duration.

flu-specific drugs called neuraminidase inhibitors. That is, they are designed to interfere with the action of the NA (neuraminidase) proteins that help viruses spread through the body. The drugs must be given very soon after infection in order to stop its spread; they do not kill the virus, but slow its progress while the body's immune system actually kills the virus particles.

These drugs are relatively expensive to produce and not available today in stockpiles large enough to treat the populations of whole countries. Therefore, despite the existence of effective antiviral drugs, the World Health Organization warns that a 1918-type flu pandemic could still be a global disaster.

■ Impacts and Issues

As described above, the 1918 flu virus is no longer extinct. In 2005, scientists at the Centers for Disease Control and Prevention (a U.S. government group) in Atlanta, Georgia, reconstructed live virus from RNA fragments recovered from tissue dating to the original pandemic. This caused some controversy. Most scientists agreed that prevention of a future flu pandemic could be aided by studying live 1918 virus. However, some also argued that resurrecting the 1918 virus itself created an unacceptable risk; if the virus were to escape from the laboratories that were using it to infect mice, monkeys, and tissue cultures, it could cause another global pandemic all by itself. Others argued that publishing the RNA information for the virus might enable sophisticated terrorists to re-create the virus as a weapon. An emergency meeting of the U.S. National Science Advisory Board for Biosecurity was called before publication of the virus data in 2005, and the board decided that the benefits of the work outweighed the risks. While it may be unlikely that the 1918 flu will escape from captivity and cause a global pandemic, WHO and other expert groups warn that a new virus might evolve naturally with properties similar to those of the 1918 flu.

By 2007, an H5N1 virus causing a variety of avian flu had been circulating in Asia for several years and was causing increasing international concern as it moved into Africa, Russia, and Europe. The present form of the virus, which was highly dangerous to humans, could only be contracted directly from birds, or by intimate association of family members or health care providers with a person sick with Avian Flu. Human to human transmission by routine contact had not been documented as of April 2007, making that form of H5N1 an unlikely candidate for a human pandemic. However, if the properties of this virus are modified by re-assortment or mutation (always an ongoing process) so that it can spread quickly among humans, it is possible to cause a global pandemic with millions of casualties. As of 2004, WHO estimated that such a pandemic would cause at least two to seven million deaths worldwide and perhaps over 50 million—comparable to the 1918 pandemic. Such large numbers of deaths are possible because the modern antiviral drugs that are effective against influenza would not be available in large enough supply, and a targeted vaccine, if one could be developed before the pandemic fulminated (reached its peak), could not be manufactured in sufficient quantities quickly enough to vaccinate enough of the population to prevent the pandemic.

■ Primary Source Connection

The influenza pandemic of 1918 killed more people than any other epidemic in recorded history, including the bubonic plague pandemic of the fourteenth century known as the Black Death. The flu moved too quickly for public health authorities to adequately respond. In both military and civilian life, hospital resources were strained by the sheer number of persons sick with influenza. Physicians and nurses were overwhelmed and in short supply. Quarantine measures were enacted, but did little to stem the spread of the disease. Mortuaries were overcrowded. One Army physician, known only as "Roy," documented his observations of the epidemic at the base hospital at Camp Devens, Massachusetts, in the letter below. The letter was found years later and now resides in the archives at the University of Michigan.

Camp Devens Letter

Camp Devens, Mass.

Surgical Ward No 16

29 September 1918

(Base Hospital)

My dear Burt,

It is more than likely that you would be interested in the news of this place, for there is a possibility that you will be assigned here for duty, so having a minute between rounds I will try to tell you a little about the situation here as I have seen it in the last week.

As you know I have not seen much Pneumonia in the last few years in Detroit, so when I came here I was somewhat behind in the niceties of the Army way of intricate diagnosis. Also to make it good, I have had for the last week an exacerbation of my old "ear rot" as Artie Ogle calls it, and could not use a Stethoscope at all, but had to get by on my ability to "spot" 'em thru my general knowledge of pneumonias. I did well enough, and finally found an old Phonendoscope that I pieced together, and from then on was all right. You know the Army regulations require very close locations etc.

Camp Devens is near Boston, and has about 50,000 men, or did have before this epidemic broke loose. It also has the Base Hospital for the Div. of the N. East. This epidemic started about four weeks ago, and has developed so rapidly that the camp is demoralized and all ordinary work is held up till it has passed. All assemblages of soldiers taboo.

These men start with what appears to be an ordinary attack of La Grippe or Influenza, and when brought to the Hosp. they very rapidly develop the most viscous type of Pneumonia that has ever been seen. Two hours after admission they have the mahogany spots over the cheek bones, and a few hours later you can begin to see the cyanosis extending from their ears and spreading all over the face, until it is hard to distinguish the coloured men from the white. It is only a matter of a few hours then until death comes, and it is simply a struggle for air until they suffocate. It is horrible. One can stand it to see

IN CONTEXT: EPIDEMIC NUMBERS

In 2005, the world's population totalled about 6.5 billion people—more than three times greater than the 1918 population. An influenza pandemic with mortality rates similar to those seen in the 1918 epidemic could kill an estimated 150 million people.

one, two, or twenty men die, but to see these poor devils dropping like flies sort of gets on your nerves. We have been averaging about 100 deaths per day, and still keeping it up. There is no doubt in my mind that there is a new mixed infection here, but what I don't know.

My total time is taken up hunting rales, rales dry or moist, sibilant or crepitant or any other of the hundred things that one may find in the chest, they all mean but one thing here—Pneumonia—and that means in about all cases death.

The normal number of resident Drs. here is about 25 and that has been increased to over 250, all of whom (of course excepting me) have temporary orders—"Return to your proper Station on completion of work." Mine says "Permanent Duty," but I have been in the Army just long enough to learn that it doesn't always mean what it says. So I don't know what will happen to me at the end of this.

We have lost an outrageous number of nurses and Drs., and the little town of Ayer is a sight. It takes Special trains to carry away the dead. For several days there were no coffins and the bodies piled up something fierce, we used to go down to the morgue (which is just back of my ward) and look at the boys laid out in long rows. It beats any sight they ever had in France after a battle. An extra long barracks has been vacated for the use of the morgue, and it would make any man sit up and take notice to walk down the long lines of dead soldiers all dressed and laid out in double rows. We have no relief here, you get up in the morning at 5.30 and work steady till about 9.30 P.M., sleep, then go at it again. Some of the men of course have been here all the time, and they are TIRED.

If this letter seems somewhat disconnected, overlook it, for I have been called away from it a dozen times the last time just now by the Officer of the Day, who came in to tell me that they have not as yet found at any of the autopsies any case beyond the Red. Hepatitis stage. It kills them before they get that far.

I don't wish you any hard luck, Old Man, but I do wish you were here for a while at least. It's more comfortable when one has a friend about. The men here are all good fellows, but I get so damned sick of pneumonia that when I go to eat I want to find some fellow who will not "Talk Shop" but there ain't none nohow. We eat it,

"SPANISH FLU" OR "LA GRIPPE:" AN EFFICIENT KILLER

The 1918 influenza outbreak was called the "Spanish Flu" or "La Grippe." The moniker came from the some 8 million influenza deaths that occurred in Spain in one month at the height of the outbreak. Ironically, more recent research has demonstrated that the strain of influenza that ravaged Spain was different from that which spread influenza around the world.

Recent research has demonstrated that the particular strain of virus was one that even an efficiently functioning immune system was not well equipped to cope with. A mutation produced a surface protein on the virus that was not immediately recognized by the immune system; this contributed to the ability of the virus to cause an infection.

live it, sleep it, and dream it, to say nothing of breathing it 16 hours a day. I would be very grateful indeed if you would drop me a line or two once in a while, and I will promise you that if you ever get into a fix like this, I will do the same for you.

Each man here gets a ward with about 150 beds (mine has 168) and has an Asst. Chief to boss him, and you can imagine what the paper work alone is—fierce—and the Govt. demands all paper work be kept up in good shape. I have only four day nurses and five night nurses (female), a ward-master, and four orderlies. So you can see that we are busy. I write this in piecemeal fashion. It may be a long time before I can get another letter to you, but will try.

This letter will give you an idea of the monthly report which has to be in Monday. I have mine most ready now. My Boss was in just now and gave me a lot more work to do so I will have to close this.

Goodbye old Pal,

"God be with you till we meet again"

Keep the Bouells open.

(Sgd) Roy.

Roy

"CAMP DEVENS LETTER." *BRITISH MEDICAL JOURNAL* (DECEMBER 22–29, 1979).

SEE ALSO *Avian Influenza; H5N1 Virus; Influenza; Influenza Pandemic of 1957; Influenza, Tracking Seasonal Influences and Virus Mutation; Pandemic Preparedness; Viral Disease.*

BIBLIOGRAPHY

Books

Corsby, Alfred W. *America's Forgotten Pandemic.* New York: Cambridge University Press, 2003.

Duncan, K. *Hunting the 1918 Flu: One Scientist's Search for a Killer Virus.* Toronto: University of Toronto Press, 2003.

Kolata, Gina. *Flu: The Story of the Great Influenza Pandemic of 1918 & the Search for the Virus That Caused It.* Upland, PA: Diane Pub. Co., 2001.

Periodicals

Holmes, Edward C. "1918 and All That." *Nature.* 303 (2004): 1787–1788.

Johnson, Niall P.A.S. "Updating the Accounts: Global Mortality of the 1918–1920 'Spanish' Influenza Pandemic." *Bulletin of the History of Medicine.* 76 (2002): 105–115.

Kaiser, Jocelyn. "Resurrected Influenza Virus Yields Secrets of Deadly 1918 Pandemic." *Science.* 310 (2005): 28029.

Koelle, Katia, et al. "Epochal Evolution Shapes the Phylodynamics of Interpandemic Influenza A (H3N2) in Humans." *Science.* 314(2006): 1898–1903.

Laver, Graeme, and Elspeth Garman. "The Origin and Control of Pandemic Influenza." *Science.* 293 (2001): 1776–1777.

Loo, Yueh-Ming, and Michael Gale Jr. "Fatal Immunity and the 1918 Virus." *Nature.* 445 (2007): 18–19.

Mills, Christina E., James M. Robins, and March Lipsitch. "Transmissibility of 1918 Pandemic Influenza." *Science.* 432 (2004): 904–906.

Smith, Kerri. "Concern as Revived 1918 Flu Virus Kills Monkeys" *Nature.* 445 (2007): 237.

Tumpey, Terrence M., et al. "Characterization of the Reconstructed 1918 Spanish Influenza Pandemic Virus." *Science.* 310 (2005): 77–80.

Web Sites

National Vaccine Program Office, United States Department of Health and Human Services. "Pandemics and Pandemic Scares in the 20th Century." <http://www.hhs.gov/nvpo/pandemics/flu3.htm#10> (accessed January 23, 2007).

The White House (U.S. Government). "National Strategy for Pandemic Influenza." November 1, 2005 <http://www.whitehouse.gov/homeland/pandemic-influenza.html> (accessed January 23, 2007).

U.S. Department of Health and Human Services. "PandemicFlu.org/AsianFlu.org." August 24, 2006 <http://www.pandemicflu.gov> (accessed January 25, 2007).

Larry Gilman

Influenza Pandemic of 1957

■ Introduction

The 1957 influenza pandemic was the second-greatest influenza pandemic in the twentieth century. It killed approximately one to two million people worldwide, including about 70,000 in the United States. The first influenza pandemic of the twentieth century, in 1918–19, killed between 20 and 100 million people worldwide and about 675,000 in the United States; the third, in 1968, killed about 700,000 people worldwide and 34,000 in the United States. Influenza ("flu" for short) is a viral infection of the respiratory system that is spread either by contact or by droplets of mucus or saliva ejected into the air by a cough or sneeze. Symptoms of flu include cough, muscle aches, vomiting, loss of appetite, fever, and, in extreme cases, death. Flu pandemics tend to occur every 10 or 11 years, but most are not as severe as those of 1918, 1957, and 1968.

■ Disease History, Characteristics, and Transmission

The flu that caused the 1957 pandemic is called Asian flu because it was first detected in China in February, 1957. United States government experts could not decide at first whether a 1918-style disaster was in the making and did not want to alarm the public, so the Surgeon General

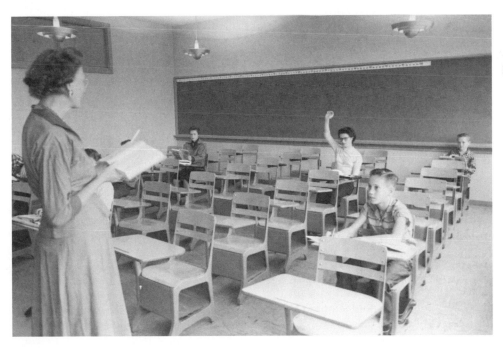

A Dallas schoolteacher conducts class with 7 of her 30 students present during the 1957 influenza pandemic. © *Bettmann/Corbis.*

WORDS TO KNOW

CAPSID: The protein shell surrounding a virus particle.

MUTATION: A mutation is a change in an organism's DNA that occurs over time and may render it less sensitive to drugs which are used against it.

PANDEMIC: Pandemic, which means all the people, describes an epidemic that occurs in more than one country or population simultaneously.

REASSORTMENT: A condition resulting when two or more different types of viruses exchange genetic material to form a new, genetically different virus.

VIRION: A virion is a mature virus particle, consisting of a core of ribonucleic acid (RNA) or deoxyribonucleic acid (DNA) surrounded by a protein coat. This is the form in which a virus exists outside of its host cell.

are given code names to distinguish them. These names are based on two of the 11 proteins found in the capsid, hemagglutinin (HA) and neuraminidase (NA). HA and NA each occur in a variety of forms which are given numbers by biologists. A virus having a type 2 HA protein and a type 2 NA protein is an H2N2 virus. The virus that caused the 1957 pandemic was an H2N2 virus.

Mutations (changes) occur in viral RNA, changing the capsid proteins in new viruses. When enough of these changes happen, the immune system's memory of its previous encounter with flu is no longer useful; the new, changed virus is not recognized as soon as it appears, and so has a chance to cause an infection before the body destroys it. Viruses can also change by reassortment. Reassortment can happen when two different types of virus infect the same cell at the same time. The new viruses that the cell manufactures may contain RNA from both types. The 1957 H2N2 virus probably arose through reassortment of a virus originating in birds (an avian influenza) and a virus already easily transmitted among humans.

■ Scope and Distribution

Today, the strain of H2N2 influenza A virus that caused the 1957 pandemic exists only in laboratory cultures. Other H2N2 viruses exist in the wild.

■ Treatment and Prevention

No antiviral drugs existed in 1957. A vaccine was created for this flu but was not available to most people. Treatment, as for the common cold, consisted mostly of rest, fluids, and staying warm. Antibiotics—drugs that kill only bacteria—are sometimes given to flu patients to fight secondary bacterial infections but do not treat the flu itself.

Today, vaccination remains the first line of defense against any flu outbreak, but several antiviral drugs are available. Efforts are sometimes made to prevent the origin of 1957-type flu viruses by preventing people who have virus infections from working around or slaughtering birds while sick. The goal is to lessen the chances that reassortment will occur in cells infected by an avian virus from the birds and a virus already easily transmitted among humans.

■ Impacts and Issues

Unlike the Spanish flu pandemic of 1918–1920, international strategies to report and respond to pandemic threats gave many nations advance warning of the new pandemic. Soon after the virus was identified in China, several nations were able to develop and produce vaccines to stem the spread of the illness. In addition to limited vaccination programs, many of the same quarantine techniques that were used to combat the 1918 pandemic were used again in 1957. Since children and families with young children were disproportionately

recommended that flu vaccinations be given only through ordinary doctor-patient channels. The pandemic did spread through the United States, however, starting in the late spring and peaking in October 1957. A second wave of infections, mostly affecting the elderly, occurred in January and February 1958. About 69,800 people died of the Asian flu in the United States (In a typical year, as of the early 2000s, about 36,000 people die of flu each year in the United States. However, the U.S. population was much smaller in 1957, so the death rate from the pandemic was relatively much higher.) Flu costs billions of dollars even in a non-pandemic year because of hospitalizations and lost work time.

Influenza is caused by a virus. Viruses are tiny clusters of molecules called virions or virus particles. Each influenza virion consists of an out shell or capsid made of proteins (a kind of complex molecule used by all living things) and an inner core of RNA (ribonucleic acid). A virion attaches to a cell using capsid proteins. It then injects its RNA into the cell. The cell's mechanisms cannot tell viral RNA from its own RNA, and manufacture proteins according to the instructions in the viral RNA. These molecules assemble themselves into new virus particles. New influenza viruses escape from the host cell by budding off from the cell membrane.

There are three types of flu, namely influenza A, B, and C. Influenza A viruses are also called avian viruses because they live in birds as well as in human beings. The 1957 flu virus was an influenza A virus. Influenza A viruses affected, many schools and libraries closed temporarily to prevent the spread of the flu within local communities. Such measures helped limit the spread of the flu among children, but the disease reemerged in early 1958. Most of the victims of the "second wave" of the pandemic were elderly.

In 2005, it was found that quality-control kits containing live Asian flu virus had been sent to 6,000 labs in 19 countries. To prevent the reintroduction of the 1957 pandemic flu virus into the general population, efforts were overseen by the World Health Organization (WHO) to track down and destroy all the virus samples. No outbreak occurred.

SEE ALSO *Avian Influenza; H5N1; Influenza; Influenza Epidemic of 1918; Influenza, Tracking Seasonal Influences and Virus Mutation; Viral Disease.*

BIBLIOGRAPHY

Books

Goldsmith, Connie. *Influenza: The Next Pandemic?* New York: Twenty-First Century Books, 2006.

Periodicals

Altman, Lawrence K. "Flu Samples, Released in Error, Are Mostly Destroyed, U.S. Says." *New York Times.* April 22, 2005.

Check, Erika. "Heightened Security After Flu Scare Sparks Biosafety Debate." *Nature.* 432 (2005): 943.

Ferguson, Neil M. "Ecological and Immunological Determinants of Influenza Evolution." *Nature.* 4222 (2003): 428-433.

Laver, Graeme and Elspeth Garman. "The Origin and Control of Pandemic Influenza." *Science.* 293 (2001): 1776–1777.

Web Sites

National Vaccine Program Office, United States Department of Health and Human Services. "Pandemics and Pandemic Scares in the 20th Century." <http://www.hhs.gov/nvpo/pandemics/flu3.htm#10> (accessed January 23, 2007).

U.S. Department of Health and Human Services. "PandemicFlu.org/AsianFlu.org." August 24, 2006 <http://www.pandemicflu.gov> (accessed January 25, 2007).

The White House (U.S. Government). "National Strategy for Pandemic Influenza." November 1, 2005 <http://www.whitehouse.gov/homeland/pandemic-influenza.html> (accessed January 23, 2007).

Larry Gilman

Influenza, Tracking Seasonal Influences and Virus Mutation

■ Introduction

Influenza is an important disease because of the rapidity with which epidemics spread, the widespread morbidity, and the severity of complications, including viral and bacterial pneumonias. During major epidemics, severe illness and death occur, mainly among the elderly and people with compromised immune systems. In the United States, between 10,000 and 40,000 people die each year from influenza complications. However, in the 1918 pandemic, most of those who died were young and healthy adults. Given the potential for serious complications and high mortality rates with influenza, it is critical that public health agencies develop a system for tracking influenza epidemics from their origin each year in order to mount defensive measures such as vaccines and educational programs for potential victims.

■ Disease History, Characteristics, and Transmission

Influenza is an acute viral disease of the respiratory tract characterized by fever, headache, myalgia (muscle aches),

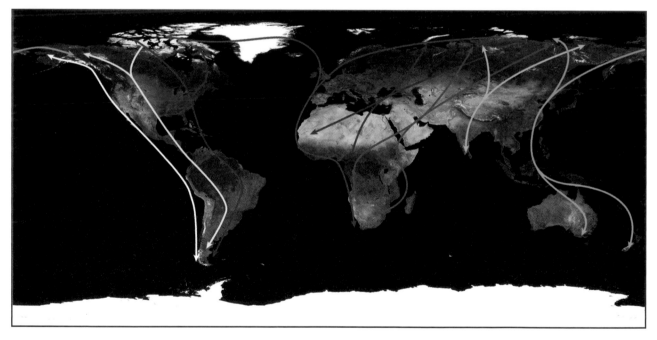

Bird migration routes are superimposed on this satellite map of the world. Many birds migrate on a seasonal basis from one area to another. The most common pattern is for birds to breed in the northern hemisphere's temperate or Arctic regions, and then migrate to the tropics or the temperate region of the southern hemisphere, avoiding the winter of the northern hemisphere. The different routes (flyways) are colored: Pacific Americas (white); Mississippi Americas (yellow); Atlantic Americas (red); East Atlantic (pink); Black Sea and Mediterranean (purple); East Africa and West Asia (blue); Central Asia (turquoise); and East Asia and Australian (green). It is thought that diseases such as avian flu can be spread along bird migratory routes. *SPL/Photo Researchers, Inc.*

prostration, nasal inflammation and discharge, sore throat, and cough. Cough can often be severe and protracted, but other manifestations are usually self-limiting, with recovery in two to seven days. The recognition of influenza is usually based on epidemiological characteristics as part of a general epidemic; otherwise it is difficult to distinguish influenza from a severe cold or other viral respiratory diseases such as viral pneumonia. Viral pneumonia can also be caused by influenza virus, although gastrointestinal tract symptoms (nausea, vomiting, diarrhea) have been reported in about 25% of children in school outbreaks. The spread of influenza virus is predominantly airborne among crowded populations in confined spaces, especially school buses and barracks. Transmission may also occur by indirect contact, as the influenza virus may persist for hours, particularly in cold and dry weather. The viral incubation period is short; usually one to three days. Influenza is communicable for about three to five days after onset in adults and up to a week in young children.

There are three types of influenza virus currently recognized: types A, B, and C. Type A includes three subtypes (H1N1, H2N2, and H3N2) that have been associated with widespread epidemics and pandemics. Type B has been associated with regional or widespread epidemics. Type C is typically associated with sporadic cases and minor localized outbreaks. The viral type is determined by the antigenic properties of two relatively stable structural proteins, the nucleoprotein and the matrix protein.

The emergence of a completely new subtype, the process of known as antigenic shift, occurs at unpredictable intervals and only with type A viruses. Viruses characterized by antigenic shift are responsible for the pandemics that result from the unpredictable recombination (new combinations of genetic material) of human and swine or avian (usually duck) antigens. Relatively minor antigenic changes—known as "drift"—of type A and type B viruses that are responsible for frequent epidemics and regional outbreaks occur constantly, necessitating periodic (almost annually) reformulation of influenza vaccine. During the past 125 years, pandemics occurred in 1889, 1918, 1957, and 1968.

■ Scope and Distribution

Once an epidemic is underway, case attack rates range from 10% to 20% in the general population and can range up to 50% in confined populations such as boarding schools, military bases, or nursing homes. Influenza epidemics caused by type A viruses, type B viruses, or both occur in the United States almost every year. In temperate zones, epidemics usually occur in winter. In the tropics, they often occur during the rainy season, but outbreaks or sporadic cases may occur in any month. Influenza also occurs naturally in swine, horses, mink, and seals, and in many domestic and wild bird species all

WORDS TO KNOW

ANTIGENIC DRIFT: Antigenic drift describes the gradual accumulation of mutations in genes (e.g. in genes coding for surface proteins) over a period of time.

COHORTING: Cohorting is the practice of grouping persons with like infections or symptoms together in order to reduce transmission to others and keep patients under close observation for a particular condition.

EPIDEMIC: From the Greek *epidemic*, meaning "prevalent among the people," is most commonly used to describe an outbreak of an illness or disease in which the number of individual cases significantly exceeds the usual or expected number of cases in any given population.

REASSORTMENT: A condition resulting when two or more different types of viruses exchange genetic material to form a new, genetically different virus.

PANDEMIC: Pandemic, which means all the people, describes an epidemic that occurs in more than one country or population simultaneously.

PROSTRATION: A condition marked by nausea, disorientation, dizziness, and weakness caused by dehydration and prolonged exposure to high temperatures; also called heat exhaustion or hyperthermia.

over the world. Transmission between species and reassortment (exchanging genetic material inside a host) of influenza A viruses have been reported to occur between swine, humans, ducks, and turkeys. The human influenza viruses responsible for the 1957 and 1968 pandemics contained gene segments closely related to those of avian influenza viruses.

Humans are the primary reservoir for human infections, though mammalian reservoirs such as swine and avian reservoirs such as ducks are likely sources of new human subtypes thought to emerge through genetic reassortment. New virulent subtypes cause pandemic influenza by spreading through a population that has little or no immunity because of lack of exposure to the new viral surface antigens.

When a new viral subtype appears, all children and adults are equally susceptible except for individuals who have lived through earlier epidemics of the same subtype. Infection produces immunity to the specific infecting virus but the duration of immunity depends on the degree of antigenic drift and the number of previous infections. Flu vaccines produce responses that are specific for the included viruses and also boost responses to related strains to which the individual has been exposed before. Attack rates tend to be age specific; people that have lived long enough to experience earlier epidemics of the same subtype usually have at least partial immunity years later, and this partial immunity protects them from closely related subtypes.

■ Treatment and Prevention

Treatment

Because any outbreak of influenza has important and sometimes catastrophic implications, all cases must be reported to local health authorities in order to assist disease surveillance. The identity of the disease agent by viral subtype as determined by laboratory testing should be provided if possible. Although annual vaccination is the primary strategy for preventing complications of influenza virus infections, the CDC notes that antiviral medications with activity against influenza viruses can be effective for the chemoprophylaxis and treatment of influenza. Four licensed influenza antiviral agents are available in the United States: amantadine, rimantadine, zanamivir, and oseltamivir. These treatments should be started within 48 hours of the onset of symptoms. Influenza A virus resistance to amantadine and rimantadine can emerge rapidly during treatment. On the basis of antiviral testing results conducted at the CDC and in Canada indicating high levels of resistance, the CDC recommends that neither amantadine nor rimantadine be used for the treatment or chemoprophylaxis of influenza A in the United States until susceptibility to these antiviral medications has been re-established among circulating influenza A viruses. Oseltamivir (Tamiflu^{TM}) may have caused delirium in some pediatric patients.

Since influenza is usually self-limiting in healthy adults under age 65, the CDC generally advises against personal stockpiling of the drugs. Federal and state health authorities and healthcare institutions are creating stockpiles of antiviral influenza medications for persons at greatest risk for complications from influenza. A potential consequence of personal stockpiling is depletion of existing supplies of antivirals so that they will not be available to those persons who most need them. In addition, widespread personal stockpiling and inappropriate use of antivirals (e.g., as a daily regimen regardless of the degree of influenza risk) might compound the risk for influenza by creating conditions for the emergence of resistant strains of influenza. Widespread resistance to oseltamivir could be catastrophic in the event of an avian flu pandemic on the scale of the 1918 pandemic.

Prevention

Influenza vaccination remains the cornerstone for the control and treatment of influenza, and antiviral influenza medications should serve as an adjunct to vaccine. In addition, the public and healthcare personnel need to be trained to avoid unprotected coughs and sneezes as well as proper handwashing. Patient isolation is impractical in most cases because of the viral incubation period during which victims are infectious without symptoms. However, during an epidemic it would be desirable to isolate patients, especially infants and children, by putting them in the same room ("cohorting") during the first five to seven days of illness.

Immunization may provide 70% to 80% protection against infection in healthy young adults when the vaccine antigen closely matches circulating viruses. Vaccine programs have been less successful in preventing disease, but have reduced the hospitalization of people over 65 for complications such as pneumococcal pneumonia by 30% to 50%. The CDC recommends that influenza vaccination for the elderly be supplemented with immunization against pneumococcal pneumonia. Immunization can benefit any individual, but it should especially be considered for emergency responders, people performing essential services, and military personnel.

Influenza vaccine should be provided each year before influenza is expected in the community (November through March in the United States). Travelers should be immunized attending on the different seasonal patterns of influenza in various parts of the world. The single dose suffices for persons with prior exposure to Influenza A and B. Two doses of vaccine one month apart are required for younger persons with no previous immunization history. Routine immunization programs should be directed primarily at those with the greatest risk of serious complications or death, and those who might spread infection to them, such as Health Care personnel and household contacts of high-risk people.

Tracking

Influenza is a disease that is under surveillance by the World Health Organization (WHO); the following procedure is recommended:

1. Influenza epidemics within a country should be reported to the WHO.

2. The viral subtype should be reported and prototype strains should be submitted to one of the three WHO centers for reference and research on influenza (Atlanta, London, and Melbourne). Throat secretion specimens, aspirates, and paired blood samples may also be sent to any WHO-recognized national influenza center.

3. Conduct epidemiological studies and promptly identify viruses at the national health agencies.

4. Ensure sufficient commercial and/or governmental facilities for the production of adequate quantities of vaccine and programs for vaccine administration to high-risk people and essential personnel.

In view of the seriousness of the threat of an avian flu pandemic, the stockpiling of adequate supplies of antiviral medications should be added to this list of national health agency responsibilities.

■ Impacts and Issues

Recent news media publicity regarding the possibility of another avian flu epidemic on the scale of the 1918 pandemic stimulated many members of the public to purchase, privately stockpile, and consume pharmaceutical products, especially oseltamivir, as a way to ward off a supposed "imminent" outbreak of H5N1 influenza. This consumption amounted to a waste of valuable antiviral supplies and has increased the probability of the emergence of resistant viral strains. During treatment, drug resistant viruses may emerge late in the course of therapy and be transmitted to others. Therefore, the cohorting of people on antiviral therapy should be considered, especially in closed populations with many high-risk individuals. Antibiotics should be administered only if patients develop bacterial complications. However, if government agencies are to ask individuals to forgo private stockpiles of antivirals, government must assure adequate supplies of antivirals for the public in case of a severe outbreak of type A influenza. In the case of a severe outbreak, aggregations of people in emergency shelters should be avoided, since this will favor outbreaks of the disease if the virus is introduced.

SEE ALSO *H5N1; Influenza; Pandemic Preparedness; Public Health and Infectious Disease.*

BIBLIOGRAPHY

Books

Heymann, David L. *Control of Communicable Diseases Manual*, 18th ed. Washington, DC: American Public Health Association, 2004.

Web Sites

Centers for Disease Control and Prevention. "Antiviral Medications for Influenza." <http://www.cdc.gov/flu/professionals/treatment> (accessed June 13, 2007).

Centers for Disease Control and Prevention. "Increased Antiviral Medication Sales before the 2005-06 Influenza Season—New York City." <http://www.cdc.gov/mmwr/preview/mmwrhtml/mm5510a3.htm> (accessed June 13, 2007).

Kenneth LaPensee

Isolation and Quarantine

■ Introduction

Isolation and quarantine are two strategies that can be used to control the spread of a disease that is contagious (easily passed from person-to-person). Both approaches are minimize the exposure of other people to infected persons.

Isolation and quarantine are not the same. Isolation is more common than quarantine and used for someone who is known to have a disease. Quarantine is used for someone who has been exposed to a disease or disease-causing agent, but who is not currently displaying symptoms and who may not necessarily become ill.

Isolation and quarantine may be voluntary. For example, during the 2003 outbreak of Severe Acute Respiratory Syndrome (SARS) in Toronto, Canada, over 15,000 people were asked to voluntarily quarantine themselves for 10

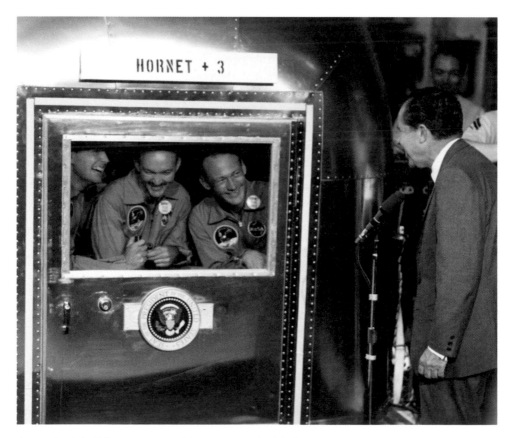

Quarantined *Apollo* 11 astronauts Neil Armstrong, Michael Collins, and Edwin E. Aldrin Jr. receive a welcome home from President Richard Nixon after completing their mission to the moon in 1969.   *© Corbis.*

days during the height of the outbreak. During a voluntary quarantine, people may elect to remain at home, forgo public gatherings, and curtail travel on airplanes, busses, trains, and other forms of public transit. However, if an outbreak involves a disease that is judged by public health authorities to be a severe contagious threat, isolation or quarantine may be imposed by law. In the United States, only disease threats that are listed in an Executive Order by the President qualify for government-imposed quarantine.

■ History and Scientific Foundations

The concept of quarantine dates back to the 14th century, when ships arriving in Venice from regions where plague was occurring were required to anchor in the harbor for forty days before the crew were permitted to go ashore. The word quarantine is derived from the Italian *quaranta giorni*, meaning forty days.

In the United States, federal legislation governing the imposition of quarantine was first enacted in 1878 in response to outbreaks of yellow fever. Then the quarantine powers of the federal government were minimal and did not override state and local government public health practices. The federal government assumed more responsibility for quarantine in 1892, in response to outbreaks of cholera.

While states continue to have powers to issue quarantines for illnesses within their borders, the federal government has had responsibility for quarantine on a national scale since the implementation of the 1944 Public Service Act. In 1967, the federal responsibility for the imposition and enforcement of quarantine was transferred to the Centers for Disease Control and Prevention (CDC), where it has remained. The Division of Global Migration and Quarantine is responsible for the nationwide system of quarantine stations (as of 2006 there were 18, with two more slated to open during 2007).

Both quarantine and isolation are designed to protect the larger community from people known to be infected with a contagious disease deemed to be a public health threat (isolation) or people who have had contact with someone who has become ill with the disease and so who may themselves be infected while not yet displaying symptoms (quarantine). Those in isolation can be treated while at the same time minimizing the chance that the disease will spread. People under quarantine can be monitored for symptoms of the disease; if symptoms do not appear within a certain time (10 days is typical, since voluntary compliance with a quarantine becomes difficult after that) then the quarantine can be lifted.

■ Applications and Research

Isolation and quarantine are public health responses to an illness outbreak. Of these, isolation is common, being

practiced daily in most hospitals, particularly since the appearance and increasing prevalence of tuberculosis and disease causing bacteria that are resistant to multiple antibiotics (an example is methicillin resistant *Staphylococcus aureus*, or MRSA). A common site in hospitals nowadays are posted warnings restricting visitation to a ward room housing a patient with a contagious infection.

Isolation is a standard procedure. In contrast, quarantine is less common and is more of a drastic measure to control an infectious disease. While it can be useful in controlling an illness outbreak, quarantine can leave lasting effects on those involved. A study conducted on some of those who were quarantined during the 2003 SARS (severe acute respiratory syndrome) outbreak in Toronto, Canada, documented symptoms of posttraumatic stress disorder and depression in about 30% of study respondents.

■ Impacts and Issues

Quarantine can affect civil liberties. Imposed quarantines may restrict freedoms of movement and assembly. Schools, restaurants, businesses, means of transit, and public spaces may be closed. The degree to which civil liberties are curtailed in response to an epidemic may be controversial, and whenever possible, quarantine is a voluntary measure. In the event of an imposed quarantine, government entities, law enforcement, media, and public health organizations should provide as much information as possible to those affected by a quarantine.

Isolation and quarantine can also affect someone's privacy, since of necessity the community will need to know who is being contained. This lack of privacy can even include revealing a person's medical history. Thus, isolation and quarantine are considered carefully and not undertaken without a demonstrated and immediate need to do so.

In the United States, an Executive Order of the president identifies quarantinable diseases and authorizes government action to implement quarantines, restrict

IN CONTEXT: EFFECTIVE RULES AND REGULATIONS

In the United States, [42 U.S.C. 247d] Sec. 319(a) of the Public Health Service Act allows the Health and Human Services (HHS) Secretary to declare a public health emergency and "take such action as may be appropriate to respond" including quarantine, prevention of disease, treatment recommendations, research, etc. if "the Secretary determines, after consultation with such public health officials as may be necessary, that (1) a disease or disorder presents a public health emergency; or (2) a public health emergency, including significant outbreaks of infectious diseases or bioterrorist attacks, otherwise exists, the Secretary may take such action as may be appropriate to respond to the public health emergency, including making grants, providing awards for expenses, and entering into contracts and conducting and supporting investigations into the cause, treatment, or prevention of a disease or disorder as described Any such determination of a public health emergency terminates upon the Secretary declaring that the emergency no longer exists, or upon the expiration of the 90-day period beginning on the date on which the determination is made by the Secretary, whichever occurs first. Determinations that terminate under the preceding sentence may be renewed by the Secretary (on the basis of the same or additional facts), and the preceding sentence applies to each such renewal. Not later than 48 hours after making a determination under this subsection of a public health emergency (including a renewal), the Secretary shall submit to the Congress written notification of the determination."

travel, and detain persons to stop the spread of certain infectious diseases. Executive Order 13295 lists cholera, diphtheria, infectious tuberculosis, plague, smallpox, yellow fever, and viral hemorrhagic fevers (such as Ebola, Marburg, and others) as quarantinable. In 2003, following an outbreak in Asia, SARS was added to the list. The growing threat of H5N1 virus and possible pandemic influenza prompted the Department of Health and Human Services (HHS) to request its addition to the list. On April 3, 2005, U.S. President George W. Bush amended Executive Order 13295, identifying pandemic influenza as quarantinable in the United States.

Increased movement of peoples worldwide—through migration, travel, or war—has prompted the need for better international protocols for preventing the spread of infectious diseases. Quarantine across national borders is problematic, sometimes complicated by war, political tensions, different languages, health, and legal systems. Over the past several decades, national governments and international agencies have worked to develop a global network of disease reporting. Increased communication about outbreaks of infectious diseases help nations prepare for disease threats and enact preventative measures within

their own borders. The United Nations World Health Organization (WHO) and other non-governmental organizations (NGOs), such as Doctors Without Borders, also report and respond to infectious disease outbreaks. International agencies and NGOs typically work with national and local governments to implement disease treatment and prevention strategies, including recommendations of isolation or voluntary or imposed quarantine.

Many of the newest international epidemic identification and national quarantine protocols were tested during the intercontinental SARS outbreak in 2003. Italian physician Carlo Urbani (1956–2003) identified the new illness when asked to travel to a Vietnamese hospital to look at a patient thought to have a new strain of influenza. Urbani diagnosed the patient, an American businessman, as suffering from a new, and possibly highly contagious disease. Urbani notified the WHO, CDC, and Vietnamese national health officials, recommending isolation of patients, quarantine of SARS-exposed healthcare workers, and screening of travelers. Urbani himself contracted SARS, and after developing symptoms while aboard an airline flight to Bangkok, Thailand, relayed the need for his own isolation upon landing. Urbani died shortly thereafter of SARS-related complications. However, his rapid identification of the disease and notification of international health authorities, and the concerted efforts of health officials in implementing screening, isolation, and quarantine, stemmed the spread of the disease and saved many lives.

SEE ALSO *Contact precautions; Influenza Pandemic of 1918; Personal Protective Equipment; Standard Precautions.*

BIBLIOGRAPHY

Books

Barry, John M. *The Great Influenza: The Epic Story of the Deadliest Plague In History.* New York: Viking, 2004.

Rothstein, Mark A. *Quarantine And Isolation: Lessons Learned from Sars: A Report to the CDC.* Darby PA: Diane Publishing, 2003.

Tierno, Philip M. *The Secret Life of Germs: What They Are, Why We Need Them, and How We Can Protect Ourselves Against Them.* New York: Atria, 2004.

Periodicals

Day, Troy, Andrew Park, Neal Madras, Abba Gumel, and Jianhong Wu. "When is quarantine a useful control strategy for emerging infectious diseases?" *American Journal of Epidemiology.* 163 (2006): 479-485.

Hawryluck, Laura, Wayne L. Gold, Susan Robinson, Stephen Pogorski, Sandra Galea, and Rima Styra. "SARS control and psychological effects of quarantine, Toronto, Canada." *Emerging Infectious Diseases.* 10 (2004): 1206–1212.

Brian Hoyle

Japanese Encephalitis

■ Introduction

Encephalitis is an inflammation of the brain that is most often caused by a virus. The Japanese encephalitis virus (JEV) is the leading cause of viral encephalitis in Asia, but the infection is relatively rare in the West. Although only a minority of cases of Japanese encephalitis causes symptoms, such as headache, seizures and paralysis, the disease is potentially fatal, and there can be long-lasting disability among survivors. There is no cure for Japanese encephalitis, but there are vaccines available. Countries that vaccinate their populations against JEV, including Japan, tend to have fewer cases of encephalitis than those where vacci-

nation is less routine, such as in India and Vietnam. Vaccination is often recommended for travelers, especially if they expect lengthy stays in rural endemic areas (where the disease occurs consistently within a specific region/locality). People who intend to reside in an area where JEV is endemic also need vaccination to protect themselves.

■ Disease History, Characteristics, and Transmission

Japanese encephalitis virus (JEV) is a flavivirus, a type of single-stranded RNA virus that is related to the St. Louis

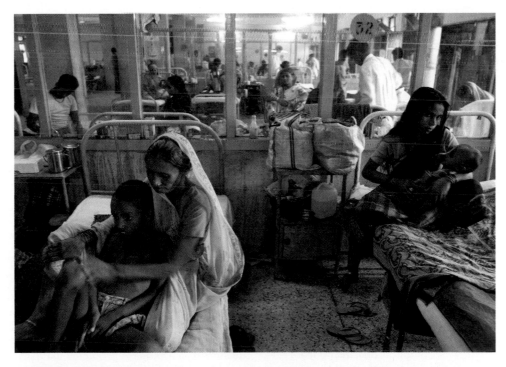

At a medical college in India in 2005, mothers cradle their children who are afflicted with Japanese encephalitis. In northern India, the largest outbreak of the disease in decades struck more than 5,000 people and claimed over 1,300 lives. *AP Images.*

WORDS TO KNOW

ARTHROPOD-BORNE DISEASE: A disease caused by one of a phylum of organisms characterized by exoskeletons and segmented bodies.

ENDEMIC: Present in a particular area or among a particular group of people.

INCUBATION PERIOD: Incubation period refers to the time between exposure to disease causing virus or bacteria and the appearance of symptoms of the infection. Depending on the microorganism, the incubation time can range from a few hours (an example is food poisoning due to *Salmonella*) to a decade or more (an example is acquired immunodeficiency syndrome, or AIDS).

MORBIDITY: The term "morbidity" comes from the Latin word "morbus," which means sick. In medicine it refers not just to the state of being ill, but also to the severity of the illness. A serious disease is said to have a high morbidity.

RESERVOIR: The animal or organism in which the virus or parasite normally resides.

encephalitis virus and West Nile virus. The incubation period of JEV is 5–15 days, and persons with symptoms will usually have a history of exposure to mosquitoes in an endemic area in Asia. Most JEV infections are subclinical, that is, the infected person has no symptoms or only mild symptoms, such as headache and fever. One person with JEV in 250 will develop acute (rapid-onset) symptoms, including headache, neck stiffness, stupor, disorientation, tremor, seizures, paralysis, and even coma. Japanese encephalitis can be difficult to distinguish from the other types of viral encephalitis; tests of blood or cerebrospinal fluid can give a definitive diagnosis if this is needed. The mortality rate among the symptomatic cases is between 10% and 30%, and is higher where there is only limited access to intensive care facilities which may be required if paralysis leads to breathing or feeding problems. Up to 30% of survivors of Japanese encephalitis are left with morbidity (complications) including long-term disabilities such as movement problems, changes in behavior, blindness, and seizures. Because intensive care is often needed in Japanese encephalitis to help the patient feed and breathe, there may also be various complications arising from the bacterial infections, such as pneumonia and urinary tract infection, that are common to any patient requiring incubation for breathing, elimination, or nutrition.

Japanese encephalitis is an arthropod-borne virus, and is transmitted through the bite of the rice paddy-breeding *Culex* mosquito, which is why the disease tends to occur mainly in rural areas. Mosquitoes become infected with JEV through feeding on the natural animal reservoirs of JEV, which are wild birds and domestic pigs. Once JEV has been transmitted to a human host, through a mosquito bite, it may spread through the body and reach the brain. The transmitting mosquitoes prefer to bite humans outdoors and are at their most active during the evening and night. JEV cannot be transmitted via direct person-to-person contact.

■ Scope and Distribution

Children and the elderly are the most likely to develop the symptomatic form of Japanese encephalitis. The disease is endemic in the countries of the Indian sub-continent, South East Asia, and North East Asia, including Japan. It is transmitted by *Culex* mosquitoes living in rural rice-growing and pig-farming regions, breeding in flooded rice fields, marshes, and standing water around rice fields. Research has shown that most people in endemic areas have been exposed to JEV, even though they may not have had any symptoms of encephalitis. The rate of symptomatic disease in an endemic area is estimated at about one per 150,000 of the population.

Japanese encephalitis is seasonal, as might be expected from a disease transmitted by mosquitoes whose activity depends upon temperature. In temperate regions, it occurs from June to September; in the sub-tropics, the season is extended from April to October, and in tropical regions, Japanese encephalitis occurs all year round. In the United States, just 12 cases were recorded between 1978 and 1993, and these were among expatriates, travelers, or military personnel returning from parts of the world where Japanese encephalitis is endemic. Currently, the rate of infection among U.S. citizens remains at less than one case per year. In endemic areas, it is those living in rural areas that are most at risk; the disease tends to occur less frequently in towns and cities. In general, the risk of travelers contacting JEV infection is low, but much depends on where they are residing and the length of potential exposure.

■ Treatment and Prevention

As of early 2007, there are no specific anti-viral drugs effective against JEV. Treatment of Japanese encephalitis involves supportive treatment dealing with the symptoms of the disease. For instance, anticonvulsant drugs can be used to treat seizures. Intensive care is often needed, if neurological problems like paralysis set in, to provide feeding and airway support. There are a number of vaccines against JEV, some of which are only available in Asia. One of these is a vaccine composed of killed JEV that sometimes causes adverse reactions, but can be used to protect those who intend an extended stay of more than a month to an area where Japanese encephalitis is endemic. If a traveler is sleeping in a rural area where JEV is endemic, then avoiding mosquito exposure is crucial by using bednets treated with the proven mosquito repellent and insecticide DEET (diethyltoluamide). It is best to avoid the outdoors during the evenings and at night, and to stay in well-screened rooms. However, only certain *Culex* species transmit JEV and only a small number of these mosquitoes are infected. Among those travelers who are infected with a JEV-bearing mosquito bite, only one in 50 to one in 1,000 will become ill with JEV.

■ Impacts and Issues

Travelers are still considered to be at low risk of contracting Japanese encephalitis. Interest in vacations to Asia has been on the increase in recent years, therefore, there are potentially more people at risk of exposure to JEV. Advice on precautions and prevention changes frequently, so those traveling to countries such as Vietnam, Japan, India, or almost anywhere in Asia are recommended to seek travel health advice from their physician prior to departure. Vaccination may or may not be recommended, depending on the traveler's specific plans, but advice on reducing exposure to mosquitoes should always be heeded.

There is a clear need for improved and cheaper vaccines against JEV. This may enable whole populations at risk to be protected. Where vaccination is practiced as routine, such as China, Korea and Japan, have tended not to have the epidemics that still occur in India, Nepal and Myanmar, where vaccination is not yet the norm. In May 2006, the World Health Organization (WHO) adopted a 10-year strategy to increase immunization coverage worldwide for several preventable diseases, including Japanese encephalitis. Advanced clinical trials of a new vaccine for children are also underway in India. In the meantime, it also appears that the range of JEV may be extending and may continue to do so with global warming and increased frequency of international travel.

There have been two outbreaks of Japanese encephalitis in Australia—one in 1995, on islands in the Torres Strait and another in 1998 on the Cape York Peninsula.

In 2004, JEV was found in mosquitoes in the Cape York Peninsula, indicating an ongoing risk from Japanese encephalitis.

SEE ALSO *African Sleeping Sickness (Trypanosomiasis); Arthropod-borne Disease; Climate Change and Infectious Disease; Mosquito-borne Diseases; St. Louis Encephalitis; West Nile.*

BIBLIOGRAPHY

Books

Mackenzie, J.S., et al. *Japanese Encephalitis and West Nile Viruses* New York: Springer, 2002.

Web Sites

Centers for Disease Control and Prevention (CDC) Division of Vector-Borne Infectious Diseases. "Japanese Encephalitis Fact Sheet." June 21, 2001 <http://www.cdc.gov/ncidod/dvdbid/ jencephalitis/facts.htm> (accessed July 20, 2007).

World Health Organization. "Japanese Encephalitis." <http://www.who.int/immunization/topics/ japanese_encephalitis/en/index.html> (accessed March 25, 2007).

Susan Aldridge

Kawasaki Syndrome

Introduction

Kawasaki syndrome is a disease of unknown cause that can affect children of any age, but tends to be most prevalent in children younger than five years of age. The disease causes acute symptoms including fever, rash, swelling, irritations in the eyes and around the mouth, and red or peeling hands and feet. In more serious cases, Kawasaki syndrome can lead to heart complications such as congestive heart failure, along with coronary artery dilations and aneurysms, both of which increase the risk of heart attacks. Kawasaki is the leading cause of acquired heart disease in children, with around 20% of children with Kawasaki syndrome developing aneurysms (thinned, weakened areas of arteries) within two weeks if the condition is not treated.

Kawasaki syndrome occurs worldwide, with a higher occurrence in Japan. It is treatable using an administration of aspirin, or via a treatment known as gamma globulin (a group of proteins in blood plasma that contains many antibodies). Due to the risk of heart complications being enhanced when treatment is delayed or not given, treatment is vital to prevent complications arising. As its causes are unknown, there is no known way to prevent contracting Kawasaki syndrome.

Disease History, Characteristics, and Transmission

Kawasaki syndrome was first described by Tomisaki Kawasaki in Japan in 1967. The disease mostly affects children and has become the most common cause of heart disease in children from developed countries. The cause of this disease is unknown although suggested causes include exposure to a toxin, exposure to chemicals used in carpet cleaning, and exposure to an airborne pathogen. The incidence of Kawasaki syndrome is also higher in Japan, and within the United States, the incidence is greatest in individuals of Asian and Pacific Island descent. This suggests that there may be a genetic component that predisposes individuals to the disease.

After acquiring Kawasaki syndrome, patients develop acute (rapid onset) symptoms. These include: fever; rash; swelling of the hands and feet; swollen lymph nodes; irritation and inflammation of the mouth, lips, and tongue; red eyes; and red palms of the hands and soles of the feet. Chronic symptoms include coronary artery dilatations and aneurysms, which leads to an increased chance of a heart attack.

Since the cause of the disease is unknown, little is known about the transmission of Kawasaki syndrome. However, it is known that the disease is not contagious.

Scope and Distribution

Kawasaki syndrome was first diagnosed in Japan, and the highest incidence of this disease remains in Japan. However, Kawasaki syndrome occurs worldwide. In the United States, around 4,000 children are diagnosed with the condition each year.

Children under the age of five years are at greatest risk of developing Kawasaki syndrome. In 2000, within the United States, 77% of all children being treated for Kawasaki syndrome were under five years of age, and peak prevalence occurred in children aged 18–24 months. However, older children, including teenagers, also develop the disease. Worldwide, cases of Kawasaki syndrome are uncommon before age six months, and this is thought to be due to the protective action of maternal antibodies.

Incidence of Kawasaki syndrome also appears to be influenced by sex and race. Males tend to be more prone to developing the disease, as are children of Asian or Pacific Island descent. Studies have also shown that Kawasaki syndrome in the United States is linked to socioeconomic status, with the disease more common in families with a high median household income.

Most incidences of Kawasaki syndrome occur during winter or early spring, suggesting that the disease may have a winter-spring seasonality.

■ Treatment and Prevention

People who have developed Kawasaki syndrome require hospitalization during which time they are treated with aspirin and an intravenous treatment known as gamma globulin (IVGG). IVGG treatment contains antibodies and comes from donor blood. This treatment is given for 8 to 12 hours and acts to decrease fever and to lower the risk of heart complications. Aspirin is also administered for both its anti-inflammatory action and to lower fever. In the majority of cases where treatment is given within 10 days after disease onset, recovery from acute symptoms is complete and heart problems are unlikely. However, the risk of developing heart problems increases the longer the patient goes without treatment.

Although recovery of the acute symptoms of Kawasaki syndrome is possible without treatment, the risk of heart problems is significant. Approximately 20–25% of children may develop enlargement of the heart and its arteries if left without treatment. This increases the likelihood of heart problems, and other complications such as arthritis, meningitis, and death. As the cause of this disease is unknown, there is no definitively known way to prevent contracting the disease.

■ Impacts and Issues

Kawasaki syndrome has become the leading cause of acquired heart problems in children less than five years of age who live in developed countries. Kawasaki syndrome now has this number one distinction after the incidence of scarlet fever (along with the rheumatic heart disease that often accompanied it) has dropped dramatically due to the introduction of antibiotics in the 1940s.

As there is no current prevention against contracting Kawasaki syndrome, it is important that patients be identified and treated as soon as possible. Furthermore, the risk of heart disease and other medical complications increases when treatment is not administered or when treatment is delayed. This is another reason why rapid administration of treatment is necessary.

Determining the cause of the disease would increase the likelihood of being able to control and prevent Kawasaki syndrome. Research has been conducted since the disease was first diagnosed in 1967. However, the specific cause for the disease remains unknown. In addition, it remains unknown whether the disease is caused by reaction to a chemical or toxin, or is a classic infectious disease of bacterial or viral origin. Current research points to an infectious trigger for the disease, but many scientists consider an autoimmune component (a condition where the body's immune system falsely interprets

WORDS TO KNOW

ANTIBODY: Antibodies, or Y-shaped immunoglobulins, are proteins found in the blood that help to fight against foreign substances called antigens. Antigens, which are usually proteins or polysaccharides, stimulate the immune system to produce antibodies. The antibodies inactivate the antigen and help to remove it from the body. While antigens can be the source of infections from pathogenic bacteria and viruses, organic molecules detrimental to the body from internal or environmental sources also act as antigens. Genetic engineering and the use of various mutational mechanisms allow the construction of a vast array of antibodies (each with a unique genetic sequence).

ACUTE: An acute infection is one of rapid onset and of short duration, which either resolves or becomes chronic.

AUTOIMMUNITY: Autoimmune diseases are conditions in which the immune system attacks the body's own cells, causing tissue destruction. Autoimmune diseases are classified as either general, in which the autoimmune reaction takes place simultaneously in a number of tissues, or organ specific, in which the autoimmune reaction targets a single organ. Autoimmunity is accepted as the cause of a wide range of disorders, and is suspected to be responsible for many more. Among the most common diseases attributed to autoimmune disorders are rheumatoid arthritis, systemic lupus erythematosis (lupus), multiple sclerosis, myasthenia gravis, pernicious anemia, and scleroderma.

GAMMA GLOBULIN: Gamma globulin is a term referring to a group of soluble proteins in the blood, most of which are antibodies that can mount a direct attack upon pathogens and can be used to treat various infections.

PREVALENCE: The actual number of cases of disease (or injury) that exist in a population.

its own tissues as foreign and attacks them) to be an important factor in the development of the disease. Kawasaki syndrome presents researchers with the challenge of solving a mysterious link between infectious disease and autoimmunity.

SEE ALSO *Childhood Infectious Diseases, Immunization Impacts; Demographics and Infectious Disease; Immune Response to Infection.*

BIBLIOGRAPHY

Periodicals

Pemberton M.N., I.M. Doughty, R.J. Middlehurst, and M.H. Thornhill. "Recurrent Kawasaki Disease." *British Dental Journal.* 186 (1999): 6, 270–271.

Web Sites

Centers for Disease Control and Prevention. "Kawasaki Syndrome." Jan. 10, 2006 <http://www.cdc.gov/ncidod/diseases/kawasaki/index.htm> (accessed February 28, 2007).

Kawasaki Disease Foundation. "Kawasaki Disease Foundation: Caring for Precious Hearts." <http://www.kdfoundation.org/> (accessed February 28, 2007).

Maryland Department of Health and Mental Hygiene. "Kawasaki Disease Fact Sheet." May 2002 <http://edcp.org/factsheets/kawasaki.html> (accessed February 28, 2007).

Koch's Postulates

■ Introduction

Koch's postulates are a set of principles that guide scientific efforts to establish the cause of an infectious disease. Koch's postulates are named after the German physician Robert Koch (1843–1910), who was the first scientist to identify several important pathogens (disease-causing agents). The postulates named after him require a series of observational and experimental conditions to be satisfied before it can be concluded that a particular microorganism causes a certain disease. Because of advances in microbiology over the last century, Koch's postulates have been revised, but they remain relevant to modern research. For example, they have been extended to include non-living molecular causes of disease such as prions.

■ History and Scientific Foundations

Robert Koch was a German medical researcher. He is today famous not only for formulating Koch's but for using them to identify the pathogens that cause some of the deadliest diseases that afflict humankind, including anthrax, cholera, and tuberculosis. Along with the French physician Louis Pasteur (1822–1895), he is considered one of the pioneers of bacteriology (the study of bacteria). Working at home in an improvised laboratory, without assistance from any university, rich patron, or government agency, Koch proved that anthrax is caused by a bacterium—the first occasion on which a disease was shown to be caused by a specific microorganism. Koch received a Nobel Prize in medicine in 1905.

Koch's postulates are four rules for deciding whether the scientific evidence warrants concluding that a certain microorganism is the cause of a disease. They are as follows:

1. The organism must be found in all animals that have the disease, not present in healthy animals.

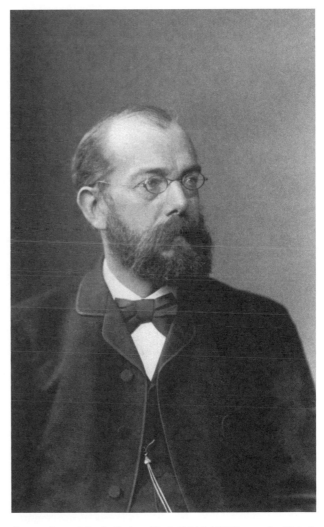

German bacteriologist Robert Koch (1843–1910) won the Nobel Prize in 1905. *The Library of Congress.*

2. It must be possible to isolate the organism from a diseased animal and grow it in pure culture (a non-living nutritional medium in a container).

465

WORDS TO KNOW

CULTURE: A culture is a single species of microorganism that is isolated and grown under controlled conditions. The German bacteriologist Robert Koch first developed culturing techniques in the late 1870s. Following Koch's initial discovery, medical scientists quickly sought to identify other pathogens. Today bacteria cultures are used as basic tools in microbiology and medicine.

ETIOLOGY: The study of the cause or origin of a disease or disorder.

PATHOGEN: A disease-causing agent, such as a bacteria, virus, fungus, etc.

GERMAN PHYSICIAN ROBERT KOCH, PIONEER OF BACTERIOLOGY

In 1880, German physician Robert Koch (1843–1910) accepted an appointment as a government advisor with the Imperial Department of Health in Berlin. His task was to develop methods of isolating and cultivating disease-producing bacteria and to formulate strategies for preventing their spread. In 1881 he published a report advocating the importance of pure cultures in isolating disease-causing organisms and describing in detail how to obtain them. The methods and theory espoused in this paper are still considered fundamental to the field of modern bacteriology and set the foundation for the first three postulates in what were later described as Koch's postulates. The fourth postulate was added by the plant biologist E.F. Smith in 1905.

3. It must then be possible to infect a healthy animal with the organisms grown in culture.

4. The organism must then be isolated again from the experimentally infected animal.

Using the principles that were later named in his honor, students of Koch in the late nineteenth century quickly identified the bacteria that cause bubonic plague, diphtheria, gonorrhea, leprosy, syphilis, tetanus, typhoid, and several other diseases.

The power of Koch's postulates as an aid to science, scientists have pointed out, comes not from their rigid application, but from their encouragement of a spirit of scientific rigor. They serve as guidelines—not absolute rules—for collecting the scientific evidence that will prove what the cause of a given disease is. Exceptions to Koch's postulate numerous; for example, many pathogens, including those that cause giardiasis, polio, and AIDS, can be carried asymptomatically, which violates the first postulate. That is, these pathogens can sometimes live and reproduce in an individual without making that individual sick. Koch's original first postulate has, therefore, been clarified, in practice, to "The organism must be found in all animals that have the disease." Also, not all pathogens can grow in pure culture, as the second postulate requires; viruses and prions, for example, can only reproduce with the help of living cells.

■ Impacts and Issues

New infectious diseases are emerging at the rate of about one per year, but it is often difficult to discover the cause of a particular infectious disease. Koch's postulates, therefore, remain relevant today. According to the editors of the journal *Nature Reviews Microbiology*, writing in 2006, "more than 120 years after they were first proposed, Koch's postulates still remain the gold standard for any investigation that sets out to prove the etiology (origin or cause) of an infectious disease."

One modern example of fulfilling Koch's postulates involves the Australian physician Barry Marshall and his work with the bacterium *Helicobacter pylori*. Marshall, a gastroenterologist, studied the bacteria in the 1980s, after a colleague noticed that *H. pylori* was present in the stomachs of patients with gastrointestinal ulcers and not present in patients without ulcers. Marshall set out to determine if *H. pylori* caused stomach ulcers, and eventually succeeding in growing it in the laboratory. Lacking human test subjects, Marshall first determined that his stomach was without disease, then infected himself by drinking a mixture containing *H. pylori*. After about a week, Marshall began vomiting, and an endoscopy (examination with a thin, flexible, camera-mounted cable) proved he had developed severe inflammation in the lining of his stomach, from which *Helicobacter pylori* was recovered. By satisfying Koch's postulates, Marshall had proven that *H. pylori* could cause disease in humans. This revolutionized the treatment of stomach ulcers, which were until this time, considered caused by stress and excess stomach acid. By the mid 1990s, scientists recognized that stomach ulcers were caused by an infectious agent, and could be successfully treated with antibiotics. Marshall was awarded the Nobel Prize for his discovery in 2005.

Koch's postulates were also been cited in the 1980s in the long and acrimonious debate between the great majority of scientists and American virologist Peter Duesberg (1936–) and a few others over whether AIDS is in fact caused by HIV. Duesberg has long maintained that HIV does not cause AIDS (he claims that recreational and other drugs do). For some years, he argued that HIV had not been shown to be the cause of AIDS according to the standards of Koch's postulates. In the mid–1990s, however, many researchers indicated that all of Koch's postulates had finally been fulfilled and that HIV had indeed been proved to be the cause of AIDS.

SEE ALSO *Bacterial Disease; Culture and Sensitivity;* Helicobacter pylori.

BIBLIOGRAPHY

Books

Brock, Thomas D. *Robert Koch, A Life in Medicine and Bacteriology.* Madison, WI: Science Tech Publishers, 1988.

Periodicals

Cohen, Jon. "Fulfilling Koch's Postulates." *Science.* 266(1994):1647.

Editorial. "Following Koch's Example." *Nature Reviews Microbiology.* 3(2005):906.

Vacomo, V., et al. "Natural History of *Bartonella* Infections (An Exception to Koch's Postulate)." *Clinical and Diagnostic Laboratory Immunology.* 9(2002):8–18.

Web Sites

National Institute of Allergy and Infectious Disease, National Institutes of Health (U.S. Government). "HIV/AIDS: Koch's Postulates Fulfilled." September, 1995 <http://www.nIald.nih.gov/ Publications/hivaids/12.htm> (accessed February 1, 2007).

Larry Gilman

CHALLENGES TO KOCH'S POSTULATES

Since the proposal and general acceptance of the postulates, they have proven to have a number of limitations. For example, infections organisms such as some the bacterium *Mycobacterium leprae*, some viruses, and prions cannot be grown in artificial laboratory media. Additionally, the postulates are fulfilled for a human disease-causing microorganism by using test animals. While a microorganism can be isolated from a human, the subsequent use of the organism to infect a healthy person is unethical. Fulfillment of Koch's postulates requires the use of an animal that mimics the human infection as closely as is possible.

Another limitation of Koch's postulates concerns instances where a microorganism that is normally part of the normal flora of a host becomes capable of causing disease when introduced into a different environment in the host (e.g., *Staphylococcus aureus*), or when the host's immune system is malfunctioning (e.g., *Serratia marcescens*).

Despite these limitations, Koch's postulates remain useful in clarifying the relationship between microorganisms and disease.

Kuru

■ Introduction

Kuru is a progressive, fatal, brain disease which was discovered in the 1950s by the American physician Carleton Gajdusek among the Fore (fore-ay) people of the eastern highlands of New Guinea. The name *kuru* means trembling with fear in the Fore dialect and refers to the tremor that is characteristic of the disease. Gajdusek went on to win the Nobel Prize in medicine in 1976 for his research, which suggested that the disease was linked to the ritualistic handling or consumption of human brain tissue during funeral ceremonies. Kuru is one of a group of rare brain diseases called the transmissible spongiform encephalopathies (TSEs), which also includes Creutzfeldt-Jakob disease (CJD). Postmortem studies show that TSEs lead to the development of tiny holes in brain tissue, giving it a "spongy" appearance. Kuru has now disappeared, as the Fore stopped the funeral practices that led to its spread.

■ Disease History, Characteristics, and Transmission

Kuru affected the cerebellum, which is the area at the base of the brain that controls coordinated movement. Accordingly, the symptoms of kuru included ataxia, or unsteadiness, tremor, stiffness, rigidity, and slurred speech. Persons with kuru did not usually suffer from memory loss or dementia until a later stage of the disease, or at all, although mood changes were common. Eventually, victims of kuru would become unable to stand or eat and they would slip into a comatose state. Death, from starvation or pneumonia would usually occur between three and nine months after the onset of symptoms.

Transmission of kuru occurred by exposure to infected brain tissue. The Fore custom was to remove the brains of the deceased during a funeral, possibly for ritualistic cooking and eating. The task of handling the brain fell to women relatives who were probably infected through any cuts or sores on their skin, or by actually consuming tissue. The women could also transmit the infection to their children through unwashed hands over the next several weeks. Once the disease entered the Fore food chain, it reached epidemic proportions. TSEs, like kuru and CJD are unusual because the infective

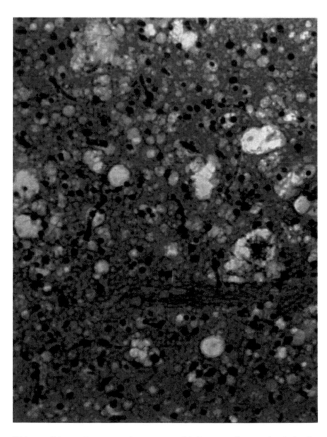

Taken with an electron microscope, this image of a monkey's brain shows it being infected with kuru prion. Between the rounded nuclei of the nerve cells (green) are tiny vacuole spaces typical of the disease's dark spots. *Phanie/Photo Researchers, Inc.*

■ Treatment and Prevention

There was no treatment for kuru and, at the present time, there is also no treatment for any TSE. Prevention of kuru meant stopping the funerary practices that allowed exposure to the infective prion. After this happened, in 1959, occasional cases still arose because of the long incubation time of the disease. The disease was first described in 1957 and the Fore people said that it appeared only a few years before this. No one knows how kuru first arose. It is possible that a few cases of a TSE crossed the species barrier from an animal with a similar disease and was spread by the consumption of infected tissue.

■ Impacts and Issues

Kuru has both cultural and scientific significance. Decimated Fore populations in the twentieth century endured upheaval to their communities and customs. Because more women than men died from the disease, Fore men were sometimes executed by village rulers in order to even out the population. When scientists first considered the disease to be triggered by a genetic susceptibility in the 1950s, the Australian government restricted the movements of the Fore to their own villages in an attempt to prevent intermarriage with islanders considered not susceptible. After Gajdusek discovered that kuru was caused by an infectious agent, the custom of honoring the dead by cannibalizing their tissue and brains ceased out of necessity. There has not been a case of kuru among the Fore in those born since cannibalism was eliminated.

Kuru might have remained as no more than a medical curiosity, had it not turned out to be a TSE. The infective agent in all TSEs, including CJD, is neither a bacterium nor a virus, but an entity known as a prion, which is best described as an infectious protein. A prion is an abnormally shaped version of a protein that occurs naturally in the brain. When the normal prion protein comes into contact with the abnormal version, it is converted into the abnormal version and can go on to corrupt other normal prion protein molecules. This cascade of damage then spreads throughout the brain. Interest in kuru was heightened with the emergence of variant CJD in the United Kingdom in the mid–1990s. The clinical course of kuru resembles that of variant CJD, rather than classical CJD. Both are spread through consumption of exposure to infected tissue and both may have arisen in the population in a similar way. Kuru could have started from a TSE that jumped the species barrier from an unknown animal host. Variant CJD is the human form of bovine spongiform encephalopathy, a TSE of cattle thought to have started when scrapie, a sheep TSE, entered cattle feed. Therefore, rare as TSEs are, it is worthwhile studying their pathology, as

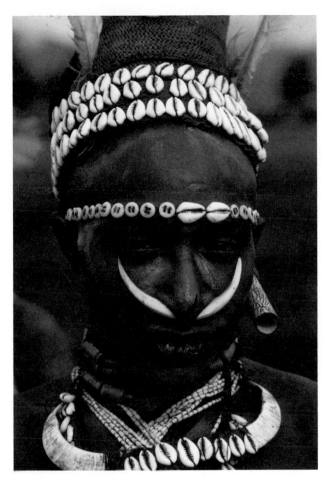

An Iwan warrior in New Guinea wears a bone through his nose in commemoration of his tribe's past cannibal practices. The fatal prion disease kuru, once associated with cannibalism, has largely disappeared from New Guinea. *© Charles & Josette Lenars/Corbis.*

agent is a kind of infectious protein called a prion, rather than a bacterium or virus. The long incubation time of kuru, which can be up to 40 years, meant that new cases continued to appear even as the disease itself began to die out once the funerary practices were abolished.

■ Scope and Distribution

Kuru was always confined to the Fore people who lived in the eastern highlands of New Guinea. They were isolated from Western civilization and from other natives by very mountainous terrain and disease has never been found elsewhere. Women and children of either sex seemed to be most at risk in the early years. Later, when adults exposed as children began to develop the disease, it affected men and women equally. During the 1950s and 1960s, it reached epidemic proportions and wiped out the population of many Fore villages.

WORDS TO KNOW

EMERGING DISEASE: New infectious diseases such as SARS and West Nile virus, as well as previously known diseases such as malaria, tuberculosis, and bacterial pneumonias that are appearing in forms that are resistant to drug treatments, are termed emerging infectious diseases.

ENCEPHALOPATHY: Any abnormality in the structure or function of the brain.

INCUBATION PERIOD: Incubation period refers to the time between exposure to disease causing virus or bacteria and the appearance of symptoms of the infection. Depending on the microorganism, the incubation time can range from a few hours (an example is food poisoning due to *Salmonella*) to a decade or more (an example is acquired immunodeficiency syndrome, or AIDS).

PRIONS: Prions are proteins that are infectious. Indeed, the name prion is derived from "proteinaceous infectious particles." The discovery of prions and confirmation of their infectious nature overturned a central dogma that infections were caused by intact organisms, particularly microorganisms such as bacteria, fungi, parasites, or viruses. Since prions lack genetic material, the prevailing attitude was that a protein could not cause disease.

circumstances could conspire to allow the emergence of a new type of this fatal brain disease.

SEE ALSO *Bovine Spongiform Encephalopathy ("Mad Cow" Disease); Creutzfeldt-Jakob Disease-nv; Prion Disease.*

BIBLIOGRAPHY

Books

Wilson, Walter R., and Merle A. Sande. *Current Diagnosis & Treatment in Infectious Diseases.* New York: McGraw Hill, 2001.

Web Sites

Jansen, Paul A. *eMedicine.* "Kuru" Oct 15, 2005. <http://www.emedicine.com/med/topic1248.htm> (accessed March 19, 2007).

National Institute of Neurological Disorders and Stroke. "Kuru Information Page." Feb 14, 2007. <http://www.ninds.nih.gov/disorders/kuru/kuru.htm> (accessed March 19, 2007).

Lassa Fever

■ Introduction

Lassa fever is an animal-borne (zoonotic) virus that is transmitted via contact with contaminated rat urine or feces. Rural regions of the West African countries Nigeria, Sierra Leone, Guinea, and Liberia known as the "Lassa belt" experience intermittent ongoing outbreaks of Lassa fever. Following infection with Lassa virus, 80% of persons remain symptom free, or develop mild symptoms, while the remaining 20% develop a more severe illness. Symptoms increase in severity as infection progresses, with neurological problems and sometimes death occurring in the later stages. Lassa fever is treated via antiviral drugs in addition to symptom management. As no vaccine is available, prevention methods focus on avoiding contaminated material, avoiding rats, and taking precautions while in close contact with infected people.

Following peace agreements within endemic countries previously upset by civil unrest, progress has been made in the treatment and prevention of Lassa fever. Furthermore, work is underway to improve diagnostic testing for Lassa fever, as well as to discover a vaccine for the virus.

■ Disease History, Characteristics, and Transmission

Lassa fever was first described in the 1950s, although the virus responsible for the infection was not identified until

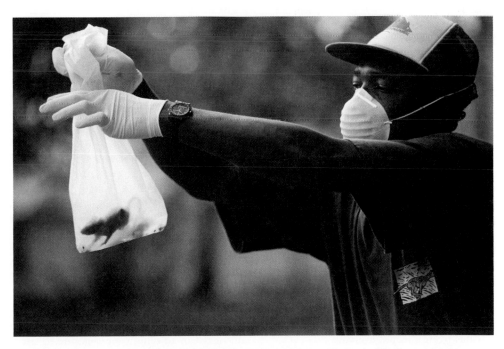

In Sierra Leone, a rat is trapped to provide information about Lassa fever, a highly dangerous virus carried by such rodents. © *Karen Kasmauski/Corbis.*

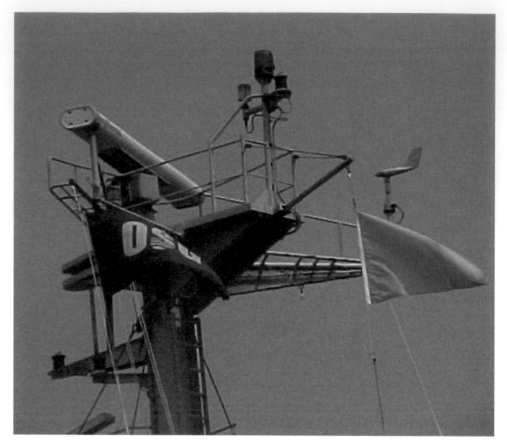

In September 2004, the ship *Overseas Marilyn* waits off the coast of Galveston, Texas, flying a yellow quarantine flag. The ship and 20 crew members were held under a voluntary quarantine as health officials investigated the death of one of the crew. Lassa fever, a virus common in West Africa, was suspected.   *AP Images.*

1969, when missionary nurses in Nigeria, West Africa, died from an infection caused by a virus identified as the Lassa virus. Lassa virus is a member of the Arenaviridae family and is transmitted to humans via contact with infected urine or droppings of certain species of rats.

Rats from the genus *Mastomys* are the reservoirs of Lassa virus. They are efficient hosts due to their high frequency of breeding and large number of offspring. Furthermore, they tend to colonize human habitats, increasing the chances of human exposure. *Mastomys* rats become infected with Lassa virus, but do not become ill from it. Humans become infected following exposure to infected rat excreta, either directly or indirectly. The virus is transmitted when humans touch objects or eat food that is contaminated with rat excreta, or when excreta comes in contact with cuts and sores. In addition, inhaling small particles of excreta in the air transmits the virus, as does consuming infected rats as food. Lassa fever is also transmitted between humans. This occurs following contact with infected body fluids such as blood, excretions, secretions, and tissues from infected humans.

Lassa fever is asymptomatic or mild in 80% of infected people. However, the remaining 20% experience severe disease in which many organs within the body are affected. Symptoms include fever, aches, vomiting, diarrhea, conjunctivitis (inflammation, redness of the conjunctiva of the eye), facial swelling, protein in the urine, and mucosal (mucous membranes such as in the nose and mouth) bleeding. Symptoms increase in severity as the disease progresses, leading to neurological problems such as hearing loss, tremors, and coma in the later stages. Symptoms usually take one to three weeks to appear, and generally last for one to four weeks. Mortality rates have been estimated to be 1% in total, and up to 15% in hospitalized patients. In fatal cases, death usually occurs within two weeks following the arise of symptoms.

■ Scope and Distribution

Lassa fever occurs predominantly in West Africa. While it is endemic (occurs naturally) in certain regions, such as Guinea, Liberia, Sierra Leone, and Nigeria, the disease may exist in adjoining regions due to the wide distribution of the host rodent species. Imported cases of Lassa fever have been reported from the United States where, in both cases, the patients were travelers who had returned from endemic regions of West Africa.

The number of annual infections within West Africa is estimated to be between 100,000 and 300,000, and annual deaths from the disease number about 5,000. As disease surveillance for Lassa fever is not uniformly undertaken, these estimates are rudimentary and subject to error. According to the Centers for Disease Control and Prevention (CDC), Lassa fever tends to be restricted to the rural regions of West Africa, particularly in areas where humans live in close proximity to the rats that are the main reservoir of the virus. Infections have also occurred as a consequence of laboratory exposure elsewhere in the world.

The people who tend to be most at risk of infection with Lassa virus are those who reside in areas with high densities of *Mastomys* rats, or those who come in contact with infected humans. Therefore, populations living in rural areas in which rat populations are high, as well as hospital staff in these areas, are at the greatest risk. However, hospital staff greatly reduce their risk by taking preventative measures including standard and isolation precautions in order to avoid contact with the virus.

■ Treatment and Prevention

Lassa fever is treated using the anti-viral drug ribavirin. This drug has been shown to be effective against early stages of Lassa fever, but does not appear to be as effective if given during the later stages of the illness. In addition to drug treatment, patients should also receive supportive care. This includes caring for the fever symptoms, and maintaining fluid and electrolyte balance, along with blood pressure and oxygenation levels.

There is no vaccine for Lassa fever, and thus, prevention consists mainly of avoiding contact with potentially contaminated materials. Contamination from rat excreta can be avoided by discouraging rats from human living quarters through removing garbage from the home, keeping cats, and maintaining clean living quarters. Furthermore, keeping food stored in rodent-proof containers prevents food becoming contaminated with infected rat excreta. People in close contact with infected persons, such as family members and health care workers can prevent contact with blood and body fluids by taking precautions such as wearing gloves, gowns, face shields, and masks while in contact with the person.

Complete eradication of *Mastomys* is unlikely to occur due to their high prevalence in endemic areas. Therefore, avoidance rather than eradication appears to be the most effective way of preventing infection via rat excreta. In order to achieve avoidance, good hygiene practices are being promoted within infected communities.

■ Impacts and Issues

The symptoms of Lassa fever are common to a variety of viral fevers, and thus diagnosis is difficult and often requires diagnostic testing that can be both expensive and time consuming. Therefore, improved testing procedures would lead to increased accuracy of diagnosis and a more accurate idea of infection prevalence. Research is also being completed to develop a vaccine for Lassa fever.

Changing the cultural attitudes among traditional peoples of Sierra Leone about the nature of Lassa fever presents a continuing challenge to workers in the London-based charity Merlin's Lassa fever group. Many traditional people in Sierra Leone still consider Lassa fever an inevitable fact of life, and are hesitant to invest in efforts to reduce exposure to rats when other diseases such as malaria remain ever-present, and are often not distinguished from Lassa fever when a person becomes ill. Workers with Merlin and other agencies continue to travel from village to village, conducting education campaigns that explain the particular connection between rats and Lassa fever, and discouraging trapping, eating, and sharing living areas with rats.

Exportation of Lassa fever, as well as many other diseases such as malaria and typhoid occurs when travelers pass through endemic areas and become infected. This creates the threat that these diseases will become introduced to areas previously unaffected by these diseases.

The Lassa virus is also considered a potential candidate for use as an agent of bioterrorism.

SEE ALSO *Airborne Precautions; Animal Importation; Antiviral Drugs; Malaria; Rapid Diagnostic Tests for Infectious Diseases; Travel and Infectious Disease; Typhoid Fever; Vaccines and Vaccine Development; War and Infectious Disease.*

WORDS TO KNOW

ENDEMIC: Present in a particular area or among a particular group of people.

RESERVOIR: The animal or organism in which the virus or parasite normally resides.

SPECIAL PATHOGENS BRANCH: A group within the U.S. Centers for Disease Control and Prevention (CDC) whose goal is to study highly infectious viruses that produce diseases within humans.

ZOONOSES: Zoonoses are diseases of microbiological origin that can be transmitted from animals to people. The causes of the diseases can be bacteria, viruses, parasites, and fungi.

IN CONTEXT: ERADICATION PROGRAM EFFECTIVENESS

Control of Lassa fever has been set back by civil unrest within endemic countries such as Guinea, Liberia, and Sierra Leone. However, peace initiatives have led to steps being taken by these three countries to develop prevention and coping strategies for Lassa virus. These developments have been led by the formation of the Mano River Union Lassa Fever Network, which has begun enhancing diagnostic testing, improving clinical management, and performing environmental control. In addition, better care facilities are being constructed for patients suffering from Lassa fever.

SOURCE: *World Health Organization (WHO)*

BIBLIOGRAPHY

Books

Arguin, P.M., P.E. Kozarsky, and A.W. Navin. *Health Information for International Travel 2005–2006.* U.S. Department of Health and Human Services, 2005.

Web Sites

Centers for Disease Control and Prevention. "Lassa Fever." December 3, 2004 <http://www.cdc.gov/ncidod/dvrd/spb/mnpages/dispages/lassaf.htm> (accessed February 22, 2007).

tanford University. "Lassa Fever Virus." 2005 <http://www.stanford.edu/group/virus/arena/2005/LassaFeverVirus.htm> (accessed February 22, 2007).

World Health Organization. "Lassa Fever." April 2005 <http://www.who.int/mediacentre/factsheets/fs179/en/> (accessed February 22, 2007).

Legionnaire's Disease (Legionellosis)

■ Introduction

Legionellosis refers to a disease caused by a type of bacteria called *Legionella*. Most commonly, the responsible organism is *Legionella pneumophila*.

The bacteria are normal residents of freshwater creeks, ponds, and lakes. They can also be present in the water supply inside buildings, where they have entered the air via tiny water droplets from ventilation or water ducts.

There are two forms of Legionellosis. The first is a more severe pneumonia that is known as Legionnaire's disease. The second includes a milder type of pneumonia and is called Pontiac fever.

■ Disease History, Characteristics, and Transmission

Legionellosis was first apparent in July 1976. At that time, an outbreak of pneumonia occurred during an American Legion convention being held at the Belle-vue-Stratford Hotel in Philadelphia, Pennsylvania. Ultimately, 221 veterans were sickened during the outbreak. Thirty-four of these people eventually died of the infection, which was later dubbed Legionnaire's disease.

The disease outbreak caused national alarm, since it was feared to be the start of an epidemic of Swine Flu, which was at the time affecting Asia. However, an investigation conducted by the United States Centers for Disease Control and Prevention (CDC) determined that the Philadelphia outbreak was due to a newly discovered bacterium, which was eventually named *L. pneumophila*.

The outbreak was traced to bacteria growing in the hotel's cooling tower. Later, investigators showed that the bacterium is capable of growth as a surface-adherent structure called a biofilm. It is likely that bits of the biofilm broke off and were sucked into the hotel's ventilation system, where the bacteria were inhaled. Other outbreaks have been traced to biofilms growing on showerheads and in contaminated drinking water.

Legionellosis is an example of an opportunistic infection—an infection that is caused in some people by a bacterium that normally does not cause harm. For example, studies have determined that 5 to 10% of Americans contain *Legionella* antibodies even though they have not developed Legionellosis. However, in people whose immune systems are less capable of fighting off an infection, the bacteria can cause disease. Pneumonia due to *Legionella* comprises 2 to 15% of all pneumonia cases in U.S. hospitals, according to the CDC.

The majority of Legionellosis—over 90% of cases—is caused by *L. pneumophila*. *L. micdadei* can also cause legionellosis, especially in people who are immuno-compromised.

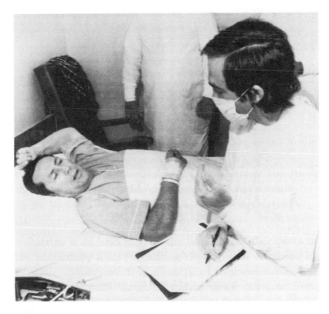

Medical doctor (right) with the Centers for Disease Control and Prevention (CDC) interviews Thomas Payne in a Pennsylvania hospital in 1976. Paine was one of the Legionnaires who became ill after attending a convention in Philadelphia. *AP Images.*

WORDS TO KNOW

BIOFILM: Biofilms are populations of microorganisms that form following the adhesion of bacteria, algae, yeast, or fungi to a surface. These surface growths can be found in natural settings such as on rocks in streams, and in infections such as can occur on catheters. Microorganisms can colonize living and inert natural and synthetic surfaces.

OPPORTUNISTIC INFECTION: An opportunistic infection is so named because it occurs in people whose immune systems are diminished or are not functioning normally; such infections are opportunistic insofar as the infectious agents take advantage of their hosts' compromised immune systems and invade to cause disease.

IN CONTEXT: REAL-WORLD RISKS

The Coordinating Center for Infectious Diseases/Division of Bacterial and Mycotic Diseases states that:

- Each year, between 8,000 and 18,000 people are hospitalized with Legionnaires' disease in the U.S. However, many infections are not diagnosed or reported, so this number may be higher. More illness is usually found in the summer and early fall, but it can happen any time of year.
- Legionnaires' disease can be very serious and can cause death in 5% to 30% of cases. Most cases can be treated successfully with antibiotics (drugs that kill bacteria in the body), and healthy people usually recover from infection.
- People most at risk of getting sick from the bacteria are older people (usually 65 years of age or older), as well as people who are smokers, or those who have a chronic lung disease (like emphysema).
- People who have weak immune systems from diseases like cancer, diabetes, or kidney failure are also more likely to get sick from Legionella bacteria. People who take drugs to suppress (weaken) the immune system (like after a transplant operation or chemotherapy) are also at higher risk.

SOURCE: *Coordinating Center for Infectious Diseases/Division of Bacterial and Mycotic Diseases, Centers for Disease Control and Prevention (CDC)*

Approximately 10,000 to 40,000 Americans acquire Legionnaires' disease every year, and 8,000 to 18,000 require hospitalization. The people who are the most likely to become ill are over age 50. The risk is greater for those with diminished immune system function due to illness, diabetes, cigarette smoking, and who are taking immunosuppressing drugs. Legionnaires' disease can occur in children, but is not normally considered a disease of childhood. Children who are at risk are those who are on a respirator to assist with breathing, and those whose immune systems are impaired due to recent surgery or drug treatment. Curiously, those infected with the human immunodeficiency virus or who have developed acquired immunodeficiency syndrome (AIDS, also cited as acquired immune deficiency syndrome) do not appear to be at higher risk than others, although when contracting the disease, their symptoms are often more severe.

Legionnaire's disease is caused by inhaling *Legionella* suspended in minute water droplets, or by aspirating *Legionella* bacteria, which occurs when particles bearing the bacteria escape the gag reflex and fall directly into the respiratory tract. The bacteria can be naturally found in bodies of fresh water and whirlpool spas (the source of the first outbreak of Pontiac fever), where they can be dispersed into the air by the action of wind and waves. As well, the bacteria growing within biofilms in stagnant water at the intake of air conditioning cooling towers, humidifiers, faucets, shower heads, and even the water misters in supermarket produce departments can slough off and be carried on water droplets. Person-to-person transmission has not been demonstrated.

When inhaled or aspirated, *Legionella* bacteria enter the lungs. Normally, as bacteria enter the lungs they are engulfed and dissolved by cells called alveolar macrophages. However, *Legionella* are able to grow and divide inside the macrophages. Eventually, the infected macrophages burst, releasing the bacteria, which infect other macrophages and continuing the cycle of infection.

The symptoms of legionellosis develop 2 to 10 days after inhalation of the bacteria. At first, the symptoms include a feeling of tiredness, headaches, fever, chills, aching muscle, and a loss of appetite. A fever of up to 104°F (40°C) can develop. A dry and hacking cough also develops; it can change to a cough that involves the release of bloody mucus. The pneumonia affects breathing in about 50% of people and can cause chest pain in about 30% of those who get the infection. Some people develop a decreased heart rate, which can be dangerous when combined with the decreased breathing capability of the lungs.

In addition to pneumonia, legionellosis can involve other areas of the body. Other, less common complications include diarrhea, nausea with vomiting, abdominal pain, kidney failure and impaired urine production (which allows the build up of toxic by-products of body processes), and diminished mental capacity.

Pontiac fever is a milder form of legionellosis, which does not involve the lower respiratory tract. The symptoms, which are flulike and which typically appear within two days of exposure to the bacteria, include fever, headache, muscle aches, and fatigue. The infection passes within a few days and often, persons do not seek medical treatment.

Scope and Distribution

Legionellosis can occur almost anywhere in the world. A 2003 survey conducted by the 36-country European Working Group for *Legionella* Infections found the disease in 34 of the member nations. As one example, scientists investigating the May 1980 eruption of Mt. St. Helens became ill, likely with *L. pneumophila* found in ponds on the hillside.

Treatment and Prevention

Cases of legionellosis that occur as part of an outbreak are usually diagnosed more quickly than isolated cases. Diagnosis is complicated by the fact that the early symptoms and appearance of the chest in an x-ray are similar to other types of bacterial or viral pneumonia. Prompt diagnosis and treatment results in a better prognosis for persons with legionellosis. Death occurs about 5% of the time for previously healthy individuals and almost 25% of the time for people who were already ill or whose immune system was impaired when they contracted the disease. In severe cases that require mechanical assistance for breathing and kidney function, the death rate can be over 65%.

Legionellosis can be diagnosed by detecting antibodies to *L. pneumophila* produced by the immune system. A number of tests use the antibodies to detect the bacteria. For example, the antibodies can be linked to a fluorescent probe, and when samples are treated with the fluorescent antibody, *L. pneumophila* will appear as bright objects upon microscopic examination. Other tests can detect the presence of protein components of the bacteria in the urine, or the presence of the bacterial genetic material in urine and other body fluid.

Legionellosis is treated with antibiotics. As the bacteria reproduce inside host cells, the antibiotics must be capable of penetrating into the host cells. Typically, levofloxacin or azithromycin are used. Prompt antibiotic therapy leads to a complete recovery in the majority of cases.

Legionellosis is prevented by keeping ductwork, pipes, cooling towers, showerheads, and other potential breeding spots clean and free of stagnant water. In reality, this sort of vigilance can be difficult to maintain

IN CONTEXT: EFFECTIVE RULES AND REGULATIONS

The Centers for Disease Control and Prevention (CDC) states that "a person diagnosed with Legionnaires' disease in the workplace is not a threat to others who share office space or other areas with him or her. However, if you thought that there your workplace was the source of the person's illness, contact your local health department."

SOURCE: *Centers for Disease Control and Prevention (CDC)*

unless a mandated and inspection schedule is imposed and documentation required.

As of 2007, there is no vaccine for legionellosis.

Impacts and Issues

In the aftermath of the Philadelphia outbreak, regulations governing the cleaning and monitoring of air conditioning systems in public places were changed to minimize the development of *L. pneumophila*.

Legionellosis has the most impact in places where people gather and which are ventilated or have shower facilities; examples include indoor recreation centers, pools, spas, hotels, and hospitals. The latter is especially important since ill people are even more susceptible to the infection. Construction workers can also be at increased risk, since the bacteria may be dispersed into the air during excavation of the site.

In contrast to diseases such as bacterial meningitis and AIDS, there is no indication that poorer regions of the world are any more at risk than the more wealthy developed world. Indeed, the association of legionellosis with facilities such as hospitals and hotels has made the disease more of a problem in developed countries.

SEE ALSO *Opportunistic Infection; Water-borne Disease.*

BIBLIOGRAPHY

Books

Betsy, Tom and James Keogh. *Microbiology Demystified*. New York: McGraw-Hill Professional, 2005.
McCoy, William F. *Preventing Legionellosis*. London: IWA Publishing, 2006.

Websites

www.Legionella.org <http://www.legionella.org/> (accessed March 6, 2007).

Brian Hoyle

Legislation, International Law, and Infectious Diseases

Introduction

While national infectious disease laws and legislation are essential, globalization demands increasingly international solutions as epidemic diseases do not respect national boundaries. International cooperation among national governments and between governments and international non-government agencies (NGOs) is facilitated by a basic set of international public health and infectious disease laws.

The body of international infectious disease law is composed of different types of agreements among nations, including: treaties, accords, conventions, and agreements. Also, nations may contribute to international infectious disease law by participating in international organizations such as the United Nations, World Trade Organization, or World Bank. Furthermore, several nations may sponsor or aid the missions of various NGOs, agreeing to let their members assess and respond to infectious disease outbreaks within their national borders.

History and Policy Response

The earliest attempts at systematized government responses to epidemic disease arose out of the persistent threat of plague in Europe. Quarantine (the confinement of persons who have been exposed to a disease, but do not show symptoms of the disease) was widely used to control epidemic plague. From the time of the Black Death, during which one-third of Europe's population perished from the plague, those who could afford to leave densely plague-infested cities often retreated to residences in the countryside. This exodus from the cities may have saved some from being exposed, but also helped spread the disease. After the Black Death, many small municipalities forbade entry to those fleeing the cities. In rural Italy, a Catholic priest wrote the Vatican asking for a decree permitting monasteries to close their doors on plague victims and refugees. Instead, the Church viewed plague as punishment for peoples' sins and instructed non-cloistered orders of lower-level clergy across Europe to minister and aid the sick.

When epidemic plague struck England in 1665, the royal government left the city. The mayor and alderman

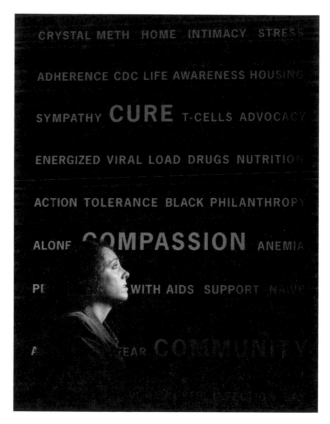

A social worker who counsels HIV patients stands by a poster in the lobby of her Chicago office. In 2006, Illinois joined 38 other states in tracking HIV cases using infected patients's names. Previously, such data were tracked anonymously. Many believe this method of tracking the disease will discourage people from being tested and treated for the virus that causes AIDS. *AP Images.*

478

were left in charge of governing the city through the epidemic. Isolation and quarantine were again employed. Businesses, public spaces, restaurants, and inns were closed—churches, however, remained open, undermining the efficacy of the health laws. The city government hired physicians and regulated burial practices, criminalizing the dumping of bodies into the River Thames. Some plague-infested inns and public housed were ordered burned. When the plague escaped the confines of London to the village of Eyam, the villagers isolated the sick and quarantined the village. Nearly 75% of its inhabitants died, but surrounding villages were largely spared from the epidemic.

The often-conflicting laws—the result of a lack of understanding about disease transmission—proved limitedly effective against plague. While it was never epidemic in London after the Great Fire of 1666, plague continued to arise periodically in European cities until the late eighteenth century. The disappearance of epidemic plague was less a victory for infectious disease law and more likely the result of diminishing numbers of its vector—the decline of black rat populations and their plague-carrying fleas. When epidemic cholera hit Europe in the 1830s, officials looked to the historical example of public health measures and laws enacted to combat plague as a foundation.

The genesis of modern infectious disease law is often traced to the cholera pandemic in Europe from 1829 to 1851. From 1816 to 1826, a cholera pandemic spread through India, Southeast Asia, and China. Three years after the pandemic subsided in China, it reached parts of Europe. In 1831 and 1832, cholera was epidemic in several of Europe's major cities. In 1849, cholera again spread through several European, and then U.S., cities. Many historians note that the time period was one of rapidly increasing immigration and trade, a dangerous situation for infectious disease. Medicine and modern scientific research were newly emerging, but scientific knowledge of disease had limitedly progressed in the preceding century. The cholera epidemics prompted substantial change in medicine, public health, and infectious disease law.

In 1954, John Snow identified polluted public water supplies as the source of cholera. Snow advocated radical changes in sanitation and water safety, persuading the London city government to approve construction of new water systems and enact laws protecting the water supply. Sanitation and hygiene laws, championed by the growing sanitation and public health movement, helped reduce incidence of cholera and other water-borne diseases.

In 1851, the First International Sanitary Conference convened in Paris, France—cholera identification and prevention was a primary concern of the attendees. Pandemic cholera spurred diplomacy between nations. England and France both sent public health officials to medical academies and hospitals abroad to study the disease and possible treatments. Infectious disease and sanitation laws that proved effective in one location were

WORDS TO KNOW

EPIDEMIC: From the Greek *epidemic*, meaning "prevalent among the people," is most commonly used to describe an outbreak of an illness or disease in which the number of individual cases significantly exceeds the usual or expected number of cases in any given population.

GERM THEORY OF DISEASE: The germ theory is a fundamental tenet of medicine that states that microorganisms, which are too small to be seen without the aid of a microscope, can invade the body and cause disease.

ISOLATION: Isolation, within the health community, refers to the precautions that are taken in the hospital to prevent the spread of an infectious agent from an infected or colonized patient to susceptible persons. Isolation practices are designed to minimize the transmission of infection.

LATENT INFECTION: An infection already established in the body but not yet causing symptoms, or having ceased to cause symptoms after an active period, is a latent infection.

PANDEMIC: Pandemic, which means all the people, describes an epidemic that occurs in more than one country or population simultaneously.

QUARANTINE: Quarantine is the practice of separating people who have been exposed to an infectious agent but have not yet developed symptoms from the general population. This can be done voluntarily or involuntarily by the authority of states and the federal Centers for Disease Control and Prevention.

VECTOR: Any agent, living or otherwise, that carries and transmits parasites and diseases. Also, an organism or chemical used to transport a gene into a new host cell.

often adopted elsewhere. From 1851 to 1900, ten international sanitary conferences met to discuss the international impacts of infectious disease. Eight international conventions were drafted, though few were adopted into force by national governments.

By the dawn of the twentieth century, science drove infectious disease law. The professionalization of medicine and scientific training of physicians in universities,

IN CONTEXT: SABIN HEALTH LAWS

Florence Sabin (1871–1953) was the first woman to graduate from the Johns Hopkins Medical School. She then became the first woman appointed to a full professorship at Johns Hopkins and was elected the first woman president of the American Association of Anatomists. After becoming the first lifetime woman member of the National Academy of Sciences, Sabin ultimately expanded her work to include research on understanding the pathology and immunology of tuberculosis.

Sabin's methods of blood analysis became important indictors of various disease states, and her work was important in attempts to combat tuberculosis. Near the end of World War II (1939–1945), Sabin was called upon to chair a study on public health practices in her home state of Colorado. As part of her work, Sabin conducted studies on the effects of water pollution and the prevention of brucellosis in cattle, At the time, brucellosis, especially in infants, often resulted from exposure to contaminated and unpasteurized milk from diseased cows.

The result of Sabin's work was the passage of the Sabin Health Laws, which signaled a critical change in public health policy. The Sabin Health Bills mandated stringent regulations regarding infectious disease, milk pasteurization, and sewage disposal.

the wide acceptance of germ theory, and the discovery of antisepsis revolutionized public health. Infectious disease laws became more effective as researchers were better able to identify the sources of disease and understand how diseases spread. By the outbreak of World War I (1914–1918), international agencies already operated to assess sanitation conditions and identify and treat disease outbreaks across national borders. The Red Cross and Pan American Sanitary Bureau helped draft international conventions on infectious disease prevention. International treaties and agreements outlined infectious disease controls associated with trade and immigration. National governments had passed laws outlining effective isolation and quarantine measures, adopted food safety regulations, instituted comprehensive health screening for arriving immigrants and restricted entry to healthy individuals, and established national public health agencies.

After World War II (1939–1941), the availability of antibiotics and the rapid development of modern vaccines again changed the ways in which health officials were able to respond to diseases. International agreements provided for the sharing and distribution of vaccines and antibiotics. The founding of the United Nations created a global organizational structure for international public health programs and laws. The World Health Organization was created on July 22,

1946, to promulgate international public health regulations and promote public health laws worldwide.

Since the 1960s, economic and trade organizations have played an increasing role in international infectious disease laws. Free trade agreements often carry requirements that exports will meet quality and safety standards or that nations can decline imports if they pose a general health threat. Trade agreements on agricultural, animal, and food products typically stipulate regulations for disease testing, hygienic packaging, safe handling, and inspection. Sometimes, trade agreements contain public health provisions, such as aid for combating endemic parasites or infectious diseases.

Even with the rise of trade organizations and the formation of the United Nations and the WHO, public health laws remain uneven throughout the world. Most international public health laws are non-binding or difficult to enforce without total cooperation by participating nations. UN and trade organization member nations have full national sovereignty, meaning they reserve the power to adopt and enforce laws within their national borders. Adding to the inequalities in national healthcare systems, sanitation systems, and resources for combating diseases, some nations do not recognize international infectious disease conventions or do not participate in WHO-led anti-disease programs. International infectious disease conventions sometimes fail completely in conflict-torn nations, often areas where infectious disease monitoring, prevention, and response are needed most. NGOs (non-governmental organizations), such as the International Red Cross and Doctors without Borders are often effective at responding to epidemic disease in these regions.

■ Impacts and Issues

Today, laws that govern response to infectious diseases are increasingly international. Increased migration and trade has expanded the reach of once-localized diseases. While globalization has aided in the spread of some diseases, it has also opened new channels for combating infectious disease. Once the exclusive domain of local and national governments, laws governing reporting and responding to infectious diseases are increasingly international.

Infectious Disease Response, Civil Liberties, and Medical Privacy in the United States

The expansion of scientific research capabilities and computerized information systems has aided the global fight against infectious disease. Researchers and public health officials are better able to identify, study, respond to, and communicate about disease outbreaks. However, disease prevention and containment measures can impede personal civil liberties or impact personal privacy.

In the United States, Executive Order 13295 provides for government authority to detain, seize, apprehend, quarantine, or isolate persons potentially sickened by or exposed to cholera, diphtheria, emerging pandemic influenza, infectious tuberculosis, plague, severe acute respiratory syndrome (SARS), smallpox, yellow fever, and viral hemorrhagic fevers. States have passed varying forms of the Model State Emergency Health Powers Act (MSEHPA), outlining state and local epidemic disease response plans and powers. Some critics assert that governments can too greatly encroach on freedoms of travel and association in when responding to epidemic disease by instituting quarantines or isolation orders.

Several nations have responded to concerns about personal privacy by passing laws safeguarding patients' personal information. In the United States, concerns of medical privacy were addressed through the passage of the Health Insurance Portability and Accountability Act (HIPAA) in 1996. The primary aim of the legislation was to protect access to private health insurance for workers who lose or change their employment. However, the legislation also contains several provisions on privacy and security. Under HIPAA, a patient's health status, medical history, payment history for medical services, and private identifying information must be protected. While insurers still have access to some of this information to facilitate payment of patient claims, patients have greater control over how much information insurers may obtain and doctors may release. Patients must be notified of any use of their personal health information or sign a waiver.

While patient privacy advocates applaud the legislation, several researchers have asserted that HIPAA hampers the ability to conducted needed avenues of research, especially those that formerly involved studying past patient medical charts. Furthermore, some researchers have noticed a drop in follow-up survey responses, complicating research on recovery and relapse.

HIPAA does not affect the reporting of notifiable diseases to federal and state health officials. The Centers for Disease Control and Prevention (CDC) National Electronic Disease Surveillance System (NEDSS) is also unaffected as individually identifiable health information is available for public health research use without consent, but cannot include personal identifiers such as name or address.

Fighting Epidemic Disease across National Borders

There is no universally accepted international body of law. Thus, international anti-infectious disease regulation is typically the result of participation in United Nations initiatives by member nations or through voluntary cooperative efforts governed by treaty. Not all

IN CONTEXT: REAL-WORLD RISKS

In June 2007, Atlanta-based attorney Andrew Speaker flew aboard a commercial aircraft to Europe for his wedding. Before he left, Speaker consulted doctors in Atlanta, where he was diagnosed with a latent (dormant) tuberculosis (TB) infection. While he was honeymooning in Italy, scientists at the Centers for Disease Control and Prevention (CDC) identified Speaker's tuberculosis as a potentially rare, often deadly form of TB, known as XDR-TB, that is resistant to almost all known antibiotics. CDC officials contacted Speaker in Italy and instructed him not to fly home on a commercial jet and to proceed to Italian health authorities for further instructions and treatment. Speaker defied the request, flew to Canada, and entered the U.S. via New York by car. Once inside the U.S., health officials issued a federal order for isolation for Speaker, the first federal isolation order issued since the 1960s. Speaker was later flown by CDC aircraft to the national Lung Institute in Denver, Colorado, for treatment, and an international cooperative effort was launched to trace fellow passengers and air crew who came into close contact with Speaker during his international flights. Preliminary tests showed the risk for Speaker transmitting XDR-TB to others was low, but the incident highlighted the need for rapid international communication and cooperation when attempting to prevent the transmission of infectious diseases across international borders.

nations participate in or acknowledge the authority of various international laws governing infectious diseases. Other nations participate in some programs and treaties while opting out of others.

Problems may also arise when national legal systems are in conflict with international law mandates. For example, many international laws are based on the assumption that national governments have broad power over local police, health officials, and healthcare facilities. The United States often adapts international regulations to fit within its system of federalism, which delegates significant powers to state and local governments. While laws governing patient privacy or federal quarantine orders apply to the whole nation, states may enact supplemental public health laws. In contrast, many other nations have centralized public health and healthcare systems that are only governed at the national level.

As infectious disease threats, treatment options, and prevention mechanisms change, so too must international law governing disease response. On July 25, 1951, WHO member states adopted the International Sanitary Regulations, later renamed the International Health Regulations (IHR), to "ensure the maximum protection against the international spread of disease with minimum interference with world traffic." IHR guidelines require that nations notify other countries about disease outbreaks within their borders, maintain accurate records about such outbreaks, establish public health protocols at national points of entry and exit (such as border crossings or airports), and that substantial restrictions on trade for disease-prevention be based on scientific evidence of a public health concern. Nations may require vaccine certificates or health screenings of travelers and immigrants, and adopt hygiene, disinfection, isolation, or quarantine protocols at points of entry as needed. Diseases that the IHR guidelines currently address include cholera, yellow fever, plague, smallpox, polio, severe acute respiratory syndrome (SARS), and new strains of human influenza.

Many aspects of the IHR remain difficult to enforce. Member nations have adopted several provisions of the IHR, while abandoning others. National laws governing reporting of diseases are sometimes not as stringent, or nations have failed to report epidemics. The annual World Health Assembly approved revised IHR in May 2005, addressing these issues and updating the list of targeted diseases to include new threats such as SARS and pandemic influenza. The revised regulations, which were accepted by the United States in December 2006, took effect in June 2007.

SEE ALSO *CDC (Centers for Disease Control and Prevention); Economic Development and Disease; Isolation and Quarantine; World Health Organization (WHO).*

BIBLIOGRAPHY

Books

Fidler, David P. *International Law and Infectious Diseases.* Oxford: Clarendon Press, 1999.

Fluss, Sev S. "International Public Health Law: An Overview," *Oxford Textbook of Public Health*, 3rd ed. Roger Detels, Walter W. Holland, James McEwen, and Gilbert S. Omenn, eds. Oxford: Oxford University Press, 1997.

Hays, J.N. *The Burdens of Disease: Epidemics and Human Response in Western History.* New Brunswick, New Jersey: Rutgers University Press, 1998.

Roemer, Ruth. "Comparative National Public Health Legislation," *Oxford Textbook of Public Health*, 3rd ed. Roger Detels, Walter W. Holland, James McEwen, and Gilbert S. Omenn, eds. Oxford: Oxford University Press, 1997.

Web Sites

United States Department of Health and Human Services. "Medical Privacy—National Standards to Protect the Privacy of Personal Health Information." <http://www.hhs.gov/ocr/hipaa/> (accessed June 8, 2007).

World Health Organization. "International Health Regulations (IHR)." <http://www.who.int/csr/ihr/en/> (accessed June 8, 2007).

Adrienne Wilmoth Lerner

Leishmaniasis

Introduction

Leishmaniasis (LEASH-ma-NIGH-a-sis) is a parasitic disease caused by a protozoan of the genus *Leishmania* and spread by the bite of a sand fly. The disease is endemic in 88 countries worldwide and about 2 million cases occur each year.

Leishmaniasis usually affects people living in tropical and subtropical regions frequently exposed to the sand fly. Signs and symptoms vary depending on the form of infection, but mild cases present with skin sores on the face, arms, and legs that eventually heal with treatment. The more severe cases of visceral leishmaniasis affect organs such as the spleen and liver and may be fatal if untreated.

Treatment with drugs is usually quite effective if administered prior to significant immune damage, but, in the majority of cases, severe scarring is often unavoidable. There is no vaccine or drug available for the prevention of leishmaniasis, however, minimizing contact with the sand fly vector significantly reduces the risk of infection.

Disease History, Characteristics, and Transmission

One of the first clinical descriptions of leishmaniasis appeared in 1756, although the disease has been referenced as far back as the first century AD. The name leishmaniasis was given to the disease in 1901 when a Scottish doctor identified the causative organism as being the protozoa *Leishmania*.

Leishmaniasis has several forms, each with varying symptomatic presentation and clinical severity. Cutaneous leishmaniasis is the most common form. It is characterized by skin sores over the face, arms, and body, which may be painful or painless. Glands near the sores may be swollen. The sores usually develop within a few weeks of infection, and may leave severe scarring.

Visceral leishmaniasis is the most serious form of the disease. It affects organs, such as the liver and spleen,

and presents symptoms such as persistent chronic fever, fatigue, scaly/gray skin, weight loss, anemia, and enlarged spleen or liver. In developing countries, this form of leishmaniasis may have a 100% fatality rate within two years if untreated.

Mucocutaneous leishmaniasis often occurs if the cutaneous (skin) form is untreated. In this form of the disease, the skin sores spread and may cause partial or total destruction of mucous membranes found in the nose, mouth, and throat. These mucosal sores often leave patients with severe facial deformities.

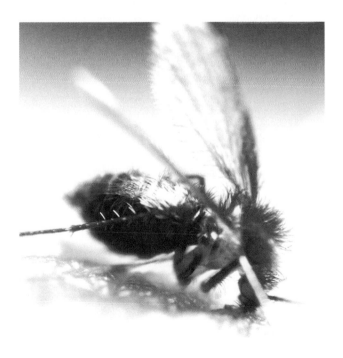

In this macrophotograph, a sand fly (*Lutzomyia longipalpis*) feeds on a human. The sand fly is a vector for leishmaniasis, a disease that causes a breakdown of tissues in humans. *Sinclair Stammers/Photo Researchers, Inc.*

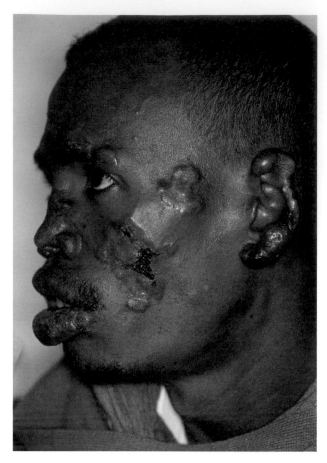

A man displays multiple disfiguring skin lesions caused by infection with *Leishmania*. The disease closely resembles a form of leprosy and is often misdiagnosed.   *Andy Crump, TDR, WHO/Photo Researchers, Inc.*

Leishmaniasis is transmitted by the bite of about 30 species of the phlebotomine sand fly, which are most active between dusk and dawn. Only female sand flies are capable of spreading the disease after infecting themselves by ingesting host blood containing the protozoa. Hosts of the parasite include dogs, foxes, jackals, and rodents. After 4 to 25 days within the sand fly, the protozoon transforms and completes its lifecycle upon being re-injected into a new host. Transmission is possible between humans through blood transfusions or the use of contaminated needles.

■ Scope and Distribution

There are an estimated twelve million cases of leishmaniasis globally. It is found in 88 countries around the world and is most common in tropical and subtropical regions of Africa, South America, and Asia. Within these regions, over 350 million people are at risk of contracting the disease. Each year there are over 1.5 million new cases of cutaneous leishmaniasis and more than 500,000 cases of visceral leishmaniasis.

The geographic distribution of the disease is limited by the suitability of habitat for the sand fly, their ability to remove blood from the host and transfer it to another, and the role the flies play in completing the life cycle of the infecting protozoa. Over 90% of global cases of visceral leishmaniasis are found in India, Bangladesh, Nepal, Sudan, and Brazil. These regions offer tropical and subtropical climates and provide the perfect conditions for phlebotomine sand flies to live, breed, and successfully transmit the disease.

People at greatest risk of contracting leishmaniasis are those living, working, or visiting those areas where sand flies are found, and there is a notably higher incidence of infection in rural areas than in urban areas. There is no indication of transmission between pregnant women and unborn children, although contaminated blood or needles can spread of disease.

Leishmaniasis is rarely occurs in the United States, but some cases of skin sores arising from cutaneous leishmaniasis have been reported in rural areas of southern Texas. As of 2007, no cases of visceral leishmaniasis have been reported in the United States.

■ Treatment and Prevention

Leishmaniasis is caused by parasitic infection and treatment with drugs is usually effective if applied prior to immune system damage. In some parts of the world, the parasite has become resistant to traditional drug treatments and, as a result, new drugs must be constantly developed to maintain effectiveness. In some cases of drug resistant visceral leishmaniasis, it may be necessary to remove the patient's spleen.

The sores caused by cutaneous leishmaniasis may lead to unsightly scarring if not treated, and severe cases of mucocutaneous leishmaniasis may require reconstructive surgery to repair damage to facial tissues. Because the disease is parasitic, there may be reactivation of infection after the initial signs and symptoms disappear. Previous infection does not provide any form of immunity against future infection.

There is no vaccine or drug available to prevent leishmaniasis, but transmission may be avoided by limiting exposure to the sand fly vector that carries the disease. Sand flies are most active from dusk to dawn, and it is best to limit outdoor activities during these times in areas where the disease occurs. Protective clothing, such as long-sleeved shirts and long pants, can reduce the amount of exposed skin and prevent fly bites. If the sleeping area is not well screened or air-conditioned, a bed net that has been soaked in or sprayed with insecticide should be used. Dogs and rodents should be kept away from sleeping areas. When exposure to sand flies is unavoidable, it is beneficial to use a strong insect repellent and spray sleeping areas with insecticides, if possible.

In addition to undertaking individual prevention, governments may implement public health measures. While avoidance of the vector is helpful in preventing individual cases, a reduction in animals harboring infection will have a greater impact on preventing the spread of disease. Public awareness is important to ensure that communities are working towards the same goal and following similar guidelines to reduce sand fly populations and animal reservoirs.

■ Impacts and Issues

The impacts of a widespread condition such as leishmaniasis are evident at the community level and also across countries and continents. One of the significant physical effects of leishmaniasis infection is the severe scarring caused by the sores that develop on the face, legs, and arms. In some communities affected by the disease, social prejudices exist towards people with these unattractive scars and in some situations people with disabling disfigurations become social outcasts. This may cause division within communities and may eventually lead to social breakdown.

On a larger scale, human-caused environmental changes are having an impact on natural habitats and as a result are increasing the risk of human exposure to the sand fly vector. Activities, such as dam building, mining, deforestation, irrigation, and conversion of land to cultivation, permanently alter the conditions under which the vectors exist naturally and create new opportunities for vector contact. Although it was previously a disease associated with poverty stricken, rural areas, leishmaniasis has successfully adapted to the urban environment. The movement of large groups from rural to urban areas, in addition to the worldwide urbanization, is also adding to this effect.

When war breaks out in areas where leishmaniasis is endemic, the disease can have an international impact. The deployment of foreign troops to these regions places those soldiers at increased risk of contracting the disease, despite extensive measures taken to prevent sand fly contact. The deployment of United States troops to Iraq in 2003 and 2004 resulted in 237 cases of leishmaniasis out of a force of about 200,000 soldiers. Soldiers fighting in Iraq have dubbed the disease "Baghdad Boil." When these foreign soldiers return to their home countries, they potentially create a portal of entry for the parasite to move into previously unaffected zones, thus aiding the worldwide spread of leishmaniasis. While these countries generally are able to implement stringent preventative measures among their troops to protect them from infection, there remains a potential risk of spreading the disease to new areas.

Co-infection of HIV and leishmaniasis also is common. HIV infection increases the risk of leishmaniasis infection, while leishmaniasis causes an increase in the

WORDS TO KNOW

CUTANEOUS: Pertaining to the skin.

PROTOZOA: Single-celled animal-like microscopic organisms that live by taking in food rather than making it by photosynthesis and must live in the presence of water. (Singular: protozoan.) Protozoa are a diverse group of single-celled organisms, with more than 50,000 different types represented. The vast majority are microscopic, many measuring less than measuring less than 5 one thousandth of an inch (0.005 millimeters), but some, such as the freshwater Spirostomun, may reach 0.17 inches (3 millimeters) in length, large enough to enable it to be seen with the naked eye.

VECTOR: Any agent, living or otherwise, that carries and transmits parasites and diseases. Also, an organism or chemical used to transport a gene into a new host cell.

VISCERAL: Visceral means pertaining to the viscera. The viscera are the large organs contained in the main cavities of the body, especially the thorax and abdomen; for example, the lungs, stomach, intestines, kidneys, or liver.

progression of HIV to AIDS. In Europe, the primary way in which leishmaniasis is transmitted is through sharing of intravenous needles. The World Health Organization considers co-infection of HIV and leishmaniasis to be a significant concern, since it could lead to spread of the disease into previously non-endemic areas. In 1998, the World Health Organization and UNAID implemented the Programme for the Surveillance and Control of Leishmaniasis to monitor leishmaniasis/HIV co-infection, improve response capability, and ensure that epidemics are detected and contained.

SEE ALSO *AIDS (Acquired Immunodeficiency Syndrome); Blood Supply and Infectious Disease; Emerging Infectious Diseases; HIV; Host and Vector; Parasitic Diseases; War and Infectious Disease; World Health Organization (WHO).*

BIBLIOGRAPHY

Books

Mandell, G.L., J.E. Bennett, and R. Dolin. *Principles and Practice of Infectious Diseases.* Vol. 2. Philadelphia: Elsevier, 2005.

IN CONTEXT: PERSONAL RESPONSIBILITY AND PROTECTION

The Centers for Disease Control and Prevention (CDC), Division of Parasitic Diseases recommends that the "best way for travelers to prevent leishmaniasis is by protecting themselves from sand fly bites." and that to decrease their risk of being bitten, travelers should:

- Stay in well-screened or air-conditioned areas as much as possible. Avoid outdoor activities, especially from dusk to dawn, when sand flies are the most active.
- When outside, wear long-sleeved shirts, long pants, and socks. Tuck your shirt into your pants.
- Apply insect repellent on uncovered skin and under the ends of sleeves and pant legs. Follow the instructions on the label of the repellent. The most effective repellents are those that contain the chemical DEET (N,N-diethylmetatoluamide). The concentration of DEET varies among repellents. Repellents with DEET concentrations of 30-35% are quite effective, and the effect should last about 4 hours. Lower concentrations should be used for children (no more than 10% DEET). Repellents with DEET should be used sparingly on children from 2 to 6 years old and not at all on children less than 2 years old.
- Spray clothing with permethrin-containing insecticides. The insecticide should be reapplied after every five washings.
- Spray living and sleeping areas with an insecticide to kill insects.
- If you are not sleeping in an area that is well screened or air-conditioned, use a bed net and tuck it under your mattress. If possible, use a bed net that has been soaked in or sprayed with permethrin. The permethrin will be effective for several months if the bed net is not washed. Keep in mind that sand flies are much smaller than mosquitoes and therefore can get through smaller holes. Fine-mesh netting (at least 18 holes to the inch; some sources say even finer) is needed for an effective barrier against sand flies. This is particularly important if the bed net has not been treated with permethrin. However, it may be uncomfortable to sleep under such a closely woven bed net when it is hot.
- NOTE: Bed nets, repellents containing DEET, and permethrin should be purchased before traveling and can be found in hardware, camping, and military surplus stores.

SOURCE: *Centers for Disease Control and Prevention (CDC)*

Web Sites

American Academy of Dermatology. "Researchers Urge Soldiers and Civilians Returning from Iraq to Be Aware of 'Baghdad Boil.'" June 30, 2005. <http://www.aad.org/aad/Newsroom/Researchers+Urge+Soldiers+and+civilians+returning.htm> (accessed February 26, 2007).

Centers for Disease Control. "Leishmania Infection." April 1, 2004. <http://www.cdc.gov/ncidod/dpd/parasites/leishmania/default.htm> (accessed February 26, 2007).

Deployment Health Clinical Center. "Leishmaniasis." June 21, 2004. <http://www.pdhealth.mil/leish.asp> (accessed February 26, 2007).

World Health Organization. "Leishmaniasis: Background Information." 2007. <http://www.who.int/leishmaniasis/en/> (accessed February 26, 2007).

World Health Organization. "Surveillance and Control of Leishmaniasis." 2007. <http://www.who.int/leishmaniasis/surveillance/en/> (accessed February 26, 2007).

Leprosy (Hansen's Disease)

■ Introduction

Leprosy, also known as Hansen's disease, is a chronic (long-term) disease caused by infection with the bacillus *Mycobacterium leprae* (*M. leprae*). The disease was greatly feared for many centuries because of the extreme disfigurement it can cause; it is widely known today from references to *Tzaraath* in the Hebrew Bible, translated as "leprosy," although the translation probably included a wide range of skin diseases. Leprosy is treatable by combination drug therapy, and eradication campaigns are under way in Africa, India, Brazil, and other places where the disease remains common.

Leprosy does not, as commonly assumed, cause fingers, toes, and noses to drop off: this is a side effect of the disease's attack on the peripheral nerves. Loss of sensation makes patients unable to respond to minor injuries and infections in their fingers, toes, and elsewhere, and it is

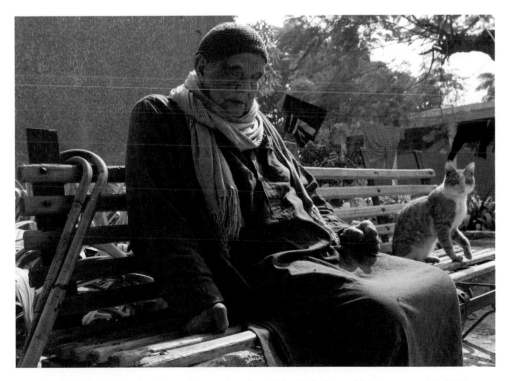

A resident in a leprosarium in Egypt sits on a bench outside the facility, which was created in 1932. Although he was cured from Hansen's disease, also known as leprosy, the resident has remained at the center since 1944. Like hundreds of other cured patients, he opted to stay there due to the social stigma surrounding the disease. The facility houses the largest leper colony in the Middle East. *Khaled Desouki/ AFP/Getty Images.*

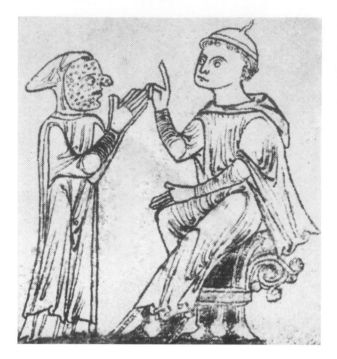

A man with leprosy (c. 1200) is pictured on the left in this illustration from a manuscript by early medical writer Roger of Salerno. The man's face is covered with sores. *Hulton Archive/Getty Images.*

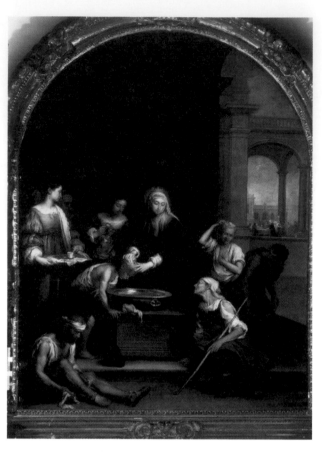

Saint Elizabeth of Hungary (1207–1231), also known as Elizabeth of Thuringia, is shown caring for the sick and those suffering from leprosy. *Giraudon/Art Resource, NY.*

these secondary causes that lead to the characteristic loss of body parts. However, leprosy can also cause puffy, deforming lesions on the face and elsewhere, as well as a number of other symptoms.

■ Disease History, Characteristics, and Transmission

History

Leprosy has been recognized for thousands of years in Asia, Egypt, and India. According to genetic data collected in recent years, *M. leprae* first probably infected human populations in East Africa over 100,000 years ago. From there, the disease spread to other parts of the world by hitchhiking on repeated waves of human migration. Leprosy is thought to have been brought to Europe by Greek soldiers returning from the conquest of India by Alexander the Great (356–323 BC); it is first mentioned explicitly in Roman records dating to 62 BC, coinciding with the return of troops from western Asia.

Particularly in the Middle Ages, when Arab invasions and the Crusades brought renewed rates of leprosy to Europe from Africa and the Middle East, the disease was intensely feared throughout Europe. People afflicted by leprosy were termed "lepers," a term now disfavored as it implies social stigma. By the 1100s approximately 19,000 asylums or leper-houses had been established by

monks and nuns to isolate and care for the victims of the disease. Persons with leprosy not confined to the leper-houses were required to give warning of their approach by sounding a wooden clapper, and were forbidden to enter churches, inns, mills, or bakeries, to touch or dine with persons without leprosy, or to walk on narrow pathways (where people coming the other way might have to touch them). Thanks to these stringent isolation measures—or possibly because of reduced frequency of the genes causing vulnerability to leprosy, leprosy slowly decreased in Europe and had become rare there by the 1600s.

Leprosy was probably spread to West Africa by European traders or colonialists, since the variety found there closely resembles that found in Europe. From West Africa it was brought to Caribbean and South America by the slave trade in the eighteenth century. The European variety is that found in North America and was introduced by colonialism and emigration. In the 1700s and 1800s, for example, immigrants from Scandinavia, where a leprosy epidemic was occurring at the time, brought the disease with them to the Midwestern United States.

In 1873, Norwegian physician The Gerhard Henrik Armauer Hansen (1841–1912) showed that leprosy is caused by a bacillus, later named *M. leprae*. Hansen did not actually identify the objects he saw in his microscope as bacteria, but noted that he found them in the tissues of all persons suffering from the disease. Initially, his discovery was given little attention. In 1879, he shared tissue samples with German physician Albert Neisser (1855–1916), who identified the bacteria and attempted to claim credit for their discovery.

Despite the identification of *M. leprae* as the cause of leprosy, progress on creating a treatment for the disease was slow. Until about 1940, treatment was by injection of oil derived from the chaulmoogra nut, a traditional remedy. Numerous injections forced the oil under the skin, a painful procedure, and today physicians do not assume that this treatment resulted in significant permanent benefit. In 1921, the U.S. Public Health Service built a research and live-in treatment center for leprosy in Carville, Louisiana. Carville researchers announced the discovery of an effective anti-leprosy drug, Promin, in 1941. Promin—a sulfone drug—still required numerous painful injections.

In the 1950s, another drug, dapsone, became available in pill form. Dapsone was highly effective but *M. leprae* began to evolve resistance to the drug over the next decade. Given alone, it would not have remained effective for more than a few decades. In the 1970s, the first multi-drug therapy (MDT) for leprosy was developed, blending dapsone with other drugs to prevent the development of resistance. In 1981, the World Health Organization (WHO) endorsed an MDT regimen consisting of dapsone, rifampin, and clofazimine. This mixture continues to be used today. Like the drug cocktails used to fight human immunodeficiency virus, MDT for leprosy exploits the fact that it is more difficult for a microorganism to evolve resistance to a several agents at once than to evolve resistance to each agent separately or in series.

For years, an obstacle to a fuller scientific understanding of *M. leprae* was the fact that it apparently impossible to grow the bacillus in pure culture (growing cells in a prepared medium) in the laboratory. Also, its population doubling time in tissue is the longest of any known bacterium, from 13 to 20 days (compared to about 20 minutes for *Escherichia coli*, the dominant bacterium in the human digestive tract). Until the early 1970s, *M. leprae* was not known to thrive in any laboratory animal; it grew only in humans and, in relatively small numbers, in the footpads of mice. In 1971, however, researchers discovered that the nine-banded armadillo (a mammal native to South America and now also found across the southern United States) can be infected with *M. leprae*. Having acquired the disease from human sources, many armadillos in the wild now have leprosy. About five percent of armadillos in Louisiana show

WORDS TO KNOW

ALLELE: Any of two or more alternative forms of a gene that occupy the same location on a chromosome.

CULTURE: A culture is a single species of microorganism that is isolated and grown under controlled conditions. The German bacteriologist Robert Koch first developed culturing techniques in the late 1870s. Following Koch's initial discovery, medical scientists quickly sought to identify other pathogens. Today bacteria cultures are used as basic tools in microbiology and medicine.

DROPLET TRANSMISSION: Droplet transmission is the spread of microorganisms from one space to another (including from person to person) via droplets that are larger than 5 microns in diameter. Droplets are typically expelled into the air by coughing and sneezing.

ENDEMIC: Present in a particular area or among a particular group of people.

ERADICATION: The process of destroying or eliminating a microorganism or disease.

LATENT: A condition that is potential or dormant, not yet manifest or active, is latent.

MULTI-DRUG THERAPY: Multi-drug therapy is the use of a combination of drugs against infection, each of which attacks the infective agent in a different way. This strategy can help overcome resistance to anti-infective drugs.

RESISTANCE: Immunity developed within a species (especially bacteria) via evolution to an antibiotic or other drug. For example, in bacteria, the acquisition of genetic mutations that render the bacteria invulnerable to the action of antibiotics.

symptoms of the disease and about 20% probably are infected with *M. leprae*.

Characteristics

Mycobacterium leprae is a rod-shaped bacterium about 1—8 µm long and .2–.5 µm wide. Bacteria of the genus Mycobacterium are characterized by an unusually thick, multi-layered cell wall, which helps make them resistant to antibiotics (drugs that kill bacteria). Both the bacterium that causes tuberculosis (*Mycobacterium tuberculosis*) and *Mycobacterium leprae* are in this genus.

M. leprae infects the mucus membranes, nerves, and skin. It tends not to invade deeper tissues because it thrives at temperatures slightly lower than that of the body core; the armadillo's low body temperature is thought to be one reason *M. leprae* can infect that species as well as humans. *M. leprae* has a particular affinity for nerve cells, which is why loss of feeling can be a symptom of leprosy.

Leprosy causes a spectrum of disease, from mild to severe. Progression of the disease is slow, with incubation times of a few years to 30 years. About 90% of persons with leprosy experience loss of temperature sensation of some part of the body (e.g., fingers) as their first symptom: that is, the patient cannot sense hot and cold with parts of their body. This often happens before any lesions or spots appear. Ability to sense pain is lost next, and then the ability to sense deep pressure. The inability to sense pain allows otherwise trivial injuries or irritations to go unchecked, often leading to infections, injuries, and loss of tissue. The progress of leprosy is divided into four stages:

1. Intermediate leprosy. In this early, mildest form, some spots (lesions) may appear on the skin. Patients with low susceptibility may defeat the infection without assistance at this stage.

2. Tuberculoid leprosy. Large pale spots called macules may appear on the skin. These lesions lack sensation. Nerves are infected, and may thicken and cease to function.

3. Borderline leprosy. In this stage, skin lesions are present and numerous. They may now take the form protruding nodules or sunken lesions that are sometimes described as appearing punched-out.

4. Lepromatous leprosy. This is the most developed and severe form of the disease. Lesions are numerous and more severe (that is, more protruding or deeper-set) than in the earlier stages. The eyes may become involved, leading to pain, light-sensitivity, glaucoma, and blindness. The testicles may atrophy.

Deepening nerve damage may lead to partial paralysis. Any of the three earlier stages of leprosy may regress to less severe stages, but not this stage.

For purposes of treatment, leprosy is separated into two types, paucibacillary and multibacillary. In paucibacillary leprosy, there are no more than five skin lesions on the patient and the number of *M. leprae* bacteria in the body is small, approximately less than a million. A skin smear shows no *M. leprae*. (A skin smear is a obtained by making a small cut in the most prominent lesion and scraping tissue from it. The sample is then placed on a microscope slide, stained with a substance that highlights the presence of *M. leprae*, and examined to see if any of the bacteria are present.) Most leprosy infections are of this type. In multibacillary leprosy, a skin smear is positive and there are more than five lesions. All more severe and advanced cases of leprosy are in the multibacillary category.

Transmission

The mode of transmission of leprosy remains uncertain. Most experts state that the disease is probably transmitted by mucus and saliva droplets produced by sneezing and coughing. People who have close contact with people with active, untreated infection are at risk for contracting the disease and so, more generally, is anyone living in a country where the disease is endemic. Experts speculate that insect bites, some animals, and bacilli in soil may also spread the disease, but none of these routes has been proved.

Only about 10% of the human population is vulnerable to infection by *M. leprae*; and of those persons, only about half will develop detectable disease. Susceptibility to infection by *M. leprae* has been shown to be associated with a person's genetic makeup, namely the possession of certain alleles (alternative forms of a gene) for a specific area of human DNA also shared by the Parkinson's disease gene *PARK2* and its co-regulated gene *PACRG*. The mechanism by which these alleles make persons more susceptible to leprosy is not yet known.

■ Scope and Distribution

Between one and two million people worldwide have been disabled by leprosy. In many countries, leprosy has been virtually eliminated. It still exists in over 100 countries, however, combining the cases in Angola, Brazil, India, Madagascar, Mozambique, Nepal, and Tanzania together account for over 95% of all cases. India accounts for 70% of cases and Brazil has the world's highest per-capita leprosy rate. In the United States, only a few dozen cases occur each year.

Treatment and Prevention

Prevention of leprosy was traditionally through isolation of victims from the uninfected. Conventional antibiotics such as penicillin have never been effective against *M. leprae*. However, the MDT combination of dapsone, rifampin, and clofazimine first developed in the late 1970s has proved highly effective. The primary drug in this combination is dapsone, which inhibits bacterial growth by preventing the formation of folic acid. Rifampin acts by inhibiting the bacterial enzyme RNA polymerase, which is needed for cell functioning. It is always used in combination with another drug. The third drug, clofazimine, inhibits bacterial growth by binding to DNA and so interfering with transcription and replication.

For paucibacillary leprosy, a two-drug MDT consisting of dapsone and rifampin is given for six months; for multibacillary leprosy, the full three-drug MDT is given for two years. MDT is given out in calendar-marked blister packs to patients, who must take the pills at home on a regular schedule.

Impacts and Issues

International efforts to eliminate leprosy have been under way since 1991, when the 49th World Health Assembly (the body which governs the World Health Organization) resolved to eliminate leprosy as a public health problem by 2000, defined as reducing the worldwide prevalence rate to less than 1 in 10,000 persons. In 1999, WHO formed the Global Alliance for the Elimination of Leprosy, based in India, with a strategy of early detection, MDT treatment, and eliminating the stigma historically attached to persons with leprosy. The global elimination goal was met, but rates remain significantly higher in the countries listed above. At an annual new-case rate of less than 1 per 10,000, India alone could register as many as 100,000 new cases a year. The U.S.-based company that makes the three anti-leprosy drugs, Novartis, is in partnership with the Global Alliance for the Elimination of Leprosy and supplies them at no cost.

The genome of *M. leprae* was sequenced in 2000, aiding researchers who are attempting to develop new anti-leprosy drugs and vaccines.

The impact of leprosy on the infected symptomatic individual has historically been severe. Furthermore, isolation and shunning of persons with Hansen's disease (use of the alternate name Hansen's disease today is intended to reduce social stigma associated with the term leprosy, although both terms are correct) did not end with the Middle Ages. Loss of one's job, social standing, family position, and the like continue to be common consequences in many societies for persons with leprosy.

In 2006, a worrisome problem was discovered; the drugs being given for the AIDS virus, which already infects about 38 million people in the undeveloped

---

IN CONTEXT: SCIENTIFIC, POLITICAL, AND ETHICAL ISSUES

The stubbornness of the leprosy stigma was underlined in Japan in 2001, when a court ruled that the Japanese government owed millions of dollars in compensation to leprosy patients who had been confined and abused in leper colonies since the 1950s. The colonies or centers were established under the 1953 Leprosy Prevention law (repealed in 1996) that forced all persons with leprosy, including children, to move to those locations. According to a Japanese government commission that studied the leper colonies, patients were sterilized—surgically rendered unable to have children—forced to have abortions, and treated as research subjects. Infanticide was also practiced. All this continued for decades after outpatient treatment with anti-leprosy drugs became available in 1960. "For 60 years, I was not treated as a human," one former patient, Mamoru Kunimoto, said. The fact that the government apologized rather than disputing the court's ruling, he said, "has given me back my humanity."

---

world, can make silent or asymptomatic leprosy become symptomatic. Patients on AIDS drugs are reporting ulcers or are losing sensation in toes and fingers as their latent (dormant) leprosy becomes active. This is something of a medical paradox; AIDS itself, which weakens the immune system, has not caused latent leprosy to become active, but the treatment for AIDS has.

Finally, as with all drug treatments for infectious disease, the evolution of drug resistance by *M. leprae* is a concern. Resistance to all major anti-leprosy drugs has been reported worldwide, particularly for dapsone. However, reports of relapse after MDT have been rare, and resistance to leprosy drugs is not yet considered a major problem.

Primary Source Connection

In January 2006 in New Delhi, India, Yohei Sasakawa, chairman of The Nippon Foundation, published a Global Appeal to End Stigma and Discrimination against People Affected by Leprosy. The text of that appeal was issued in the names of 12 world leaders and Nobel Peace Prize laureates.

The Nippon Foundation, a non-governmental organization, founded in 1962, supports research and programs for the betterment of people's lives around the world. With a special focus on developing countries, the foundation is active in issues dealing with human resources development, hunger alleviation, public health, and help for the disabled.

GLOBAL APPEAL TO END STIGMA AND DISCRIMINATION AGAINST PEOPLE AFFECTED BY LEPROSY

Leprosy is among the world's oldest and most dreaded diseases. Without an effective remedy for much of its long history, it often resulted in terrible deformity. It was also thought to be extremely communicable. Patients were abandoned, forced to live in isolation and discriminated against as social outcasts.

In the early 1980s, an effective cure for leprosy became available. Multidrug therapy has successfully treated over 14 million people to date. Contrary to popular belief, leprosy is extremely difficult to contract. With prompt diagnosis and treatment, it can be medically cured within 6 to 12 months without risk of deformity.

Yet fear of leprosy remains deep-rooted. Misguided notions endure — that it is "highly contagious," "incurable" and "hereditary." Some even regard it as "a divine punishment."

Ignorance and misunderstanding result in prejudice and discriminatory attitudes that remain firmly implanted as custom and tradition.

Consequently, patients, cured persons and their entire families suffer stigma and discrimination. This limits their opportunities for education, employment and marriage, and restricts their access to public services.

Fearful that by speaking out they will invite further discrimination, for long years people affected by leprosy, including their families, have been cowed into silence. Such silence reinforces the stigma that surrounds them.

The world has remained indifferent to their plight for too long.

Article 1 of the Universal Declaration of Human Rights states that "All human beings are born free and equal in dignity and human rights." This article, however, is meaningless to people affected by leprosy, who continue to suffer discrimination.

We appeal to the UN Commission on Human Rights to take up this matter as an item on its agenda, and request that it issue principles and guidelines for governments to follow in eliminating all discrimination against people affected by leprosy.

We further urge governments themselves to seriously consider this issue and act to improve the present situation with a sense of urgency.

Finally, we call on people all over the world to change their perception and foster an environment in which leprosy patients, cured persons and their families can lead normal lives free from stigma and discrimination.

January 29, 2006

Oscar Arias
Former President of Costa Rica
Nobel Peace Prize Laureate

Jimmy Carter
Former President of the United States of America
Nobel Peace Prize Laureate

The Dalai Lama
Nobel Peace Prize Laureate

El Hassan bin Talal
Prince of the Jordanian Hashemite Royal Dynasty

Václav Havel
Former President of the Czech Republic

Luiz Inácio Lula da Silva
President of the Federative Republic of Brazil

Olusegun Obasanjo
President of the Federal Republic of Nigeria

Mary Robinson
Former President of Ireland
Former UN High Commissioner for Human Rights

Yohei Sasakawa
Chairman, The Nippon Foundation

Desmond Tutu
Archbishop Emeritus of Cape Town
Nobel Peace Prize Laureate

R. Venkataraman
Former President of India

Elie Wiesel
President, The Elie Wiesel Foundation for Humanity
Nobel Peace Prize Laureate

Contact The Nippon Foundation (http://www.nippon-foundation.or.jp or fax 813-6229-5602) for more information

In 2006 various humanitarian leaders signed the "Global Appeal to End Stigma and Discrimination Against People Affected by Leprosy." The signers—including former U.S. President Jimmy Carter, spiritual leader the Dali Lama, and Archbishop Desmond Tutu—asked the UN Commission on Human Rights, as well as governments and people throughout the world, to end stigma and discrimination against people with leprosy. *The Nippon Foundation.*

BIBLIOGRAPHY

Books

Demaitre, Luke. *Leprosy in Premodern Medicine: A Malady of the Whole Body.* Baltimore, MD: Johns Hopkins University Press, 2007.

Gould, Tony. *A Disease Apart: Leprosy in the Modern World.* New York: St. Martin's Press, 2005.

Periodicals

McNeil Jr., Donald G. "Worrisome New Link: AIDS Drugs and Leprosy." *New York Times.* October 24, 2006.

Mira, Marcelo, et al. "Susceptibility to Leprosy is Associated with *PARK2* and *PACRG*." *Nature.* 427(2004):636-40.

Monot, Marc, et al. "On the Origin of Leprosy." *Science.* 308(2005):1040–1042.

Web Sites

British Broadcasting Corporation. "Koizumi Apologises for Leper Colonies." May 25, 2001 <http://news.bbc.co.uk/2/hi/asia-pacific/1350630.stm> (accessed February 6, 2007).

Centers for Disease Control and Prevention. "Hansen's Disease (Leprosy)." October 12, 2005 <http://www.cdc.gov/ncidod/dbmd/diseaseinfo/hansens_t.htm> (accessed February 6, 2007).

International Leprosy Association. "Global Project on the History of Leprosy." October 10, 2003 <http://www.leprosyhistory.org/english/englishhome.htm> (accessed February 6, 2007).

World Health Organization, United Nations. "Leprosy." 2007 <http://www.who.int/topics/leprosy/en/> (accessed February 6, 2007).

Leptospirosis

Introduction

Leptospirosis is a disease that is caused by bacteria from the genus *Leptospira*. It is considered an emerging disease and is found worldwide. Leptospirosis often goes undiagnosed, since the symptoms of this disease are similar to those of a number of other diseases, including influenza. For this reason, the prevalence of the disease is unknown.

Infection occurs when humans come in contact with freshwater, soil, or vegetation that is contaminated with the urine of an infected animal. The bacteria pass from the urine into the human body via mucosal linings, such as the linings of the eyes, nose, or mouth; through broken skin; or orally, when food or water is ingested. Illness develops, usually within 10 days, and is characterized by fever, aches, vomiting, diarrhea, and jaundice. Treatment with antibiotics leads to successful recovery, although, in some cases, a second phase can occur with more severe symptoms. During this second phase, known as Weil's disease, patients suffer more severe symptoms that may include kidney failure, liver failure, or meningitis. Weil's disease occurs in around 10% of cases.

Leptospirosis occurs mainly in the tropics, although it is a worldwide disease found both in rural and urban regions of developed and developing countries. There is no vaccine for this disease, and prevention efforts focus on avoiding contact with anything that may have been contaminated with the bacteria. Risk is highest for people who work or spend time outdoors, in freshwater, or with animals.

Disease History, Characteristics, and Transmission

Leptospirosis was first recognized in 1886 by the German scientist Adolf Weil (1848–1916). The cause of the disease was not identified until about 40 years later, during the 1920s, when both Japanese and German scientists discovered that bacteria were responsible. Leptospirosis is caused by leptospires, which are disease-causing bacteria in the genus *Leptospira*. The primary agent causing leptospirosis is *Leptospira interrogans*.

Scope and Distribution

Leptospirosis most commonly occurs in the tropics, although it is present in temperate regions. Leptospires

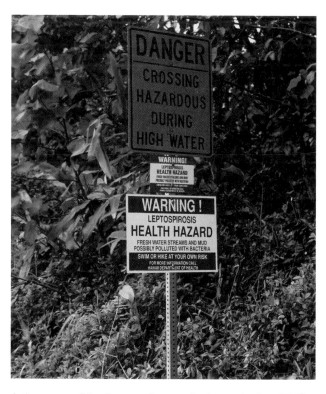

A sign warns of the dangers of contracting leptospirosis or Weil's disease from a contaminated water source. Leptospirosis is caused by *Leptospira* bacteria, which are excreted in the urine of rats and other rodents. The presence of rodent urine in water can lead to infections in humans, dogs, and cattle. *Simon Fraser/Photo Researchers, Inc.*

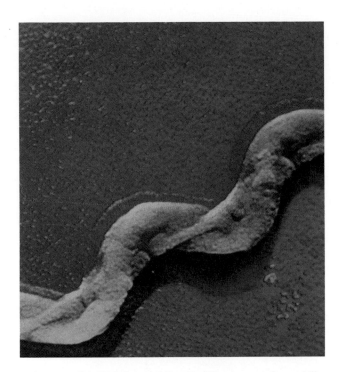

In humans, the spiral-shaped *Leptospira* bacteria cause fever, chills, aches, eye inflammation, and a skin rash. The disease can also cause damage to the liver, kidneys, and nervous system. *Omikron/Photo Researchers, Inc.*

WORDS TO KNOW

JAUNDICE: Jaundice is a condition in which a person's skin and the whites of the eyes are discolored a shade of yellow due to an increased level of bile pigments in the blood resulting from liver disease. Jaundice is sometimes called icterus, from a Greek word for the condition.

LEPTOSPIRE: Also called a leptospira, a leptospire is any bacterial species of the genus *Leptospira*. Infection with leptospires causes leptospirosis.

WEIL'S DISEASE: Weil's disease, named after German doctor Adolf Weil (1848–1916), is a severe form of leptospirosis or seven-day fever, a disease caused by infection with the corkscrew-shaped bacillus *Leptospira interrogans*.

thrive best in warm temperatures and moist conditions. They are transmitted by wild and domestic animals including rodents, dogs, cattle, horses, and pigs. Therefore, people who spend a great deal of time outdoors, or with animals, are more likely to contract leptospirosis. This includes veterinarians, military personnel, farmers, and sewer workers. In addition, people taking part in outdoor recreational activities, such as camping or water sports, are also at higher risk, since they are more likely to come in contact with urine-contaminated water.

Leptospirosis occurs worldwide but tends to be underreported in most countries, since it is often overlooked during diagnosis. This is due to the similarities between symptoms of leptospirosis and those of other tropical diseases. As a result, the global prevalence of this disease is unknown. However, increases in the occurrence of this disease were observed in Germany between 1962 and 2003. These increases are thought to be a result of more frequent travel, increases in freshwater recreational activities, and higher rat populations in cities.

■ Treatment and Prevention

Patients with leptospirosis can recover without treatment, although recovery may take several months, and lack of treatment may lead to complications. Treatment is usually administered as soon as possible and involves a course of antibiotics. A range of antibiotics can be used, including doxycycline, penicillin, ampicillin, and amoxicillin. Recovery can take from three days to several weeks. However, in most cases recovery is complete. More severe complications arise when the patient does not receive antibiotics or if the patient develops the second phase of the illness.

There is no vaccine for leptospirosis, so prevention is best achieved by avoiding contaminated water, soil, or vegetation, particularly in areas with infected or potentially infected animals. Clothing, such as boots or waders, will provide protection during recreational activities, and gloves will provide protection when handling animals. Taking antibiotics while traveling through infected areas may also help prevent severe infections from developing, if people become contaminated.

■ Impacts and Issues

Leptospirosis is becoming more common and has been recognized as an emerging infectious disease by the United States Directors of Health Promotion and Education. Since this disease occurs in both developed and developing countries and in both urban and rural areas, it has become globally important.

Despite the high likelihood of recovery following treatment, there is still a significant mortality rate for leptospirosis. This is largely due to delayed diagnosis, since the disease is hard to recognize. In addition, due to the lack of a vaccine, avoidance of the bacteria remains the best prevention method. This avoidance depends on

IN CONTEXT: PERSONAL RESPONSIBILITY AND PROTECTION

As of April 2007, the CDC states that "No vaccine is available to prevent leptospirosis in the United States. Travelers who might be at an increased risk for the disease should be advised to consider preventive measures such as wearing protective clothing and minimizing contact with potentially contaminated water. Such travelers also might benefit from chemoprophylaxis (a course of treatment prior to exposure that reduces risk or impact of disease). Until further data become available, CDC recommends that travelers who might be at increased risk for leptospirosis be advised to consider chemoprophylaxis begun 1 to 2 days before exposure and continuing through the period of exposure."

Individuals should always seek advice from their personal physician with regard to specific medications and doses.

SOURCE: *Centers for Disease Control and Prevention. Health Information for International Travel 2005–2006. Atlanta: US Department of Health and Human Services, Public Health Service, 2005.*

the maintenance of rigorous sanitation methods, which is not always possible in developing countries or in countries experiencing war or other social upheavals. Therefore, contamination still occurs frequently.

The chance of exposure to contaminated sources is exacerbated during floods, outdoor activity, or in animal-populated regions. In 1995, widespread flooding in Nicaragua spread the bacteria, and more than 2,000 people contracted leptospirosis. At least 13 of those with the disease died. Two years later, nine Americans became infected while white-water rafting in Costa Rica. In addition, growing rat populations, especially in inner cities, increase public exposure to leptospirosis when water systems and sewers become contaminated. This has been suggested as one cause of the higher levels of leptospirosis seen in Germany during 1962–2003.

SEE ALSO *Bacterial Disease; Emerging Infectious Diseases; Meningitis, Bacterial; Personal Protective Equipment; Travel and Infectious Disease; War and Infectious Disease; Water-borne Disease.*

BIBLIOGRAPHY

Books

Mandell, G. L., J. E. Bennett, and R. Dolin. *Principles and Practice of Infectious Diseases.* 6th ed. Philadelphia: Elsevier, 2004.

World Health Organization. *Human Leptospirosis: Guidance for Diagnosis, Surveillance and Control.* Malta: World Health Organization, 2003.

Periodicals

Jansen, A., et al. "Leptospirosis in Germany, 1962–2003." *Emerging Infectious Diseases* 11 (2005): 1048–1054.

Web Sites

Directors of Health Promotion and Education. "Leptospirosis." <http://www.dhpe.org/infect/Lepto.html> (accessed March 1, 2007).

Centers for Disease Control and Prevention. "Leptospirosis." October 12, 2005. <http://www.cdc.gov/ncidod/dbmd/diseaseinfo/leptospirosis_g.htm> (accessed March 1, 2007).

Lice Infestation (Pediculosis)

■ Introduction

Of the many parasites that can infest humans, one of the most common is the louse, a wingless insect. There are several types of lice that infect humans, usually classified as one of three species. These are the head louse (*Pediculus humanus capitis*), which infests only the head; the body louse *Pediculus humanus corporis*), which lives in clothing near the skin; and the crab louse or pubic louse (*Phthirus pubis*), which mostly infests the groin. Infestation with lice is called pediculosis (ped-ih-q-LO-sis). Recently some biologists have argued that the head louse and body louse may be different varieties of a single species. Head and body lice can interbreed in captivity, but do not do so on the human body.

■ Disease History, Characteristics, and Transmission

Human lice can exist only on human beings; they die in about 24 hours if they are removed from the body. Lice also infest humans' nearest evolutionary cousins, the chimpanzees and gorillas, but these lice belong to a different species than those that infest humans. As apes and humans continued to evolve over the last few million years, their lice evolved along with them.

The female head or body louse lays several eggs a day. Lice eggs are called nits (the source of the word "nitpick") and are cemented to the hair or, in the case of body lice, to clothing fibers. The eggs take 7–10 days to hatch. A female louse can start laying eggs 7–10 days after hatching. A louse bites through the skin to suck blood from its host about five times a day.

On a healthy host, lice can cause itching, rash, fever, headaches, and fatigue, but are rarely life-threatening. However, body lice can act as carriers of more serious diseases. Three types of disease can be transmitted by body lice to the humans that they bite, namely relapsing fever (caused by the bacterium *Borrelia recurrentis*),

trench fever (caused by the bacillus *Bartonella quintana*), and—most seriously—typhus (caused by *Rickettsia prowazekii*).

Lice spread by crawling from one host to another or through the transfer of eggs. The majority of head lice are spread by head to head contact or, more rarely, by coming into contact with objects that have picked up eggs from the hair, such as combs, pillows, hats, hair ties, and the like. Body lice are spread through body contact or shared clothing and bedding. Pubic lice are spread primarily through sexual contact or other body contact.

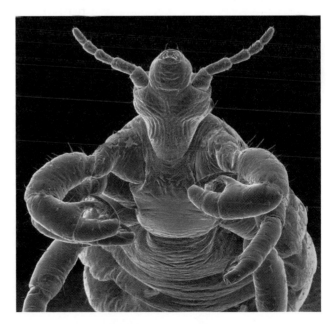

A colored scanning electron micrograph (SEM) shows the blood-sucking human body louse, *Pediculus humanus corporis*. At the upper center is the head of the louse, with its two antennae and biting mouthparts (at top). The three pairs of legs each terminate in a powerful curved claw for gripping. *David Scharf/Photo Researchers, Inc.*

WORDS TO KNOW

PARASITE: An organism that lives in or on a host organism and that gets its nourishment from that host. The parasite usually gains all the benefits of this relationship, while the host may suffer from various diseases and discomforts, or show no signs of the infection. The life cycle of a typical parasite usually includes several developmental stages and morphological changes as the parasite lives and moves through the environment and one or more hosts. Parasites that remain on a host's body surface to feed are called ectoparasites, while those that live inside a host's body are called endoparasites. Parasitism is a highly successful biological adaptation. There are more known parasitic species than nonparasitic ones, and parasites affect just about every form of life, including most all animals, plants, and even bacteria.

IN CONTEXT: REAL-WORLD RISKS

The Division of Parasitic Diseases (DPD), Centers for Disease Control and Prevention (CDC) recommends that "for children under 2 years old, remove crawling bugs and nits by hand. If this does not work, ask your child's health care provider for treatment recommendations. The safety of head lice medications has not been tested in children 2 years of age and under."

SOURCE: *Centers for Disease Control and Prevention*

■ Scope and Distribution

Throughout history, lice infestation has been common in most populations. Dead lice and eggs have been found on Egyptian mummies and Roman bodies buried under volcanic ash at Pompeii. About 6–12 million people acquire head lice in the United States each year; smaller numbers acquire body or pubic lice.

The head louse is still found worldwide at all levels of society. Head lice are extremely common in developing countries. In Western industrialized countries, outbreaks are often associated with schoolchildren.

With the Industrial Revolution and the spread of bathing technology through much of the modern world—indoor plumbing, soap, shampoo, laundry machines, and detergent—the body louse has become less common. Today human body lice are found mostly in situations where poor hygiene, overcrowding, and wearing the same clothing for extended periods are more common—whether these be entire countries or impoverished groups, such as the homeless, in richer countries.

■ Treatment and Prevention

Prevention of lice infestation is accomplished by treating those who are infested and by environmental control (cleaning objects that may have picked up eggs). The two methods of treating lice infestation are pesticides (chemicals that kill insects or other pests) and physical removal of the lice via lice combs. The pesticides most often used are permethrin and pyrethrins, followed by malathion or lindane. However, as is common with pesticides, heavily exposed populations of lice have evolved resistance to these chemicals. The U.S. National Pediculosis Association advises against the use of pesticides on any person with pre-existing illnesses such as severe asthma, epilepsy, cancer, or AIDS. Fine-toothed steel combs can also be used to remove head lice and nits from hair.

■ Impacts and Issues

According to studies reported in the *Annals of the New York Academy of Sciences* in 2006, lice and louse-borne disease were being increasingly reported among homeless and poor inner-city populations in industrialized countries such as the United States, France, Holland, and Russia.

Wars and social breakdown can lead to large outbreaks of lice, as can any condition where people exist in crowded areas without acess to sanitation and clean clothing. A large outbreak of typhus occurred in several refugee camps in Burundi in 1997 where most of the inhabitants were louse-infested.

The safety of the pesticides used in standard anti-lice products is questioned by the American Pediculosis Association, which has campaigned for the use of fine-toothed combs as the treatment of choice in removing lice. Some individuals can have allergic reactions to the pesticides used to treat pediculosis.

SEE ALSO *Parasitic Diseases; Typhoid Fever; Typhus.*

BIBLIOGRAPHY

Periodicals

Elston, Dirk M. "Drugs Used in the Treatment of Pediculosis." *Journal of Drugs in Dermatology* 4.2 (March-April 2005): 207–211.

Raoult, Didier, and Véronique Roux. "The Body Louse as a Vector of Reemerging Human Diseases." *Clinical Infectious Diseases* 29 (1999): 888–911.

Wade, Nicholas. "What a Story Lice Can Tell." *New York Times* (October 5, 2004).

Witkowski, Joseph A., and Lawrence Charles Parish. "Pediculosis and Resistance: The Perennial Problem." *Clinics in Dermatology* 20 (2002): 87–92.

Web Sites

The National Pediculosis Association. "Welcome to Headlice.org." 2007. <http://www.headlice.org/> (accessed January 22, 2007).

IN CONTEXT: EFFECTIVE RULES AND REGULATIONS.

Schools and daycare facilities often exclude children for 24 hours after treatment for head lice, or they maintain a "no-nit policy" that excludes treated children until nits are not visible upon inspection of the scalp. Evidence shows these policies often result in the needless loss of instructional time. Usually by the time a case of head lice is discovered, the possibility of transmission to others has already existed for at least a month, and pesticide treatment quickly kills both adult lice and nits. Also, killed nits may temporarily remain in the hair after treatment.

Listeriosis

■ Introduction

Listeriosis is an infection that is caused by eating food that is contaminated by the bacterium *Listeria monocytogenes*. The infection, which can be serious, primarily affects pregnant women, infants, and immunocompromised people (those whose immune systems are not functioning as efficiently as is normal).

■ Disease History, Characteristics, and Transmission

The bacterium *Listera monocytogenes* is a normal inhabitant of soil and water. Vegetables can become contaminated with the bacterium, if soil or manure clings to them. Humans can then become infected if the contaminated vegetables are not properly washed before eating.

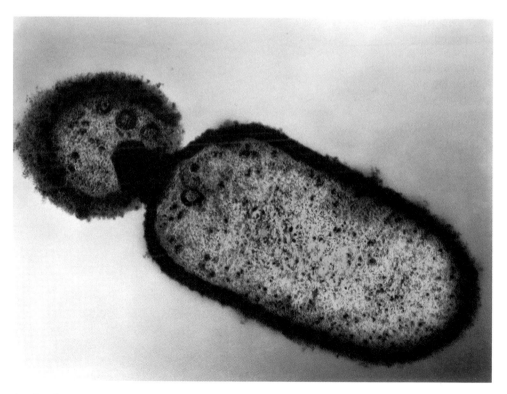

A colored transmission electron micrograph (TEM) shows *Listeria monocytogenes* bacterium (center to bottom right). It is dividing by a process of unequal cell growth known as budding. Its progeny, or daughter cell, is seen at the upper left. It causes listeriosis, a form of food poisoning that results in abdominal pains, fever, and diarrhea.   *Dr Kari Lounatmaa/Photo Researchers, Inc.*

Foods other than vegetables also can become contaminated, since animals, such as cattle, can harbor the bacterium without any ill effects. Meat and dairy products may become contaminated unknowingly. Infection can result, if the meat is eaten raw or is cooked improperly and if unpasteurized milk is consumed. Other foods that can be contaminated by *L. monocytogenes* include cheeses (particularly those made with unpasteurized milk) and processed meats that are unrefrigerated for a time sufficient for contaminating bacteria to multiply. In contrast to some bacterial infections, where a large number of living bacteria need to be consumed to cause illness, relatively few *L. monocytogenes* need to be eaten to cause listeriosis.

Symptoms of listeriosis include flulike fever, nausea, and vomiting, as well as abdominal cramping, diarrhea, and headache. The symptoms may appear within a few days after eating the contaminated foods, but also can appear 2–3 months later. In people whose immune systems are compromised, the infection can progress to a lethal blood infection (sepsis) or brain infection. Infections during pregnancy can lead to infection of the newborn, as well as to miscarriage, stillbirth, or premature birth.

■ Scope and Distribution

Listeriosis has become a significant health threat. In the United States, for example, approximately 2,500 people are sickened with listeriosis each year. Of these, about 500 die, representing a mortality (death) rate of 20%.

Pregnant women are about 20 times more likely to acquire listeriosis than are other adults. In addition, immunocompromised individuals, who cannot as easily fight off infections, are susceptible to listeriosis. The proper functioning of the immune system may be impaired by certain diseases, including diabetes, cancer, kidney disease, and acquired immunodeficiency syndrome (AIDS, also cited as acquired immune deficiency syndrome), as well as by advanced age, and certain drugs, such as those taken by transplant patients to reduce the likelihood of transplant rejection. Listeriosis also can occur in individuals whose immune systems are functioning normally, but the infection is usually not nearly as serious.

■ Treatment and Prevention

L. monocytogenes is easily killed by pasteurization—a process during which a product is held at a certain temperature for a certain length of time to kill most bacteria without altering the chemistry or taste of the product. However, some foods can become contaminated after they have been processed, but before they are packaged for sale. Delicatessen-style meat and hot

WORDS TO KNOW

IMMUNOCOMPROMISED: A reduction of the ability of the immune system to recognize and respond to the presence of foreign material.

PASTEURIZE: To subject a substance to pasteurization, a process where fluids such as wine and milk are heated for a predetermined time at a temperature that is below the boiling point of the liquid. The treatment kills any microorganisms that are in the fluid but does not alter the taste, appearance, or nutritive value of the fluid.

SEPSIS: Sepsis refers to a bacterial infection in the bloodstream or body tissues. This is a very broad term covering the presence of many types of microscopic disease-causing organisms. Sepsis is also called bacteremia. Closely related terms include septicemia and septic syndrome. According to the Society of Critical Care Medicine, severe sepsis affects about 750,000 people in the United States each year. However, it is predicted to rapidly rise to one million people by 2010 due to the aging U.S. population. Over the decade of the 1990s, the incident rate of sepsis increased over 91%.

dogs are two common examples. The bacteria can remain alive and capable of causing infection during transport of the product to the supermarket, sale, and consumption.

A number of common-sense precautions can prevent listeriosis. Thoroughly cooking beef, pork, and poultry is sufficient to kill any *L. monocytogenes* that may contaminate the product. Washing vegetables removes bacteria. When storing food, uncooked meat should not be allowed to come into contact with vegetables, food that is already cooked, or prepared foods. All items used in the preparation of uncooked foods should be thoroughly washed before re-use to avoid transferring *L. monocytogenes* to other foodstuffs. While cheeses made from unpasteurized milk (such as Brie, Camembert, and feta) are preferred by some people, and the consumption of unpasteurized milk is sometimes advocated as a healthy alternative, there is a risk to these practices, since they increase the likelihood of exposure to the bacteria. Finally, prepared foods should be eaten promptly, since *L. monocytogenes*, in contrast to most other disease-causing bacteria, can slowly grow at temperatures above 39°F (4°C). A malfunctioning refrigerator can also create conditions in which the bacteria can grow.

IN CONTEXT: EFFECTIVE RULES AND REGULATIONS

Government agencies such as the U.S. Food and Drug Admin-istration and the U. S. Department of Agriculture monitor food regularly in an attempt to reduce contamination of food by the Listeria bacterium and other infectious agents. Food monitoring and plant inspection are key monitoring and prevention tools, recalls can also be issued for contaminated or suspect food.

■ Impacts and Issues

Listeriosis can be a serious infection and, in the case of pregnant women, it can lead to miscarriage, stillbirth, premature delivery, or infection in the newborn. Although pregnant women in the United States are not routinely tested for infection with the bacteria that causes listeriosis, many health care providers recommend that pregnant women avoid consuming unpasteurized milk products and ready-to-eat deli-type meat products unless they are reheated until steaming hot.

From 1996–2002, the rate of listeriosis cases in the United States fell by 35%. This is attributed to aggressive sampling and testing programs by government meat inspectors, and education designed to raise awareness about the dangers of *L. monocytogenes*, especially among at-risk groups, such as pregnant women. In 2003, the U.S. Food Safety and Inspection Service established new regulations for scrutiny at plants that make or process ready-to-eat meat and poultry products. The rule also encourages plants to install new technologies to elimi-nate or reduce the growth of *L. monocytogenes*.

Researchers are working on "smart packaging" that may help reduce the sale and consumption of contami-nated foods, such as deli meats. One type of this pack-aging incorporates molecules that recognize surface components of *L. monocytogenes*. These molecules are combined with other molecules that change color in the presence of the bacterium, and this color change can alert consumers that the product is contaminated.

SEE ALSO *Bacterial Disease; Food-borne Disease and Food Safety.*

BIBLIOGRAPHY

Books

DiClaudio, Dennis. *The Hypochondriac's Pocket Guide to Horrible Diseases You Probably Already Have.* New York: Bloomsbury, 2005.

Rosaler, Maxine. *Listeriosis (Epidemics).* New York: Rosen Publishing Group, 2003.

Ryser, Elliot T., and Elmer H. Marth. *Listeria, Listeriosis, and Food Safety.* 3rd ed. Boca Raton: CRC, 2007.

Brian Hoyle

Liver Fluke Infections

■ Introduction

Liver fluke infections are the result of infestation by parasitic worms known as liver flukes. There are two main types of liver fluke infections, Fascioliasis and Pisthorchiasis. Although each infection is caused by different species of flukes, they share similarities in characteristics and transmission. Humans become infected when they ingest the cysts containing parasitic forms of the flukes. These cysts open in the digestive system and release the parasites. Humans most often ingest the cysts after drinking contaminated water or eating raw or undercooked food that contains the cysts.

Infection can be asymptomatic or can be either acute or chronic. Mild cases of both Fascioliasis and Opisthorchiasis result in tiredness, fever, aches, swollen liver, abdominal pain, and rash. Symptoms of chronic forms include exacerbated versions of the acute symptoms with possible diarrhea, nausea, swelling of the face, blockage of the bile ducts, and sometimes complications such as migration of flukes to other regions in the body. Administration of one of a variety of antihelminthic drugs is usually effective, with recovery likely to occur.

Fascioliasis occurs worldwide, while Opisthorchiasis generally occurs in regions of Asia. Increased cases of liver fluke infection have been reported in China, argued to be a consequence of an increase in the consumption of raw foods.

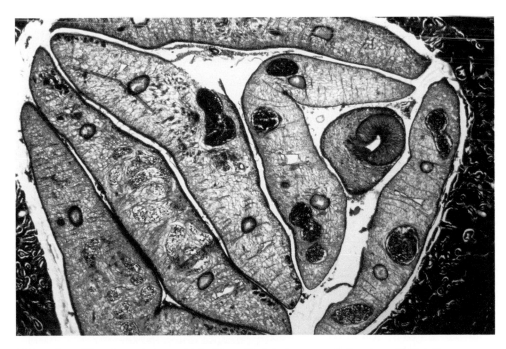

This section of liver tissue shows multiple *Clonorchis sinensis*, commonly known as Chinese liver flukes. *Pr. Bouree/Photo Researchers, Inc.*

WORDS TO KNOW

ANTIHELMINTHIC: Antihelminthic drugs are medicines that rid the body of parasitic worms.

ASYMPTOMATIC: A state in which an individual does not exhibit or experience symptoms of a disease.

CYST: Refers to either a closed cavity or sac or the stage of life of some parasites during which they live inside an enclosed area. A stage in a protozoan's life when it is covered by a tough outer shell and has become dormant.

HELMINTH: A representative of various phyla of worm-like animals.

LARVAE: Immature forms (wormlike in insects; fishlike in amphibians) of an organism capable of surviving on its own. Larvae do not resemble the parent and must go through metamorphosis, or change, to reach the adult stage.

PARASITE: An organism that lives in or on a host organism and that gets its nourishment from that host. The parasite usually gains all the benefits of this relationship, while the host may suffer from various diseases and discomforts, or show no signs of the infection. The life cycle of a typical parasite usually includes several developmental stages and morphological changes as the parasite lives and moves through the environment and one or more hosts. Parasites that remain on a host's body surface to feed are called ectoparasites, while those that live inside a host's body are called endoparasites. Parasitism is a highly successful biological adaptation. There are more known parasitic species than nonparasitic ones, and parasites affect just about every form of life, including most all animals, plants, and even bacteria.

TREMATODES: Commonly known as flukes; a class of worms characterized by flat, oval-shaped bodies.

■ Disease History, Characteristics, and Transmission

Liver fluke infections are caused by liver flukes, which are a type of helminth or parasitic worm. There are two main diseases that affect humans infected with liver flukes: Fascioliasis, or liver fluke infection, and Opisthorchiasis, or Chinese liver fluke infection.

Liver flukes belong to a specific group of parasitic worms known as flukes, or trematodes. Fascioliasis is caused by species of fluke from the genus *Fasciola*, namely one species, *Fasciola hepatica*, the sheep liver fluke. The life cycle of this fluke is as follows: eggs released from host's feces into water; larvae from the eggs infect snails; snails release larvae, which forms cysts containing infective parasite stages, onto vegetation; humans ingest cysts when they eat the vegetation (for example, watercress). The cysts then break open in the human digestive tract and the flukes enter the liver and destroy tissue. Opisthorchiasis is caused by a species of fluke from the genus *Clonorchis* or *Opisthrochis*, namely *C. sinensis*, *O. viverrini*, or *O. felineus*. These flukes have a similar lifecycle to the sheep liver fluke, except, rather than being encysted on plants, they are encysted inside fish. Humans then consume the fish and become infected.

■ Scope and Distribution

Liver fluke infections occur worldwide, though the distribution of Fascioliasis and Opisthorchiasis differs. Fascioliasis is known to occur worldwide, occurring in both temperate and tropical regions. *F. hepatica* infections have been reported in Europe, the Middle East, and Asia. *F. gigantica* infections have been reported in Asia, Africa, and Hawaii. In general, Fascioliasis is closely connected to regions where sheep and cattle are raised. Sheep and cattle are natural hosts for liver flukes, and thus are likely to transmit the parasite to humans in close contact with the animals or their water supply.

Opisthorchiasis occurs in areas of Asia and Europe. In particular, *O. viverrini* infections have been reported from northeast Thailand, Laos, and Kampuchea. *O. felineus* infections have been reported mostly in Europe and Asia. Almost all of China contains infections of *O. sinensis*.

In China, health officials reported a 75% increase in the number of cases of liver fluke from 2001 to 2004. The cause of the increase has been attributed to an increased desire to consume raw or undercooked seafood and meat, both of which are a source of liver flukes. As a consequence of this increase in infections, there has also been an increase in the number of cases in which a liver disorder has developed due to the flukes.

■ Treatment and Prevention

Treatment for liver fluke infections is achieved through administration of medications. There are a number of effective drugs, including triclabendazole, praziquantel, bithionol, albendazole, and mebendazole. Treatment of infection caused by *Fasciola hepatica* usually involves triclabendazole or bithionol. Use of praziquantel has been ineffective in some cases and is thus not recommended by the CDC to be used to treat *F. hepatica* fluke infections. Opisthorchiasis fluke infections can be effectively treated using praziquantel, which is the preferred treatment as suggested by the Centers for Disease Control and Prevention (CDC). These medications act to eradicate the parasite. Praziquantel works by paralyzing the flukes' attachment apparatus, which disables them from remaining attached to the host's blood vessels. This leads to the death of the parasites and eventually the infection dissipates.

On occasions, treatment using the above mentioned drugs may cause side effects such as diarrhea, dizziness, or headache. However, full recovery is likely to occur following treatment. In some cases, liver damage resulting from the attachment of flukes to tissue may make patients vulnerable to other infections. Treatment may be required for several days or weeks depending on the type of fluke causing the infection.

There are no vaccines against liver fluke, thus avoidance of these parasites is the best method of prevention. Avoidance can be achieved by boiling or purifying drinking water, ensuring freshwater fish and vegetation is cooked thoroughly prior to consumption, and eradicating or controlling snails as they are an intermediate host for flukes.

■ Impacts and Issues

Liver flukes are transmitted to humans via consumption of raw meat, fish, and vegetation. Therefore, the food habits of humans have strong implications for the prevalence of liver fluke infections. In China, an increase in the consumption of raw or undercooked meat and seafood resulted in a large increase in the number of people infected with liver flukes. During the years 2001–2004, Chinese health officials reported a 75% increase in fluke infections, highlighting the possibility that increased consumption of food potentially containing liver flukes is causing increased infection.

The liver fluke *F. hepatica*, also known as the sheep liver fluke, often infects livestock such as sheep, cattle, and pigs. This creates issues for the beef, lamb, and pork industries, as the flukes can do extensive damage to the animals, and can be a source of infection for human populations. Prevention of liver fluke infection in livestock requires routine worming of animals, as well as the implementation of snail control methods such as exclusion of animals from snail-infested regions, or drainage of water bodies containing snails. The disease is likely to occur in wet areas where snails are present. If snails are absent, so too are these flukes due to their dependence on snails.

Incidence of liver flukes are greatest in areas that lack adequate sanitation and water purification resources. Increased sanitation practices, including proper disposal and treatment of human and livestock wastes, prevention of water source contamination by fecal mat-

IN CONTEXT: DISEASE IN DEVELOPING NATIONS

In taxonomic terms, liver flukes belong to the the class Trematoda, which is then subdivided into two orders of obligate parasites, Digenea and Monogenea. Obligate parasites are those that are unable to live independently of a host. The trematodes of importance to human disease are part of the Digenea order and include blood, tissue, and intestinal flukes. All are mainly found in developing nations located in tropical and subtropical regions. Flukes are rarely a natural problem in temperate climatic zones.

ter, and safer food storage and preparation practices, could dramatically reduce the occurrence of disease caused by all helminths. However, the World Health Organization (WHO) notes that over one billion people worldwide do not have access to clean, uncontaminated water. Coupled with a diet rich in the foods that most often carry liver flukes, unsanitary conditions make liver flukes difficult to prevent in underdeveloped regions.

SEE ALSO *Food-borne Disease and Food Safety; Helminth Disease; Lung Fluke (Paragonimus) Infection; Opportunistic Infection; Parasitic Diseases.*

BIBLIOGRAPHY

Web Sites

Cambridge University. "Fasciola hepatica: The Liver Fluke." Oct. 5, 1998 <http://www.path.cam.ac.uk/~schisto/OtherFlukes/Fasciola.html#minorFasc> (accessed February 23, 2007).

Cambridge University. "Opisthorchis sinensis: The Chinese Liver Fluke." Oct. 5, 1998 <http://www.path.cam.ac.uk/~schisto/OtherFlukes/Opisthorchis.egg.html> (accessed February 23, 2007).

Centers for Disease Control (CDC). "Fascioliasis." May 6, 2004 <http://www.dpd.cdc.gov/dpdx/html/Fascioliasis.htm> (accessed February 23, 2007).

Centers for Disease Control (CDC). "Opisthorchiasis." May 6, 2004 < http://www.dpd.cdc.gov/dpdx/HTML/Opisthorchiasis.htm> (accessed May 2, 2007).

Meat Promotion Wales. "Liver Fluke." <http://www.hybucigcymru.org.uk/content.php?nID=206&lID=1> (accessed February 23, 2007).

ProMED-Mail. "Food-borne Parasitic Infections Increase in China." May 18, 2005 <http://www.promedmail.org/pls/promed/f?p=2400:1202:997653105689672184::NO::F2400_P1202_CHECK_DISPLAY,F2400_P1202_PUB_MAIL_ID:X,28969> (accessed February 23, 2007).

Lung Fluke (Paragonimus) Infection

■ Introduction

Lung fluke infection, or paragonimiasis, is a potentially serious illness that is caused by over 30 species of trematodes (parasitic flatworms) of the genus *Paragonimus*. Among the more than 10 species reported to infect humans, the most common is *P. westermani*, found in tropical and subtropical regions of the Far East.

Lung flukes are not transmitted from person to person. Humans contract paragonimiasis when they eat inadequately cooked or pickled flesh that is infected. Most reported cases result from consuming raw freshwater crabs or crayfish. However, some species of lung fluke occur only in domestic or wild animals. Humans can contract the illness from consuming the raw flesh of these creatures. *Paragonimus* infect wild boars, wild and domestic canids, wild and domestic felids, raccoons, mongooses, rats, and weasels.

■ Disease History, Characteristics, and Transmission

Until the last quarter of the twentieth century, the public health importance of lung fluke infections was grossly underestimated. As a result, knowledge of the epidemiology of some species of fluke is still limited.

Both snails and crustaceans serve as intermediate hosts of the parasitic flatworms that cause paragonimiasis. Lung fluke eggs hatch in freshwater into miracidia (early-stage larvae), which penetrate the snails. The miracidia develop into very short-tailed cercariae (larvae in the final free-swimming stage) that penetrate and form cysts in the gills or muscles of freshwater crayfish and crabs. Humans or other animals then consume the raw infected crustaceans. The eggs hatch in the duodenum and the young flukes penetrate the gut wall, and eventually, the pleural cavity. Within two to three weeks, the worms, which are hermaphroditic (having both male and female reproductive organs), penetrate beneath the lungs where they meet and cross-fertilize. Adult tremat-

odes become partly encapsulated in the lung tissues of their definitive host, where they lay eggs. The eggs pass into the alveoli. They are then passed in sputum (matter coughed up from the respiratory tract) or swallowed and are passed later in feces. Eggs that reach water hatch and begin the cycle again. The time from infection to oviposition is 65–90 days.

Lung fluke infections can be serious illnesses. Onset of symptoms generally occurs between six and ten weeks after infection. A classical symptom is bloody sputum in which eggs can be found. Other symptoms include cough, difficulty breathing, diarrhea, abdominal pain, fever, and hives. The infection is often mistaken for pulmonary tuberculosis. The parasite can migrate from the lungs to other organs including the brain and striated muscles. Lung flukes that become localized in the brain can create major neurological symptoms. Humans infected with *Paragonimus* usually display symptoms of epilepsy for the first time in adult life. Infections can persist for years, with some cases reported in which people suffered for twenty to forty years.

■ Scope and Distribution

At the start of the twenty-first century, over 21 million people worldwide were estimated by tropical disease specialists to be infected with lung fluke. *Paragonimus westermani* is the most common parasite responsible for human infection in the Far East, where it has a large range of mammalian reservoirs. Human infections with *P. heterotremus* are well known in Thailand and with *P. pulmonalis* in the Far East. *P. africanus* and *P. uterobilateralis* are distributed among humans in West Africa. *P. mexicanus* affects people in parts of Central and South America.

The best method of avoiding infection is to only consume properly cooked food. The preferred treatment is praziquantel tablets with bithionol tablets as an alternative drug. Praziquantel stops worms from developing or multiplying in the body.

■ Impacts and Issues

Paragonimiasis once tended to be limited to regions where the appropriate crustaceans formed part of the human diet in one culinary delicacy or another. However, the rise of a global cuisine has contributed to the spread of lung flukes. In 2006, two people who consumed live, imported, freshwater crabs in an Orange County, California, restaurant contracted paragonimiasis.

The invasion of nonnative species into American and Canadian waters poses a further threat to human health. The mitten crab, *Eriocheir sinensis*, was first spotted in fisheries on the west coast in 1992. This Yellow Sea native is a Chinese delicacy and crabs were imported live to markets in Los Angeles and San Francisco before California outlawed their possession. A female can carry from 250,000 to 1 million eggs. The crabs, adept on land, climb easily over levees as they migrate upstream. Mitten crabs can carry lung fluke, though no infected crabs have been detected in North American waters.

SEE ALSO *Helminth Disease; Parasitic Diseases.*

BIBLIOGRAPHY

Books

Peters, Wallace, and Geoffrey Pasvol. *Tropical Medicine and Parasitology.* London: Mosby, 2002.

Web Sites

International Society for Infectious Diseases. "ProMed Mail: Mitten Crab—USA and Canada." August 1, 1999. <http://www.promedmail.org/pls/promed/f?p=2400.1000> (accessed May 26, 2007).

International Society for Infectious Diseases. "ProMed Mail: Paragonimiasis from Eating Raw Imported Freshwater Crab." August 20, 2006. <http://www.promedmail.org/pls/promed/f?p=2400:1000> (accessed May 26, 2007).

WORDS TO KNOW

ALVEOLI: An alveolus (alveoli is plural) is a tiny air sac located within the lungs. The exchange of oxygen and carbon dioxide takes place within these sacs.

DEFINITIVE HOST: The organism in which a parasite reaches reproductive maturity.

INTERMEDIATE HOST: An organism infected by a parasite while the parasite is in a developmental form, not sexually mature.

OVIPOSITION: Ovum is Latin for "egg" to oviposition is to position or lay eggs, especially when done by an insect.

PLEURAL CAVITY: The lungs are surrounded by two membranous coverings, the pleura. One of the pleura is attached to the lung, the other to the ribcage. The space between the two pleura, the pleural cavity, is normally filled with a clear lubricating fluid called pleural fluid.

TREMATODES: Trematodes, also called flukes, are a type of parasitic flatworm. In humans, flukes can infest the liver, lung, and other tissues.

Lyme Disease

■ Introduction

Lyme disease is a bacterial infection caused by the spirochete (corkscrew-shaped bacterium) *Borrelia burgdorferi*. It is transmitted to humans through the bites of several kinds of ticks, including deer ticks (*Ixodes scapularis*) and the western black-legged tick (*Ixodes pacificus*) in the United States and *Ixodes ricinis*) in Europe. The untreated disease presents in two or three stages, starting with a localized infection that produces a skin rash and sometimes fever, headache, and other symptoms. The second stage may involve arthritis, neurological symptoms, such as depression and Bell's facial palsy, and meningitis (inflammation of the membranes that enclose the central nervous system). In the third stage, long-term arthritis and neurological symptoms may occur. The disease is treated using antibiotics. Earlier treatment is more effective, as the symptoms of untreated Lyme disease may take years to reverse or be irreversible. There is controversy between Lyme patient advocacy groups and many doctors about the existence of hard-to-detect, chronic Lyme infection and the advisability of treating such infections with antibiotics.

■ Disease History, Characteristics, and Transmission

History

Lyme disease has probably existed for centuries. Judging by case records, observations of what was probably Lyme disease were recorded in Germany and Scandinavia in the late nineteenth and early twentieth centuries. Examination of museum specimens of deer ticks collected in the United States has detected Lyme disease bacteria dating to the 1940s. In 1975, some mothers in the town of Lyme, Connecticut—for which the disease is named—began noticing arthritis, fatigue, erythema migrans rashes, and other symptoms in about 50 local children. Two of these women, Judith Mensch and Polly Murray, began tracking the cases by recording dates and locations. Several of the children recalled being bitten by a tick just before becoming ill. Murray called rheumatologist Allen Steer, who investigated the cases and concluded that a tick-borne pathogen was to blame for the disease.

Thus, the existence of Lyme disease was recognized and its transmission by ticks was known in 1975. However, the specific pathogen causing the disease was still unknown. In 1981, Dr. Willy Burgdorfer, working at the National Institute of Allergy and Infectious Diseases (NIAID) of the U.S. National Institutes of Health, was studying the transmission of Rocky Mountain spotted fever by ticks. Studying the microorganisms found in black-legged ticks (one of the two U.S. tick varieties that transmits Lyme disease), Burgdorfer noticed a hitherto-unknown variety of corkscrew-shaped bacterium (spirochetes) in fluids from two ticks. Within a year, this bacterium had been named *Borrelia burgdorferi* in Burgdorfer's honor.

In 1982, other researchers found *Borrelia burgdorferi* in deer ticks. By combining cultured *B. burgdorferi* bacteria with blood samples from people with Lyme disease, it was shown that the patients' blood contained an antibody specific to *B. burgdorferi*. This showed that the blood donors had been infected with *B. burgdorferi*. Finally, in 1983, researchers found *B. burgdorferi* in blood and tissue samples from patients with Lyme disease, and the proof that the bacterium caused the disease was clinched.

In the years since 1983, there has been persistent controversy over the question of whether Lyme disease can exist in a chronic form that is not detected by standard tests, causing a wide range of neurological and other symptoms that overlap with those of fibromyalgia and chronic fatigue syndrome. There is also expert disagreement over the question of whether treatment of possible chronic Lyme infection with antibiotics is good medical practice.

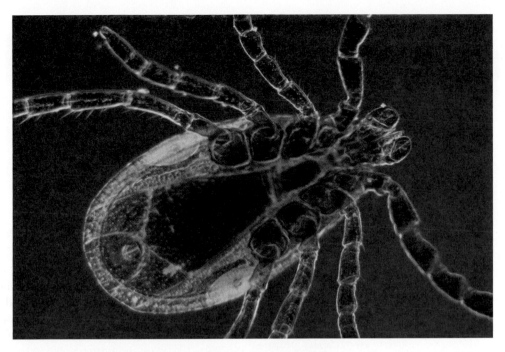

A magnified deer tick (*Ixodes scapularis*), a blood sucking arachnid, can cause disease in humans and animals. Such ticks can transmit the bacterium that causes Lyme disease.   *Kent Wood/Photo Researchers, Inc.*

Characteristics and Transmission

Lyme disease is caused by the spirochete *B. burgdorferi*, a member of the phylum Spirochaetes. Spirochetes are corkscrew- or helix-shaped bacteria. *B. burgdorferi* are about 0.2–0.5 μm wide, 3–18 μm long, and are built with a double layered structure, like a long, blunt-ended corkscrew nested within a slightly larger corkscrew of the same shape. In the space between the two layers are flagella. Each flagellum is a long, hairlike filament attached to a rotating base embedded in the outer cell wall. Many types of bacteria have flagella, but normally the flagella protrude into the bacterium's environment and are used for propulsion like tiny outboard propellers. A spirochete uses a different strategy—its internal flagella wrap lengthwise around the inner layer of the bacterium, forcing it into its characteristic corkscrew shape. Furthermore, as the flagella rotate, they cause the whole shape of the bacterium to change as if it were rotating on its axis. Just as an actual corkscrew is driven into a cork by rotating, a spirochete progresses through the medium in which it is embedded. Its corkscrewing mode of locomotion gives it a mobility advantage over other bacteria in more viscous (thicker, stickier) media.

Both syphilis and Lyme disease are caused by spirochetes. There are three common species of *B. burgdorferi*, namely *Borrelia garinii*, *Borrelia afzellia*, and *Borrelia burgdorferi* sensu stricto (meaning in the strict sense); together, these three are known as *Borrelia burgdorferi* sensu lato ("in the wide sense") or simply, for convenience, as *Borrelia burgdorferi*. *Borrelia burgdor-*

feri sensu strictu is the only Lyme strain so far found in the United States as of 2007. Three other, less-common species of *Borrelia burgdorferi* sensu lato (in the broad sense) have been discovered to cause Lyme disease in Africa, Asia, and Europe.

Lyme disease is a vector-borne disease, meaning that it is transmitted to human beings by an intermediate host (in this case a tick), not directly from other human beings. Although far from the most common infectious disease in the United States, it is the most common vector-borne disease, accounting for over 95% of reported vector-borne illness cases. The vector for Lyme disease is the deer tick, and the transmission of Lyme disease to humans is intimately involved with the life cycle of both the *B. burgdorferi* spirochete and the tick.

In the spring, tick eggs lying on the ground hatch, producing tick larvae. Each larva attaches to a small mammal, usually a mouse. Ticks attach firmly to the skin and feed on their host by sucking blood. The larval tick ingests *B. burgdorferi* from its mouse host and becomes infected: this infection does not sicken the tick. In the fall and winter, the larva drops off the mouse and becomes dormant, attaching itself to vegetation. The next spring, it molts and becomes a nymph-stage tick. The nymph attaches to a deer, mouse, or human host— its preferred host is the deer—and bites the host, transmitting Lyme disease. The tick develops to an adult form throughout the summer, living on the host. In this stage it mates. In the fall, it drops off its host and lays eggs in leaf litter on the ground (about 3,000 eggs per laying

WORDS TO KNOW

BABESIOSIS: An infection of the red blood cells caused by *Babesia microti*, a form of parasite (parasitic sporozoan).

ENDEMIC: Present in a particular area or among a particular group of people.

GRANULOCYTE: Any cell containing granules (small, grain-like objects) is a granulocyte. The term is often used to refer to a type of white blood cell (leukocyte).

HOST: Organism that serves as the habitat for a parasite, or possibly for a symbiont. A host may provide nutrition to the parasite or symbiont, or simply a place in which to live.

MENINGITIS: Meningitis is an inflammation of the meninges—the three layers of protective membranes that line the spinal cord and the brain. Meningitis can occur when there is an infection near the brain or spinal cord, such as a respiratory infection in the sinuses, the mastoids, or the cavities around the ear. Disease organisms can also travel to the meninges through the bloodstream. The first signs may be a severe headache and neck stiffness followed by fever, vomiting, a rash, and, then, convulsions leading to loss of consciousness. Meningitis generally involves two types: non-bacterial meningitis, which is often called aseptic meningitis, and bacterial meningitis, which is referred to as purulent meningitis.

NYMPH: In aquatic insects, the larval stage.

SPIROCHETE: A bacterium shaped like a spiral. Spiral-shaped bacteria, which live in contaminated water, sewage, soil, and decaying organic matter, as well as inside humans and animals.

SPOROZOAN: The fifth Phylum of the Protist Kingdom, known as Apicomplexa, comprises several species of obligate intracellular protozoan parasites classified as Sporozoa or Sporozoans, because they form reproductive cells known as spores. Many sporozoans are parasitic and pathogenic species, such as *Plasmodium falciparum, P. malariae, P. vivax, Toxoplasma gondii, Pneumocysts carinii, Cryptosporidum parvum* and *Cryptosporidum muris,* The Sporozoa reproduction cycle has both asexual and sexual phases. The asexual phase is termed schizogony (from the Greek, meaning generation through division), in which merozoites (daughter cells) are produced through multiple nuclear fissions. The sexual phase is known as sporogony (i.e., generation of spores) and is followed by gametogony or the production of sexually reproductive cells termed gamonts.

VECTOR: Any agent, living or otherwise, that carries and transmits parasites and diseases. Also, an organism or chemical used to transport a gene into a new host cell.

---

female), beginning a new two-year cycle. This is the basic ecology of Lyme disease in the northeastern and north-central United States.

In northern California and Oregon, a more complex vector ecology exists. A reservoir of *B. burgdorferi* is maintained in the wild by *Ixodes neotomaei* ticks (which do not bite humans) and the dusky-footed wood rat. A second type of tick, *Ixodes pacificus*, which usually feeds on lizards—which does not host *B. burgdorferi*—occasionally feeds on infected wood rats in its nymphal stage. Those few *Ixodes pacificus* ticks that feed on infected wood rats and then on humans can cause Lyme disease.

Once in a human host, *Borrelia burgdorferi* can cause three stages of disease. Stage 1 is the erythema migrans rash, which is centered on the site of the tick bite. There is disagreement over how common this rash is. Some experts say that less than 50% of Lyme disease patients experience it, while others say 80%. Stage 2 affects the nervous system, joints, and heart. Stage 3 is late or chronic infection.

Stage 1 (early Lyme disease). The characteristic Lyme rash is a red, inflamed patch of skin about 2 in (5 cm) or more wide. It sometimes takes on a bull's-eye form with a central clear space. The rash usually develops within 3–30 days (most often 7–14 days) of the detachment of the tick. A single spot is most common, but multiple spots may develop as the bacteria spread widely from the tick bite. Influenzalike symptoms are also common at this stage. Symptoms include joint pain, fatigue, neck pain, headache, and fever. Coughing, vomiting, and diarrhea do not happen, allowing this condition to be told apart from a real flu.

Stage 2 (early disseminated Lyme disease). Within 4–6 weeks, neurological and arthritic symptoms develop. About 15% of untreated patients develop neurological symptoms. Meningitis (inflammation of the meninges, the membranes that enclose the central nervous system)

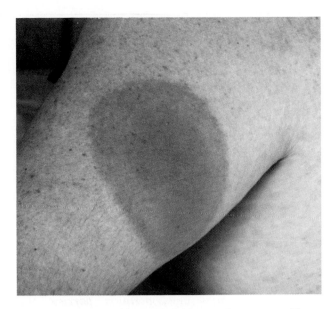

A bull's eye rash (*Erythema migrans*) is an early symptom of Lyme disease. Ticks transport the acute inflammatory disease characterized by skin changes, joint inflammation, and flu-like symptoms. *Larry Mulvehill/Photo Researchers, Inc.*

may occur, with headache and neck stiffness, Bell's palsy (partial paralysis of facial muscles), blindness due to pressure on the optic nerve (especially in children), depression, anxiety, memory loss, and more. These neurological symptoms usually go away after some weeks or months; however, the infection may remain, and in up to 5% of untreated patients may become chronic. (These figures are disputed by some physicians, who argue that the chronic rate is higher in both treated and untreated patients.) About 5% of untreated patients also develop cardiac symptoms, including atrioventricular block and inflammation of the heart. Several months into the illness, most untreated patients (about 60%) develop arthritis—joint swelling and pain, especially in large joints such as the knee. These arthritic symptoms may become chronic in some patients. Arthritis may persist in the knees even years after antibiotic therapy. In Stage 2, other common symptoms include diarrhea, shortness of breath, rapid or irregular heartbeat, testicular pain, shaking hands, frequent need to urinate, and poor sense of balance. Exactly how *Borrelia burgdorferi* causes all these symptoms remains largely unknown.

Stage 3 (chronic or late Lyme disease). According to some physicians, 30–50% of treated and untreated Lyme patients develop a disorder with several symptoms that is hard to distinguish from fibromyalgia and chronic fatigue syndrome. Symptoms include fatigue, joint paint (arthralgia), muscle pain (myalgia), and other dysfunctions of the nervous system. It should be noted that the existence of a third-stage, chronic or late form, of Lyme

disease has been controversial. Some researchers have maintained that Lyme disease is reliably eradicated by treatment with antibiotics and that cases of apparent chronic infection are actually psychiatric (mental) disorders. This controversy persists partly because laboratory tests for the presence of *B. burgdorferi* are unreliable, with many false negatives (tests showing no infection when there is infection).

One reason why Lyme disease may produce such varied symptoms is that the ticks that transmit it are also host to numerous other pathogens, and can serve as vectors for such disorders as babesiosis (infection of the red blood cells caused by the parasitic sporozoan *Babesia microti*) and human granulocytic ehrlichiosis (an infection of white blood cells caused a species of bacteria in the *Ehrlichia* genus). When more than one pathogen infects a person at a time, the result is called co-infection. Some researchers state that the majority of Lyme disease victims are probably co-infected with other organisms.

Even untreated, Lyme disease is rarely fatal.

■ Scope and Distribution

Lyme disease is a larger problem in the United States than elsewhere in the world, with about 15,000 new cases reported each year. However, most experts agree that the disease is greatly underreported and that the true number of new cases is probably more on the order of 100,000 per year. As of 2006, about 150,000 cases had been reported in the U.S. since 1976, the year after Lyme disease was officially recognized as a new disease.

There are 12 U.S. states in which Lyme disease is most commonly found: Connecticut, Delaware, Maine, Maryland, Massachusetts, Minnesota, New Jersey, New Hampshire, New York, Pennsylvania, Rhode Island, and Wisconsin. Lyme disease is endemic (normally occurs), with incidences as high as 3%, in parts of these states. About 70% of persons who contract Lyme disease catch it from a tick picked up in their own backyard; most of the remaining 30% acquire ticks while hiking or walking in woods or fields away from home.

■ Treatment and Prevention

Lyme disease is treated primarily with antibiotics. Which antibiotics are used depends on disease stage, symptoms, and allergic reactions. If Lyme disease is diagnosed early—as often happens when a person visiting his physician displays a characteristic rash and or flulike symptoms and reports a tick bite—treatment is a 14- to 21-day course of oral (swallowed) antibiotics, most often doxycycline, clarithomycin, or amoxicillan. Treatment success at this stage is about 95% (although some researchers state that a much higher percentage of patients than 5% go on to develop a chronic form of the disease).

IN CONTEXT: PERSONAL RESPONSIBILITY AND PROTECTION

The Division of Vector Borne Infectious Diseases at Centers for Disease Control and Prevention (CDC) states that to reduce risks of contracting Lyme Disease that you should:

- Avoid areas with a lot of ticks. Ticks prefer wooded and bushy areas with high grass.
- Take extra precautions when ticks that transmit Lyme disease are most active.
- If you do enter a tick area, walk in the center of the trail to avoid contact with overgrown grass, brush, and leaf litter.
- Keep ticks off your skin. Properly use insect repellent with 20% - 30% DEET on adult skin and clothing to prevent tick bite. Effective repellents are found in drug, grocery and discount stores. Permethrin is another type of repellent. It can be purchased at outdoor equipment stores that carry camping or hunting gear. Permethrin kills ticks on contact! One application to pants, socks, and shoes typically stays effective through several washings. Permethrin should not be applied directly to skin. For details on permethrin visit the National Pesticide Information Center.
- Wear long pants, long sleeves, and long socks to keep ticks off your skin. Light-colored clothing will help you spot ticks more easily. Tucking pant legs into socks or boots and tucking shirts into pants help keep ticks on the outside of clothing. If you'll be outside for an extended period of time, tape the area where your pants and socks meet to prevent ticks from crawling under your clothes.
- Check your skin and clothes for ticks every day!
- If a tick is attached to your skin for less than 24 hours, your chance of getting Lyme disease is extremely small. But just to be safe, monitor your health closely after a tick bite and be alert for any signs and symptoms of tick-borne illness.

SOURCE: *Division of Vector Borne Infectious Diseases at Centers for Disease Control and Prevention (CDC), Division of Vector Borne Infectious Diseases*

For Stage 2 (early disseminated) Lyme disease, the same agents are used but in large doses. In this case they are given intravenously (by needle, into a vein) rather than in pill form. If the heart is inflamed, penicillin G also may be used. Supportive medicines may be given for specific symptoms, such as pain relievers for arthritis symptoms and antidepressants for neurological symptoms, such as depression and anxiety.

Lyme disease is prevented by avoiding infected ticks. Particularly in spring, areas that are known to be infested with ticks should be avoided. Light-colored clothing makes it easier to spot ticks and remove them before they bite. Wearing long-sleeved shirts, tucking pants

into socks, and applying insect repellents containing DEET (n,n,diethyl-m-toluamide) or treated with permethrin can decrease the chances of a tick bite. Promptly removing a tick that has attached is important, because *B. burgdorferi* usually does not infect the host until 36 hours after tick attachment. Ticks should be removed by gripping them right next to the skin with tweezers and pulling: the body of the tick should never be squeezed or irritated by heat or chemicals while the tick is attached, as this will drive its stomach contents into the skin and increase the chances of infection.

Many of the ticks acquired by people engaged in outdoor activity in the northeast United States, where 90% of all Lyme disease cases have been reported, are dog ticks (*Dermacentor variabilis*), which cannot transmit Lyme disease. The Lyme-transmitting deer tick *Ixodes scapularis* is notably smaller than a dog tick. Even if one is bitten by a tick, it is not necessary to seek treatment for Lyme disease unless flulike symptoms or the characteristic erythema migrans rash appear.

As of early 2007, no vaccine for Lyme disease was available.

■ Impacts and Issues

Lyme disease has become the most common vector-borne inflammatory disease in the United States thanks to changing human activities. In the nineteenth century, the central and northeastern United States were largely deforested and deer populations were eliminated or greatly reduced by hunting and habitat loss over large areas. After food production shifted elsewhere, these regions have largely reforested, and deer populations, along with the ticks that infest them, have rebounded. At the same time, greater numbers of human beings have been brought into contact with ticks by living in suburban developments and enjoying outdoor recreations such as hiking.

A 79 percent-effective vaccine for Lyme disease, LYMErix, was placed on the market in 1999. It was withdrawn in 2002, however, because of low sales. Low demand was caused by a combination of the vaccine's high cost ($50 per inoculation), its inconvenience (three shots were needed over a year), and fears that the vaccine might trigger permanent arthritis or neurological problems. Debate among experts over whether LYMErix was sufficiently safe remains fierce to this day. As of 2007, a European company was developing a vaccine that is intended to work for a wider range of *B. burgdorferi* species and to avoid the possible health dangers of the LYMErix vaccine.

Lyme disease is a notoriously contentious subject, dividing patient advocacy groups from many physicians. This is partially due to the fact that Lyme disease has no definitive, predictable course. Some infected persons show no symptoms; others show symptoms, are debilitated for a time, and are successfully treated; still others are left with permanent disabilities from the disease. Disagreements, often angry, persist on whether long-term Lyme infection exists, what its symptoms and proper treatment are (if any), and whether Lyme disease is diagnosed too much or too little. As Lyme disease is argued to be drastically under-reported—both Lyme disease patient groups and the CDC claim that the number of cases meeting CDC diagnostic criteria is about 10 times greater than the number actually counted in official figures—the total economic and personal impact of the disease is hard to estimate.

Finally, patient advocacy groups argue that Lyme disease research is greatly underfunded compared to that for other diseases such as West Nile virus, although there were eight times more reported Lyme disease cases than West Nile virus cases in 2005. This is with only the reported number, but since the CDC states that there may be 10 times more cases of Lyme disease each year that meet CDC diagnostic standards than are reported, the underfunding situation is much worse than it seems from official numbers. Advocates for greater attention to Lyme disease introduced Federal Lyme Bill HR 741, the Lyme & Tick-Borne Disease Prevention, Education & Research Act of 2007, which would allot $100 million over a five-year period for research, prevention, and other measures to combat Lyme disease. As of March, 2007, the House of Representatives had not voted on the bill.

■ Primary Source Connection

Travel advisories are maintained by most developed countries in an effort to provide citizens with information about health and safety hazards while traveling abroad. In the United States, the Centers for Disease Control and Prevention (CDC) maintains a Traveler's Health website at <http://www.cdc.gov/travel/> that features vaccination recommendations and other health information for specific countries and destinations. In the newspaper article below, the author discusses recommendations, including Lyme disease prevention, made by foreign governments for its citizens traveling to the United States. It should be again noted that the LYMErix vaccine mentioned in the article is no longer available.

Travel Advisories: Wait 'Til You Hear What They Say about Us

You've checked the travel advisories, gotten a few vaccinations and stocked up on Imodium and antimalarials.

Now, you're off on that exotic vacation.

But what about travelers heading here, to the good old U.S.A.?

PETS CAN CONTRACT LYME DISEASE, TOO

The tiny deer ticks that harbor Lyme disease bacteria can also transmit the disease to many pets, including dogs, horses, and occasionally, cats. Although a vaccine against Lyme exists for dogs, reducing the opportunity for ticks to bite an animal remains the front line of defense against Lyme disease in pets. Veterinarians recommend that pet owners:

- Walk dogs and ride horses on cleared trails.
- Use an approved anti-tick and flea product specific to dogs, cats, and horses.
- Groom horses daily, checking for ticks, especially near the head, throat area, belly, and under the tail.
- Remove brush and woodpiles from horse pastures.
- Mow lawns and pastures, keeping grass short.
- Examine dogs and cats regularly for ticks, especially pets that spend time both indoors and outdoors.
- Watch for symptoms of Lyme disease in pets, including fever, limping, loss of appetite, and fatigue in dogs and cats, and weight loss, swollen joints, muscle tenderness, and intermittent lameness in horses.

They get travel advisories, too. The advisories aim to keep U.S.-bound tourists, students and workers safe from our health hazards.

Most international health and travel organizations agree that travelers risk little in the United States by drinking the tap water or eating food bought from street vendors.

But they warn about West Nile encephalitis, an illness that is passed on to humans by infected mosquitoes, who in turn, are infected by birds. West Nile virus can cause flu-like symptoms and is especially worrisome for adults over 50, who are at a greater risk for developing serious complications.

"Use insect repellent accordingly" and "stay in during dusk and dawn hours," Great Britain's travel Web site advises.

Visitors from Japan, where U.S. beef is banned, worry about bovine spongiform encephalopathy, better-known as "mad cow disease." One Washington-state cow was found to have the brain-wasting disease in 2003.

"They are very afraid of mad cow disease in Japan," said Chigusa Suzuki, a Japanese editor and translator living in New York City. "But once they get to the United States, the fear disappears and they go to a steakhouse. They want the American experience and that includes having a steak."

Travelers to the United States also are warned about Lyme disease, which is passed on by ticks.

Many international travel Web sites recommend being watchful for tick bites or even considering a three-dose vaccine of LYMErix if tourists plan on spending a lot of time in U.S. forests.

The U.S. Centers for Disease Control, which advises U.S. travelers heading to foreign lands, reassures people coming here: "There are, of course, health risks, but in general, the precautions required are minimal," its Web site says.

But often, health dangers that are of little concern to people actually living in the United States seem most pressing for visitors from afar. For instance, while you might not worry about contracting rabies, the illness can be spotted on nearly every international health advisory Web site.

The United Kingdom's Department of Health Web site warns travelers to the United States to be especially wary of rabies and to "avoid being bitten by any animal."

That's good advice for any traveler, of course.

Maureen Mckinney

MCKINNEY, MAUREEN. "TRAVEL ADVISORIES: WAIT 'TIL YOU HEAR WHAT THEY SAY ABOUT US." *DAILY HERALD* (ARLINGTON HEIGHTS, IL) MARCH 21, 2005.

SEE ALSO *Arthropod-borne Disease; Climate Change and Infectious Disease; Emerging Infectious Diseases; Mosquito-borne Disease; Rocky Mountain Spotted Fever; Vector-borne Disease; Zoonoses.*

BIBLIOGRAPHY

Books

Edlow, Jonathan A. *Bull's Eye: Unraveling the Medical Mystery of Lyme Disease.* New Haven, CT: Yale University Press, 2004.

Vanderhoof-Forschner, Karen. *Everything You Need to Know About Lyme Disease and Other Tick-Borne Disorders.* 2nd ed. New York: Wiley, 2003.

Periodicals

Donta, Sam. "Late and Chronic Lyme Disease: Symptom Overlap with Chronic Fatigue Syndrome and Fibromyalgia." *Medical Clinics of North America* 86 (2002): 341–349.

Hayes, Edward B., and Joseph Piesman. "How Can We Prevent Lyme Disease?" *New England Journal of Medicine* 348 (2003): 2424–2429.

Ramamoorthi, Nandhini, et al. "The Lyme Disease Agent Exploits a Tick Protein to Infect the Mammalian Host." *Nature* 436 (July 28, 2005): 573–577.

Steere, Allen C. "Lyme Disease." *New England Journal of Medicine* 345 (2001): 115–123.

Wormser, Gary P. "Early Lyme Disease." *New England Journal of Medicine* 354 (2006): 2794–2800.

Web Sites

American Lyme Disease Foundation. "Home Page." September 22, 2006. <http://www.aldf.com/> (accessed February 7, 2007).